Portable LPN

The All-in-One Reference for Practical Nurses

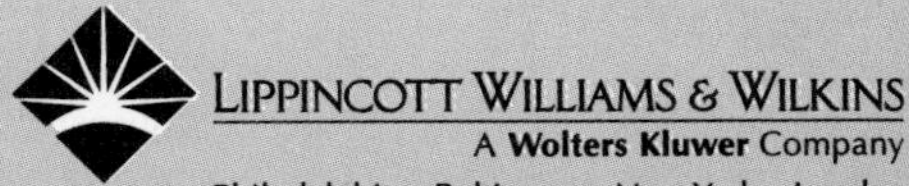

STAFF

Publisher
Judith A. Schilling McCann, RN, MSN

Editorial Director
William J. Kelly

Clinical Director
Joan Robinson, RN, MSN

Senior Art Director
Arlene Putterman

Editorial Project Manager
Sean Webb

Clinical Project Managers
Kathryn Henry, RN, BSN, CCRC;
Carol A. Saunderson, RN, BA, BS

Editor
Catherine E. Harold

Copy Editors
Kimberly Bilotta (supervisor),
Heather Ditch, Carolyn Peterson,
Pamela Wingrod

Designers
Will Boehm (book design),
Linda Franklin (project manager)

Digital Composition Services
Diane Paluba (manager),
Joyce Rossi Biletz, Donna S. Morris

Manufacturing
Patrica K. Dorshaw (director),
Beth J. Welsh

Editorial Assistants
Megan L. Aldinger, Karen J. Kirk,
Linda K. Ruhf

Design Assistant
Georg Purvis, 4th

Indexer
Deborah Tourtlotte

PLPN011205 — D
07 06 05   10 9 8 7 6 5 4 3 2 1

Library of Congress
Cataloging-in-Publication Data
Portable LPN: the all-in-one reference for practical nurses.
p. ; cm.
Includes bibliographical references and index.
1. Practical nursing — Handbooks, manuals, etc. I. Lippincott Williams & Wilkins.
[DNLM: 1. Nursing, Practical — methods — Handbooks. WY 49 P8385 2006]
RT62.P67 2006
610.73 — dc22
ISBN 1-58255-581-8 (alk. paper) 2005025760

Contents

Contributors and consultants

Ruth A. Barkley-Arnold, LPN
Case Manager Nurse Specialist
Aetna
Blue Bell, Pa.

Janice W. Chapman, RN, MSN
Instructor of Nursing
Site Coordinator
Health Careers Department
Reid State College
Atmore, Ala.

Shirley Lyon Garcia, RN, BSN
Nursing Program Director, PNE
McDowell Technical Community College
Marion, N.C.

Aaron Pack, LPN
Staff Nurse
Norman (Okla.) Regional Hospital

Noel C. Piano, RN, MS
Instructor
Lafayette School of Practical Nursing
Williamsburg, Va.

Elaine M. Rissel-Muscarella, RN, BSN
Health Care Services Specialist
Erie 2 Chautauqua-Cattaraugus BOCES School of Nursing
Ashville, N.Y.

Lauren R. Roach, LPN, HCS-D
Manager of Office Operations
Good Samaritan Home Care Services, LLC
Vincennes, Ind.

June Fonda Sager, LPN
Field Nurse
Guardian Home Care
Athens, Ga.

Kendra S. Seiler, RN, MSN, CNOR
Nursing Instructor
Rio Hondo Community College
Whittier, Calif.

Betty Sims, RN, MSN
Nurse Consultant
Board of Nurse Examiners
Austin, Tex.
Adjunct Faculty
St. Philips College
San Antonio, Tex.

Collette M. Swan, RN, MSN
Director and Instructor of Nursing
South Seattle Community College

Audrey E. Taleff, MSN, FNP
Family Nurse Practitioner
Waianae Coast Comprehensive Health Care
Adjunct Faculty, LPN Program
Leeward Community College
Waianae, Hawaii

1 Patient mobility, hygiene, comfort, and safety

This chapter covers the fundamental procedures needed to ensure patient mobility, hygiene, comfort, and safety. Each entry begins with a brief introduction and, where appropriate, a description of equipment preparation. The entry then provides implementation tips to help you perform each procedure efficiently and effectively. Each entry also includes sections on special considerations and documentation. No matter which procedure you're performing, make sure to follow standard nursing protocol.

Standard nursing protocol

Standard nursing protocol should be followed before, during, and after each procedure.

Before a procedure

- Verify the physician's order.
- Ensure patient privacy.
- Introduce yourself to the patient by giving your name, title, and role.
- Check the patient's I.D. bracelet and ask for his name, when possible, to confirm his identity.
- Explain the procedure and rationale in language familiar to the patient.
- Gather the needed equipment.
- Wash your hands before each new patient contact.
- Put on clean gloves.
- Adjust the bed to an appropriate height.
- Lower the side rail nearest you, if needed.

During a procedure

- Encourage patient involvement whenever possible.
- Monitor the patient's tolerance of the procedure. Watch for signs of discomfort or fatigue.

After a procedure

- Help the patient into a comfortable position.
- Remove or dispose of soiled supplies and equipment appropriately.
- Wash your hands.
- Place items the patient may need within reach.
- Place the call bell within reach, and make sure the patient knows how to use it.
- Raise the side rails, if appropriate, and place the bed in its lowest position.
- Store unused or reusable supplies and equipment.
- Document the procedure, the patient's response, and expected and unexpected outcomes.

Body mechanics and transfer techniques

Passive range-of-motion exercises

- In passive range-of-motion (ROM) exercises, a nurse, physical therapist, or caregiver moves the patient's joints through their full range of motion.
- Passive ROM exercises are used for patients with temporary or permanent loss of mobility, sensation, or consciousness.
- These exercises improve or maintain joint mobility, help prevent contractures, and increase circulation to the affected part.
- To perform passive ROM exercises properly, you must recognize the patient's limits of motion and support all joints during movement.
- These exercises are contraindicated in patients with infected joints, acute thrombophlebitis, severe arthritic joint inflammation, or recent trauma with possible hidden fractures or internal injuries.

Implementation tips

- Follow the standard nursing protocol described at the start of the chapter.
- Determine which joints need ROM exercises, and ask the physician or physical therapist about limitations or precautions for specific exercises.
- The exercises described below are designed to move all of the patient's joints, but they don't have to be performed in the order given or all at once. You can schedule them over the course of a day, whenever the patient is in the most convenient position.
- Remember to perform all exercises slowly, gently, and to the end of the normal ROM or to the point of discomfort, but no further.
- At the end of each exercise, return the involved area to a neutral position. (See *Glossary of joint movements*, page 4.)
- Support each joint by holding the areas distal and proximal to it.

Exercising the neck

- Support the patient's head with your hands and extend the neck, flex the chin to the chest, and tilt the head laterally toward each shoulder.
- Rotate the head from right to left, rotate the head in a circular motion, and gently bend the head to extend the neck.

Exercising the shoulders

- Support the patient's arm in an extended, neutral position; then extend the forearm and flex it back.
- Abduct the arm outward from the side of the body, and adduct it back to the side.
- Rotate the shoulder so the arm crosses the midline, and bend the elbow so the hand touches the opposite shoulder.
- Return the shoulder to a neutral position and, with elbow bent, push the arm backward for complete external rotation.

Exercising the elbow

- Place the patient's arm at his side with his palm facing up.
- Flex and extend the arm at the elbow.

Exercising the forearm

- Stabilize the patient's elbow, and then rotate the hand to bring the palm up (supination).
- Rotate it back again to bring the palm down (pronation).

Exercising the wrist

- Stabilize the forearm, and flex and extend the wrist.
- Then rock the hand sideways for lateral flexion, and rotate the hand in a circular motion.

Exercising the fingers and thumb

- Extend the patient's fingers, and then flex the hand into a fist; repeat extension and flexion of each joint of each finger and thumb separately.
- Spread two adjoining fingers apart (abduction), and then bring them together (adduction).
- Oppose each fingertip to the thumb, and rotate the thumb and each finger in a circle.

Exercising the hip and knee

- Fully extend the patient's leg.
- Bend the hip and knee toward the chest, allowing full joint flexion, and then return to the extended position.
- Next, move the straight leg sideways, out and away from the other leg (abduction), and then back, over, and across it (adduction).
- Rotate the straight leg toward and then away from the midline.

Glossary of joint movements

Joints should be exercised to the point of discomfort, but not pain. Move them in the intended direction of function, hold the position for a few seconds, and then return to the rest position.

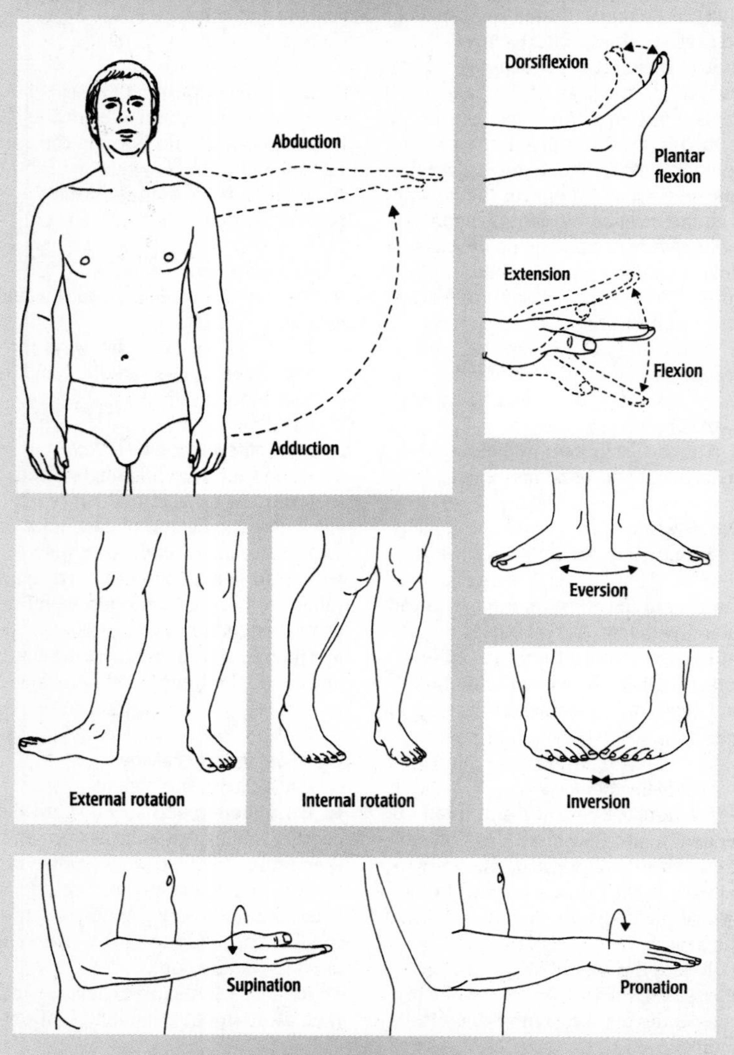

Exercising the ankle

◆ Bend the patient's foot so the toes push upward (dorsiflexion).
◆ Then bend the foot so the toes push downward (plantar flexion).
◆ Rotate the ankle in a circle.
◆ Invert the ankle so the sole faces the midline; then evert the ankle so the sole faces away from the midline.

Exercising the toes

◆ Flex the patient's toes toward the sole, and then extend them back toward the top of the foot.
◆ Spread two adjoining toes apart (abduction), and then bring them together (adduction).

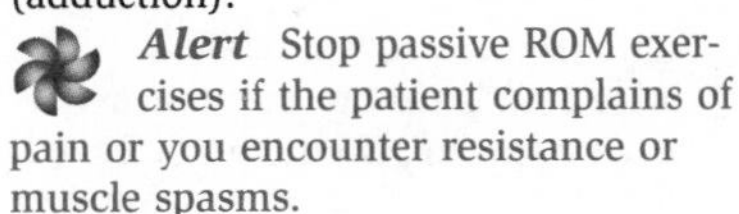

Alert Stop passive ROM exercises if the patient complains of pain or you encounter resistance or muscle spasms.

Special considerations

◆ Because joints begin to stiffen within 24 hours of disuse, start passive ROM exercises as soon as possible and perform them at least every 4 hours — even while bathing or turning the patient.
◆ Ensure proper body mechanics, and repeat each exercise at least five times.
◆ Patients who need prolonged bed rest or limited activity but who aren't profoundly weak can be taught to perform ROM exercises on their own (called active ROM), or they may benefit from isometric exercises.
◆ If a disabled patient needs long-term rehabilitation after discharge teach a family member or caregiver to perform passive ROM exercises and consult a physical therapist for follow-up care.

Documentation

◆ Record which joints were exercised; whether active or passive ROM was performed; whether the patient had edema, pressure areas, pain from the exercises, or limited ROM; and the patient's tolerance of the exercises.

Transfer from bed to stretcher

◆ This is one of the most common transfers you'll encounter.
◆ Depending on the patient's size and condition and your physical abilities, you may need help from one or more coworkers to accomplish it.
◆ Techniques for performing this transfer include the straight lift, carry lift, lift sheet, and sliding board.

Alert Before attempting a transfer, review the principles of body mechanics. Consider using additional staff when transferring heavier patients.

Implementation tips

◆ Follow the standard nursing protocol described at the start of the chapter.
◆ To prevent injury, remember to use good body mechanics with all transfers.
◆ Tell the patient that you're going to move him onto a stretcher.
◆ Adjust the bed to the same height as the stretcher. Lock the bed and stretcher wheels to ensure the patient's safety.
◆ Move I.V. lines and other tubing out of the way, and make sure there's no danger of them pulling loose.

Four-person straight lift

◆ Place the stretcher parallel to the bed.
◆ One team member stands at the center of the outside edge of the stretcher, and another stands at the patient's head.
◆ The two other team members stand next to the outside edge of the bed — one at the center and the other at the patient's feet.

◆ Slide your arms, palms up, under the patient while the other team members do the same. This way, the people in the center support the patient's buttocks and hips, the person at the head of the bed supports the patient's head and shoulders, and the person at the foot supports the patient's legs and feet.
◆ On a count of three, everyone lifts the patient several inches, moves him onto the stretcher, and slides their arms out from under him. Keep movements smooth to minimize patient discomfort and avoid muscle strain by team members.

Four-person carry lift
◆ Place the stretcher perpendicular to the bed, with the head of the stretcher at the foot of the bed.
◆ All four team members line up on the same side of the bed as the stretcher, with the tallest member at the patient's head and the shortest at his feet. The person at the patient's head is the team leader and gives the lift signals.
◆ Everyone flexes their knees and slides their hands, palms up, under the patient until he rests securely on their upper arms. Make sure the patient is adequately supported at the head and shoulders, buttocks and hips, and legs and feet.
◆ On a count of three, everyone straightens their knees and rolls the patient onto his side, against their chests. This reduces strain on the lifters and allows them to hold the patient for several minutes if needed.
◆ Together, the team members step back, with the person holding the patient's feet moving the farthest. Everyone moves forward to the side of the stretcher and, on a count of three, lowers the patient onto the stretcher by bending their knees and sliding their arms out from under the patient.

Four-person lift sheet transfer
◆ Position the bed, stretcher, and team members for the straight lift.
◆ Each team member grasps the edges of the sheet close to the patient — a position that allows a firm grip, provides stability, and spares the patient undue feelings of instability.
◆ On a count of three, everyone lifts or slides the patient onto the stretcher in a smooth, continuous motion to avoid muscle strain and minimize patient discomfort.

Sliding-board transfer
◆ Place the stretcher parallel to the bed.
◆ Stand next to the bed while a coworker stands next to the stretcher.
◆ Reach over the patient and pull the far side of the bed sheet toward you to turn the patient slightly on his side. Your coworker then places the sliding board beneath the patient, making sure the board bridges the gap between stretcher and bed.
◆ Ease the patient onto the sliding board and release the sheet. Your coworker then grasps the near side of the sheet at the patient's hips and shoulders and pulls him onto the stretcher in a smooth, continuous motion. Your coworker then reaches over the patient, grasps the far side of the sheet, and logrolls him toward her.
◆ Remove the sliding board as your coworker returns the patient to the supine position.

Special considerations
◆ After all transfers, position the patient comfortably on the stretcher, apply safety straps, and raise and secure the side rails.
◆ When transferring an immobile or obese patient from bed to stretcher, first lift and move him, in increments, to the edge of the bed. Then rest for a few seconds, repositioning the patient

if needed, and lift him onto the stretcher. If the patient can bear weight on his arms or legs, two or three coworkers can perform this transfer.

Documentation

◆ Record the time and, if needed, the type of transfer in your notes.

Transfer from bed to wheelchair

◆ For a patient with little or no lower-body sensation or one-sided weakness, immobility, or injury, the transfer from bed to wheelchair may require partial support to full assistance — initially by at least two people.
◆ After transfer, proper positioning helps prevent excessive pressure on bony prominences and the skin breakdown that may result.

Implementation tips

◆ Follow the standard nursing protocol described at the start of the chapter.
◆ Use good body mechanics during the transfer to prevent injury.
◆ Place the wheelchair parallel to the bed, facing the foot of the bed, and lock its wheels. Make sure the bed wheels are also locked and that the bed is in its lowest position.
◆ Remove the wheelchair footrests to avoid interfering with the transfer.
◆ With the patient in a supine position, obtain a baseline pulse rate and blood pressure.
◆ Help the patient into appropriate clothing, nonslip footwear, and ordered braces or assistive devices.
◆ Raise the head of the bed, and let the patient rest briefly to adjust to posture changes and decrease postural hypotension. Then bring him to the dangling position. If the patient could have cardiovascular instability, recheck his pulse rate and blood pressure. To prevent falls, don't proceed until his vital signs stabilize.
◆ Ask the patient to move toward the edge of the bed and, if possible, to place his feet flat on the floor. Stand in front of the patient, blocking his toes with your feet and his knees with yours to keep his knees from buckling.
◆ Flex your knees slightly, place your arms around the patient's waist, and tell him to place his hands on the edge of the bed. To prevent back strain, don't bend at your waist.
◆ Ask the patient to push himself off the bed and to support as much of his own weight as possible. At the same time, straighten your knees and hips, raising the patient as you straighten your body.
◆ Supporting the patient as needed, pivot toward the wheelchair, keeping your knees against his. Tell the patient to grasp the farthest armrest of the wheelchair with his closest hand, and to back up so that the backs of his legs touch the wheelchair.
◆ Help the patient lower himself into the wheelchair by flexing your hips and knees, but not your back. Instruct him to reach back and grasp the other wheelchair armrest as he sits to avoid abrupt contact with the seat.
◆ To check cardiovascular stability, check the patient's pulse rate and blood pressure. If the systolic blood pressure drops by 20 mm Hg or more, or the diastolic blood pressure drops by at least 10 mm Hg, the patient has orthostatic hypotension. The pulse rate may increase by 20 beats or more as well. Recheck the patient's status after 3 minutes until vital signs are stable and the patient is asymptomatic.
◆ If the patient can't position himself correctly, help him move his buttocks against the back of the chair so that the ischial tuberosities, not the sacrum, provide the base of support.

◆ Put the footrests back on the wheelchair, and place the patient's feet flat on the footrests, pointed straight ahead. Then position the knees and hips with the correct amount of flexion and in appropriate alignment. If appropriate, use elevating leg rests to flex the patient's hips at more than 90 degrees; this position relieves pressure on the popliteal space and places more weight on the ischial tuberosities.
◆ Position the patient's arms on the wheelchair's armrests with shoulders abducted, elbows slightly flexed, forearms pronated, and wrists and hands in the neutral position. If needed, support or elevate the patient's hands and forearms with a pillow to prevent dependent edema.

Special considerations

◆ If the patient starts to fall during the transfer, ease him to the closest surface — bed, floor, or chair. Never stretch to finish the transfer. Doing so can cause loss of balance, falls, muscle strain, and other injuries to you and the patient.
◆ If the patient has one-sided weakness, place the wheelchair on his unaffected side. Instruct the patient to pivot and bear as much weight as possible on the unaffected side. Support the affected side because the patient will tend to lean to this side. To prevent slumping in the wheelchair, use pillows to support a hemiplegic patient's affected side.

Documentation

◆ Record the time of transfer, the amount of assistance needed, and the patient's tolerance of the transfer.

Common patient positions

◆ Proper patient positioning maintains functional body alignment, ensures patient safety, promotes respiration and circulation, relieves pressure, and aids in administering treatment. (See *Positioning patients*.)

Assistive devices

Canes

◆ For a patient who's occasionally unsteady or has one-sided weakness or joint pain or pressure, a cane can provide balance and support for walking. It also reduces fatigue and strain on weight-bearing joints.
◆ Canes aren't appropriate for patients with bilateral weakness; they should use crutches or a walker.
◆ Although wooden canes are available, aluminum canes are most common. They come in three types and provide varying levels of support.
◆ The standard design with a half-circle handle provides the least support. It's used by patients who need only slight assistance with walking.
◆ The T-handle cane has a straight handle with grips and a bent shaft. It's used by patients with hand weakness and provides greater stability than a standard cane.
◆ Three- or four-footed (quad) canes are used by patients with poor balance or one-sided weakness and an inability to hold onto a walker with both hands.

Preparation of equipment

◆ To function properly, a cane must be the correct height for the patient.
◆ A poorly fitted cane can cause the patient to lose his balance and fall. If a cane is too short, the patient will have to drop his shoulder out of alignment to use it. If the cane is too long, he'll have to raise his shoulder, making it difficult to support his weight.

Positioning patients

This table lists various positions in which patients may be placed. These positions may be used for comfort, but proper positioning also maintains functional body alignment and safety, promotes respiration and circulation, relieves pressure, and aids in administering treatment.

POSITION	INDICATIONS	IMPLEMENTATION	RATIONALE
Dorsal recumbent (supine)	◆ Spinal cord injury ◆ Urinary catheter insertion ◆ Vaginal examination	◆ Place the patient on his back with the knees slightly flexed. ◆ Place a pillow beneath his head for comfort.	◆ Immobilizes the spine
Trendelenburg's	◆ Shock ◆ Cystic fibrosis	◆ Position the patient in a supine position with his feet elevated 30 to 40 degrees higher than his head.	◆ Promotes postural drainage and venous return
Reverse Trendelenburg's	◆ Cervical traction ◆ Post lower extremity-vessel surgery	◆ Elevate the head of the bed and lower the feet.	◆ Provides counterbalance for traction ◆ Promotes blood flow to the lower extremities
Prone	◆ Immobilization ◆ Acute respiratory distress syndrome ◆ Post lumbar puncture or myelogram	◆ Place the patient on his stomach with the head turned to one side. ◆ Position the arms at the side or above the head. ◆ Make sure that the legs are extended.	◆ Enables examination of the back and spine ◆ Promotes gas exchange
Lateral (side-lying)	◆ Post abdominal surgery ◆ Coma ◆ Pressure ulcer ◆ Enema or rectal irrigation	◆ Place the patient on his side, with his weight being mostly supported by the lateral aspect of the lower scapula and the lower ileum. ◆ Support with pillows.	◆ Promotes safety ◆ Prevents atelectasis, pressure ulcers, and aspiration of food and secretions

(continued)

Positioning patients *(continued)*

POSITION	INDICATIONS	IMPLEMENTATION	RATIONALE
Sims'	◆ Coma ◆ Rectal injuries	◆ Position the patient on his side with a small pillow beneath his head. ◆ Flex one knee toward the abdomen, with the other knee only slightly flexed. ◆ Place one arm behind the body and the other in a comfortable position. Support with pillows.	◆ Enables examination of the back and rectum ◆ Prevents pressure ulcers and atelectasis
Elevation of extremity	◆ Thrombophlebitis ◆ Post cast application ◆ Edema ◆ Post surgery on limb	◆ Use the bed controls to elevate the legs, or use pillows to elevate the arms and legs.	◆ Promotes circulation and comfort ◆ Enables examinations and procedures
Fowler's	◆ Head injury, cranial surgery, increased intracranial pressure (ICP) ◆ Post abdominal surgery ◆ Dyspnea ◆ Vomiting ◆ Post thyroidectomy ◆ Post eye surgery	◆ Elevate the head of the bed to 45 degrees and raise the bed section under the patient's knees, flexing the knees *slightly.*	◆ Enables examination ◆ Immobilizes the spine ◆ Promotes drainage, cardiac output, and ventilation ◆ Prevents aspiration of food and secretions
Semi-Fowler's	◆ Head injury, cranial surgery, increased ICP ◆ Post abdominal surgery ◆ Dyspnea ◆ Vomiting ◆ Post thyroidectomy ◆ Post eye surgery	◆ Elevate the head of the bed to 30 degrees and raise the bed section under the patient's knees, flexing the knee *slightly.*	◆ Promotes drainage, cardiac output, and ventilation ◆ Prevents aspiration of food and secretions

Positioning patients *(continued)*

POSITION	INDICATIONS	IMPLEMENTATION	RATIONALE
High Fowler's	◆ Head injury, cranial surgery, increased ICP ◆ Dyspnea, respiratory distress ◆ Feeding (during and after meals) ◆ Hiatal hernia	◆ Elevate the head of the bed to 90 degrees and raise the bed section under the patient's knees, flexing the knees *slightly.*	◆ Promotes drainage, cardiac output, and ventilation ◆ Prevents aspiration of food and secretions
Lithotomy	◆ Perineal or rectal procedure	◆ Place the patient on his back (either flat or with the head slightly elevated). ◆ Knees should be flexed at right angles and feet placed in stirrups.	◆ Enables examination of the pelvis

◆ To fit properly, the handle of the cane should be level with the greater trochanter and allow about 15 degrees of flexion at the elbow.

◆ Ask the patient to hold the cane on his unaffected side 4″ to 6″ (10 to 15 cm) from the base of his little toe. If the cane is aluminum, adjust its height by depressing the metal button on the shaft and raising or lowering the handle. If the cane is wooden, you'll have to remove the rubber tip, have any excess length sawed off, and reapply the rubber tip.

Implementation tips

◆ Follow the standard nursing protocol described at the start of the chapter.

◆ Explain how to walk with a cane, and show the patient how to do it.

◆ Tell the patient to hold the cane on his unaffected (strong) side, close to his body. This position moves weight away from the involved side, promotes a steady gait, and keeps the patient from leaning toward the cane.

◆ Teach the patient to move the cane and affected (weak) leg together, and then move the strong leg by itself.

◆ Urge the patient to keep the length and timing of each step equal rather than making one step long and slow and the other short and quick.

◆ After showing the patient how to walk with the cane, have him try it. If needed, coordinate practice sessions with the physical therapy department.

Patient teaching tip Urge the patient to keep good posture and to look ahead, not down, while using a cane.

Using stairs

STAIRS WITH A RAILING

◆ The patient may hold the cane in whichever hand he prefers and use the railing for support.

◆ To go up the stairs, the patient should lead with the strong leg and follow with the weak leg.

◆ To go down the stairs, he should lead with the weak leg and follow with the strong one.
◆ Help the patient remember by giving him this reminder sentence: "The strong go up; the weak go down."

STAIRS WITHOUT A RAILING

◆ If the stairs have no railing, the patient should use the standard walking technique, but he should move the cane just before moving the affected leg.
◆ To go up the stairs, the patient should hold the cane on his strong side, step with the strong leg, advance the cane, and then move the weak leg.
◆ To go down the stairs, he should hold the cane on his strong side, advance the cane, step with the weak leg, and then move the strong leg.

Using a chair

◆ To teach the patient to sit down, stand by his affected side, and tell him to place the backs of his legs against the edge of the chair seat. Then tell him to move the cane away from his body and to reach back with both hands to grasp the chair's armrests. Supporting his weight on the armrests, he can then lower himself onto the seat.
◆ While he's seated, he should keep the cane hooked on the armrest or the chair back.
◆ To teach the patient to get up, stand by his affected side, and tell him to unhook the cane from the chair and hold it in his stronger hand as he grasps the armrests. Then tell him to move his strong foot slightly forward, to lean slightly forward, and to push against the armrests to raise himself upright.
◆ Tell the patient not to lean on the cane when sitting or rising from the chair to prevent falls.
◆ Supervise the patient each time he gets in or out of a chair until you're both certain he can do it alone.

Special considerations

◆ To prevent falls during the learning period, guard the patient carefully by standing on his stronger side, slightly behind him, and placing one foot between his feet and the other to the outside of his stronger leg. If needed, use a walking belt.

Documentation

◆ Record the type of cane used, the amount of guarding needed, the distance walked, and the patient's understanding and tolerance of cane walking.

Crutches

◆ Crutches let the patient support himself with his hands and arms, shifting weight away from one or both legs. Usually, crutches are used for patients who have leg injuries or weakness.
◆ To use crutches successfully, the patient needs balance, stamina, and upper-body strength.
◆ The type of crutches selected, and the walking gait used, depend on the patient's condition.
◆ Three types of crutches are commonly used. Standard aluminum or wooden crutches are used by a patient with a sprain, strain, or cast. These crutches require stamina and upper-body strength.
◆ Aluminum forearm crutches are for patients, such as paraplegics, who use a swing-through gait. These crutches have a collar that fits around the forearm and a horizontal handgrip for support.
◆ Platform crutches provide padded arm surfaces and are used by arthritic patients and those who can't bear weight through their wrists.

Implementation tips

◆ Follow the standard nursing protocol described at the start of the chapter.

◆ Consult with the patient's physician and physical therapist to coordinate rehabilitation orders and teaching.

◆ Make sure the crutches fit the patient properly. (See *Fitting a patient for a crutch.*)

◆ Find out which gait the patient will be using. Describe it to him. Then show him how to do it.

◆ If needed to help prevent falls, place a walking belt around the patient's waist while you teach him.

◆ To start, position the crutches and have the patient shift his weight from side to side. Then, if possible, place him in front of a full-length mirror so he can see the process of walking while he learns it.

Four-point gait

◆ A patient who can bear weight on both legs may use the four-point gait.

◆ Teach this sequence: right crutch, left foot, left crutch, right foot.

◆ Suggest that the patient count out the steps to help develop the rhythm of the gait.

◆ Tell him to make sure each step (crutch and foot) is of equal length.

◆ This is the safest gait because three points are always in contact with the floor. However, the four-point gait requires more coordination than others because the patient is constantly shifting his weight.

◆ If the patient masters this gait, he may be able to use the faster two-point gait.

Two-point gait

◆ If a patient has weak legs but good coordination and arm strength, teach the two-point gait.

◆ This is the most natural crutch-walking gait because it mimics walking, with alternating swings of the arms and legs.

◆ Tell the patient to advance the right crutch and left foot together, followed by the left crutch and right foot together.

Three-point gait

◆ If the patient can bear only partial or no weight on one leg, teach the three-point gait.

◆ Tell him to advance the affected (weak) leg and both crutches by 6" to 8" (15 to 20 cm) while supporting his weight on the unaffected (strong) leg.

Fitting a patient for a crutch

Position the crutch so it extends from a point 4" to 6" (10 to 15 cm) to the side and 4" to 6" in front of the patient's feet to 1½" to 2" (4 to 5 cm) below the axillae (about the width of two fingers). Then adjust the handgrips so the patient's elbows are flexed at a 15-degree angle when he's standing with the crutches in the resting position.

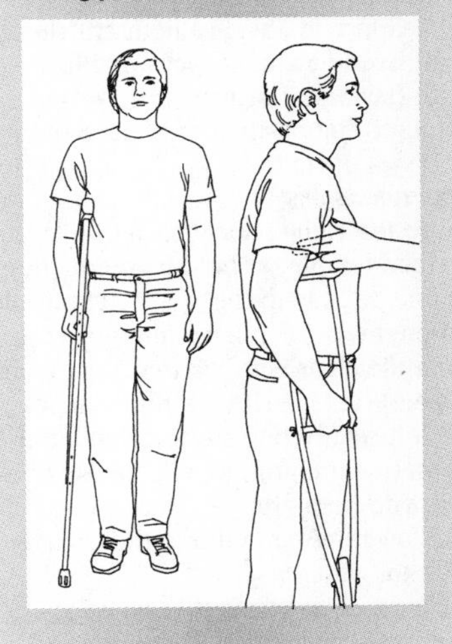

◆ Then tell him to bring the strong leg forward while supporting most of his weight on the crutches and some of it on the weak leg, if possible.

◆ Stress the importance of taking steps of equal length and duration with no pauses.

Swing gaits

◆ If the patient has paralysis of the hips and legs, teach the swing-to or swing-through gaits. These are the fastest gaits.

◆ Tell him to advance both crutches and then to swing his legs into line with (swing-to) or beyond (swing-through) the position of the crutches.

Chairs and stairs

◆ To teach the patient to get up from a chair, tell him to hold both crutches in one hand with the tips resting firmly on the floor. Then have him push up from the chair with his free hand while supporting himself with the crutches.

◆ To teach him to sit down, tell him to reverse the process, supporting himself with both crutches in one hand and lowering himself into the chair with the other.

◆ To teach the patient to go up stairs using a three-point gait, tell him to step up with the strong leg while supporting his weight with both crutches and the weak leg on the lower step. Then he can move the crutches and weak leg up.

◆ To teach him to go down stairs, tell him to step down with both crutches and the weak leg. Then he can follow with the strong leg.

◆ To help him remember, give him this reminder sentence: "The strong go up; the weak go down."

Special considerations

◆ If time permits, urge the patient to perform arm- and shoulder-strengthening exercises to prepare for crutch walking.

◆ Find out from the physician or physical therapist if you can teach the patient two walking techniques — one fast and one slow. That way, he can switch between them to reduce muscle fatigue and adapt to various walking conditions.

Complications

◆ If the patient has a chronic condition, the swing-to and swing-through gaits can lead to atrophy of the hips and legs unless he routinely performs appropriate therapeutic exercises.

◆ Caution the patient against habitually leaning on his crutches because prolonged pressure on the axillae can damage the brachial nerves, causing brachial nerve palsy.

Documentation

◆ Record the type of gait used, the patient's weight-bearing status, the amount of assistance needed, the distance walked, and the patient's tolerance of the crutches and gait.

Walkers

◆ A walker is a three-sided metal frame with four legs and handgrips. The patient stands in the open side of the frame and is supported on three sides.

◆ A walker offers greater stability and security than other walking aids. It's used for patients with too little strength or balance for crutches or a cane and for patients who need frequent rest periods.

◆ The standard walker is for patients with one- or two-sided weakness and patients who can't bear weight on one leg. This walker requires arm strength and balance.

◆ For extremely weak or poorly coordinated patients, wheels may be placed on the two front legs of a standard walker. That way, the patient can roll the walker forward instead of having to lift it. However, because wheels can increase the risk of falling, they must be used with caution.

◆ For patients who have to use stairs without double handrails, a stair walker may be helpful. It has an extra set of handles that extend toward the patient on the open side. To use this walker, the patient needs good arm strength and balance.

◆ A patient with very weak legs may prefer a rolling walker, which has four wheels and may also have a seat.

◆ For a patient with very weak arms, a reciprocal walker may be best. It lets the patient move one side of the walker at a time.

Preparation of equipment

◆ Obtain the prescribed walker, and make sure it's adjusted properly to the patient's height.

◆ Standing comfortably in the walker with his hands on the grips, the patient's elbows should be flexed at a 15-degree angle.

◆ To adjust the height of the walker, turn it upside down. Push the button on the shaft of one leg, adjust the leg length by sliding the shaft in or out, and then release the button. Then do the same for the other legs. Make sure the walker is level when you're finished.

Implementation tips

◆ Follow the standard nursing protocol described at the start of the chapter.

◆ Help the patient stand in the walker, and tell him to hold the handgrips firmly and equally. Stand behind him; if he has one affected leg, stand closer to that leg.

Standard walker

◆ If the patient has one weak leg, tell him to move the walker 6″ to 8″ (15 to 20 cm) forward and to step into the walker with the weak leg first. Then he should follow with the strong leg, supporting himself on his arms. Urge him to take equal strides.

◆ If the patient has equal strength in both legs, tell him to move the walker 6″ to 8″ forward and to step into it with either leg.

◆ If the patient can't use one leg at all, tell him to move the walker 6″ to 8″ forward and to swing into it, supporting his weight on his arms.

◆ Also teach the patient how to sit down and get up from a chair safely. (See *Sitting and standing using a walker*, page 16).

Reciprocal walker

◆ For a reciprocal walker, teach the two-point gait.

◆ Instruct the patient to stand with his weight evenly on his legs and the walker. Stand behind him, slightly to one side.

◆ Tell him to move the walker's right side and his left foot at the same time. Then have him move the walker's left side and his right foot at the same time.

◆ You may also teach the four-point gait.

◆ Tell the patient to stand with his weight evenly on his legs and the walker. Stand behind him, slightly to one side.

◆ Tell him to move the right side of the walker forward, followed by his left foot. Next, have him move the left side of the walker forward, followed by his right foot.

Wheeled or stair walker

◆ If the patient is using a wheeled or stair walker, reinforce the physical therapist's instructions.

Sitting and standing using a walker

Sitting down

◆ First, tell the patient to stand with the back of his stronger leg against the front of the chair, his weaker leg slightly off the floor, and the walker directly in front.

◆ Tell him to grasp the armrests on the chair one arm at a time while supporting most of his weight on the stronger leg. (In the illustrations, the patient has left leg weakness.)

◆ Tell the patient to lower himself into the chair and slide backward. After he's seated, he should place the walker beside the chair.

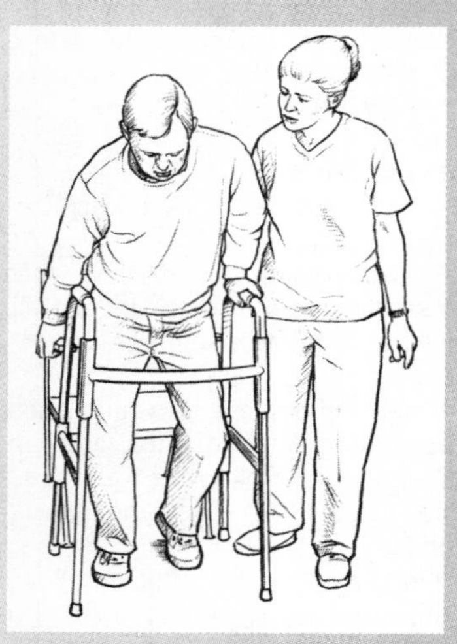

Getting up

◆ After bringing the walker to the front of the patient's chair, tell him to slide forward in the chair. Placing the back of his stronger leg against the seat, he should then advance the weaker leg.

◆ Next, with both hands on the armrests, the patient can push himself to a standing position. Supporting himself with the stronger leg and the opposite hand, the patient should grasp the walker's handgrip with his free hand.

◆ Then the patient should grasp the free handgrip with his other hand.

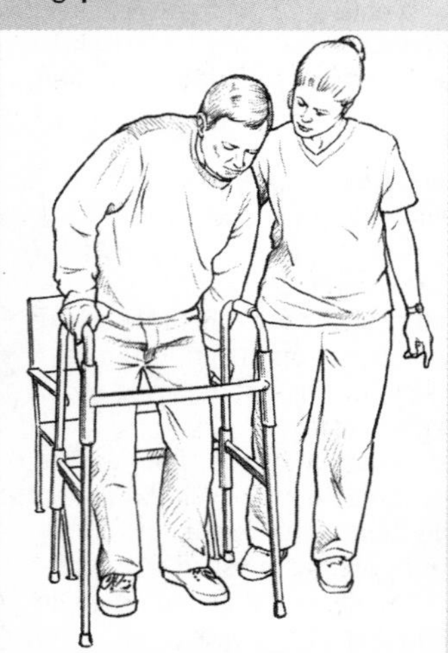

◆ Stress the need for caution.

Special considerations

◆ If the patient starts to fall, support his hips and shoulders to help him stay upright if possible. If not, ease him slowly to the closest surface — bed, floor, or chair.

Documentation

◆ Record the type of walker and attachments used, the patient's weight-bearing status, the degree of guarding needed, the distance walked, and the patient's tolerance of walking.

Supplemental bed equipment

◆ Certain equipment can promote the bedridden patient's comfort and help

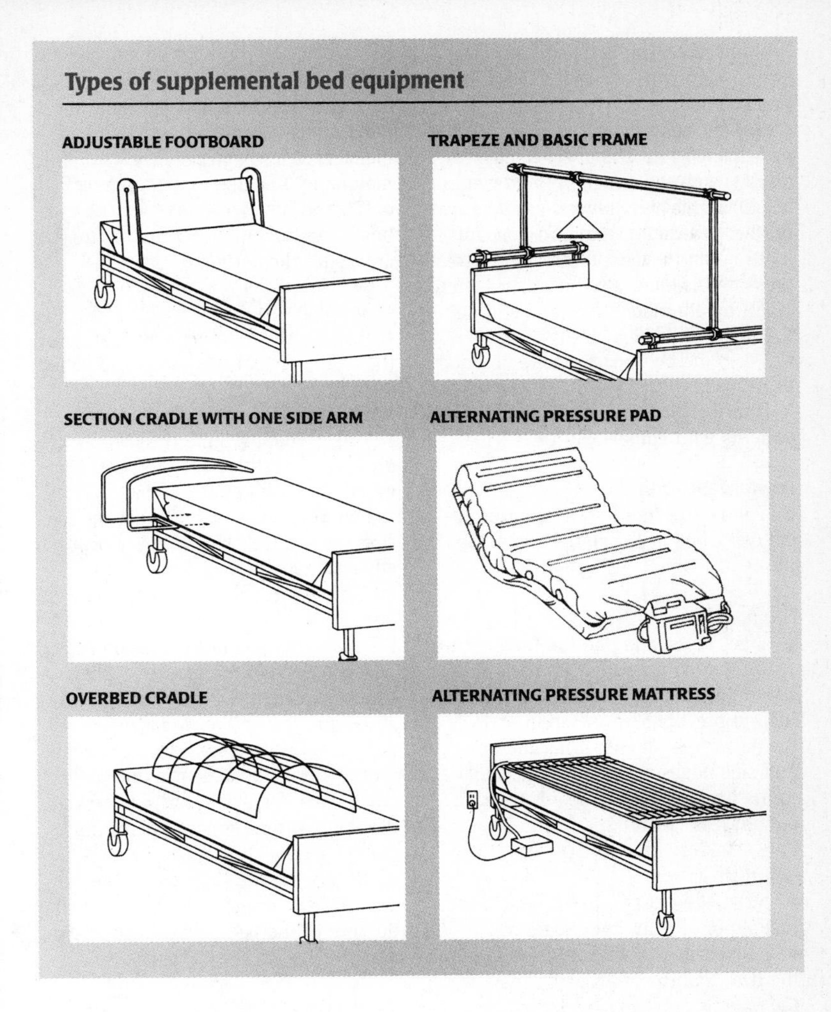

prevent pressure ulcers and other complications of immobility. (See *Types of supplemental bed equipment*.)

◆ A wooden or hard plastic footboard keeps the feet in proper alignment and helps prevent footdrop. It can also be used to lift the bed linens off the patient's feet.

◆ A foot cradle — a horizontal or arched bar over the end of the bed — lifts linens off the patient's feet, preventing skin irritation and breakdown. This is especially helpful in patients with peripheral vascular disease or neuropathy.

◆ A metal overbed cradle, a cage-like frame placed on top of the mattress, lifts bed linens off a patient with burns, open wounds, or a wet cast.

◆ A basic metal frame and trapeze (a metal triangle that hangs from the frame) help a patient with arm strength lift himself off the bed — for exercise and to help with bed-making and bed-pan positioning.

◆ An alternating pressure pad (a vinyl pad divided into chambers filled with air or water and attached to an electric pump) or mattress places less pressure on the skin than a standard hospital mattress and is used to prevent or treat pressure ulcers. It also stimulates circulation by alternately inflating and deflating its chambers.

◆ A simple bed board, made of wood or canvas-covered wood, can be used to firm the mattress and is helpful for patients with spinal injuries.

Implementation tips

◆ Follow the standard nursing protocol described at the start of the chapter.

Footboard

◆ First, cover and pad the footboard with a folded drawsheet or bath blanket to cushion the hard footboard and help to prevent skin irritation and breakdown. To do so, bring the top and side edges of the sheet or blanket to the back of the footboard, miter the corners, and secure them. Don't leave any wrinkles where the patient's feet will rest.

◆ Move the patient up in the bed to make room for the footboard.

◆ Loosen the top linens at the foot of the bed, and then fold them back over the patient to expose his feet.

◆ Based on the design of the footboard, you may lift the mattress at the foot of the bed and place the lip of the footboard between the mattress and the bedsprings. Or you may secure the footboard under both sides of the mattress.

◆ Adjust the footboard so the patient's feet rest comfortably against it. If it isn't adjustable, tuck a folded bath blanket between the board and the patient's feet.

◆ Unless the footboard has side supports, place a sandbag, a folded bath blanket, or a pillow beside each foot to maintain 90-degree foot alignment.

◆ Extend the top linens over the footboard, tuck them under the mattress, and miter the corners.

Foot cradle

◆ Loosen the top linens at the foot of the bed, and fold them over the patient or to one side.

◆ For a one-piece cradle, slide one side arm under the mattress so the cradle arches over the bed, and place the other side arm under the mattress on the opposite side. Then adjust the tension rods so they rest securely over the edge of the mattress.

◆ For a sectional cradle with two side arms, first slide the side arms under the mattress. Secure the tension rods over the edge of the mattress. Then carefully place the arch over the bed and connect it to the side arms.

◆ For a sectional cradle with one side arm, connect the side arm and arched cradle bar. Then slide the side arm under the mattress on one side of the bed.

◆ Unfold the top linens over the cradle, tuck them under the mattress at the foot of the bed, and miter the corners.

Overbed cradle

◆ Loosen and remove the top linens.

◆ Carefully lower the cradle onto the bed, over the patient. Secure it in place by wrapping roller gauze around both sides of the cradle, pulling the gauze taut, and attaching it to the bedsprings.

◆ Cover the cradle with the top linens, tuck them under the mattress at the foot of the bed, and miter the corners.

Basic frame and trapeze

◆ Ideally, an orthopedic technician will attach a frame and trapeze to the patient's bed.

◆ If an orthopedic technician isn't available, get help to attach these devices to the bed as needed.

◆ Make sure the trapeze hangs within easy reach so the patient won't need to strain to reach it.

Alternating pressure pad or mattress

◆ If possible, transfer the patient from his bed to a chair or stretcher. Get help for the transfer, if needed.

◆ Strip the linens from the bed. Then inspect the plug and electrical cord of the device for defects. Don't use the unit if it appears damaged.

◆ Replace the mattress with the alternating pressure mattress or unfold the pad on top of the regular mattress with the correct side facing up.

◆ Place the motor on a linen-saver pad on the floor or on a footstool near the mattress outlets — far enough away to avoid being tripped over. Connect the tubing securely to the motor and to the mattress outlets, and plug the cord into an electrical outlet. Turn the motor on.

◆ After several minutes, watch how the chambers fill and empty. Make sure the tubing has no kinks.

◆ Place a bottom sheet over the pad or mattress, and tuck it in loosely. To keep the tubing open, don't miter the corner where the tubing attaches.

◆ Don't place too many layers of drawsheets or linen-saver pads between the alternating pressure pad or mattress and the patient because these decrease the effectiveness of the alternating pressure device.

◆ Position the patient comfortably in the bed, cover him with the top linens, and tuck them in loosely.

◆ If the pad or mattress becomes soiled, clean it with a damp cloth and mild soap, and dry it well. To avoid causing damage, don't use alcohol or sharp items such as safety pins.

◆ When the patient no longer needs the pad or mattress, or the patient is discharged, turn the motor off, disconnect the tubing, and unplug the cord from the wall outlet. Remove the pad or mattress from the bed and either discard it or follow your facility's policy for cleaning and storing it.

◆ Coil the tubing and electrical cord, and strap them to the motor. Return the motor unit to the central supply department.

Bed board

◆ Transfer the patient from his bed to a stretcher or a chair. Obtain assistance if necessary.

◆ Strip the linens from the bed.

◆ If the bed board consists of wooden slats encased in canvas, lift the mattress at the head of the bed and center the board over the bedsprings to prevent it from jutting out and causing accidental injury. Unroll the slats to cover the bedsprings at the head of the bed. Then lift the mattress at the foot of the bed and unroll the remaining slats.

◆ If the bed board consists of one solid or two hinged pieces of wood, lift the mattress on one side of the bed and center the board over the bedsprings.

◆ After positioning the bed board, replace the linens. Then return the patient to bed.

Special considerations

◆ For an overbed or foot cradle, place the patient in bed before positioning and securing the device, and remove the device before the patient gets out of bed. This helps ensure proper placement and avoid patient injury.

◆ When turning or positioning the patient on his side, make sure the tension rod of the foot cradle doesn't rest against his skin; if it does, it could cause pressure and skin breakdown.

◆ If you're using a bed board with a plastic-covered mattress, remember that the plastic may slide easily over the board. When transferring the patient from a stretcher to the bed, have a coworker stand on the opposite side of the bed to stabilize it.

◆ If the bottom sheet isn't wide enough to cover both a standard and a specialty mattress (such as a foam mattress), use two bottom sheets. Cover the standard mattress with one sheet. Then cover the foam mattress with a second sheet and tuck it between the standard and foam mattresses.

◆ You may need two top sheets to cover the patient when you're using a footboard, foot cradle, or bed cradle.

Documentation

◆ Record the type of supplemental bed equipment used, the time and date of use, and the patient's response to treatment.

Special beds

Low–air-loss therapy bed

◆ Low–air-loss therapy beds are made of segmented, inflatable air cushions that relieve pressure, help prevent and treat skin breakdown, and minimize pain.

◆ You may use such a bed for patients with skin grafts or surgical flaps, pressure ulcers, edema, or advanced arthritis as well as oncology and transplant patients.

◆ Low–air-loss therapy beds circulate cool air, which helps to evaporate moisture and reduce temperature, thereby reducing excess skin moisture and preventing maceration.

◆ Some models pulsate to promote circulation or rotate to ease turning, mobilize secretions, and prevent pulmonary complications.

◆ The low–air-loss therapy bed can't be used for a patient with an unstable cervical, thoracic, or lumbar fracture.

Rotation bed

◆ Because of their constant motion, rotation beds — such as the Roto Rest — promote postural drainage and peristalsis and help prevent the complications of immobility.

◆ These beds rotate from side to side like a cradle. They reach 62 degrees of elevation and full side-to-side turning about every 4½ minutes.

◆ Because the bed holds the patient motionless, it's especially helpful in spinal cord injury, multiple trauma, stroke, multiple sclerosis, coma, severe burns, hypostatic pneumonia, atelectasis, or other unilateral lung problems that cause poor ventilation and perfusion.

◆ Rotation beds aren't used for a patient with severe claustrophobia, an unstable cervical fracture without neurologic deficit, or complications of immobility.

◆ Some rotation beds, such as the Roto Rest, allow use of cervical traction devices and tongs. They also may provide variable angles of rotation, a fan, access for X-rays, and supports and clips for chest tubes, catheters, and drains.

Air-fluidized therapy bed

◆ Originally designed for managing burns, the air-fluidized therapy bed is now used for patients with other conditions, such as pressure ulcers, wounds, and surgical flaps and grafts. By allowing harmless contact between the bed's surface and grafted sites, the bed promotes comfort and healing.

◆ The traditional bed is a large tub that supports the patient on a thick layer of silicone-coated microspheres.

Another version combines the air-fluidized section with a low–air-loss or cushioned section. A monofilament polyester filter sheet covers the microspheres, allowing moisture to pass through.

◆ Warmed air from a blower beneath the bed passes through the microspheres and can be adjusted to help control hypothermia and hyperthermia. The resulting fluid-like surface reduces pressure on the skin, easing capillary blood flow, helping prevent pressure ulcers, and promoting wound healing.

◆ Special controls let you change various areas of the bed to best suit the patient's needs.

◆ The air-fluidized therapy bed can't be used for a patient with an unstable spine. It usually shouldn't be used for patients who can't expel pulmonary secretions because the lack of back support impairs productive coughing. Some models come with adjustable back and leg supports to promote positioning.

Special considerations

Low–air-loss therapy bed

◆ Every 2 hours, encourage coughing and deep breathing, turn or reposition the patient, and examine the patient's skin.

◆ If the bed rotates, make sure invasive lines and tubes are secured at the correct angle to minimize the risk of binding, disconnecting, or dislodging.

◆ To position a bedpan, deflate the seat portion of the bed, roll the patient away from you, and place the bedpan on the turning sheet. Then reposition the patient. To remove the bedpan, hold it steady, roll the patient away from you, and remove it. Then reinflate the seat portion of the bed.

◆ Don't use pins or clamps to secure sheets or tubing because they may puncture the bed and cause air loss.

Rotation bed

◆ If the patient develops cardiac arrest while on the bed, perform cardiopulmonary resuscitation after taking the bed out of gear, locking it in horizontal position, removing the side arm support and the thoracic pack, lifting the shoulder assembly, and dropping the arm pack. You won't need a cardiac board because of the bed's firm surface.

◆ Lock the bed in the extreme lateral position for access to the back of the head, thorax, and buttocks through the appropriate hatches. Clean the mattress and nondisposable packs during patient care, rinse them thoroughly to remove all soap residue, and make sure they are completely dry. When replacing the packs and hatches, take care not to pinch the patient's skin between the packs.

◆ Expect increased drainage from any pressure ulcers for the first few days the patient is on the bed because the motion helps debride necrotic tissue and improves local circulation.

◆ Schedule and perform daily range-of-motion exercises, as ordered, because the bed allows full access to all extremities without disturbing spinal alignment.

◆ For female patients, tape an indwelling urinary catheter to the thigh before bringing it through the perineal hatch. For a male patient with spinal cord lesions, tape the catheter to the abdomen and then to the thigh to facilitate gravity drainage. Hang the drainage bag on the clips provided, and make sure it doesn't get caught between the bed frames during rotation.

◆ If the patient has a tracheal or endotracheal tube with mechanical ventilation, attach the tube support bracket between the cervical pack and the arm packs. Tape the connecting T tubing to the support and run it beside the patient's head and off the center of the table to help prevent reflux of condensation.

◆ For a patient with pulmonary congestion or pneumonia, suction secretions more often during the first 12 to 24 hours on the bed because the motion will increase drainage.

◆ For maximum effectiveness, the bed should rotate for 20 of each day's 24 hours. Don't stop the bed for more than 30 minutes.

Age alert Older adults are especially prone to sensory distress from the constant motion of a rotation bed. Provide emotional support.

Air-fluidized therapy bed

◆ Monitor the patient's fluid and electrolyte status because this bed promotes evaporative water loss. Because of this drying effect, always cover a mesh graft for the first 2 to 8 days, as ordered.

◆ If the patient has excessive upper respiratory tract dryness, use a humidifier and mask as ordered. Encourage coughing and deep breathing every 2 hours or according to facility policy. Monitor intake and output, and encourage fluids as permitted.

◆ For a patient on prolonged bed rest, watch for hypocalcemia and hypophosphatemia.

◆ To place a bedpan, roll the patient away from you, place the bedpan on the flat sheet, and push it into the microspheres. Then reposition the patient. To remove the bedpan, hold it steady and roll the patient away from you. Turn off the air pressure and remove the bedpan. Then turn the air on and reposition the patient.

◆ Don't secure the filter sheet with pins or clamps because they may puncture the sheet and release microspheres. Holes or tears may be repaired with iron-on patching tape.

◆ Sieve the microspheres monthly or between patients to remove any clumped microspheres. Handle them carefully to avoid spills; spilled microspheres may cause falls.

◆ Treat a soiled filter sheet and clumped microspheres as contaminated items; handle them according to facility policy.

◆ Change the filter sheet and operate the unit unoccupied for 24 hours between patients.

◆ Examine the patient's skin and reposition him every 2 hours. Specialty beds don't eliminate the need for frequent monitoring and position changes.

◆ For cardiopulmonary resuscitation, an emergency STOP/DEFLATE button immediately stops the action of the bed.

Documentation

Low–air-loss therapy bed

◆ Record the duration of therapy and the patient's response to it.

◆ Document the condition of the patient's skin, including the presence of pressure ulcers and other wounds.

◆ Document the patient's comfort level and tolerance of rotational angles, as applicable.

Rotation bed

◆ Record a baseline skin examination, changes in the patient's condition, degree of bed rotation, and the patient's response to therapy.

◆ Note turning times and ongoing care on the flowchart.

Air-fluidized therapy bed

◆ Record the duration of therapy and the patient's response to it.

◆ Document the condition of the patient's skin, pressure ulcers, and other wounds.

Hygiene and comfort

Bed bath

◆ A complete bed bath cleans the skin, stimulates circulation, provides mild exercise, and promotes comfort. Bathing also allows examination of skin condition, joint mobility, and muscle strength.
◆ Depending on the patient's overall condition and duration of hospitalization, he may have a complete or partial bath daily.
◆ A partial bath — including hands, face, axillae, back, genitalia, and anal region — can replace the complete bath for the patient with dry, fragile skin or extreme weakness, and can supplement the complete bath for the diaphoretic or incontinent patient.

Implementation tips

◆ Follow the standard nursing protocol described at the start of the chapter.
◆ Adjust the temperature of the patient's room to prevent drafts.
◆ Determine the patient's preference for soap or other hygiene aids because some patients are allergic to soap or lotions.
◆ Test the water temperature carefully with your elbow to avoid scalding or chilling the patient; the water should feel comfortably warm.
◆ Change the water as often as needed to keep it warm and clean.
◆ Before and after you wash an area, keep it covered with a bath blanket to provide warmth and privacy.
◆ Fold the washcloth around your gloved hand to form a mitt while bathing the patient. This keeps the cloth warm longer and avoids dribbling water on the patient from the cloth's loose ends.
◆ When washing a patient's face, start with the eyes. Work from the inner to the outer canthus, and don't use soap. Use a separate section of the washcloth for each eye to avoid spreading ocular infection.
◆ If the patient tolerates soap, apply it to the cloth, and wash the rest of his face, ears, and neck, using firm, gentle strokes.
◆ Thoroughly rinse all areas washed with soap because residual soap can cause itching and dryness.
◆ When bathing a patient's arm, use long, smooth strokes and move from wrist to shoulder, to stimulate venous circulation.
◆ To improve circulation, maintain joint mobility, and preserve muscle tone, move the body joints through their full range of motion during the bath.
◆ If possible, soak the patient's hands in the basin to remove dirt and soften nails.
◆ When bathing a patient's legs, move from ankle to hip to stimulate venous circulation.
◆ Don't massage the leg. Leg massage may dislodge any existing thrombus and possibly cause a pulmonary embolus.
◆ Bathe the anal area from front to back to avoid contaminating the perineum.
◆ Observe overall skin condition and color during the bath to check peripheral circulation.
◆ Use firm strokes to avoid tickling the patient.
◆ Dry all areas thoroughly, taking special care in skin folds and creases.
◆ When changing the bath water, lower the bed and raise the side rails to ensure patient safety.
◆ When the bath is completed, dress the patient in a clean gown, and remake the bed or change the linens.

◆ If the patient tolerates deodorant, apply it.
◆ Use warm lotion to massage the patient's back; cold lotion can startle the patient and cause muscle tension and vasoconstriction.
◆ During a back massage, pay special attention to bony prominences. Check for redness, abrasions, and pressure ulcers.
◆ Carry soiled linens to the hamper with outstretched arms. To avoid spreading microorganisms, don't let soiled linens touch your clothing.

Special considerations

◆ A bag bath involves the use of 8 or 10 premoistened, warmed, disposable cloths (in a plastic bag or prepackaged pouch container) that contain a no-rinse surfactant instead of soap. A bag bath saves time compared to the conventional bed bath because no rinsing is required.
◆ Before using them, warm the prepackaged cloths in a microwave or special warming unit supplied by the manufacturer.
◆ Use a separate cloth to wash each part of the patient's body.
◆ Don't wash a trauma or rape victim until she has been examined by a physician and, possibly, the police. Washing may remove important evidence (powder burns or body fluids) that may be needed later in court.

Documentation

◆ Record the date and time of the bed bath on the flowchart.
◆ Note the patient's tolerance for the bath, his range of motion, and his self-care abilities, and report unusual findings.

Tub baths and showers

◆ Tub baths and showers provide personal hygiene, stimulate circulation, and reduce tension for the patient. They also let you see the patient's skin condition and check joint mobility and muscle strength.
◆ If not precluded by the patient's condition or safety considerations, privacy during bathing promotes the patient's sense of well-being by letting him take charge of his own care.
◆ Patients who are recovering from recent surgery, who are emotionally unstable, or who have casts or dressings in place usually need a physician's permission for a tub bath or shower.

Implementation tips

◆ Follow the standard nursing protocol described at the start of the chapter.
◆ Taking care to respect his privacy, help the patient bathe, as needed; he may appreciate help washing his back.
◆ If you can safely leave the patient alone during a bath or shower, do so. Place the call bell within easy reach, and show the patient how to use it.
◆ Ask the patient to leave the door unlocked for his safety, but assure him that you'll post an "Occupied" sign on the door. Stay nearby in case of emergency, and check on the patient every 5 to 10 minutes.
◆ Dry the floor of the bathing area well to prevent slipping.
◆ Make sure the tub or shower is cleaned and disinfected before and after a bath or shower.

For a bath

◆ Position a chair next to the tub to help the patient get in and out and to provide a seat if he becomes weak.
◆ Place a bath blanket over the chair to cover the patient if he gets chilled.

For a shower

◆ Place a nonskid chair in the shower to provide support and give the patient a place to sit down while washing his

legs and feet, reducing the risk of falling
- Cover the floor of the shower with a nonskid mat if it doesn't have nonskid strips.
- Place a towel mat next to the bathing area.
- Move electrical appliances, such as hair driers and heaters, from the patient's reach to prevent electrical accidents.
- Adjust water flow and temperature just before the patient gets into the shower.

Special considerations
- If you're giving a tub bath to a patient who has a cast or dressing on an arm or leg, wrap the limb in a clear plastic bag. Secure the bag with tape, being careful not to constrict circulation. Tell the patient to dangle the arm or leg over the edge of the tub to keep it out of the water.
- Urge the patient to use safety devices, bars, and rails when bathing.
- Because bathing in warm water causes vasodilation, the patient may feel faint. If so, open the drain or turn off the shower. Cover the patient's shoulders and back with a bath towel, and instruct him to lean forward in the tub and to lower his head. Or, help him out of the shower onto a chair, lower his head, and call for help. Never leave the patient unattended. When the patient recovers, help him to bed and monitor his vital signs.

Documentation
- Describe the patient's skin condition in your notes, and record any discoloration or redness.

Hair care
- Hair care includes combing, brushing, and shampooing.
- Combing and brushing stimulate scalp circulation, remove dead cells and debris, and distribute hair oils to produce a healthy sheen.
- Shampooing removes dirt and old oils and helps prevent skin irritation.
- Frequency of hair care depends on the length and texture of the patient's hair, the duration of hospitalization, and the patient's condition. Usually, hair should be combed and brushed daily and shampooed according to the patient's normal routine. Typically, no more than 1 week, or perhaps 2 weeks, should elapse between washings.
- Shampooing is contraindicated in patients with a recent craniotomy, depressed skull fracture, conditions that require intracranial pressure monitoring, or other cranial involvement.

Implementation tips
- Follow the standard nursing protocol described at the start of the chapter.

Combing and brushing
- Make sure the comb and brush are clean by washing them in hot, soapy water. The comb should have dull, even teeth to prevent scratching the scalp.
- If the hair is tangled, rub alcohol or oil on the strands to loosen them.
- Part hair into small sections for easier handling. Comb one section at a time, working from the ends toward the scalp to remove tangles.
- Anchor each section of hair above the area being combed to avoid hurting the patient. After combing, brush vigorously.
- Style the hair as the patient prefers. Braiding long or curly hair helps prevent snarling.

Shampooing a bedridden patient's hair
- Place a wastebasket on a linen-saver pad on the floor or on a footstool

How to make a shampoo trough

To make a shampoo trough, roll a bath blanket, towel, or drawsheet into a log. Shape the log into a "U" and place it in a large plastic bag. Arrange the bag under the patient's head, with the end of the bag extending over the edge of the bed and into a bucket on the floor, as shown below. Proceed with the shampooing as you would with a shampoo tray.

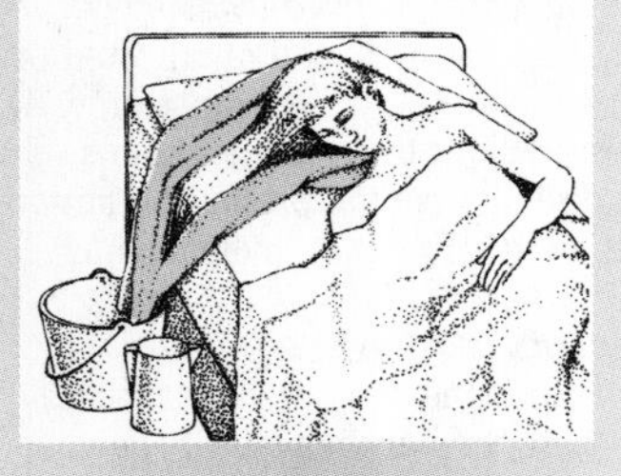

near the head of the bed. The pail or container catches wastewater from the shampoo tray. Another option is to make a shampoo trough. (See *How to make a shampoo trough.*)

◆ Lower the head of the bed until it's horizontal, and remove the patient's pillow, if allowed.

◆ Place a bath towel and linen-saver pad together, and position them around the patient's neck and over her shoulders. This protects the patient from moisture and pads her neck against pressure from the shampoo tray.

◆ Place the shampoo tray under the patient's head with her neck in the U-shaped opening. Arrange the bath blanket and towel so the patient is comfortable.

◆ Adjust the shampoo tray to carry wastewater away from the patient's head, and place the drainage tubing in the pail. Tuck a folded towel or drawsheet under the opposite side of the shampoo tray to promote drainage, if needed.

◆ When shampooing, place cotton in the patient's ears to keep moisture out of them.

◆ Rub shampoo into the patient's hair with your fingertips. Vigorous rubbing stimulates the scalp and may also help the patient relax.

◆ Rinse all shampoo from the patient's hair, and towel dry. Remove the cotton from the patient's ears after shampooing and rinsing.

Special considerations

◆ When giving hair care, check the patient's scalp carefully for signs of scalp disorders or skin breakdown, particularly if the patient is bedridden. Make sure that each patient has her own comb and brush to avoid cross-contamination.

◆ If you don't have a shampoo tray and can't devise a trough, place pillows under the patient's shoulders to elevate her head, and use a basin. Because a standard basin doesn't have a drainage spout, empty it frequently to prevent overflow.

Documentation

◆ Record the date, time, and patient's response to the shampoo on the flowchart.

◆ Note hair characteristics and distribution. Describe any hair and scalp abnormalities.

Shaving

◆ Performed with a straight, safety, or electric razor, shaving is part of most male patients' daily care. Besides reducing bacterial growth on the face, shaving promotes patient comfort by removing whiskers that can itch and irritate the skin and produce an unkempt appearance.

◆ Because nicks and cuts are most common with a straight or a safety razor, use an electric razor if the patient has a clotting disorder or is having anticoagulant therapy.
◆ Shaving may be contraindicated if the patient has a facial skin disorder or wound.

Implementation tips

◆ Follow the standard nursing protocol described at the start of the chapter.
◆ Unless contraindicated, place a conscious patient in the high Fowler's or Fowler's position.
◆ If the patient is unconscious, raise his head to keep soap and water from running behind it.

Using a straight or a safety razor

◆ Make sure the blade is sharp, clean, even, and rust-free. If needed, insert a new blade securely into the razor. A razor may be used more than once, but only by the same patient.
◆ Drape a bath towel around the patient's shoulders, and tuck it under his chin to protect the bed from moisture and to catch falling whiskers.
◆ Using a washcloth, wet the patient's entire beard with warm water. Let the warm cloth soak his beard for at least 1 minute to soften the whiskers.
◆ After putting on gloves, apply shaving cream to the patient's beard. If you're using soap, rub to form a lather.
◆ Gently stretch the patient's skin taut with one hand and shave with the other, holding the razor firmly. Ask the patient to puff his cheeks or turn his head, as needed, to shave hard-to-reach areas.
◆ Begin at the sideburns and work toward the chin using short, firm, downward strokes in the direction of hair growth. This reduces skin irritation and helps prevent nicks and cuts.
◆ Rinse the razor often to remove whiskers. Apply more warm water or shaving cream to the patient's face, as needed, to maintain adequate lather.
◆ Shave across the chin and up the neck and throat. Use short, gentle strokes for the neck and the area around the nose and mouth to avoid skin irritation.

Using an electric razor

◆ If you're using an electric razor, check its cord for fraying or other damage that could create an electrical hazard.
◆ If the razor isn't double-insulated or battery operated, use a grounded three-pronged plug.
◆ Using a circular motion and pressing the razor firmly against the skin, shave each area of the patient's face until smooth.

Special considerations

◆ If the patient is conscious, ask about his usual shaving routine. Although shaving in the direction of hair growth is most common, the patient may prefer the opposite direction.
◆ Don't share patients' shaving equipment to prevent cross-contamination.
◆ Shaving may be contraindicated if the patient is on anticoagulant therapy (for example, post–tissue plasminogen activator, heparin infusion).

Complications

◆ Cuts and abrasions are the most common complications of shaving and may warrant application of antiseptic lotion.

Documentation

◆ If applicable, record nicks or cuts resulting from shaving.

Eye care

◆ When paralysis or coma impairs or eliminates the corneal reflex, frequent eye care aims to keep the exposed cornea moist and to prevent ulceration and inflammation.
◆ Application of saline-saturated gauze pads over the eyelids moistens the eyes. Commercially available eye ointments and artificial tears also lubricate the corneas, but a physician's order is required for their use.

Implementation tips
◆ Follow the standard nursing protocol described at the start of the chapter.
◆ To remove secretions or crusts on the eyelids or eyelashes, soak a cotton ball in sterile normal saline solution. Then gently wipe the patient's eye, working from the inner canthus to the outer canthus to keep debris and fluid out of the nasolacrimal duct.
◆ To prevent cross-contamination, use a fresh cotton ball for each wipe until the eye is clean.
◆ To prevent irritation, avoid using soap on the patient's eyes.
◆ After cleaning the eyes, instill artificial tears or apply eye ointment, as ordered, to keep them moist.
◆ Soak gauze or eyepads in sterile normal saline solution, place them over the eyelids, and secure them with hypoallergenic tape. Change gauze pads, as needed, to keep them well saturated.

Special considerations
◆ Although eye care isn't a sterile procedure, asepsis should be maintained as much as possible.

Documentation
◆ Record the time and type of eye care in your notes. If applicable, chart the use of eyedrops or ointment in the patient's medication record.
◆ Document unusual crusting or excessive or colored drainage.

Contact lens care

◆ Illness or emergency treatment may require that you insert or remove and store a patient's contact lenses. Proper handling and lens care techniques help prevent eye injury and infection as well as lens loss or damage.
◆ Although all contact lenses float on the corneal tear layer, appropriate lens-handling techniques depend in large part on which type of lenses the patient wears. Rigid lenses typically have a smaller diameter than the cornea; soft lens diameter typically exceeds that of the cornea. Because they're larger and more pliable, soft lenses tend to mold themselves more closely to the eye for a more stable fit than rigid lenses.
◆ Although most patients remove and clean their lenses daily, some wear lenses overnight or for several days (sometimes up to a month) without removing them for cleaning. Still other patients wear disposable lenses, which means that they replace old lenses with new ones at regular intervals (a few days to a few months), possibly without removing them for cleaning between replacements.

Implementation tips
◆ Follow the standard nursing protocol described at the start of the chapter.

Inserting rigid lenses
◆ Wet one lens with solution. Gently rub it between your thumb and index finger, or place it on your palm and rub it with your opposite index finger. Rinse well with the solution, leaving a small amount in the lens.

◆ Place the lens, convex side down, on the tip of the index finger of your dominant hand.
◆ Instruct the patient to gaze upward slightly. Separate the eyelids with your other thumb and index finger, and place the lens directly and gently on the cornea. You need not press it to the eye; the tear film will attract it naturally at the first touch.

Inserting soft lenses
◆ Place the lens, convex side down, on the tip of the index finger of your dominant hand.
◆ To see if the lens is inside out, bend it between your thumb and index finger or fill it with saline or soaking solution. If the lens tends to roll inward or the edge points slightly inward, it's oriented correctly. If the edge points outward or the lens tends to collapse over your fingertip, it's probably inside out and should be reversed.
◆ Instruct the patient to gaze upward slightly. Separate the eyelids with your other thumb and index finger, and place the lens on the sclera, just below the cornea. Then, slide the lens gently upward with your finger until it centers on the cornea.

Removing rigid or soft lenses
◆ If a commercial lens storage case isn't available, place enough sterile normal saline solution into two small medicine cups to submerge a lens in each one.
◆ Make sure containers are labeled with the correct patient identification and will be stored properly in a safe location.
◆ To avoid confusing the left and right lenses, which may have different prescriptions, mark one cup "L" and the other cup "R" and place the corresponding lens in each cup. (See *Removing a patient's contact lenses,* page 30.)

Cleaning lenses
◆ If the patient can't tell you how to clean his lenses properly, remember that all lens types require two steps: cleaning and disinfection.
◆ Cleaning involves rubbing the lens with a surfactant solution designed to remove most surface deposits. The cleaning step may also include use of an enzyme agent to remove protein deposits against which surfactant cleaners are typically ineffective.
◆ Disinfection, which doesn't require rubbing, may be accomplished through chemical means or by heat.
◆ If you must clean a patient's lenses, use only his own solutions. This minimizes the risk of allergic reactions to substances included in other solution brands.
◆ Never touch the nozzle of a solution bottle to the lens, your fingers, or anything else to avoid contaminating the solution in the bottle.

Special considerations
◆ If the patient's eyes appear dry or you have trouble removing a lens from an eye, instill several drops of sterile normal saline solution, and wait a few minutes before trying again to remove the lens. This process minimizes the risk of corneal damage. If you still can't remove the lens easily, notify the physician.
◆ Avoid instilling eye medication while the patient is wearing contact lenses. The lenses could trap the medication, possibly causing eye irritation or lens damage.
◆ Don't let soft lenses, which are 40% to 60% water, dry out. If they do, soak them in sterile normal saline solution and they may return to their natural shape.
◆ If an unconscious patient comes into the emergency department, check for contact lenses by opening each eyelid and searching with a small flash-

Removing a patient's contact lenses

Contact lens removal techniques depend largely on the type of lenses the patient wears and how readily they come off of the eye. For successful removal of soft and rigid lenses, follow the steps outlined below. If you have trouble removing lenses manually, try using a specially made suction cup.

Soft lenses
With the patient looking up and his upper lid raised, use your dominant index finger to slide the lens onto the lower cornea. Pinch the lens between your index finger and thumb to remove it (as shown below)

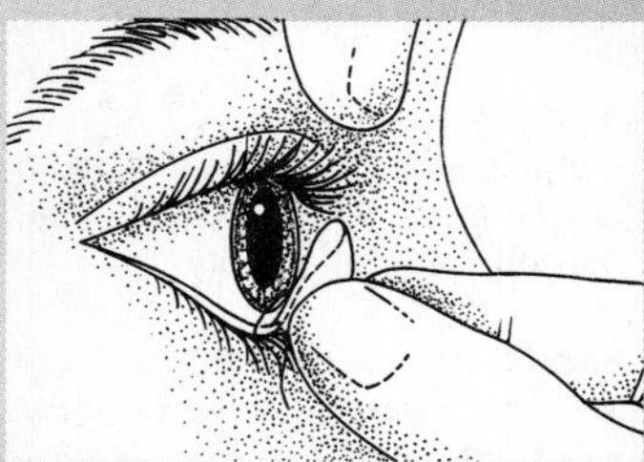

Rigid lenses
Place one thumb on each eyelid and move the lids toward each other, pressing gently against the eyeball. When the lids meet the lens edges, the suction breaks and the lens is released (as shown below). Catch the lens in your lower hand or remove it from the patient's lashes.

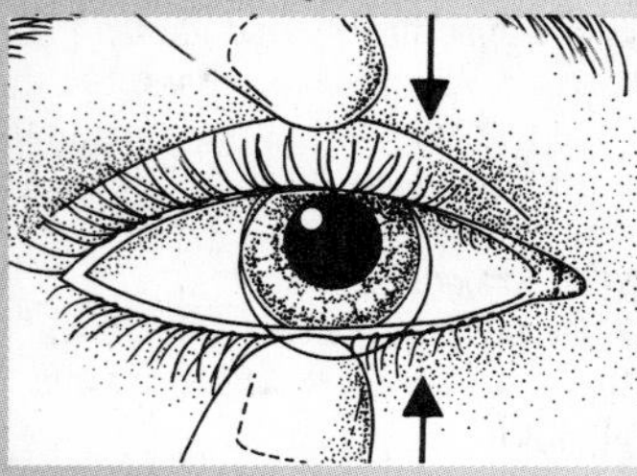

Using a suction cup
Separate the lids with your nondominant hand. Squeeze the suction cup with your dominant hand, and place it gently against the lens (as shown below). Open your fingers slightly to create suction between the lens and the cup. Rock the lens gently to remove it.

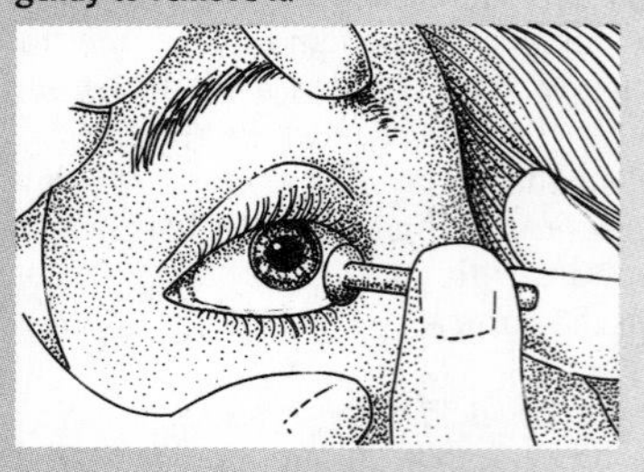

light. If you detect lenses, remove them immediately because tears can't circulate freely beneath the lenses with eyelids closed, possibly leading to corneal oxygen depletion or infection.

◆ If a patient can't care for his lenses adequately during hospitalization, urge him to send them home with a family member. If you aren't sure how to care for the lenses in the interim, store them in sterile normal saline solution until a family member can take them home.

Documentation

◆ Record eye condition before and after removing lenses; the time of lens insertion, removal, and cleaning; the location of stored lenses; and, if applicable, the removal of lenses from the facility by a family member.

Ear and hearing aid care

◆ Avoid drying or cleaning ears with sharp objects such as bobby pins. A soft cotton swab should be used after bathing to dry excess liquid and remove softened earwax.

◆ Adjusting to a hearing aid takes patience, practice, and hours of wear. Several weeks or even months may pass before your patient feels completely comfortable.

◆ Once the patient learns how, inserting, removing, and caring for a hearing aid will become just another daily routine.

Implementation tips

Inserting a hearing aid

◆ Wash your hands.

◆ Make sure the hearing aid is turned off and the volume is turned all the way down.

◆ Examine the earmold to determine whether it's for the right or left ear. Then line up the parts of the earmold with the corresponding parts of the external ear.

◆ Rotate the earmold slightly forward, and insert the canal portion.

◆ Gently push the earmold into the ear while rotating it backward. Adjust the folds of the ear over the earmold, if needed. The earmold should fit snugly and comfortably.

◆ After inserting the earmold, adjust other parts of the hearing aid as needed. For example, place a behind-the-ear hearing aid over the ear.

◆ Finally, set the switch to the ON position and slowly turn the volume halfway up.

◆ Teach the patient how to insert his hearing aid, and watch his technique.

Adjusting to a hearing aid

◆ To help your patient adjust to his hearing aid, tell him to start by wearing it for only short periods at a time. For example, he could wear it for 2 to 4 hours for the first 2 days and then increase the wearing time by 2 hours each day until he feels comfortable adjusting to the new sounds heard.

◆ Once the patient is comfortable wearing the aid, urge him to wear it as much as possible.

◆ Tell the patient to try to block out background sounds when listening to conversations. This takes practice. If the background noise gets too annoying, tell him to turn down the volume and watch the speaker's face closely. In a large group, tell him to stay as close to the speaker as possible.

◆ Suggest that the patient talk to only one person at a time until he gets used to the hearing aid. Urge him to experiment in difficult situations — for example, with loud music playing in the background.

Removing a hearing aid

◆ Set the switch to the OFF position and lower the volume.

◆ Remove the earmold by rotating it forward and pulling outward.

◆ Remove or unclip the hearing-aid case. After removing the hearing aid, store it in a safe place.

◆ Teach the patient how to remove his hearing aid, and watch his technique.

Cleaning the earmold

◆ Tell your patient to keep the earmold clean and free of excess wax to prevent infection and keep the device working properly.

◆ To clean a body aid, detach the earmold from the receiver. For a behind-the-ear hearing aid, detach the earmold where its tubing meets the hook of the hearing-aid case, if possible. Don't remove the hearing aid if glue or a small metal split ring secures the earmold tubing to the hearing-aid case.

◆ After detaching the earmold, soak it in a mild soapy solution; then rinse and dry it well. The patient may want to blow out excess moisture through the earmold opening.

◆ If the opening is clogged with wax or debris, use a pipe cleaner or toothpick to remove it. Avoid pushing debris into the opening.

◆ Never clean or immerse any part except the earmold in water.

◆ Don't insert sharp objects into the microphone or receiver opening. Only an audiologist or hearing-aid dealer should clean these parts.

◆ For an in-the-ear aid with a nonremovable earmold, wipe the earmold with a damp cloth.

◆ Store the dry, clean earmold in the hearing-aid case.

Special considerations

◆ Tell the patient not to turn the hearing aid volume up too high because doing so may distort sound and cause a high-pitched whistling or squealing sound. (This sound also may signal a loose-fitting earmold.)

◆ Tell the patient to avoid wearing the hearing aid outside for long periods in hot, humid, or cold weather.

◆ Never store a hearing aid near a stove or heater or on a sunny windowsill.

◆ Caution the patient not to wear the hearing aid in the rain, in the bathtub or shower, during activities that cause excessive sweating, or when using a hair dryer, hairspray, or a vaporizer.

◆ Don't drop a hearing aid on a hard surface. Work over a bed or other soft surface when changing batteries or removing the aid from the ear.

◆ Replace dead batteries with new ones of the same type. When inserting a battery, turn off the hearing aid and then match the negative (–) and positive (+) signs. If the patient wears the hearing aid 10 to 12 hours daily, the batteries probably will need to be replaced weekly. (See *Solving hearing aid problems*.)

◆ If the hearing aid won't be used for several days, remove the battery to protect the device from leakage or corrosion. Leave the battery case open. Store the aid in an airtight container with a silica-gel packet, especially in a humid climate.

◆ To clean the battery, gently rub it with a pencil eraser to remove corrosion. If the battery gets damp, dry the contacts with a cotton swab.

◆ Tell the patient to store extra batteries in the freezer to lengthen their shelf life.

◆ For pain or drainage in the ear — a sign of skin or cartilage infection, a middle-ear infection, a tumor, or an improperly fitted earmold — tell the patient to call the physician.

Documentation

◆ Record type of hearing device, which ears have aids, patient ability to self-manage hearing aid care, and any abnormalities of the ears such as excess wax accumulation.

Mouth and denture care

◆ Given in the morning, at bedtime, or after meals, mouth care entails brushing and flossing the teeth and inspecting the mouth. It removes soft plaque deposits and calculus from the teeth, cleans and massages the gums, reduces mouth odor, and helps prevent infection.

◆ By freshening the patient's mouth, mouth care also enhances the taste of food, aiding appetite and nutrition.

◆ Although an ambulatory patient usually can perform mouth care alone, a bedridden patient may need partial or full assistance. A comatose patient will need the use of suction equipment to prevent aspiration during oral care. For information about denture care, see *Dealing with dentures*, page 34.

Implementation tips

◆ Follow the standard nursing protocol described at the start of the chapter.

Solving hearing aid problems

If a hearing aid fails to operate, review the instructions in the operator's manual or consult the checklist below.

PROBLEM AND POSSIBLE CAUSES	POSSIBLE SOLUTIONS
No sound or weak sound	
◆ Incorrect battery insertion	◆ Reinsert battery.
◆ Dead battery	◆ Try a new battery.
◆ Clogged earmold opening	◆ Unclog the earmold opening.
◆ Twisted plastic tubing	◆ Untwist the plastic tubing.
◆ Switch is OFF or on T for use with telephone	◆ Switch to ON position.
◆ Volume isn't high enough	◆ Turn volume control at least one-half rotation.
Whistling or squealing sound	
◆ Incorrect earmold insertion	◆ Reinsert earmold.
◆ Volume turned too high	◆ Turn down volume.
◆ Earmold not securely snapped to a receiver of a body hearing aid. (A whistling sound is normal when the earmold isn't inserted and the hearing aid is turned on; such whistling indicates that the aid is working and that the battery is inserted correctly.)	◆ Secure earmold to receiver.

Patients capable of self-care

◆ For a bedridden patient capable of self-care, encourage him to perform his own mouth care.

◆ Watch the patient to make sure he's flossing correctly, and correct him if needed.

◆ Tell him to wrap the floss around the second or third fingers of both hands. Starting with his front teeth and without injuring the gums, he should insert the floss as far as possible into the space between each pair of teeth. Then he should clean the surfaces of adjacent teeth by pulling the floss up and down against the side of each tooth.

◆ Remind the patient to use a clean 1"(2.5 cm) section of floss for each pair of teeth.

Patients not capable of self-care

◆ Lower the head of the bed, and position the patient on his side with his face extended over the edge of the pillow to allow oral drainage and prevent fluid aspiration.

◆ If available, use oral suction equipment. If suction equipment isn't available, wipe the inside of the patient's mouth often with a gauze pad.

◆ Place a linen-saver pad under the patient's chin and an emesis basin near his cheek to absorb or catch oral drainage.

◆ Lubricate the patient's lips with petroleum jelly to prevent dryness and cracking.

◆ If needed, devise a bite-block to keep from being bitten during the procedure or to hold the patient's mouth open during oral care. Wrap a gauze pad over the end of a tongue blade,

Dealing with dentures

Prostheses made of acrylic resins, vinyl composites, or both, dentures replace some or all of the patient's natural teeth. Dentures require proper care to remove soft plaque deposits and calculus and to reduce mouth odor. Such care involves removing and rinsing dentures after meals, daily brushing and removal of tenacious deposits, and soaking in a commercial denture cleaner. Dentures must be removed from the comatose or presurgical patient to prevent possible airway obstruction.

Equipment

Start by assembling the following equipment at the patient's bedside:
◆ emesis basin ◆ labeled denture cup ◆ toothbrush or denture brush ◆ gloves ◆ toothpaste ◆ commercial denture cleaner ◆ paper towel ◆ cotton-tipped mouth swab ◆ mouthwash ◆ gauze ◆ optional: adhesive denture liner.

Preparation

◆ Wash your hands and put on gloves.

Removing dentures

◆ To remove a full upper denture, grasp the front and palatal surfaces of the denture with your thumb and forefinger. Position the index finger of your opposite hand over the upper border of the denture, and press to break the seal between denture and palate. Grasp the denture with gauze because saliva can make it slippery.

◆ To remove a full lower denture, grasp the front and lingual surfaces of the denture with your thumb and index finger, and gently lift up.

◆ To remove partial dentures, first ask the patient or caregiver how the prosthesis is retained and how to remove it. If it's held in place with clips or snaps, then exert equal pressure on the border of each side of the denture. Avoid lifting the clasps, which easily bend or break.

Oral and denture care

◆ After removing dentures, place them in a properly labeled denture cup. Add warm water and a commercial denture cleaner to remove stains and hardened deposits. Follow package directions. Avoid soaking dentures in mouthwash containing alcohol because it may damage a soft liner.

◆ Instruct the patient to rinse with mouthwash to remove food particles and reduce mouth odor. Then stroke the palate, buccal surfaces, gums, and tongue with a soft toothbrush or cotton-tipped mouth swab to clean the mucosa and stimulate circulation. Inspect for irritated areas or sores because they may indicate a poorly fitting denture.

◆ Carry the denture cup, emesis basin, toothbrush, and toothpaste to the sink. After lining the basin with a paper towel, fill it with water to cushion the dentures in case you drop them. Hold the dentures over the basin, wet them with warm water, and apply toothpaste to a denture brush or long-bristled toothbrush. Clean the dentures using only moderate pressure – to prevent scratches, and warm water – to prevent distortion.

◆ Clean the denture cup, and place the dentures in it. Rinse the brush, and clean and dry the emesis basin. Return all equipment to the patient's bedside stand.

Wearing dentures

◆ If the patient desires, apply adhesive liner to the dentures. Moisten them with water, if necessary, to reduce friction and ease insertion.

◆ Encourage the patient to wear his dentures to enhance his appearance, facilitate eating and speaking, and prevent changes in the gum line that may affect denture fit.

fold the edge in, and secure it with adhesive tape.
- Using a dental floss holder, hold the floss against each tooth and direct it as close to the gum as possible without injuring the sensitive tissues around the tooth.
- Brush the patient's lower teeth from the gum line up and the upper teeth from the gum line down. Place the brush at a 45-degree angle to the gum line, and press the bristles gently into the gingival sulcus. Use short, gentle strokes to prevent gum damage.
- If the patient is able to, have him rinse often during brushing by taking a mouthwash-water mixture through a straw. Hold the emesis basin steady under his cheek, and wipe his mouth and cheeks with tissues as needed.
- After brushing the patient's teeth, dip a cotton-tipped mouth swab into the mouthwash solution. Gently stroke the gums, buccal surfaces, palate, and tongue to clean the mucosa and stimulate circulation.
- Check the patient's mouth for cleanliness and tooth and tissue condition.

Special considerations
- Use sponge-tipped mouth swabs to clean the teeth if the patient has sensitive gums. These swabs produce less friction than a toothbrush but don't clean as well.
- Clean the mouth of a toothless comatose patient by wrapping a gauze pad around your index finger, moistening it with mouthwash, and gently swabbing the oral tissues.
- Remember that mucous membranes dry quickly if the patient breathes through his mouth or is receiving oxygen therapy. Moisten his mouth and lips regularly with moistened sponge-tipped swabs or water.

Documentation
- Record the date and time of mouth care.
- Note unusual conditions, such as bleeding, edema, mouth odor, excessive secretions, or plaque on the tongue.

Back care

- Regular bathing and massage of the neck, back, buttocks, and upper arms promotes patient relaxation and allows examination of skin condition.
- Particularly important for the bedridden patient, massage causes cutaneous vasodilation, helping to prevent pressure ulcers caused by prolonged pressure on bony prominences or by perspiration.
- Gentle back massage can be performed after a myocardial infarction but may be contraindicated in patients with rib fractures, surgical incisions, or other recent traumatic injury to the back.

Implementation tips
- Follow the standard nursing protocol described at the start of the chapter.
- Determine the patient's body structure and skin condition, and then tailor the duration and intensity of the massage accordingly. Ask the patient to tell you if you're applying too much or too little pressure.
- Fold a washcloth around your hand to form a mitt. This keeps the loose ends of the cloth from dripping water onto the patient and keeps the cloth warm longer.
- Use long, firm strokes to bathe the patient's back, beginning at the neck and shoulders and moving downward to the buttocks.
- Rinse and dry well because moisture trapped between the buttocks can

How to give a back massage

Effleurage, friction, and petrissage are the three strokes used commonly when giving a back massage. Start with effleurage, go on to friction, and then to petrissage. Perform each stroke at least six times before moving on to the next, and then repeat the whole series if desired.

When performing effleurage and friction, keep your hands parallel to the vertebrae to avoid tickling the patient. For all three strokes, maintain a regular rhythm and steady contact with the patient's back to help him relax.

EFFLEURAGE

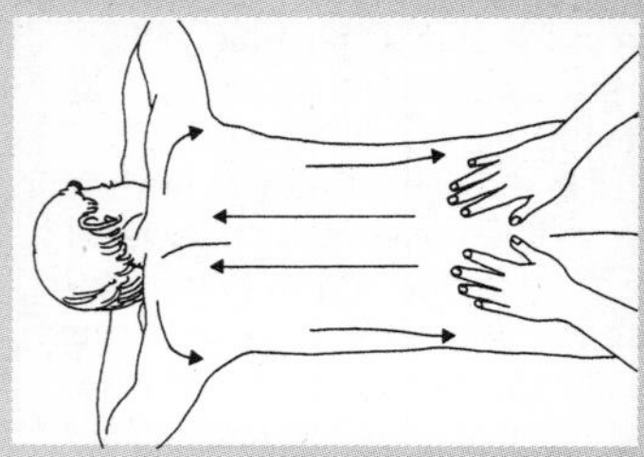

Using your palm, stroke from the buttocks up to the shoulders, over the upper arms, and back to the buttocks (as shown above). Use slightly less pressure on the downward strokes.

cause chafing and increase the risk of pressure ulcers.

- While giving back care, closely examine the patient's skin, especially the bony prominences of the shoulders, the scapulae, and the coccyx, for redness or abrasions.
- Using cold lotion could chill or startle the patient and cause muscle tension and vasoconstriction. If needed, warm the lotion by placing the bottle in a basin of warm water.
- Apply lotion to the patient's back using long, firm strokes. The lotion reduces friction, making back massage easier.
- Massage the patient's back, beginning at the base of the spine and moving upward to the shoulders. For a relaxing effect, massage slowly; for a stimulating effect, massage quickly. Alternate the three basic strokes: effleurage, friction, and pétrissage. (See *How to give a back massage*.) Add warmed lotion as needed, keeping one hand on the patient's back to avoid interrupting the massage.
- Finish the massage by using long, firm strokes.

Special considerations

- If you're giving back care at bedtime, get the patient ready for bed beforehand so the massage can help him fall asleep.
- Use fresh lotion for each patient to prevent cross-contamination.
- If the patient has oily skin, use talcum powder or lotion of the patient's choice. However, to prevent aspiration, don't use powder if the patient has an endotracheal or tracheal tube in place. Also, avoid using powder and lotion together because the combination of the two may macerate the skin.
- Give special attention to bony prominences because these areas are prone to pressure ulcers.
- Don't massage the patient's legs unless ordered because reddened legs can signal clot formation, and massage can dislodge the clot, causing an embolus.
- Develop a turning schedule and give back care at each position change.

FRICTION

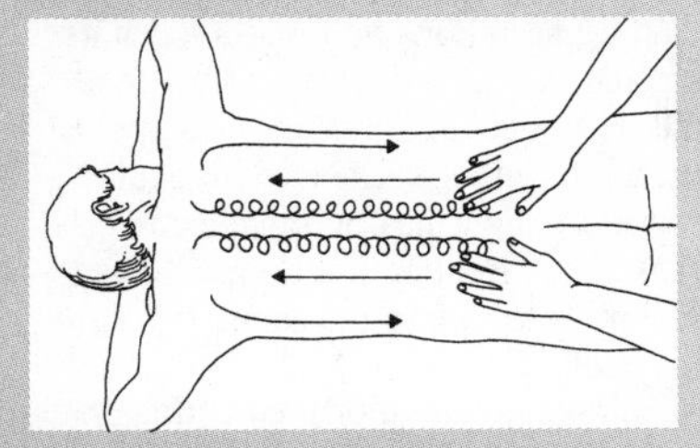

Use circular thumb strokes to move from buttocks to shoulders; then, using a smooth stroke, return to the buttocks (as shown above).

PETRISSAGE

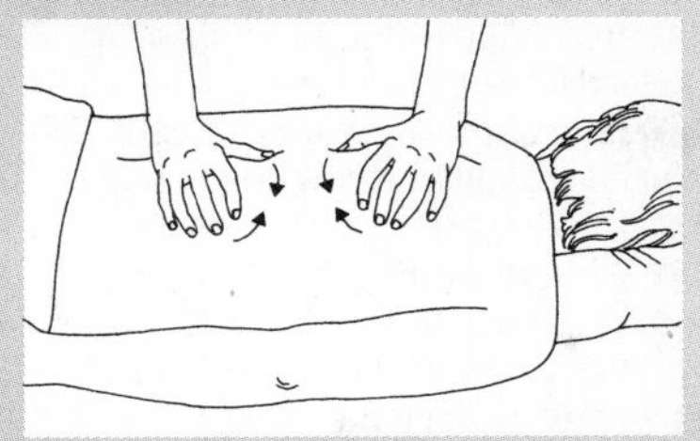

Using your thumb to oppose your fingers, knead and stroke half the back and upper arms, starting at the buttocks and moving toward the shoulder (as shown above). Then knead and stroke the other half of the back, rhythmically alternating your hands.

Documentation

◆ Chart back care on the flowchart.
◆ Record redness, abrasion, or change in skin condition in your notes.

Foot care

◆ Daily bathing of feet and regular trimming of toenails promotes cleanliness, prevents infection, stimulates peripheral circulation, and controls odor by removing debris from between toes and under toenails.
◆ Foot care is particularly important for bedridden patients and those especially susceptible to foot infection. Increased susceptibility may be caused by peripheral vascular disease, diabetes mellitus, poor nutritional status, arthritis, or any condition that impairs peripheral circulation. In such patients, proper foot care should include meticulous cleanliness and regular observation for signs of skin breakdown.
◆ Toenail trimming is contraindicated in patients with toe infections, diabetes mellitus, neurologic disorders, renal failure, or peripheral vascular disease, unless performed by a physician or podiatrist.

Implementation tips

◆ Follow the standard nursing protocol described at the start of the chapter.
◆ Test water temperature with a bath thermometer or your elbow. Patients with reduced peripheral sensation could burn their feet in overly hot water (more than 105° F [40.6° C]) without feeling any pain.
◆ Place a linen-saver pad and a towel under the patient's feet to keep the bottom bed linen dry. Then position the basin on the pad.
◆ Insert a pillow beneath the patient's knee for support, and cushion the rim of the basin with the towel to prevent pressure.
◆ Soak each foot in turn to soften the skin and toenails, loosen debris under toenails, and comfort and refresh the patient.

◆ Refill the basin with warm water to clean and soak each foot separately.
◆ While the second foot is soaking, give the first one a pedicure. Using a cotton-tipped applicator, carefully clean the toenails. Using an orangewood stick, gently remove any dirt beneath the toenails; avoid injuring subungual skin.
◆ Dry the feet thoroughly, especially between the toes, to avoid skin breakdown. Blot gently to dry because harsh rubbing may damage the skin.
◆ Apply lotion to moisten dry skin, or lightly dust water-absorbent powder between the toes to absorb moisture.
◆ Consult a podiatrist if nails need trimming.

Special considerations

◆ While providing foot care, observe the color, shape, and texture of the toenails. If you see redness, drying, cracking, blisters, discoloration, or other signs of traumatic injury, especially in patients with impaired peripheral circulation, notify the physician. Because such patients are vulnerable to infection and gangrene, they need prompt treatment.
◆ When giving a bedridden patient foot care, perform range-of-motion exercises (unless contraindicated) to stimulate circulation and prevent foot contractures and muscle atrophy.

Documentation

◆ Record the date and time of the foot care you provided in your notes.
◆ Record and report abnormal findings and nursing actions you take.

Perineal care

◆ Perineal care, which includes care of the external genitalia and the anal area, should be performed during the daily bath and, if needed, at bedtime and after urination and bowel movements.
◆ The procedure promotes cleanliness and prevents infection. It also removes irritating secretions and odors, such as smegma, a cheese-like substance that collects under the foreskin of the penis and on the inner surface of the labia.
◆ If the patient has perineal skin breakdown, frequent bathing followed by application of an ointment or cream aids healing.
◆ Following genital or rectal surgery, you may need to use sterile supplies, including sterile gloves, gauze, and cotton balls.

Implementation tips

◆ Follow the standard nursing protocol described at the start of the chapter.

Female patient

◆ To minimize exposure and embarrassment, place a bath blanket over the patient with corners head to foot and side to side. Wrap each leg with a side corner, tucking it under her hip. Then fold back the corner between her legs to expose the perineum.
◆ Ask the patient to bend her knees slightly and to spread her legs.
◆ Separate her labia with one hand and wash with the other.
◆ Use gentle downward strokes from the front to the back of the perineum to prevent intestinal organisms from contaminating the urethra or vagina.
◆ Use a clean section of washcloth for each stroke by folding each used section inward. This prevents the spread of contaminated secretions or discharge.
◆ Using a clean washcloth, rinse thoroughly from front to back because soap residue can cause skin irritation.
◆ Pat the area dry with a bath towel because moisture can also cause skin irritation and discomfort.

◆ To wash the anal area, turn the patient on her side to Sims' position, if possible, for optimal exposure. Clean, rinse, and dry the anal area, starting at the posterior vaginal opening and wiping from front to back.

Male patient

◆ Drape the patient's legs to minimize exposure and embarrassment, and then expose the genital area.
◆ Hold the shaft of the patient's penis with one hand and wash with the other.
◆ Start at the tip and work in a circular motion from the center to the periphery to avoid introducing microorganisms into the urethra. Use a clean section of washcloth for each stroke to prevent the spread of contaminated secretions or discharge.
◆ Rinse thoroughly, using the same circular motion.
◆ For an uncircumcised patient, gently retract the foreskin and clean beneath it. Rinse well but don't dry the area because moisture provides lubrication and prevents friction when replacing the foreskin. Replace the foreskin to avoid constriction of the penis, which causes edema and tissue damage.
◆ Wash the rest of the penis, using downward strokes toward the scrotum. Rinse well and pat dry with a towel.
◆ Clean the top and sides of the scrotum; rinse thoroughly and pat dry. Handle the scrotum gently to avoid causing discomfort.
◆ Turn the patient on his side. Clean the bottom of the scrotum and the anal area. Rinse well and pat dry.

Special considerations

◆ Give perineal care to a patient of the opposite sex in a matter-of-fact way to minimize embarrassment.
◆ If the patient is incontinent, first remove excess feces with toilet tissue; then position him on a bedpan. Irrigate the perineal area to remove any remaining fecal matter.
◆ After cleaning the perineum, apply ointment or cream (petroleum jelly, zinc oxide cream, or vitamin A and D ointment) to provide a barrier between the skin and excretions, and to prevent skin breakdown.

Documentation

◆ Record perineal care and any special treatment in your notes.
◆ Document the need for continued treatment, if needed, in your notes.
◆ Describe perineal skin condition and any odor or discharge.

Hour-of-sleep care

◆ Effective hour-of-sleep care prepares the patient for a good night's sleep. It meets his physical and psychological needs in preparation for sleep. It includes providing for the patient's hygiene, making the bed clean and comfortable, and ensuring safety. It also gives an opportunity to answer the patient's questions about the next day's tests and procedures and to discuss his worries and concerns.
◆ Ineffective care may contribute to sleeplessness, which can intensify patient anxiety and interfere with treatment and recovery.

Implementation tips

◆ Follow the standard nursing protocol described at the start of the chapter.
◆ If the patient is on bed rest, offer a bedpan, urinal, or commode. Otherwise, help the patient to the bathroom.
◆ Wash the patient's face and hands, and dry them well. Encourage the patient to do this himself, if possible, to promote independence.
◆ Provide toothpaste or a properly labeled denture cup and commercial denture cleaner. Help the patient with

oral hygiene as needed. If the patient prefers to wear dentures until bedtime, leave denture-care items within easy reach.
- After providing mouth care, turn the patient on his side or stomach. Wash, rinse, and dry the patient's back and buttocks. Massage well with lotion to help relax the patient.
- While providing back care, check the skin for redness, cracking, or other signs of breakdown.
- If the patient's gown is soiled or damp, provide a clean one and help him put it on, if needed.
- Check dressings, binders, antiembolism stockings, or other aids; change or readjust them as needed.
- Refill the water container, and place it and a box of facial tissues within easy reach to prevent falls if the patient needs these items.
- Straighten or change bed linens, as needed. Cover the patient with a blanket or place one within easy reach to prevent chills during the night. If the patient appears distressed, restless, or in pain, give ordered drugs, as needed.
- After making the patient comfortable, evaluate his mental and physical condition. Place the bed in a low position and raise the side rails according to facility policy.
- Place the call bell within easy reach, and instruct the patient to call you if needed.
- Tidy the patient's environment: Move all breakables from the overbed table out of his reach, and remove any equipment and supplies that could cause falls should the patient get up during the night.
- Finally, turn off the overhead light and put on the night-light.

Special considerations
- Ask the patient about his sleep routine at home and, whenever possible, let him follow it.
- Also try to observe certain rituals, such as a bedtime snack, which can aid sleep.
- A back massage, tub bath, or shower may also help relax the patient and promote a restful night. If the patient normally bathes or showers before bedtime, let him do so if his condition and physician's orders permit it.

Documentation
- Record the time and type of hour-of-sleep care in your notes. Include application of soft restraints or any other special procedures.

Physical restraints and restraint alternatives

JCAHO and OBRA standards and regulations

- The Joint Commission on Accreditation of Healthcare Organizations (JCAHO) issued major standards revisions regarding the use of restraints that went into effect on January 1, 2001.
- The Omnibus Budget Rehabilitation Act (OBRA) of 1987 also put the long-term care industry on notice that chemical and physical restraints were only to be used in cases of medical necessity, as determined by an independent health care practitioner.
- One purpose of these regulations was to reduce the use of restraints, and these revisions still remain current according to the January 2005 JCAHO standards.
- JCAHO and OBRA require that restraints be limited to emergencies in which the patient is at risk of harming himself or others, and only as a last resort after other nonphysical interventions have failed.

◆ The regulations also emphasize staff education in preventing the need for restraints.
◆ A licensed independent practitioner must conduct an initial evaluation in person within 1 hour of the precipitating event, and give an order for restraints. This order must be renewed for the continued use of restraints.
◆ According to the JCAHO, hospital policies and procedures must address the prevention of restraint use, and should also consist of a guide for restraint use when needed.
◆ The revised JCAHO standards and OBRA regulations require continuous monitoring and assessment to ensure patient safety.
◆ The patient's family must be promptly notified about the use of restraints if the patient agreed to have them informed about his care.
◆ Moreover, the patient must be informed of the conditions needed for his release from restraints. If released, a debriefing about the restraint episode must occur between the patient and staff.
◆ All documentation on restraint use should be completed according to facility policy.

Restraint use and application

◆ Soft restraints are used to limit movement to prevent a confused, disoriented, or combative patient from injuring himself or others.
◆ These restraints should be used only when less restrictive measures have failed.
◆ Vest and belt restraints, used to prevent falls from a bed or a chair, permit full movement of arms and legs.
◆ Limb restraints, used to prevent removal of supportive equipment — such as I.V. lines, indwelling catheters, and nasogastric tubes — allow only slight limb motion.
◆ Like limb restraints, mitts prevent removal of supportive equipment, keep the patient from scratching rashes or sores, and keep a combative patient from injuring himself or others.
◆ Body restraints, used to control a combative or hysterical patient, immobilize all or most of the body.
◆ When soft restraints aren't sufficient and sedation is dangerous or ineffective, leather restraints can be used. Depending on the patient's behavior, leather restraints may be applied to all limbs (four-point restraints) or to one arm and one leg (two-point restraints).
◆ The duration of restraint use is governed by federal law, state law, recommendations by accrediting bodies, and facility policy.

Implementation tips

◆ Follow the standard nursing protocol described at the start of the chapter.
◆ Obtain a physician's order for restraint, but never leave a confused or combative patient unattended while trying to secure the order. Have a colleague provide one-to-one care as needed until proper medical orders are received. You may consult the supervising RN for assistance or permission to implement restraint pending the physician's order.
◆ Make sure the restraints are the correct size, using the patient's build and weight as a guide. If you use leather restraints, make sure the straps are unlocked and the key fits the locks.
◆ If needed, get help to restrain the patient before entering his room. You may need several coworkers in an organized effort, with each person having a specific task. For example, one person may explain the procedure to the patient and apply the restraints while the others immobilize the patient's arms and legs.

Knots for securing soft restraints

When securing soft restraints, use knots that can be released quickly and easily, like those shown below. Never secure restraints to the bed's side rails.

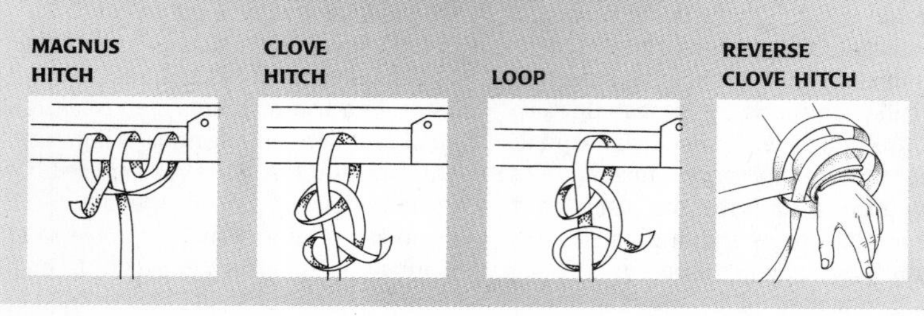

- Tell the patient what you're about to do, and describe the restraints to him. Inform him that they're being used to protect him from injury rather than to punish him. Maintain a calm, nonthreatening demeanor when applying the restraint.
- Tie all restraints securely to the frame of the bed, chair, or wheelchair and out of the patient's reach. Never secure a restraint to a bed rail or other movable part of the equipment.
- Use a bow or a knot that can be released quickly and easily in an emergency. (See *Knots for securing soft restraints*.) Never tie a regular knot to secure the straps.
- Leave 1″ to 2″ (2.5 to 5 cm) of slack in the straps to allow room for movement.

Special considerations

- Because the authority to use restraints varies among facilities, make sure you know your facility's policy. You may be able to apply restraints without a physician's order in an emergency, with the consent of the supervising RN.
- Also, know your state's regulations governing restraints. For example, some states prohibit the use of four-point restraints. Some facilities may require that a family member sign a consent form agreeing to restraints when clearly needed.
- If a patient is at high risk for aspiration, restrain him on his side.
- When loosening restraints, have a coworker on hand to help restrain the patient if needed.
- After determining the patient's behavior and condition, you may decide to use a two-point restraint to restrain one arm and the opposite leg — for example, the right arm and the left leg. Never restrain the arm and leg on the same side because the patient may fall out of bed.
- Never secure all four four-point restraints to one side of the bed because the patient may fall out of bed.
- Don't apply a limb restraint above an I.V. site because the constriction may occlude the infusion or cause infiltration into surrounding tissue.
- Never secure restraints to the side rails because someone might inadvertently lower the rail before noticing the attached restraint. This may jerk the patient's limb or body, causing discomfort or injury. Never secure restraints to the fixed frame of the bed if the patient's position will be changed.
- Don't restrain a patient in the prone position. This position limits his field

of vision, intensifies feelings of helplessness and vulnerability, and impairs respiration, especially if the patient has been sedated.

◆ Because a restrained patient has limited mobility, his nutrition, elimination, and positioning become your responsibility. Long periods of immobility can predispose a patient to pneumonia, urine retention, constipation, and sensory deprivation. To prevent pressure ulcers, reposition the patient every 2 hours, and massage and pad bony prominences and other vulnerable areas.

◆ Check the patient and the restraints every 15 to 30 minutes, and ask the patient often about elimination needs. Release the restraints every 2 hours; check the patient's pulse and skin condition, and perform range-of-motion (ROM) exercises. Document all examinations and findings.

◆ After applying a vest restraint, check the patient's respiratory rate and breath sounds regularly. Loosen the vest often, if possible, so the patient can stretch, turn, and breathe deeply.

◆ When applying a limb restraint, wrap the patient's wrist or ankle with gauze pads to reduce friction between the patient's skin and the restraint, helping to prevent irritation and skin breakdown. Stay alert for signs of impaired circulation distal to the restraint.

◆ When using mitts made of transparent mesh, check hand movement and skin color often to monitor circulation. Remove the mitts every 2 hours to stimulate circulation, and perform passive ROM exercises to prevent contractures.

◆ After applying a belt restraint, slip your hand between the patient and the belt to ensure a secure but comfortable fit. A loose belt can be raised to chest level; a tight one can cause abdominal discomfort.

◆ After applying leather restraints, check the patient regularly to give emotional support and to reassess the need for continued restraint. Check the patient's pulse rate and vital signs according to facility policy.

◆ For information regarding restraints for children, see *Types of child restraints,* page 44.

Documentation

◆ Record the behavior that warranted restraint, interventions used before the use of restraints, why they failed, when restraints were applied, the type of restraints used, how the patient's safety needs were met while restraints were in use as well as why the restraints were either continued or discontinued.

◆ Document any injuries or complications, the time and name of the physician notified, your interventions, and your actions.

◆ Record your examinations of the patient, including signs of injury, nutrition, hydration, circulation, skin integrity, range of motion, vital signs, hygiene, elimination, comfort, physical and psychological status, and readiness for removing restraints.

◆ Record your interventions to help the patient meet the conditions for removing restraints. Note that the patient was continuously monitored.

Restraint use and fall risk

◆ The use of physical restraints to prevent falls has been the subject of much debate. Although preventing falls is important, some studies have shown that restraints don't prevent serious injuries and can actually do more harm than good. One study shows that restraints on confused ambulatory nursing home residents increases falls.

◆ Restraints should be used only when all other alternatives have failed.

Types of child restraints

You may need to restrain an infant or a child to prevent injury or to facilitate examination, diagnostic tests, or treatment. If so, follow these steps:

- Provide a simple explanation, reassurance, and constant observation to minimize the child's fear.
- Explain the restraint to the parents and enlist their help.
- Reassure them that it won't hurt the child.
- Make sure that the restraint ties or safety pins are secured outside the child's reach to prevent injury.
- When using a mummy restraint, secure the infant's arms in proper alignment with the body to avoid dislocation and other injuries.

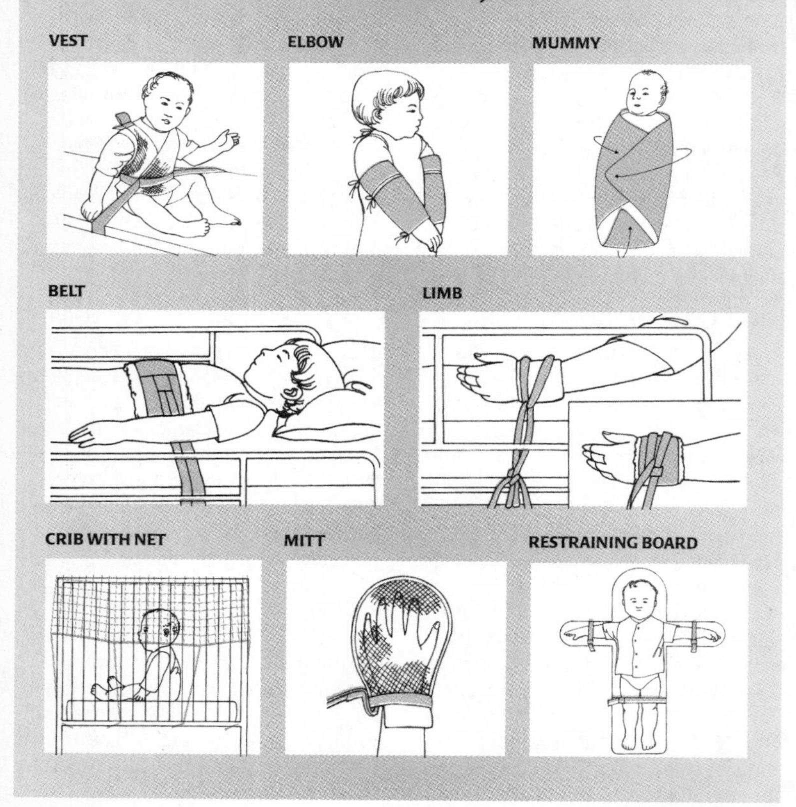

- In many cases, the cause of agitated behavior is an unmet basic need, such as toileting or pain relief. Determining the cause of the patient's behavior can lead to a simple alternative measure, such as changing his position, providing a bedpan, or giving an analgesic.

Preventing falls: Alternatives to restraints

Because restraints should be used only as a last resort, here are some alternative measures that may be used to prevent falls.

- Assist with exercises and gait training to improve the patient's leg strength.
- Teach the patient how to properly use a walker or other assistive device.
- Offer a bedpan or urinal to the patient or assist him to the toilet every 2 hours. An alternative is to assist with toileting on awakening in the morning, after meals, and when the patient goes to bed.
- Place the patient in a reclining chair or use a wedge cushion. Sit him in a place where he can be observed.
- Use bed alarms.
- Have family members, staff, or volunteers sit with the patient.
- Make sure the patient has an adequate intake of nutrition and fluids.

Alternatives to restraints

- Alternatives to restraints include developing an ambulation program, providing frequent help to the bathroom, adding daily exercise into the care plan, and encouraging staff-patient interaction. (See *Preventing falls: Alternatives to restraints*.)
- Other strategies include putting the call bell within easy reach and implementing closer monitoring.
- Such interventions as daily indoor or outdoor walks with patients, saddle-type seats to prevent sliding out of chairs, and use of volunteers to help residents aren't difficult to implement.
- The most effective interventions are typically those that reflect high-quality patient care. Other factors include education of all staff members, reassessment of patients to determine the need for restraints, support from administration, cooperation of physicians, and involvement of the patients' family members.
- Reducing the use of restraints requires an organized, planned effort to change attitudes, beliefs, practices, and policies in a health care facility. Cooperative effort at all levels can ultimately improve the quality of life for residents.

2 Vital signs

Temperature

◆ Body temperature represents the balance between heat produced by metabolism, muscular activity, and other factors and heat lost through the skin, lungs, and body wastes. A stable temperature pattern promotes proper function of cells, tissues, and organs; a change in this pattern usually signals the onset of illness.
◆ Temperature can be measured with either electronic digital, tympanic, or chemical-dot thermometers. (See *Types of thermometers.*)
◆ Oral temperature in adults normally ranges from 97° to 99.5° F (36.1° to 37.5° C); rectal temperature, the most accurate reading, is usually 1° F (0.6° C) higher; axillary temperature, the least accurate, reads 1° to 2° F (0.6° to 1.1° C) lower; and tympanic temperature reads 0.5° to 1° F (0.3° to 0.6° C) higher. (See *Comparing temperature measurement routes,* page 48.)
◆ Temperature normally fluctuates with rest and activity. Lowest readings typically occur between 4 and 5 a.m.; the highest readings occur between 4 and 8 p.m.
◆ Other factors also influence temperature, including gender, age, emotional conditions, and environment. Heightened emotions raise temperature; depressed emotions lower it. A hot external environment can raise temperature; a cold environment lowers it.
◆ Women typically have higher temperatures than men, especially during ovulation.
◆ Normal temperature is highest in neonates and lowest in elderly persons.

Implementation tips

◆ If the patient has had hot or cold liquids, chewed gum, or smoked, wait 15 minutes before taking an oral temperature.

Types of thermometers

You can take an oral, rectal, or axillary temperature with a chemical-dot device or various electronic digital thermometers. You may even have access to a tympanic thermometer. Mercury thermometers are no longer recommended because of the risk of poisoning if the glass instrument breaks.

You'll use the oral route most for adults who are awake, alert, oriented, and cooperative. For infants, young children, and confused or unconscious patients, you may need to take a rectal or tympanic temperature.

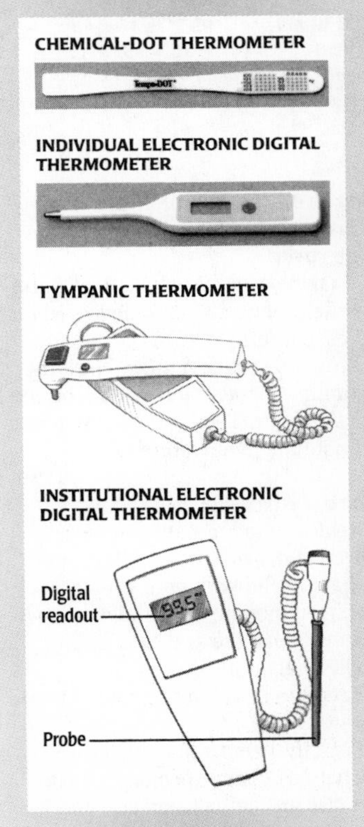

Comparing temperature measurement routes

You can take the patient's temperature four different ways. The table below compares each route.

ROUTE	NORMAL TEMPERATURE	CONSIDERATIONS
Oral	97.7° to 99.5° F (36.5° to 37.5° C)	Used for adults and older children who are awake, alert, oriented, and cooperative
Axillary (armpit)	96.7° to 98.5° F (35.9° to 36.9° C)	Used for neonates and patients with impaired immune systems when infection is a concern; less accurate because it can vary with blood flow to the skin
Rectal	98.7° to 100.5° F (37° to 38° C)	Used for infants, young children, and confused or unconscious patients; wear gloves and lubricate the thermometer
Tympanic (ear)	98.2° to 100° F (36.8° to 37.8° C)	Used for adults and children, conscious and cooperative patients, and confused or unconscious patients; provides automatic timing through a push-button device

Using an electronic thermometer

◆ Insert the probe into a disposable probe cover.

◆ If taking a rectal temperature, lubricate the probe cover to reduce friction and ease insertion.

◆ Leave the probe in place until the maximum temperature appears on the digital display. Then remove the probe and note the temperature.

Using a chemical-dot thermometer

◆ Remove the thermometer from its protective dispenser case by grasping the handle end with your thumb and forefinger, moving the handle up and down to break the seal, and pulling the handle straight out.

◆ Keep the thermometer sealed until use.

◆ Read the temperature as the last dye dot that has changed color or fired; then discard the thermometer and its dispenser case.

Using a tympanic thermometer

◆ Make sure the lens under the probe is clean and shiny. Attach a disposable probe cover.

◆ Stabilize the patient's head; then gently pull the ear straight back (for children up to age 1) or up and back (for children age 1 and older to adults).

◆ Insert the thermometer until the entire ear canal is sealed. The thermometer should be inserted toward the tympanic membrane.

◆ Then press the activation button and hold it for 1 second. The temperature will appear on the display.

Age alert For infants younger than age 6 months, instead of a tympanic reading take a rectal reading. For children ages 6 months to 3 years, the American Academy of Pediatrics recommends a rectal reading but tympanic readings are acceptable. Mercury thermometers are prohibited because of the risk of toxicity if broken.

Taking an oral temperature

◆ Put on clean gloves to prevent body fluid exposure.
◆ Position the tip of the thermometer under the patient's tongue, as far back as possible on either side of the frenulum linguae to promote contact with superficial blood vessels and obtain a more accurate reading.
◆ Instruct the patient to close his lips but to not bite down with his teeth.
◆ Leave the thermometer in place for the appropriate length of time, depending on which thermometer was used.
◆ Remove your gloves, and wash your hands.

Taking a rectal temperature

◆ Put on clean gloves to prevent body fluid exposure.
◆ Position the patient on his side with his top leg flexed, and drape him to provide privacy. Then fold back the bed linens to expose the anus.
◆ Squeeze the lubricant onto a facial tissue to prevent contamination of the lubricant supply.
◆ Lubricate about ½″ (1.3 cm) of the thermometer tip for an infant, 1″ (2.5 cm) for a child, or about 1½″ (3.8 cm) for an adult. Lubrication reduces friction and thus eases insertion.
◆ Lift the patient's upper buttock, and insert the thermometer about ½″ for an infant or 1½″ for an adult. Gently direct the thermometer along the rectal wall toward the umbilicus. This will avoid perforating the anus or rectum. It will also help ensure an accurate reading because the thermometer will register hemorrhoidal artery temperature instead of fecal temperature.
◆ Hold the thermometer in place for the appropriate length of time to prevent damage to rectal tissues caused by displacement.
◆ Carefully remove the thermometer and wipe it as necessary. Then wipe the patient's anal area to remove any lubricant or feces.
◆ Remove your gloves, and wash your hands.

Taking an axillary temperature

◆ Put on clean gloves.
◆ Because moisture conducts heat, gently pat the axilla dry with a facial tissue. Avoid harsh rubbing, which generates heat.
◆ Position the thermometer in the center of the axilla, with the tip pointing toward the patient's head.
◆ Tell the patient to grasp his opposite shoulder and to lower his elbow and hold it against his chest. This promotes skin contact with the thermometer.
◆ Axillary temperature takes longer to register than oral or rectal temperature because the thermometer isn't enclosed in a body cavity. Leave the thermometer in place for the appropriate length of time, depending on which thermometer you're using.
◆ Grasp the end of the thermometer and remove it from the axilla.
◆ Remove your gloves and wash your hands.

Special considerations

◆ Oral measurement is contraindicated in young children and infants; patients who are unconscious or disoriented; patients who must breathe through their mouth; and patients prone to seizures.
◆ Because it may injure inflamed tissue, rectal measurement is contraindicated in patients with diarrhea, bleeding tendencies, recent rectal or prostatic surgery or injury.
◆ Rectal measurement should be avoided in patients with recent myo-

Pulse points

Shown below are anatomic locations where an artery crosses bone or firm tissue and can be palpated for a pulse.

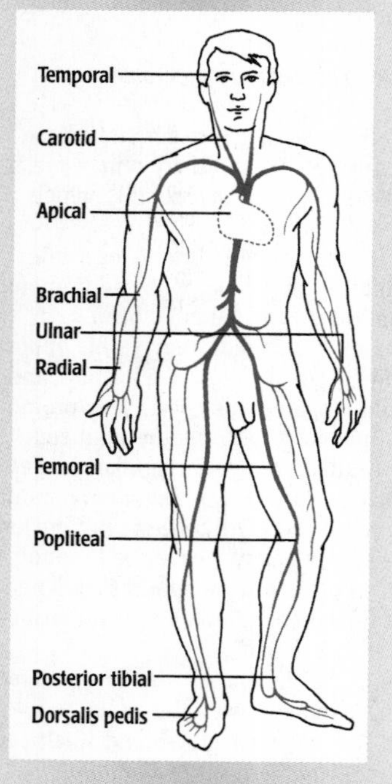

cardial infarction because anal manipulation may stimulate the vagus nerve, causing bradycardia or another rhythm disturbance.

◆ Use the same thermometer for repeated temperature measurements to avoid variations caused by equipment differences.

◆ Store chemical-dot thermometers in a cool area because exposure to heat activates the dye dots.

◆ Oral temperatures can still be measured when the patient is receiving nasal oxygen because oxygen administration raises oral temperature by only about 0.3° F (0.2° C).

Documentation

◆ Record the time, route, and temperature on the patient's chart.

Pulse

◆ Blood pumped into an already-full aorta during ventricular contraction creates a fluid wave that travels from the heart to the peripheral arteries. This recurring wave—called a *pulse*—can be palpated at locations on the body where an artery crosses over bone on firm tissue. (See *Pulse points*.)

◆ In adults and children over age 3, the radial artery in the wrist is the most common palpation site. In infants and children younger than age 3, a stethoscope is used to listen to the heart itself rather than palpating a pulse. Because auscultation is done at the heart's apex, this is called the *apical pulse.*

◆ An apical-radial pulse is taken by simultaneously counting apical and radial beats — the first by auscultation at the apex of the heart, the second by palpation at the radial artery.

◆ Some heartbeats detected at the apex can't be detected at peripheral sites. When this occurs, the apical pulse rate is higher than the radial; the difference is the pulse deficit.

◆ Pulse taking involves determining the rate (number of beats per minute), rhythm (pattern or regularity of the beats), and volume (amount of blood pumped with each beat). If the pulse is faint or weak, use a Doppler ultrasound blood flow detector if available. (See *Using a Doppler device*.)

Using a Doppler device

More sensitive than palpation for determining pulse rate, the Doppler ultrasound blood flow detector is especially useful when a pulse is faint or weak. Unlike palpation, which detects arterial wall expansion and retraction, this instrument detects the motion of red blood cells (RBCs).

◆ Apply a small amount of coupling gel or transmission gel (not water-soluble lubricant) to the ultrasound probe.

◆ Position the probe on the skin directly over the selected artery. In the illustration below left, the probe is over the posterior tibial artery.

◆ When using a Doppler model like the one in the illustration below left, turn the instrument on and, moving counterclockwise, set the volume control to the lowest setting. If your model doesn't have a speaker, plug in the earphones and slowly raise the volume. The Doppler ultrasound stethoscope shown in the illustration below right is basically a stethoscope fitted with an audio unit, volume control, and transducer, which amplifies the movement of RBCs.

◆ To obtain the best signals with either device, tilt the probe 45 degrees from the artery, being sure to put gel between the skin and the probe. Slowly move the probe in a circular motion to locate the center of the artery and the Doppler signal – a hissing noise at the heartbeat. Avoid moving the probe rapidly because this distorts the signal.

◆ Count the signals for 60 seconds to determine the pulse rate.

◆ After you've measured the pulse rate, clean the probe with a soft cloth soaked in antiseptic solution or soapy water. Don't immerse the probe or bump it against a hard surface.

DOPPLER PROBE WITH AMPLIFIER

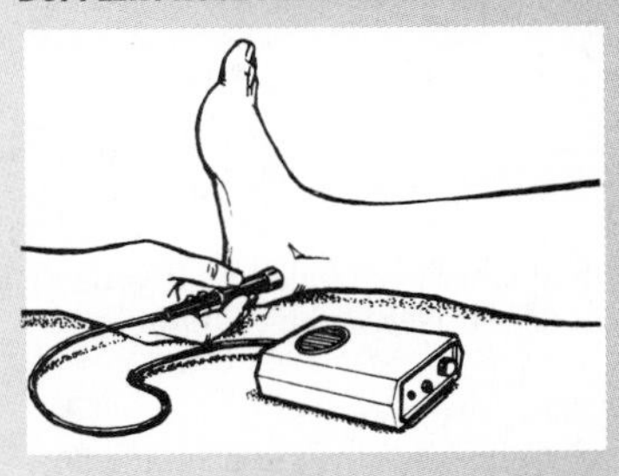

DOPPLER ULTRASOUND STETHOSCOPE

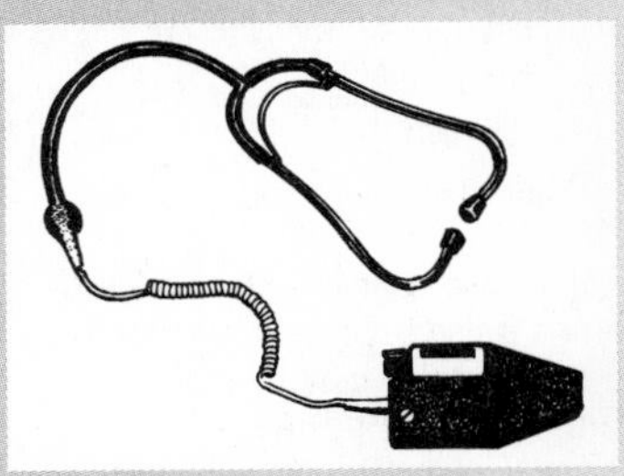

Implementation tips

◆ If you aren't using your own stethoscope, disinfect the earpieces with an alcohol pad before and after use to prevent cross-contamination.

◆ Make sure the patient is comfortable and relaxed because an awkward, uncomfortable position may affect the heart rate.

Taking a radial pulse

◆ Place the patient in a sitting or supine position, with his arm at his side or across his chest.

◆ Gently press your index, middle, and ring fingers on the radial artery, inside the patient's wrist. You should feel a pulse with only moderate pressure; excessive pressure may obstruct blood flow distal to the pulse site.

Identifying pulse patterns

TYPE	RATE	RHYTHM (PER 3 SECONDS)
Normal	60 to 80 beats/ minute; in neonates, 120 to 140 beats/minute	● ● ● ●
Tachycardia	More than 100 beats/ minute	●●●●●●●
Bradycardia	Less than 60 beats/ minute	● ● ●
Irregular	Uneven time intervals between beats (for example, periods of regular rhythm interrupted by pauses or premature beats)	●●●● ●●●

◆ Don't use your thumb to take the patient's pulse because your thumb's own strong pulse may be confused with the patient's pulse.
◆ After locating the pulse, count the beats for 60 seconds, or count for 30 seconds and multiply by 2. Counting for a full minute provides a more accurate picture of irregularities.
◆ While counting the rate, check pulse rhythm and volume by noting the pattern and strength of the beats. (See *Identifying pulse patterns*.)
◆ If you detect an irregularity, repeat the count, and note whether it occurs in a pattern or randomly. If you're still in doubt, take an apical pulse.

Taking an apical pulse

◆ Help the patient to a supine position, and drape him if needed.
◆ Warm the diaphragm or bell of the stethoscope in your hand. Placing a cold stethoscope against the skin may startle the patient and momentarily increase the heart rate.
◆ Keep in mind that the bell transmits low-pitched sounds more effectively than the diaphragm.
◆ Place the diaphragm or bell of the stethoscope over the apex of the heart

CAUSES
◆ Varies with such factors as age, physical activity, and gender (men usually have lower pulse rates than women).
◆ Accompanies stimulation of the sympathetic nervous system by emotional stress, such as anger, fear, or anxiety, or by the use of certain drugs such as caffeine. ◆ May result from exercise and from certain health conditions, such as heart failure, anemia, and fever (which increases oxygen requirements and therefore pulse rate).
◆ Accompanies stimulation of the parasympathetic nervous system by drug use, especially cardiac glycosides, and such conditions as cerebral hemorrhage and heart block. ◆ May also be present in fit athletes.
◆ May indicate cardiac irritability, hypoxia, digoxin toxicity, potassium imbalance, or sometimes more serious arrhythmias if premature beats occur frequently. ◆ Occasional premature beats are normal.

(normally located at the fifth intercostal space left of the midclavicular line).
◆ Count the beats for 60 seconds (or count for 30 seconds and multiply by 2) and note their rhythm, volume, and intensity (loudness).

Taking an apical-radial pulse
◆ Two nurses work together to obtain the apical-radial pulse; one palpates the radial pulse while the other auscultates the apical pulse with a stethoscope. Both must use the same watch when counting beats.
◆ Determine a time to begin counting. Then each nurse should count beats for 60 seconds.
◆ Calculate the pulse deficit and report significant values.

Special considerations
◆ When the peripheral pulse is irregular, take an apical pulse to measure the heartbeat more directly. Apical pulse is the most accurate pulse measurement.
◆ If the pulse is faint or weak, use a Doppler ultrasound blood flow detector, if available.
◆ If another nurse isn't available for an apical-radial pulse, hold the stethoscope in place with your hand that holds the watch while palpating the radial pulse with your other hand. You can then feel any discrepancies between the apical and radial pulses.

Documentation
◆ Record pulse rate, rhythm, and volume as well as the time of measurement. "Full" or "bounding" describes a pulse of increased volume; "weak" or "thready," decreased volume.
◆ When recording an apical pulse, include the intensity of the heart sounds.
◆ When recording an apical-radial pulse, chart the rate according to the pulse site — for example, A/R pulse of 80/76.

Blood pressure

◆ Defined as the lateral force exerted by blood on the arterial walls, blood pressure depends on the force of ventricular contractions, arterial wall elasticity, peripheral vascular resistance, and blood volume and viscosity.
◆ Systolic, or maximum, pressure occurs during left ventricular contraction and reflects the integrity of the heart, arteries, and arterioles. Diastolic, or

Positioning the blood pressure cuff

Wrap the cuff snugly around the upper arm above the antecubital area. When measuring an adult's blood pressure, place the lower border of the cuff about 1" (2.5 cm) above the antecubital space. The center of the cuff bladder should rest directly over the medial aspect of the arm. Many cuffs have an arrow for you to position over the brachial artery. Then place the bell of the stethoscope on the brachial artery at the point where you hear the strongest beats.

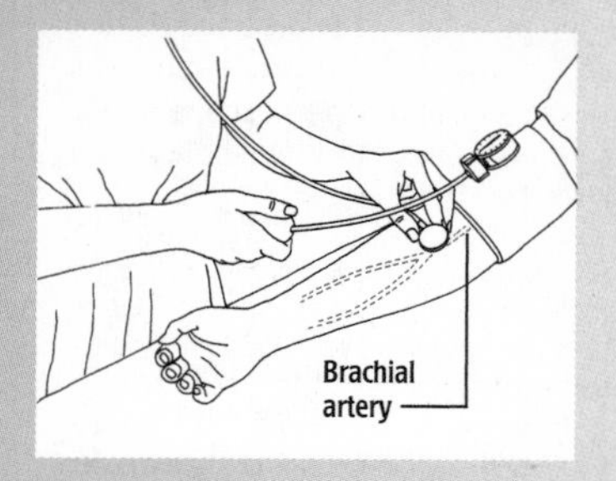

Using an electronic vital signs monitor

An electronic vital signs monitor allows you to track a patient's vital signs continually, without having to reapply a blood pressure cuff each time. In addition, the patient won't need an invasive arterial line to gather similar data.

Some automated vital signs monitors are lightweight and battery-operated and can be attached to an I.V. pole for continual monitoring, even during patient transfers. Newer models can display patient temperature and pulse oximetry as well as blood pressure. A built in printer is also available on certain models. Make sure that you know the capacity of the monitor's battery, and plug the machine in whenever possible to keep it charged.

Before using any monitor, check its accuracy. Determine the patient's pulse rate and blood pressure manually, using the same arm you'll use for the monitor cuff. Compare your results when you get initial readings from the monitor. If the results differ, call your supply department or the manufacturer's representative.

Preparing the device

- ◆ Explain the procedure to the patient. Describe the alarm system so he won't be frightened if it's triggered.
- ◆ Make sure that the power switch is off. Then plug the monitor into a properly grounded wall outlet. Secure the dual air hose to the front of the monitor.
- ◆ Connect the pressure cuff's tubing into the other ends of the dual air hose, and tighten connections to prevent air leaks. Keep the air hose away from the patient to avoid accidental dislodgment.
- ◆ Squeeze all air from the cuff, and wrap the cuff loosely around the patient's arm or leg, allowing 2 fingerbreadths between cuff and arm or leg. Never apply the cuff to a limb that has an I.V. line in place. Position the cuff's "artery" arrow over the palpated brachial artery. Then secure the cuff for a snug fit.

Setting limits

- ◆ When you turn on the monitor, it will default to a manual mode. (In this mode, you can obtain vital signs yourself before switching to the automatic mode.) Press the AUTO/MANUAL button to select the automatic minimum, pressure occurs during left ventricular relaxation and directly indicates blood vessel resistance.

◆ Blood pressure is measured in millimeters of mercury with a sphygmomanometer and a stethoscope, usually at the brachial artery (less often at the popliteal or radial artery). (See *Positioning the blood pressure cuff.*)

◆ The mercury sphygmomanometer provides the most accurate measurement of blood pressure. However, because of risks of toxicity with accidental breakage, aneroid, hybrid, or oscillometric devices are more often being used.

◆ The sphygmomanometer consists of an inflatable compression cuff linked to a manual air pump and a mercury manometer or an aneroid gauge. Electronic devices may also be used to measure blood pressure. (See *Using an electronic vital signs monitor.*)

◆ Blood pressure is lowest in the neonate and rises with age, weight gain, prolonged stress, and anxiety.

◆ Frequent blood pressure measurement is critical after serious injury, surgery, or anesthesia and during any illness or condition that threatens cardiovascular stability. Frequent mea-

---

mode. The monitor will give you baseline data for the pulse rate, systolic and diastolic pressures, and mean arterial pressure.

◆ Compare your previous manual results with these baseline data. If they match, you're ready to set the alarm limits. Press the SELECT button to blank out all displays except systolic pressure.

◆ Use the high and low limit buttons to set the specific limits for systolic pressure. (These limits range from a high of 240 to a low of 0.) You'll also do this three more times for mean arterial pressure, pulse rate, and diastolic pressure. After you've set the limits for diastolic pressure, press the select button again to display all current data. Even if you forget to do this last step, the monitor will automatically display current data 10 seconds after you set the last limits.

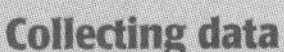

Collecting data

◆ You also need to tell the monitor how often to obtain data. Press the SET button until you reach the desired time interval in minutes. If you've chosen the automatic mode, the monitor will display a default cy-

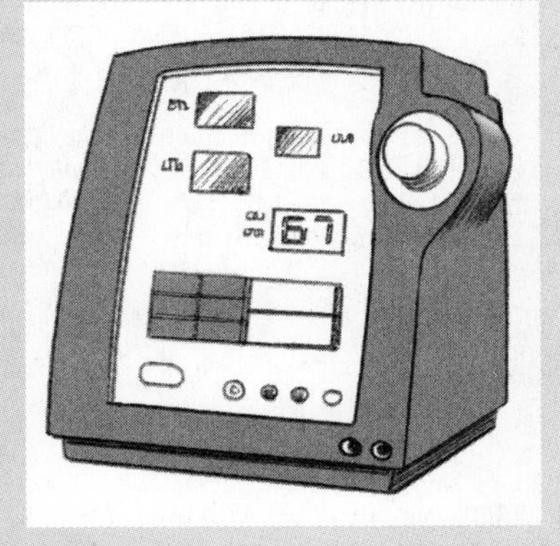

cle time of 3 minutes. You can override the default cycle time to set the interval you prefer.

◆ You can obtain a set of vital signs at any time by pressing the START button. Also, pressing the CANCEL button will stop the interval and deflate the cuff. You can retrieve stored data by pressing the PRIOR DATA button. The monitor will display the last data obtained along with the time elapsed since then. Scrolling backward, you can retrieve data from the previous 99 minutes.

Correcting problems of blood pressure measurement

Blood pressure readings can be falsely high or falsely low due to various causes. You'll need to assess the situation and respond accordingly.

PROBLEM AND CAUSES	NURSING ACTIONS
False-high reading	
◆ Cuff too small	◆ Make sure that the cuff bladder is 20% wider than the circumference of the arm or leg being used for measurement.
◆ Cuff wrapped too loosely, reducing its effective width	◆ Tighten the cuff.
◆ Slow cuff deflation, causing venous congestion in the arm or leg	◆ Never deflate the cuff more slowly than 2 mm Hg/ heartbeat, except in cases of severe bradycardia.
◆ Tilted mercury column	◆ Read pressures with the mercury column vertical.
◆ Poorly timed measurement—after patient has eaten, ambulated, appeared anxious, or flexed arm muscles	◆ Postpone blood pressure measurement or help the patient relax before taking pressures.
False-low reading	
◆ Incorrect position of arm or leg	◆ Make sure the arm or leg is level with the patient's heart.
◆ Mercury column below eye level	◆ Read the mercury column at eye level.
◆ Failure to notice auscultatory gap (sound fades out for 10 to 15 mm Hg, then returns)	◆ Estimate systolic pressure by palpation before actually measuring it. Then check this pressure against the measured pressure.
◆ Inaudible low-volume sounds	◆ Before reinflating the cuff, instruct the patient to raise the arm or leg to decrease venous pressure and amplify low-volume sounds. After inflating the cuff, tell the patient to lower the arm or leg. Then deflate the cuff and listen. If you still fail to detect low-volume sounds, chart the palpated systolic pressure.

surement may be done with an automated vital signs monitor.

◆ Measure blood pressure regularly in patients with a history of hypertension or hypotension. Yearly screening is recommended for all adults.

Implementation tips

◆ If you aren't using your own stethoscope, disinfect the earpieces with an alcohol pad before placing them in your ears to avoid cross-contamination.

◆ Carefully choose a cuff of appropriate size for the patient. An excessively narrow cuff may cause a false-high pressure reading; an excessively wide one, a false-low reading. (See *Correcting problems of blood pressure measurement.*)

◆ The patient can lie in a supine position or sit erect during blood pressure measurement. Keep the patient's arm level with the heart by placing it on a table or a chair arm or by supporting it with your hand. Don't use the patient's muscle strength to hold up the arm; tension from muscle contraction can elevate systolic pressure and distort the findings. If the artery is below heart level, you may get a false-high reading.

◆ Keep the manometer at eye level. If your sphygmomanometer has an aneroid gauge, place it level with the patient's arm.
◆ To obtain a reading in an arm (the most common site), wrap the sphygmomanometer cuff snugly around the upper arm, above the antecubital area (the inner aspect of the elbow).
◆ Locate the brachial artery (just below and slightly medial to the antecubital area) by palpation, and center the cuff bladder over the brachial artery.
◆ Center the bell of the stethoscope over the part of the brachial artery where you detect the strongest beats and hold it in place with one hand. The bell of the stethoscope transmits low-pitched arterial blood sounds more effectively than does the diaphragm.
◆ Watch the manometer while you pump the bulb until the mercury column or aneroid gauge reaches about 20 to 30 mm Hg above the point at which the pulse disappears.
◆ Slowly open the air valve and watch the mercury drop or the gauge needle descend. Release the pressure at a rate of about 2 to 3 mm Hg/second, and listen for pulse sounds (Korotkoff's sounds). These sounds, which determine the blood pressure measurement, are classified as follows:
- *Phase I.* A clear, faint tapping starts and increases in intensity to a thud or a louder tap.
- *Phase II.* The tapping changes to a soft swishing sound.
- *Phase III.* A clear, crisp tapping sound returns.
- *Phase IV (First diastolic sound).* The sound becomes muffled and takes on a blowing quality.
- *Phase V.* The sound disappears.

◆ As soon as you hear blood begin to pulse through the brachial artery, note the reading on the aneroid dial or mercury column. This sound reflects phase I (the first Korotkoff's sound) and coincides with the patient's systolic pressure.
◆ Continue to deflate the cuff, noting the point at which pulsations diminish or become muffled — phase IV (the fourth Korotkoff's sound) — and the point at which they disappear — phase V (the fifth Korotkoff's sound).
◆ Continue to listen for 10 to 20 mm Hg after the last sound, and then release any remaining air.
◆ The American Heart Association and the World Health Organization recommend documenting phases I and V in most adults. To avoid confusion and make your measurements more useful, follow this format for recording blood pressure: systolic/disappearance (for example, 120/76).

Age alert When measuring blood pressure in an infant or child, use a cuff of appropriate size. Because blood pressure may be inaudible in children younger than age 2, consider using an electronic stethoscope or Doppler to obtain a more accurate measurement.

Special considerations

◆ Don't take a blood pressure reading in the arm on the side affected by a mastectomy because it may decrease already compromised lymphatic circulation, worsen edema, and damage the arm.
◆ Likewise, don't take a blood pressure reading on an arm with an arteriovenous fistula because blood flow through the vascular device may be compromised.

Documentation

◆ Record blood pressure as systolic over diastolic pressures, along with the limb used and the patient's position.
◆ If the blood pressure was palpated or auscultated using a Doppler device, record this as well.

Respirations

◆ Controlled by the respiratory center in the lateral medulla oblongata, respiration is the exchange of oxygen and carbon dioxide between the atmosphere and body cells.
◆ External respiration, or breathing, is accomplished by the diaphragm and chest muscles and delivers oxygen to the lower respiratory tract and alveoli.
◆ Four measures of respiration — rate, rhythm, depth, and sound — reflect the body's metabolic state, diaphragm and chest-muscle condition, and airway patency.
◆ Respiratory *rate* is recorded as the number of cycles (with inspiration and expiration comprising one cycle) per minute; *rhythm*, as the regularity of these cycles; *depth*, as the volume of air inhaled and exhaled with each respiration; and *sound*, is the audible digression from normal, effortless breathing.

Implementation tips

◆ The best time to check the patient's respirations is immediately after taking his pulse rate. Keep your fingertips over the radial artery, and don't tell the patient you're counting respirations. If you tell him, he'll become conscious of his respirations and the rate may change.
◆ Count respirations by observing the rise and fall of the patient's chest as he breathes. Or, position the patient's opposite arm across his chest and count respirations by feeling its rise and fall. Consider one rise and one fall as one respiration.
◆ Count respirations for 30 seconds and multiply by 2, or count for 60 seconds if respirations are irregular to account for variations in respiratory rate and pattern.
◆ As you count respirations, be alert for and record such breath sounds as stertor, stridor, wheezing, and an expiratory grunt.
◆ *Stertor* is an inspiratory snoring sound resulting from secretions in the trachea and large bronchi. Listen for it in patients with neurologic disorders and in those who are comatose.
◆ *Stridor* is an inspiratory crowing sound that occurs with upper airway obstruction in laryngitis, croup, or the presence of a foreign body.
◆ *Wheezing* is caused by partial obstruction in the smaller bronchi and bronchioles. This high-pitched, musical sound is common in patients with emphysema or asthma.

Age alert When listening for stridor in infants and children with croup, also watch for sternal, substernal, or intercostal retractions. In infants, an expiratory grunt indicates imminent respiratory distress. In older patients, an expiratory grunt may result from partial airway obstruction or neuromuscular reflex.

◆ Observe chest movements for depth of respirations. If the patient inhales a small volume of air, record this as shallow; if he inhales a large volume, record this as deep.
◆ Observe the patient for use of accessory muscles, such as the scalene, sternocleidomastoid, trapezius, and latissimus dorsi. Using these muscles reflects weakness of the diaphragm and the external intercostal muscles — the major muscles of respiration.

Special considerations

◆ Adult respiratory rates of less than 8 or more than 40 breaths per minute are usually considered abnormal; report the sudden onset of such rates promptly. (See *Identifying abnormal respiratory patterns.*)
◆ Watch the patient for signs of dyspnea, such as an anxious facial expres-

Identifying abnormal respiratory patterns

Here are typical characteristics of the more common abnormal respiratory patterns.

Apnea
Absence of breathing; may be periodic

Apneustic respirations
Prolonged, gasping inspiration followed by extremely short, inefficient expiration

Biot's respirations
Rapid, deep breathing with abrupt pauses between each breath; equal depth to each breath

Bradypnea
Decreased rate but regular pattern of breathing

Cheyne-Stokes respirations
Breaths that gradually become faster and deeper than normal, then slower, during a 30 to 170 second period; alternates with 20 to 60 second periods of apnea

Hyperpnea
Deep breathing at a normal rate

Kussmaul respirations
Rapid, deep (resembling sighs) breathing without pauses. In adults, more than 20 breaths/minute, breathing usually sounds labored

Tachypnea
Shallow breathing with increased respiratory rate

sion, flaring nostrils, a heaving chest wall, cyanosis, or a change in level of consciousness.

◆ To detect cyanosis, look for characteristic bluish discoloration in the nail beds or the lips, under the tongue, in the buccal mucosa, or in the conjunctiva.

◆ In determining the patient's respiratory status, consider his personal and family history. Ask whether he smokes and, if so, for how many years and how much he smokes per day.

Age alert A child's respiratory rate may double in response to exercise, illness, or emotion. Normally, the rate for neonates is 30 to 80 breaths/minute; for toddlers, 20 to 40; and for children of school age and older, 15 to 25. Children usually reach the adult rate (12 to 20) at about age 15.

Documentation

◆ Record the rate, depth, rhythm, and sound of the patient's respirations.

3 Assessment

Collecting patient data

Performing a 10-minute examination

◆ You won't always want or need to examine a patient in 10 minutes. However, rapid examination is crucial when you must intervene quickly — such as when a patient's physical, mental, or emotional status changes.

◆ You may also perform a rapid examination to confirm a diagnostic finding. For example, if arterial blood gas analysis indicates a low oxygen content, you'll quickly check the patient for other signs of oxygen deprivation, such as increased respiratory rate and cyanosis.

General guidelines

◆ Try to collect the patient data not only quickly but also systematically. To save time, cover several components at once. For example, make general observations while checking the patient's vital signs or asking history questions.

◆ Be flexible. You may not use the same sequence each time. Let the patient's chief complaint and your initial observations guide your examination. Sometimes, a quick history may be impossible. Instead, you may need to rely on your observations and the patient's chart.

◆ Keep the patient calm and cooperative. If you don't know him, introduce yourself by name and title. Stay calm, and reassure him that you can help. If you can reduce his anxiety, he'll be more likely to give you accurate information.

◆ Avoid drawing quick conclusions. In particular, don't assume that the patient's current symptom is related to his admitting diagnosis.

When every minute counts, follow these steps.

Check airway, breathing, and circulation

◆ As your first priority, this step may consist of just a momentary observation. However, if a patient seems to be unconscious or is having trouble breathing, examine him more thoroughly to detect the problem and allow immediate intervention.

Make general observations

◆ Note the patient's mental status, general appearance, and level of consciousness (LOC) for clues about the nature and severity of his condition.

Check vital signs

◆ Take the patient's temperature, pulse, respiratory rate, and blood pressure. They provide a quick overview of his condition as well as valuable information about the heart, lungs, and blood vessels.

◆ The seriousness of the patient's chief complaint and your general observations of his condition will determine how extensively you measure vital signs. Vital signs are further discussed in chapter 2.

Age alert A patient's age, activity level, and physical and emotional condition may affect his vital signs. Compare your findings with the patient's baseline, if available.

Conduct the health history

◆ Using pointed questions; explore the patient's view of his chief complaint. Find out what's bothering him most. Ask him to quantify the problem. For instance, does he feel worse today than he did yesterday? Such questions will help focus your interview and examination.

◆ If you're in a hurry or the patient can't respond, use other sources, such as family members, admission forms, the medical history, and the patient's chart.

Perform the physical examination

◆ Begin by concentrating on areas related to the patient's chief complaint — the abdomen, for example, if the patient complains of abdominal pain. Compare the results with baseline data, if available.
◆ Sometimes, you may have to perform a complete head-to-toe or body systems examination — for instance, if a patient is unresponsive (yet has no breathing or circulatory problems) or is confused and, thus, unreliable.
◆ In most cases, the patient's chief complaint, your general observations, and your findings about the patient's vital signs will guide your examination.

Guidelines for an effective interview

When you have time to collect all pertinent data, begin by interviewing the patient. An effective interviewing technique will help you collect essential health history information efficiently. Use these guidelines to enhance your skills.

Be prepared

◆ Before the interview, review all available information. Read the current and, if applicable, previous clinical records. This will focus the interview, prevent the patient from tiring, and save you time.
◆ Review the information with the patient to make sure it's correct.
◆ Keep in mind that the patient's current complaint may be unrelated to his history.

Create a pleasant interviewing atmosphere

◆ Select a quiet, well lit, relaxing setting. Extraneous noise and activity can disrupt concentration, as can too much or too little light. A relaxing atmosphere eases the patient's anxiety, promotes comfort, and conveys your willingness to listen.
◆ Ensure privacy. Some patients won't share personal information if they think others can overhear. You may, however, let friends or family members remain if the patient requests it or if he needs their help.
◆ Make sure the patient feels as comfortable as possible. If he's tired, short of breath, or frightened, provide care and reschedule the interview.
◆ Take your time. If you seem rushed, you may distract the patient. Give him your undivided attention. If you have little time, focus on specific areas of interest and return later instead of hurrying through the entire interview.

Establish a good rapport

◆ Sit and chat with the patient for a few minutes before the interview. Standing may suggest that you're in a hurry, leading the patient to rush and omit important information.
◆ Explain the purpose of the interview. Emphasize how the patient benefits when the health care team has the information needed to diagnose and treat a disorder.
◆ Show your concern for the patient's story. Maintain eye contact, and occasionally repeat what he tells you. If you seem preoccupied or uninterested, he may choose not to confide in you.
◆ Urge the patient to help you to gather information to be used to develop a realistic care plan that will serve his perceived needs.

Set the tone and focus

◆ Encourage the patient to talk about his chief complaint. This helps you focus on his most troublesome signs and symptoms and lets you determine the patient's emotional state and level of understanding.

◆ Keep the interview informal but professional. Allow time for the patient to answer questions fully and to add his own perceptions.

◆ Speak clearly and simply. Avoid medical terms.

Age alert Make sure the patient understands you, especially if he's elderly. If you think he doesn't, ask him to restate what you've discussed.

◆ Pay close attention to the patient's words and actions, interpreting not only what he says but also what he doesn't say.

Age alert If the patient is a child, direct as many questions as possible to him. Rely on the parents for information if the child is very young.

Choose your words carefully

◆ Ask open-ended questions to encourage the patient to provide complete and pertinent information. Avoid yes-or-no questions.

◆ Listen carefully to the patient's answers. Use his words in your later questions to encourage him to elaborate on his signs, symptoms, and other problems.

Take notes

◆ Avoid documenting everything during the interview, but make sure to jot down important information, such as dates, times, and key words or phrases. Use these to help you recall the complete history for the medical record.

◆ If you're tape-recording the interview, obtain written consent from the patient.

Determining overall health status

◆ For a quick look at the patient's overall health, ask these questions.

- Has your weight changed? Do your clothes, rings, and shoes fit?
- Do you have nonspecific signs and symptoms, such as weakness, fatigue, night sweats, or fever?
- Can you keep up with your normal daily activities?
- Have you had any unusual symptoms or problems recently?
- How many colds or other minor illnesses have you had in the last year?
- What prescription drugs, over-the-counter drugs, or herbal supplements do you take?

Determining activities of daily living

◆ For a more complete look at the patient's health and health history, ask these questions.

Diet and elimination

- How would you describe your appetite?
- What do you normally eat in a 24-hour period?
- What foods do you like and dislike? Is your diet restricted at all?
- How much fluid do you drink during an average day? Are the beverages caffeinated or not?
- Are you allergic to any food?
- Do you prepare your meals, or does someone prepare them for you?
- Do you go to the grocery store, or does someone else shop for you?
- Do you eat snacks and, if so, what kind?
- Do you eat a variety of foods?
- Do you have enough money to purchase the groceries you need?
- When do you usually go to the bathroom? Has this pattern changed recently?
- Do you take any foods, fluids, or drugs to maintain your normal elimination patterns?

Exercise and sleep

– Do you have a special exercise program? What is it? How long have you been following it? How do you feel after exercising?
– How many hours do you sleep each day? When? Do you feel rested afterward?
– Do you fall asleep easily?
– Do you take any drugs or do anything special to help you fall asleep?
– What do you do when you can't sleep?
– Do you wake up during the night?
– Do you have sleepy spells during the day? When?
– Do you routinely take naps?
– Do you have any recurrent, disturbing dreams?
– Have you ever been diagnosed with a sleep disorder, such as narcolepsy or sleep apnea?

Recreation

– What do you do when you aren't working?
– What kind of unpaid work do you do for enjoyment?
– How much leisure time do you have?
– Are you satisfied with what you can do in your leisure time?
– Do you and your family share leisure time?
– How do your weekends differ from your weekdays?

Tobacco, alcohol, and drugs

– Do you use tobacco? If so, what kind? How much do you use each day? Each week? When did you start using it? Have you ever tried to stop?
– Do you drink alcoholic beverages? If so, what kind (beer, wine, whiskey)?
– How much alcohol do you drink each day? Each week? What time of day do you usually drink?
– Do you usually drink alone or with others?
– Do you drink more when you're under stress?
– Has drinking ever hampered your job performance?
– Do you or does anyone in your family worry about your drinking?
– Do you feel dependent on alcohol?
– Do you feel dependent on coffee, tea, or soft drinks? How much of these beverages do you drink in an average day?
– Do you use drugs that aren't prescribed by a physician (marijuana, cocaine, heroin, steroids, sleeping pills, tranquilizers)?

Determining family dynamics

◆ When determining how and to what extent the patient's family fulfills its functions, remember to ask about both the family into which the patient was born (family of origin) and, if different, the patient's current family.
◆ Because the following questions target a nuclear family — that is, mother, father, and children — you may need to modify them somewhat for other types of families, such as single-parent families, families that include grandparents, patients who live alone, or unrelated individuals who live as a family.
◆ Remember, you're determining the *patient's perception* of family function.

Affective function

◆ To determine how family members regard each other, ask these questions.
– How do the members of your family treat each other?
– How do they feel about each other?
– How do they regard each other's needs and wants?
– How are feelings expressed in your family?
– Can family members safely express both positive and negative feelings?
– What happens when family members disagree?

- How do family members deal with conflict?
- Do you feel safe in your environment?

Socialization and social placement

◆ To determine the flexibility of family responsibilities, which aids discharge planning, ask these questions.
- How satisfied are you and your partner with your roles as a couple?
- How did you decide to have (or not to have) children?
- Do you and your partner agree about how to bring up the children? If not, how do you work out differences?
- Who takes care of the children? Is this arrangement mutually satisfactory?
- How well do you feel your children are growing up?
- Are family roles negotiable within the limits of age and ability?
- Do you share cultural values and beliefs with your children?

Health care function

◆ To identify the family caregiver and thus facilitate discharge planning, ask these questions.
- Who takes care of family members when they're sick? Who makes physician appointments?
- Are your children learning about personal hygiene, healthful eating, and the importance of adequate sleep and rest?
- How does your family adjust when a member is ill and unable to fulfill expected roles?

Family and social structure

◆ To determine the value the patient places on family and other social structures, ask these questions.
- How important is your family to you?
- Do you have any friends whom you consider family?
- Does anyone other than your immediate family (for example, grandparents) live with you?
- Are you involved in community affairs? Do you enjoy the activities?

Economic function

◆ To explore money issues and their relation to power roles within the family, ask these questions.
- Does your family income meet the family's basic needs?
- Who makes decisions about family money allocation?
- If you take prescription drugs, do you have enough money to pay for them?

Performing palpation

◆ Palpation uses pressure to determine structure size, placement, pulsation, and tenderness. To perform light palpation, press gently on the skin, indenting it ½" to ¾" (1 to 2 cm). Use the lightest touch possible; too much pressure blunts your sensitivity. Close your eyes to concentrate on feeling.

Performing auscultation

◆ Auscultation of body sounds — particularly those produced by the heart, lungs, blood vessels, stomach, and intestines — detects both high-pitched and low-pitched sounds. (See *Performing auscultation*.)

Checking the skin, hair, and nails

Initial skin questions

◆ Determine if your patient has any known skin disease, such as psoriasis, eczema, or hives.

Performing auscultation

Although you can perform auscultation directly over a body area using only your ears, you'll typically perform it indirectly, using a stethoscope.

Listening for high-pitched sounds

To listen for high-pitched sounds properly, such as breath sounds and first and second heart sounds, use the diaphragm of the stethoscope. Make sure you place the entire surface of the diaphragm firmly on the patient's skin. If the area is excessively hairy, you can improve diaphragm contact and reduce extraneous noise by applying water or water-soluble jelly to the skin before auscultating.

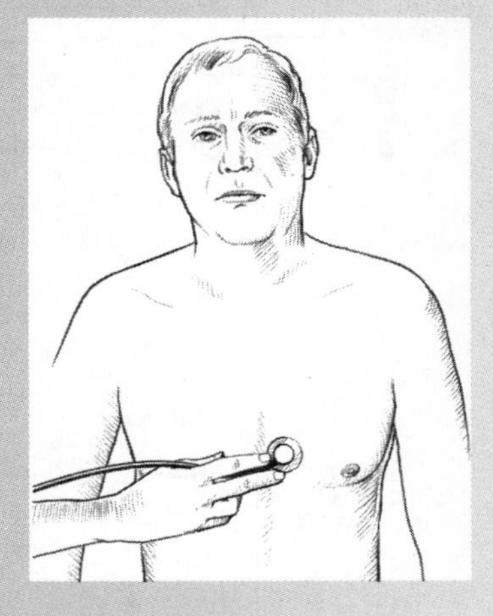

Listening for low-pitched sounds

To listen for low-pitched sounds, such as heart murmurs and third and fourth heart sounds, lightly place the bell of the stethoscope on the appropriate area. Don't exert pressure. If you do, the patient's chest will act as a diaphragm and you will miss low-pitched sounds. If the patient is extremely thin or emaciated, use a stethoscope with a pediatric chest piece.

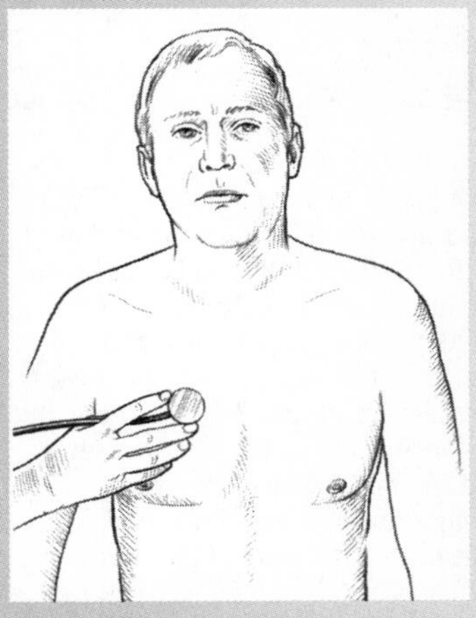

- Ask him to describe any changes in skin pigmentation, temperature, moisture, or hair distribution.
- Explore skin signs and symptoms, such as itching, rashes, or scaling. Is his skin excessively dry or oily?
- Find out if the skin reacts to hot or cold weather. If so, how?

Structure of the skin

This illustration shows a cross section of the skin and its major structures.

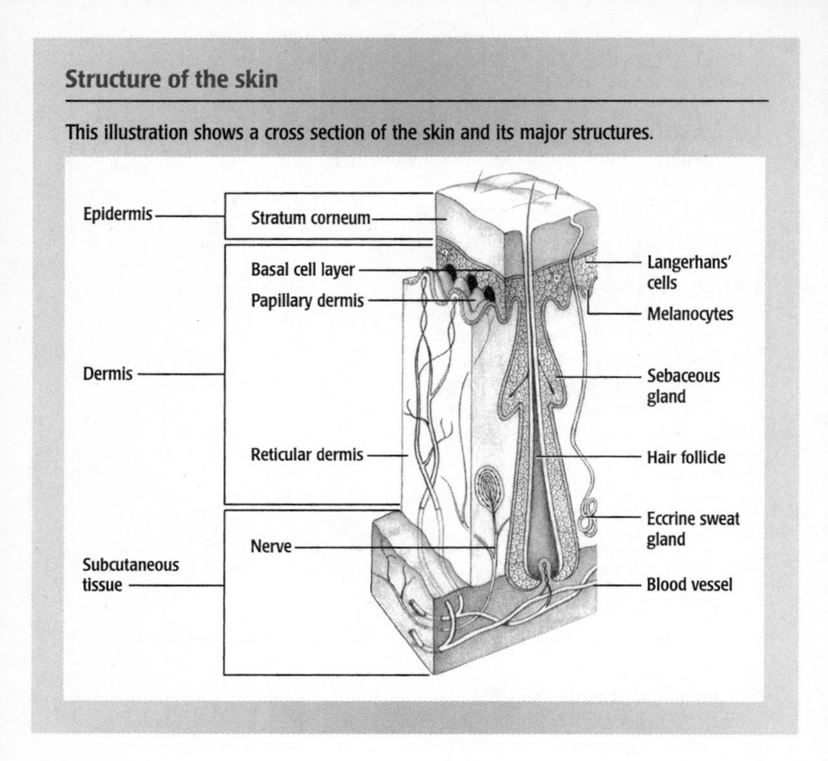

◆ Ask the patient about skin care, sun exposure, use of sun protection factor (SPF) products, SPF number used, and use of protective clothing.

◆ Ask if your patient has noticed easy bruising or bleeding, changes in warts or moles, or lumps. Ask about the presence and location of scars, sores, and ulcers. Consider how these changes might affect the various skin layers. (See *Structure of the skin*.)

Inspecting and palpating the skin

◆ Before you begin your examination, make sure that the lighting is adequate for inspection. Put on a pair of gloves. To examine the patient's skin, you'll use both inspection and palpation — sometimes simultaneously.

◆ During your examination, focus on such skin tissue characteristics as color, texture, turgor, moisture, and temperature. Evaluate skin lesions, edema, hair distribution, and fingernails and toenails.

Color

◆ Begin by systematically inspecting the skin's overall appearance. Remember, skin color reflects the patient's nutritional, hematologic, cardiovascular, and pulmonary status. (See *Evaluating skin color variations*.)

◆ Observe the patient's general coloring and pigmentation, keeping in mind racial differences as well as normal variations from one part of the body to another. Examine all exposed areas of the skin, including the face, ears, back

Evaluating skin color variations

COLOR	DISTRIBUTION	POSSIBLE CAUSE
Absent	Small, circumscribed areas	Vitiligo
	Generalized	Albinism
Blue	Around lips (circumoral pallor) or generalized	Cyanosis (*Note:* In black patients, bluish gingivae are normal.)
Deep red	Generalized	Polycythemia vera (increased red blood cell count)
Pink	Local or generalized	Erythema (superficial capillary dilation and congestion)
Tan to brown	Facial patches	Chloasma of pregnancy or butterfly rash of lupus erythematosus
Tan to brown-bronze	Generalized (not related to sun exposure)	Addison's disease
Yellow	Sclera or generalized	Jaundice from liver dysfunction (*Note:* In black patients, yellow-brown pigmentation of the sclera is normal.)
Yellow-orange	Palms, soles, and face; not sclera	Carotenemia (carotene in the blood)

of the neck, axillae, and backs of the hands and arms.

◆ Note the location of any bruising, discoloration, or erythema. Look for pallor, a dusky appearance, jaundice, and cyanosis. Ask the patient if he has noticed any changes in skin color anywhere on his body.

Texture

◆ Inspect and palpate the texture of the skin, noting thickness and mobility.

◆ Does the skin feel rough, smooth, thick, fragile, or thin? Changes can indicate local irritation or trauma, or they may be a result of problems in other body systems. For example, rough, dry skin is common in hypothyroidism; soft, smooth skin is common in hyperthyroidism.

◆ To determine if the skin over a joint is supple or taut, have the patient bend the joint as you palpate.

Turgor

◆ Checking the turgor, or elasticity, of the patient's skin helps you to evaluate hydration. To check turgor, gently squeeze the skin on the forearm. If it quickly returns to its original shape, the patient has normal turgor. If it resumes its original shape slowly or maintains a tented shape, the skin has poor turgor. (See *Evaluating skin turgor,* page 70.)

Evaluating skin turgor

To determine skin turgor in an adult, gently squeeze the skin on the forearm or sternoclavicular junction between your thumb and forefinger as shown. In an infant, roll a fold of loosely-adherent abdominal skin between your thumb and forefinger. Then release the skin.

If the skin quickly returns to its original shape, the patient has normal turgor. If it returns to its original shape slowly over 30 seconds, or maintains a tented position as shown, the skin has poor turgor.

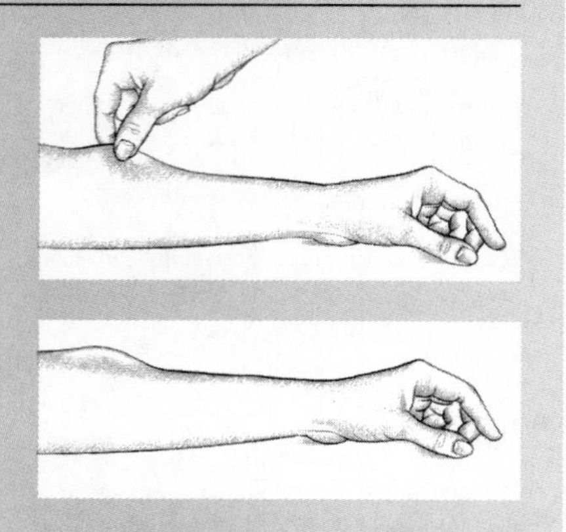

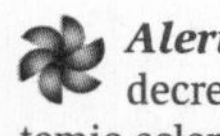

Alert Dehydration and aging decrease turgor. Progressive systemic sclerosis increases it.

◆ In an elderly patient, the skin of the forearm tends to be paper-thin, dry, and wrinkled, so it doesn't accurately represent the patient's hydration status.

◆ To accurately determine skin turgor in an elderly patient, try squeezing the skin of the sternum or forehead instead of the forearm.

Moisture

◆ Observe the skin for excessive dryness or moisture. If the patient's skin is too dry, you may see reddened or flaking areas. Elderly patients commonly have dry, itchy skin. Moisture that appears shiny may result from oiliness.

◆ If the patient is overhydrated, the skin may be edematous and spongy.

◆ Localized edema can occur in response to trauma or skin abnormalities such as ulcers. When you palpate local edema, document related discoloration or lesions.

Temperature

◆ To check skin temperature, touch the surface with the back of your hand. Inflamed skin will feel warm from increased blood flow. Cool skin results from vasoconstriction. With hypovolemic shock, for instance, the skin feels cool and clammy.

◆ Make sure to distinguish between generalized and localized warmth or coolness. Generalized warmth, or hyperthermia, is related to fever from a systemic infection or viral illness. Localized warmth occurs with a burn or localized infection. Generalized coolness occurs with hypothermia; localized coolness, with arteriosclerosis.

Skin lesions

◆ During your inspection, you may note vascular changes in the form of red, pigmented lesions. These lesions may indicate disease.

◆ Among the most common lesions are hemangiomas, telangiectases, petechiae, purpura, and ecchymoses. (See *Recognizing skin lesions.*)

Recognizing skin lesions

The illustrations below depict the most common primary and secondary lesions.

Primary lesions

Bulla Fluid-filled lesion that's more than 2 cm in diameter (also called a blister) – for example, severe poison oak or ivy dermatitis, bullous pemphigoid, second-degree burn

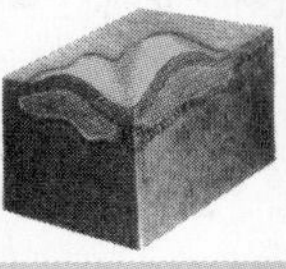

Comedo Plugged pilosebaceous duct, exfoliative, formed from sebum and keratin – for example, blackhead (open comedo), whitehead (closed comedo)

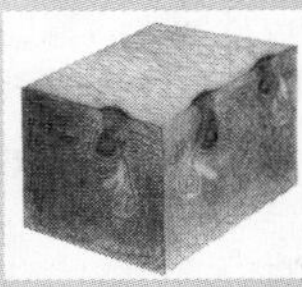

Cyst Semisolid or fluid-filled encapsulated mass extending deep into dermis (sebaceous cyst, cystic acne)

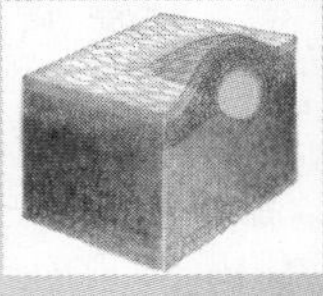

Macule Flat, pigmented, circumscribed area that's less than 1 cm in diameter – for example, freckle, rubella

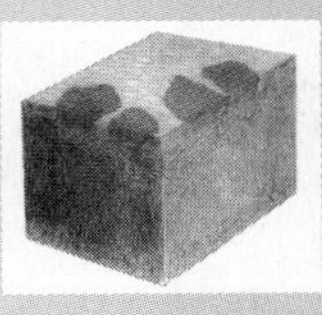

Nodule Firm, raised lesion that's deeper than a papule, that extends into the dermal layer, and 0.5 to 2 cm in diameter – for example, intradermal nevus

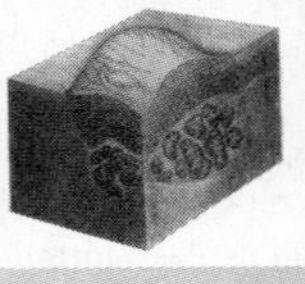

Papule Firm, inflammatory, raised lesion that's up to 0.5 cm in diameter and may be the same color as skin or pigmented – for example, acne papule, lichen planus

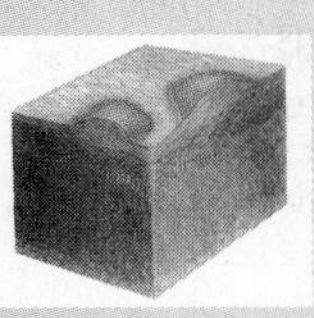

Patch Flat, pigmented, circumscribed area that's more than 2 cm in diameter – for example, herald patch (pityriasis rosea)

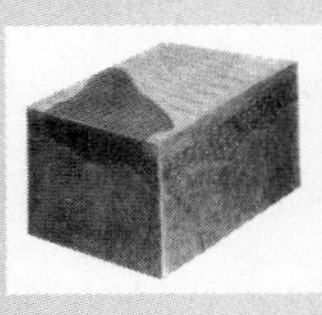

Plaque Circumscribed, solid, elevated lesion that's more than 1 cm in diameter – for example, psoriasis (Elevation over skin surface covers larger surface area in comparison with height.)

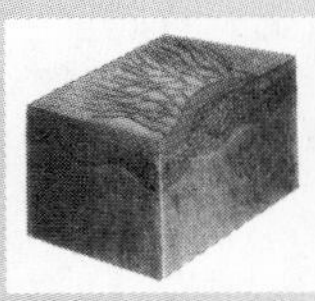

Pustule Raised, circumscribed lesion that's usually less than 1 cm in diameter and contains purulent material, making it a yellow-white color – for example, acne pustule, impetigo, furuncle

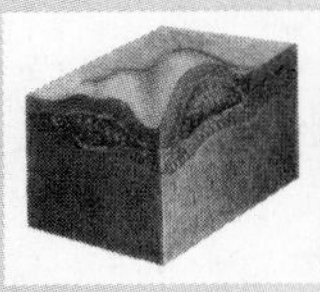

Tumor Elevated solid lesion more than 2 cm in diameter, extending into dermal and subcutaneous layers (dermatofibroma)

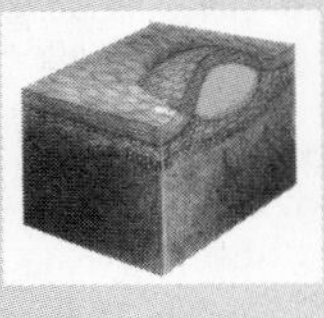

(continued)

Recognizing skin lesions *(continued)*

Primary lesions *(continued)*

Vesicle Raised, circumscribed, fluid-filled lesion that's less than 0.5 cm in diameter; for example, chickenpox, herpes simplex

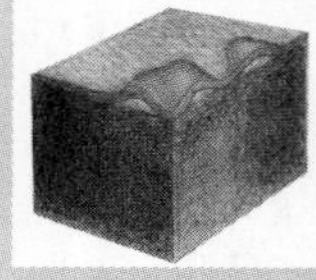

Wheal Raised, firm lesion (with intense localized skin edema) that varies in size, shape, and color (from pale pink to red) and disappears within hours – for example, hive (urticaria), insect bite

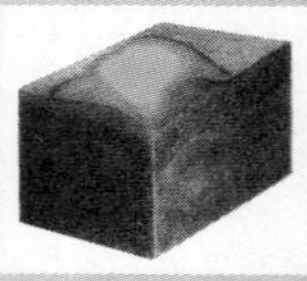

Secondary lesions

Atrophy Thinning of skin surface at the site of the disorder – for example, striae, aging skin

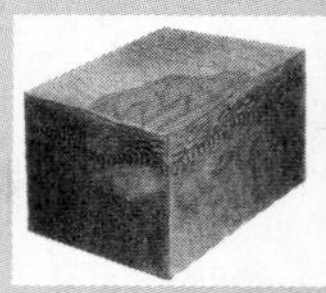

Crust Dried sebum, serous, sanguineous, or purulent exudate, overlying an erosion or weeping vesicle, bulla, or pustule – for example, impetigo

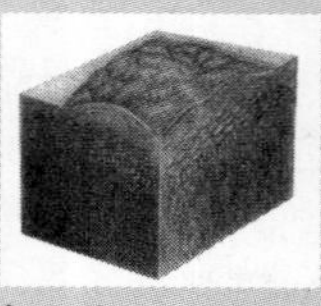

Erosion Circumscribed lesion involving loss of superficial epidermis – for example, rug burn, abrasion

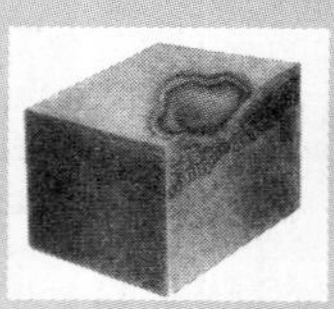

Excoriation Linear scratched or abraded areas, commonly self-induced – for example, abraded acne lesions, eczema

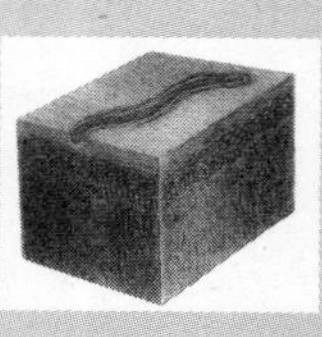

Fissure Linear cracking of the skin extending into the dermal layer – for example, hand dermatitis (chapped skin)

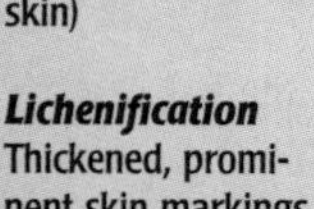

Lichenification Thickened, prominent skin markings caused by constant rubbing – for example, chronic atopic dermatitis

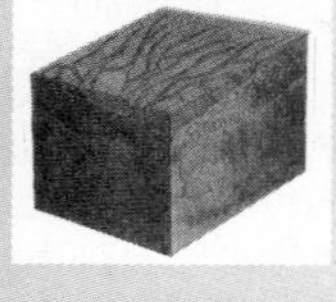

Scale Thin, dry flakes of shedding skin – for example, psoriasis, dry skin, neonate desquamation

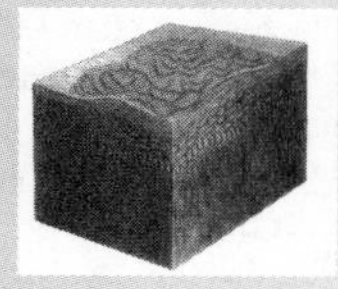

Scar Fibrous tissue (caused by trauma, deep inflammation, or surgical incision) that's red and raised when it's new, pink and flat for up to 6 weeks, and pale and depressed when it's old – for example, a healed surgical incision

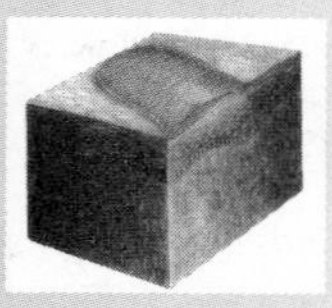

Ulcer Epidermal and dermal destruction that may extend into subcutaneous tissue and that usually heals with scarring – for example, pressure ulcer or stasis ulcer

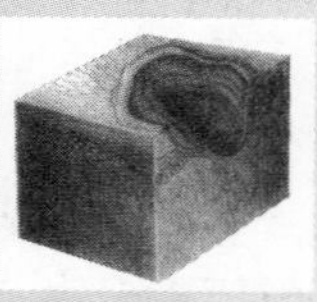

◆ You'll often see telangiectases in pregnant patients and in those with hepatic cirrhosis.

Examining dark skin

◆ Be prepared for certain color variations when examining dark-skinned patients. For example, some dark-skinned patients have a pigmented line, called Futcher's line, extending diagonally and symmetrically from the shoulder to the elbow on the lateral edge of the biceps muscle. This line is normal. Also normal are deeply pigmented ridges in the palms.
◆ To detect color variations in dark-skinned and black patients, examine the sclerae, conjunctivae, buccal mucosa, tongue, lips, nail beds, palms, and soles.
◆ A yellow-brown color in dark-skinned patients or an ash-gray color in black patients indicates pallor, which results from a lack of the underlying pink and red tones normally present in dark skin.
◆ Among dark-skinned black patients, yellowish pigmentation may not indicate jaundice. To detect jaundice in these patients, examine the hard palate and the sclerae.
◆ Look for petechiae by examining areas with lighter pigmentation, such as the abdomen, gluteal areas, and the volar aspect of the forearm. To distinguish petechiae and ecchymoses from erythema in dark-skinned patients, apply pressure to the area. Erythematous areas will blanch, but petechiae and ecchymoses won't.
◆ When you check for edema in dark-skinned patients, remember that the affected area may have decreased color because fluid expands the distance between the pigmented layers and the external epithelium. When you palpate the affected area, it may feel tight.
◆ Cyanosis can be difficult to identify in both white and black patients. Because certain factors, such as cold, affect the lips and nail beds, make sure to check the conjunctivae, palms, soles, buccal mucosa, and tongue as well.
◆ To detect rashes in black or dark-skinned patients, palpate the area to identify changes in skin texture.

Initial hair questions

◆ Determine if your patient has any hair problems, such as hair loss or increased growth and distribution of hair.
◆ Ask the patient to identify physiological factors that could cause hair disorders, such as skin infections, ovarian or adrenal tumors, increased stress, or systemic diseases, such as hypothyroidism or malignancies.
◆ If the patient isn't receiving chemotherapy or radiation therapy, ask when the patient first noticed hair loss or thinning and whether it was sudden or gradual.
◆ Ask when the patient first noticed any increase in hair growth or altered distribution of hair.
◆ Ask if the change occurred in just a few spots or all over the patient's body.
◆ Ask about medication use.
◆ Ask about itching, pain, discharge, anorexia, nausea, vomiting, altered bowel habits, urine changes, fatigue, pain, temperature intolerance, fever, or weight change.
◆ If the patient is female, find out if she has menstrual irregularities, and note her pregnancy history.
◆ If the patient is male, ask about sexual dysfunction, such as decreased libido or impotence.
◆ Ask about hair care. Does the patient often use a hot blow dryer or electric curlers? What about dye, bleach, or perms?

Hair structure

The illustration below shows a hair shaft and its associated glands.

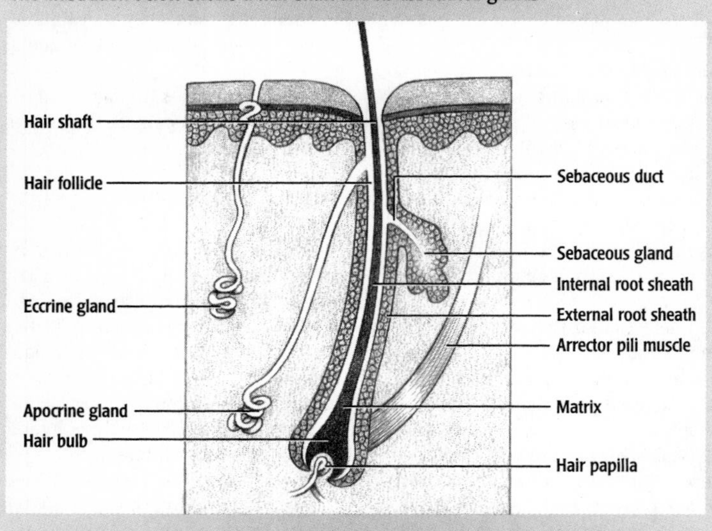

- Check for a family history of alopecia, and ask what age relatives were when they started losing hair.
- Also ask about nervous habits, such as pulling the hair or twirling it.
- Ask about dietary habits and use of supplements.

Age alert In children, alopecia may stem from chemotherapy or radiation therapy, seborrheic dermatitis (known as cradle cap in infants), alopecia mucinosa, tinea capitis, and hypopituitarism. Tinea capitis may produce a kerion lesion that's boggy, raised, tender, and hairless. Trichotillomania, a psychological disorder more common in children than adults, may produce patchy baldness with stubby hair growth from habitual hair pulling. Other causes include progeria and congenital hair shaft defects such as trichorrhexis nodosa.

Inspecting the hair

- Start by inspecting and palpating the hair over the patient's entire body, not just on his head. (See *Hair structure*.) To palpate the patient's hair, rub a few strands between your index finger and thumb.
- Note the distribution, quantity, texture, and color of the patient's hair. The quantity and distribution of head and body hair varies among patients. However, hair should be evenly distributed over the entire body.
- The texture of scalp hair also varies among patients. As a rule, hair should be shiny and smooth, not dry or brittle.
- Differences in grooming and hairstyling may affect the texture and quality of hair. Dryness or brittleness can result from harsh hair treatments or

Nail anatomy

The illustration below shows the anatomic components of a fingernail.

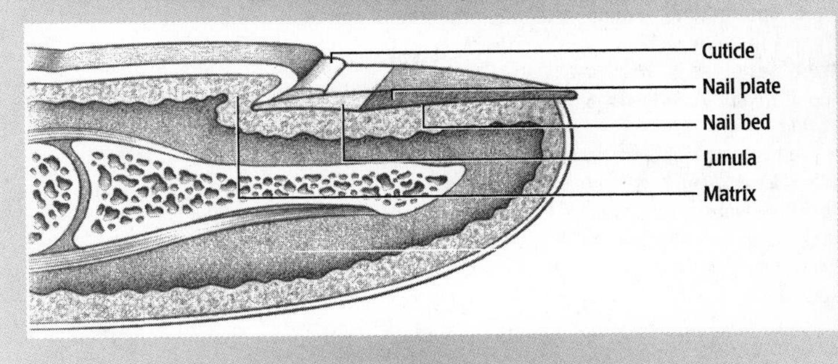

hair care products, or it might be from a systemic illness.

◆ Extremely oily hair is usually related to an excessive production of sebum or poor grooming habits.

◆ Check for patterns of hair loss and growth. If you notice patchy hair loss, look for regrowth.

◆ Examine the scalp for erythema and scaling, which may indicate dermatitis.

◆ Note areas of excessive hair growth, which may indicate a hormone imbalance or a systemic disorder such as Cushing's syndrome.

Initial nail questions

◆ Ask the patient about any changes in nail growth or color.

◆ Ask the patient about any conditions that could cause these changes, such as infection, nutritional deficiencies, systemic illnesses, or stress.

◆ Determine if the patient has had any changes in nail shape, color, or brittleness. (See *Nail anatomy*.)

◆ Ask when the patient first noticed nail changes. Were these changes sudden or gradual?

◆ Ask about other signs or symptoms, such as bleeding, pain, itching, or discharge.

◆ Ask about any history of nail problems, nail biting, or serious illness.

Inspecting the nails

◆ Checking the nails is vital for two reasons: Their appearance can be a critical indicator of systemic illness, and their overall condition tells you a lot about the patient's grooming habits and self-care.

◆ Examine the nails for color, shape, thickness, consistency, and contour. First, look at the color of the nails.

Alert Light-skinned patients typically have pinkish nails. Dark-skinned patients typically have brown nails. Brown-pigmented bands in the nail beds are normal in dark-skinned people and abnormal in light-skinned people.

Alert Thick nails are usually caused by psoriasis, fungal infections, or decreased vascular blood supply to the nailbed.

Alert In patients who smoke cigarettes, nails may turn yellow from nicotine stains. Psoriasis and fun-

Evaluating clubbed fingers

In a patient whose fingers are clubbed, suspect hypoxia. When examining a patient's fingers for early clubbing, gently palpate the bases of the nails. Normally, they'll feel firm, but in early clubbing, they'll feel springy.

To evaluate clubbing, have the patient place the first phalanges of the forefingers together. Normal nail bases are concave and create a small, diamond-shaped space when the first phalanges are opposed, as shown.

NORMAL FINGERS

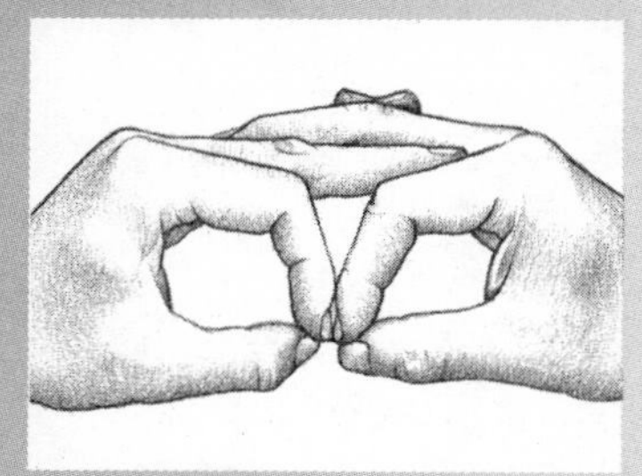

Late clubbing

In late clubbing, however, the now convex nail bases can touch without leaving a space, as shown. This condition is associated with pulmonary or cardiovascular disease. When you spot clubbed fingers, think about the possible causes, such as emphysema, chronic bronchitis, lung cancer, or heart failure.

CLUBBED FINGERS

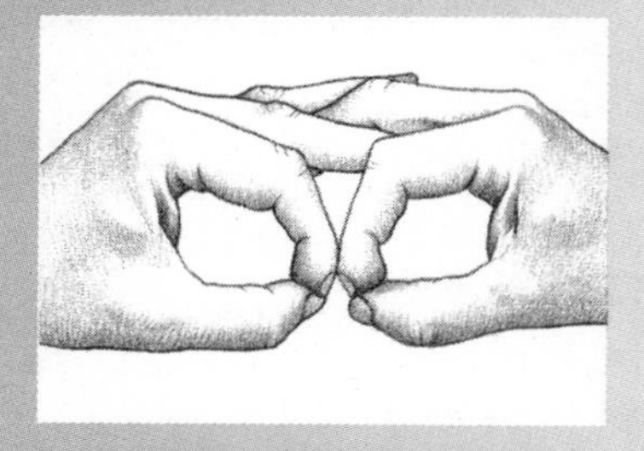

gal infections also can turn nails yellow.

◆ Nail beds can be used to determine a patient's peripheral circulation (capillary refill). Press on the nail bed and then release, noting how long the color takes to return. It should return immediately, or at most within 3 seconds.

◆ Next inspect the shape and contour of the nails. The surface of the nail bed should be either slightly curved or flat. The edges of the nail should be smooth, rounded, and clean. The normal angle of the nail base is 160 degrees. (See *Evaluating clubbed fingers*.)

Age alert In children, clubbing is most common in those with cyanotic congenital heart disease and cystic fibrosis. Surgical correction of heart defects may reverse clubbing. In elderly patients, arthritic deformities of the fingers or toes may disguise the presence of clubbing.

◆ Curved nails are a normal variation. They may appear to be clubbed until you determine that the nail angle is still 160 degrees or less.

◆ Finally, palpate the nail bed to check the thickness of the nail and the strength of its attachment to the bed.

Anatomic structures of the eye

This cross section details important anatomic structures of the eye.

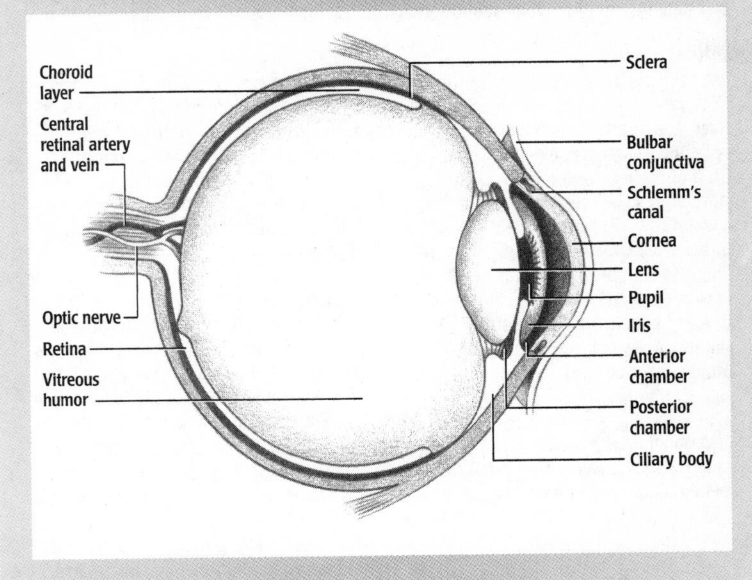

Checking the eyes, ears, nose, and throat

Initial questions

Eyes

◆ Find out when the patient had his last eye examination and whether there were any abnormalities. (See *Anatomic structures of the eye*.)

◆ Ask the patient about vision problems, such as myopia, hyperopia, blurred vision, or double vision. (See *Common eye complaints,* page 78.)

◆ Does the patient know his visual acuity? Does he wear corrective lenses?

◆ Ask if he has noticed any vision disturbances, such as rainbows around lights, blind spots, or flashing lights.

◆ Ask if he has excessive tearing, dry eyes, itching, burning, pain, inflammation, swelling, color blindness, or photophobia.

◆ Elicit any history of eye infections, eye trauma, glaucoma, cataracts, detached retina, or other eye disorders.

◆ If he's older than age 50 or has a family history of glaucoma, ask about the date and results of his last test for glaucoma.

Ears

◆ Find out if the patient has hearing problems, such as deafness, poor hearing, tinnitus, or vertigo. (See *Evaluat-*

Common eye complaints

If your patient is seeking medical attention for a vision problem, his chief complaint will probably be one of the following disorders.

Decreased visual acuity

Lack of visual acuity – the ability to see clearly – is commonly associated with refractive errors. In nearsightedness, or myopia, the eye focuses the visual image in front of the retina, causing objects in close view to be seen clearly and those at a distance to be blurry. In farsightedness, or hyperopia, the eye focuses the visual image behind the retina, causing objects in close view to be blurry and those at a distance to be clear. An abnormally shaped eyeball causes both of these problems.

Diplopia

Also called *double vision,* diplopia is caused by extraocular muscle misalignment. It occurs when the visual axes aren't directed at the object of sight at the same time.

Eye pain

A complaint of eye pain needs immediate attention because it may signal an emergency. Ask the patient what the quality, duration, frequency, and onset of the pain is; what causes it (for example, bright light); whether headaches accompany it; and what he does to relieve it.

Diseases that can cause eye pain include coma, acute angle-closure glaucoma, corneal damage (foreign body, abrasions), trauma to eye, and conjunctivitis.

Visual halos or bright light rings

Increased intraocular pressure, (IOP) as occurs in glaucoma, causes the patient to see halos and rainbows around bright lights. It can be caused by corneal edema, as a result of prolonged contact lens wear, or fluctuation in blood glucose levels in undiagnosed diabetic patients.

Night blindness

The patient may complain of poor vision when darkness descends. Night blindness, or the inability to adapt to dim light or darkness, is caused by retinal degeneration, such as retinitis pigmentosa, optic nerve disease, glaucoma, or vitamin A deficiency related to malnutrition or chronic alcoholism.

Vision loss

Your patient may complain of central or peripheral vision loss, or he may report a scotoma – a blind spot in the visual field that's surrounded by an area of normal vision. Disease in any structure of the eye can result in vision loss. The degree and location of blindness depends on the disease causing the problem and the lesion's location. The major causes of blindness in the United States are glaucoma, untreated cataracts, retinal disease, and macular degeneration.

Visual floaters

Visual floaters are specks of varying shape and size that float through the visual field and disappear when the patient tries to look at them. They're caused by small cells floating in the vitreous humor. Visual floaters require further investigation because they may indicate vitreous hemorrhage and retinal separation. A large, black floater that appears suddenly may indicate vitreous detachment.

Evaluating hearing loss

Use this table to review the causes, onset, and associated signs and symptoms of hearing loss.

TYPE AND CAUSE	ONSET	SIGNS AND SYMPTOMS
External ear		
Cerumen impaction	Sudden or gradual	Itching
Foreign body	Sudden	Discharge
Otitis externa	Sudden	Pain, discharge
Middle ear		
Serous otitis media	Sudden or gradual	Fullness, itching
Acute otitis media	Sudden	Pain, fever, upper respiratory tract infection
Perforated tympanic membrane	Sudden	Trauma, discharge
Inner ear		
Presbycusis	Gradual	None
Drug-induced loss (ototoxicity)	Sudden or gradual	Tinnitus, other adverse drug effects
Ménière's disease	Sudden	Dizziness
Acoustic neuroma	Gradual	Vertigo

ing hearing loss.) Is he abnormally sensitive to noise? Has he noticed recent changes in his hearing?

◆ Ask about ear discharge, pain, or tenderness behind the ears.

◆ Ask about frequent or recent ear infections or ear surgery.

◆ Ask the date and result of his last hearing test.

◆ Ask if he uses a hearing aid.

◆ Determine his ear-care habits, including the use of cotton-tipped applicators to remove earwax.

◆ Ask about exposure to loud noise, including the use of protective earplugs or headphones.

Nose

◆ Ask about nasal problems, including allergies, sinusitis, discharge, colds, coryza (more than four times a year), rhinitis, trauma, and frequent sneezing.

◆ Determine whether your patient has an obstruction, breathing problems, or an inability to smell. Has he had nosebleeds? Has he had a change in appetite or the sense of smell? Has he used nasal sprays?

◆ Ask if he has had surgery on his nose or sinuses. If so, ask when, why, and what type.

Visual acuity charts

The charts used most often for testing vision are the Snellen alphabet chart and the "E" chart, the latter of which is used for young children and adults who can't read. Both charts are used to test distance vision and measure visual acuity. The patient reads each chart at a distance of 20′ (6.1 m).

Recording results

Visual acuity is recorded as a fraction. The top number (20) is the distance between the patient and the chart. The bottom number is the distance from which a person with normal vision could read the line. The larger the bottom number, the poorer the patient's vision.

Age differences

In adults and children ages 6 and older, normal vision is measured as 20/20. For children younger than age 6, normal vision varies. For children age 3 and younger, normal vision is 20/50; for children age 4, 20/40; and for children age 5, 20/30.

SNELLEN ALPHABET CHART

20/200 E 200 FT 61 m 1
20/100 F P 100 FT 30.5 m 2
20/70 T O Z 70 FT 21.3 m 3
20/50 L P E D 50 FT 15.2 m 4
20/40 P E C F D 40 FT 12.2 m 5
20/30 E D F C Z P 30 FT 9.14 m 6
20/25 F E L O P Z D 25 FT 7.62 m 7
20/20 D E F P O T E C 20 FT 6.10 m 8
20/15 L E F O D P C T 15 FT 4.57 m 9
20/13 F D P L T C E O 13 FT 3.96 m 10
20/10 P E Z O L C F T D 10 FT 3.05 m 11

"E" CHART

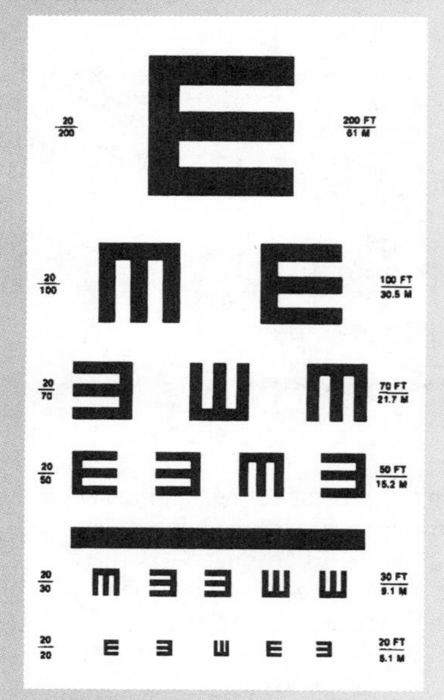

Mouth and throat

◆ Investigate whether your patient has sores in the mouth or on the tongue. Does he have a history of oral herpes infection?

◆ Find out if he has toothaches, bleeding gums, loss of taste, voice changes, dry mouth, or frequent sore throats.

◆ If the patient has frequent sore throats, ask when they occur. Do they include fever or trouble swallowing? How have the sore throats been treated medically?

Recognizing common eye disorders

During an eye examination, you may observe any of several abnormalities. These illustrations show some of those abnormal findings.

PERIORBITAL EDEMA

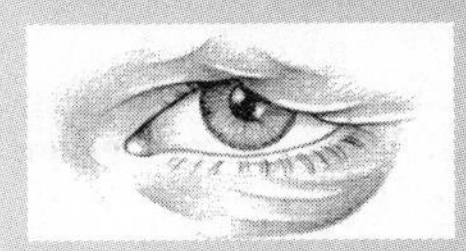

PTOSIS

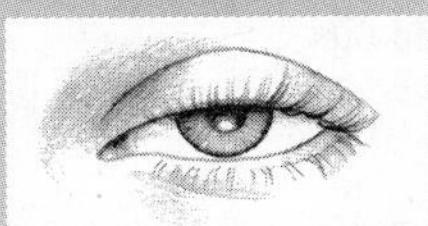

ACUTE HORDEOLUM

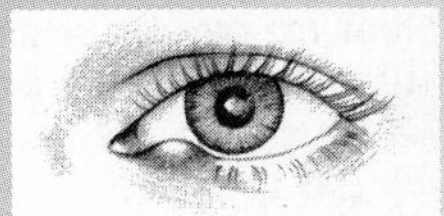

◆ Ask if the patient has ever had a problem swallowing. If so, is the trouble with solids or liquids? Is it constant or intermittent? What causes the trouble? What makes it go away?
◆ Determine whether the patient has dental caries or tooth loss. Ask if he wears dentures or bridges.
◆ Ask about the date and result of his last dental examination.
◆ Ask about his dental hygiene practices, including the use of fluoride toothpaste.

Examining the eyes

◆ Check the patient's visual acuity. (See *Visual acuity charts*.)
◆ Check the patient for eye disorders such as eye infections, eye trauma, glaucoma, cataracts, or detached retina. (See *Recognizing common eye disorders*.)

Examining the ears

◆ Begin by observing the ears for position and symmetry. The top of the ear should line up with the outer corner of the eye, and the ears should look symmetrical, with an angle of attachment of no more than 10 degrees. The face and ears should be the same shade and color. Auricles that protrude from the head, or "lop" ears, are fairly common and don't affect hearing ability.

Alert Low-set ears commonly accompany congenital disorders, including kidney problems.

◆ Inspect the auricle for lesions, drainage, nodules or redness. Pull the helix back, and note if it's tender.

Alert If the patient feels pain when you pull the ear back, he may have otitis externa. If he has crusted, indurated, or ulcerated lesions that fail to heal, they should be excised and examined. They may be basal cell or squamous cell carcinoma of the auricle, both of which are common. Advanced lesions are easy to diagnose, but small growths are commonly overlooked.

◆ Inspect and palpate the mastoid area behind each auricle.
◆ Finally, inspect the opening of the ear canal. Patients normally have varying amounts of hair and cerumen, or earwax, in the ear canal. Cerumen may be flaky and vary in color.

Alert Be alert for discharge, redness, or odor. Look for nodules or cysts. In acute otitis externa, the ear canal is often swollen, narrowed, moist, pale, tender, and sometimes, reddened. In chronic otitis externa, the ear canal is often thickened, red, and itchy. Cerumen shouldn't be impacted in the ear canal.

Examining the nostrils and sinuses

◆ To perform direct inspection of the nostrils, you'll need an otoscope.
◆ Have the patient sit in front of you and tilt his head back. Insert the tip of the otoscope into one of the nostrils.
◆ Shine the otoscope light into the nostril to illuminate the area.
◆ Note the color and patency of the nostril and the presence of exudate. The mucosa should be moist, pink to red, and free from lesions and polyps. Normally, you wouldn't see drainage, edema, or inflammation of the nasal mucosa, although some tissue enlargement is normal in a pregnant patient.
◆ When you've completed your inspection of one nostril, remove the otoscope; then inspect the other nostril.
◆ Next examine the sinuses. Remember, only the frontal and maxillary sinuses are accessible; you won't be able to palpate the ethmoidal and sphenoidal sinuses. However, if the frontal and maxillary sinuses are infected, you can assume that the other sinuses are, too.
◆ Begin by checking for swelling around the eyes, especially over the sinus area. Then palpate the frontal and maxillary sinuses for tenderness and warmth. To palpate the frontal sinuses, place your thumb above the patient's eyes, just under the bony ridges of the upper orbits, and press up. Place your fingertips on his forehead and apply gentle pressure. To palpate the maxillary sinuses, apply gentle pressure by pressing your thumbs (or index and middle fingers) up and in on each side of the nose, just below the zygomatic bone (cheekbone).

Examining the mouth, throat, and neck

◆ First, inspect the patient's lips. They should be pink, moist, symmetrical, and without lesions. Put on gloves and palpate the lips for lumps or surface abnormalities.
◆ Use a tongue blade and a bright light to inspect the oral mucosa. Have the patient open his mouth, and then place the tongue blade on top of his tongue.
◆ The oral mucosa should be pink, smooth, moist, and free from lesions and unusual odors.
◆ Next observe the gingivae, or gums: They should be pink, moist, have clearly defined margins at each tooth, and not be retracted.
◆ Inspect the teeth, noting their number, condition, and whether any are missing or crowded. If a patient is wearing dentures, ask him to remove them so you can examine his gums.
◆ Finally, inspect the tongue. It should be midline, symmetrical, moist, pink, and free from lesions. The posterior surface should be smooth, and the anterior surface should be slightly rough with small fissures. The tongue should move easily in all directions, and it should lie straight to the front at rest.
◆ Ask the patient to raise the tip of his tongue and touch his palate directly behind his front teeth. Inspect the ventral surface of the tongue and the floor of the mouth. Next, wrap a piece of gauze around the tip of the tongue and move the tongue first to one side then the other to inspect the lateral borders. They should be smooth and even-textured.

Alert Dark-skinned patients have increased pigmentation of the oral mucosa.

Age alert Elderly patients may have varicose veins on the ventral surface of the tongue.

Alert Oral cancers tend to develop under the tongue; be sure to examine this area thoroughly.

◆ Inspect the patient's oropharynx by asking him to open his mouth while you shine the penlight on the uvula and palate. You may need to insert a tongue blade into the mouth and depress the tongue. Place the tongue blade slightly off-center to avoid eliciting the gag reflex. The uvula and oropharynx should be pink and moist, without inflammation or exudates. The tonsils should be pink and shouldn't be hypertrophied.

◆ Ask the patient to say "ah," and then watch for movement of the soft palate and uvula. In cranial nerve X paralysis, when the patient says "ah," the soft palate fails to rise and the uvula deviates to the opposite side.

◆ Note any unusual breath odors.

Alert If your patient has a peritonsillar abscess, painful swallowing, and a displaced, beefy, red uvula, he probably has acute tonsillitis. This is a potential emergency because it can obstruct the airway. In this condition, a streptococcal infection spreads from the tonsils to the surrounding soft tissue.

Alert Note lumps, lesions, ulcers, or edema of the lips or tongue. Swelling of the lips and tongue could indicate angioedema, which is usually allergic in nature. Lesions and ulcerations on the lips may be related to herpes simplex infection or syphilis. Carcinoma may appear as a scaly plaque, an ulcer, or a nodular lesion — it usually affects the lower lip.

◆ Next palpate the patient's neck. Using the finger pads of both hands, bilaterally palpate the chain of lymph nodes under the patient's chin in the preauricular area; then proceed to the area under and behind the ears.

◆ Check the nodes for size, shape, mobility, consistency, and tenderness, comparing nodes on one side with those on the other.

◆ Proceed down to the trachea, normally located midline in the neck. Place your thumbs along each side of the trachea near the lower part of the neck. Check whether the distance between the trachea's outer edge and the sternocleidomastoid muscle is equal on both sides. Note any pain or tenderness.

Alert Tracheal deviation may result from a mass in the neck, a mediastinal mass, atelectasis, or pneumothorax.

◆ To palpate the thyroid, stand behind the patient and put your hands around his neck, with the fingers of both hands over the lower trachea.

◆ Ask him to swallow as you feel the thyroid isthmus. The isthmus should rise with swallowing because it lies across the trachea, just below the cricoid cartilage.

◆ Displace the thyroid to the right and then to the left, palpating both lobes for enlargement, nodules, tenderness, a gritty sensation, or a pulsation. Lowering the patient's chin slightly and turning toward the side you're palpating helps relax the muscle and facilitate examination.

Checking the respiratory system

Initial questions

◆ Inquire about dyspnea or shortness of breath. Does your patient have breathing problems after physical exertion? Ask him about pain, wheezing, paroxysmal nocturnal dyspnea, and orthopnea (for example, ask how many pillows he needs to sleep comfortably).

◆ Ask whether the patient has a cough, sputum production, hemoptysis, or night sweats.

Locations of normal breath sounds

These photographs show the normal locations of different types of breath sounds.

ANTERIOR THORAX

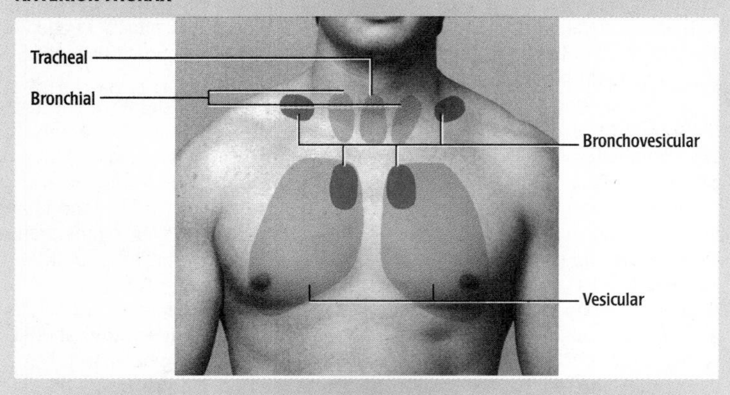

POSTERIOR THORAX

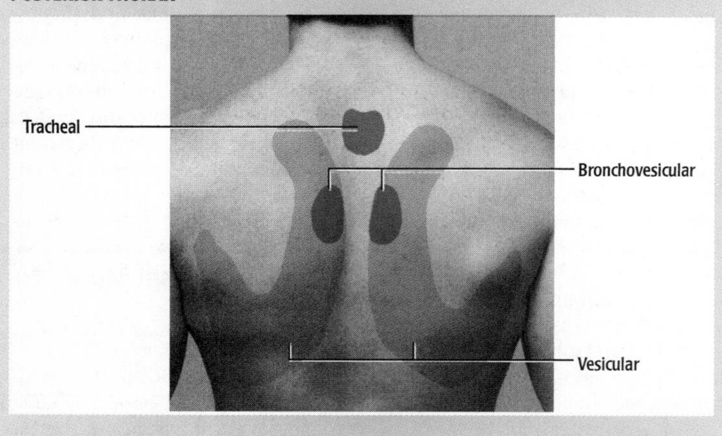

◆ Find out if he has emphysema, pleurisy, bronchitis, tuberculosis, pneumonia, asthma, or frequent respiratory tract infections.

Examining the chest

◆ Position the patient to allow access to his posterior and anterior chest. If his condition permits, have him sit on the edge of a bed or examining table or on a chair, leaning forward with his arms folded across his chest. If this

Qualities of normal breath sounds

BREATH SOUND	QUALITY	INSPIRATION-EXPIRATION RATIO	LOCATION
Tracheal	Harsh, high-pitched	I about = E	Over trachea
Bronchial	Loud, high-pitched	I<E	Over the manubrium
Bronchovesicular	Medium in loudness and pitch	I = E	Next to sternum, between scapula
Vesicular	Soft, low-pitched	I>E	Over most of both lungs

isn't possible, place him in semi-Fowler's position for the anterior chest examination. Then ask him to lean forward slightly and use the side rails or mattress for support while you quickly examine his posterior chest. If he can't lean forward, place him in a lateral position or ask another staff member to help him to sit up.

- Systematically compare one side of the chest with the other.
- First, inspect the patient's chest for obvious problems, such as draining, open wounds, bruises, abrasions, scars, and cuts. Also look for less obvious problems, such as rib deformities, fractures, lesions, or masses.
- Examine the shape of the patient's chest wall. Observe the anteroposterior and transverse diameters.
- Note the patient's respiratory pattern, watching for characteristics such as pursed-lip breathing.
- Observe the movement of the chest during respirations. It should move upward and outward symmetrically with inspiration. Factors that may affect movement include pain, poor positioning, and abdominal distention. Watch for paradoxical movement (possibly from fractured ribs or flail chest) and asymmetrical expansion (atelectasis or underlying pulmonary disease).
- Check for use of accessory muscles and retraction of intercostal spaces during inspiration (possibly indicating respiratory distress). You may notice sudden, violent intercostal retraction (airway obstruction or tension pneumothorax); retraction of the abdominal muscles during expiration (chronic obstructive pulmonary disease and other obstructive disorders); inspiratory intercostal bulging (cardiac enlargement or aneurysm); or localized expiratory bulging (rib fracture or flail chest).

Auscultating breath sounds

- Auscultation of breath sounds is an important step in physical examination. It helps you detect abnormal accumulation of fluid or mucus and obstructed air passages.
- To detect breath sounds, auscultate the anterior, lateral, and posterior thorax. Begin at the upper lobes, and move from side to side and down, comparing findings. (See *Locations of normal breath sounds* and *Qualities of normal breath sounds*.)

Abnormal breath sounds

Crackles **Intermittent, nonmusical, crackling sounds heard during inspiration; classified as fine or coarse**

Wheezes **High-pitched sounds caused by blocked airflow, heard on exhalation**

Rhonchi **Low-pitched snoring or rattling sound; heard primarily on exhalation**

Stridor **Loud, high-pitched sound heard during inspiration**

Pleural friction rub **Low-pitched, grating sound heard during inspiration and expiration; accompanied by pain**

Age alert If the patient is a child, begin just below the right clavicle, moving to the midsternum, left clavicle, left nipple, and right nipple. Listen to one full breath (inspiration and expiration) at each point.

◆ Auscultate the lungs to detect normal, abnormal, and absent breath sounds. (See *Abnormal breath sounds*.)

◆ Classify breath sounds by their location, intensity, pitch, and duration during the inspiratory and expiratory phases.

Checking the cardiovascular system

Initial questions

◆ Ask the patient about cardiac problems, such as palpitations, tachycardia or other irregular rhythms, chest pain, dyspnea on exertion, paroxysmal nocturnal dyspnea, and cough.

◆ Explore vascular problems. Does the patient experience cyanosis, edema, ascites, intermittent claudication, cold extremities, or phlebitis?

◆ Ask about orthostatic hypotension, hypertension, rheumatic fever, varicose veins, and peripheral vascular diseases.

◆ Ask when, if ever, the patient had his last electrocardiogram.

Examining the precordium

◆ First, place the patient in a supine position, with his head flat or elevated for respiratory comfort. (See *Positioning the patient for cardiac auscultation.*)

◆ If you're examining an obese patient or one with large breasts, have the patient sit upright. This position will bring the heart closer to the anterior chest wall and make pulsations more visible.

◆ If time allows, you can use tangential lighting to cast shadows across the chest. This makes it easier to see abnormalities.

◆ Standing to the patient's right (unless you're left-handed), remove the clothing covering his chest wall. Quickly identify the following anatomic sites, named for their underlying structures: sternoclavicular, pulmonary, aortic, right ventricular, epigastric, and left ventricular areas.

◆ Make a visual sweep of the chest wall, watching for movement, pulsations, and exaggerated lifts or heaves (strong outward thrusts seen at the sternal border or apex during systole).

◆ Auscultate the patient's heart sounds. (See *Auscultating heart sounds,* page 88.)

Positioning the patient for cardiac auscultation

During auscultation, you'll typically stand to the right of the patient, who is in a supine position. The patient may lie flat or at a comfortable elevation.

If the heart sounds seem faint or undetectable, try repositioning the patient. Alternate positioning may enhance the sounds or make them seem louder by bringing the heart closer to the surface of the chest. Common alternate positions include the seated, forward-leaning position and the left-lateral decubitus position.

Forward-leaning position

The forward-leaning position is best for hearing high-pitched sounds related to semilunar valve problems, such as aortic and pulmonic valve murmurs. Aortic insufficiency is sometimes heard only in the forward-leaning position. To auscultate these sounds, help the patient into the forward-leaning position and place the diaphragm of the stethoscope over the aortic and pulmonic areas in the right and left second intercostal spaces.

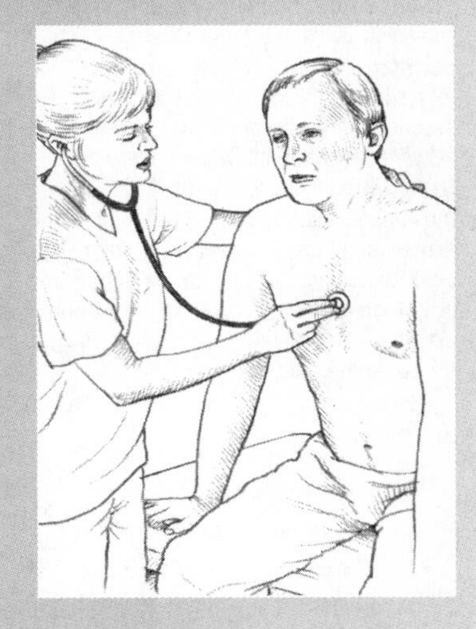

Left-lateral side-lying position

The left-lateral side-lying position is best for hearing low-pitched sounds related to atrioventricular valve problems, such as mitral valve murmurs and extra heart sounds. A mitral stenosis murmur is sometimes heard only in the left-lateral position. A pericardial rub can be heard in this position and is an abnormal finding. To auscultate these sounds, help the patient into the left-lateral side-lying position and place the bell of the stethoscope over the apical area. If these positions don't enhance the heart sounds, try auscultating with the patient standing or squatting.

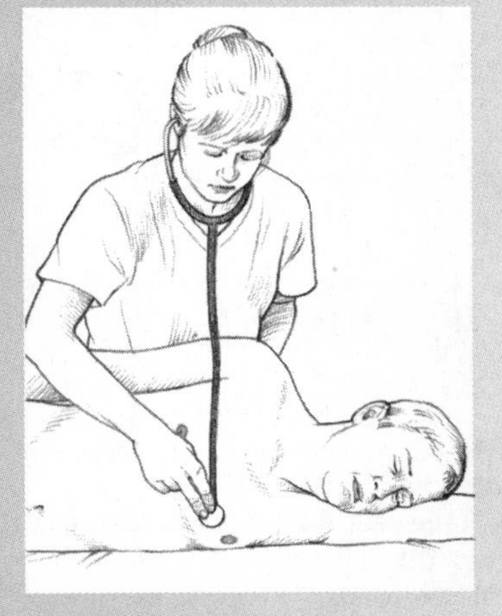

Auscultating heart sounds

Using a stethoscope with 10" to 12" (25- to 30-cm) tubing, follow these steps to auscultate heart sounds.

◆ Locate the four different auscultation sites, as illustrated at right.
◆ In the aortic area, blood moves from the left ventricle during systole, crosses the aortic valve and flows through the aortic arch. In the pulmonic area, blood ejected from the right ventricle during systole crosses the pulmonic valve and flows through the main pulmonary artery. In the tricuspid area, sounds reflect the movement of blood from the right atrium across the tricuspid valve, filling the right ventricle during diastole. In the mitral, or apical, area, sounds represent blood flow across the mitral valve and left ventricular filling during diastole.

◆ Begin auscultation in the aortic area, placing the stethoscope in the second intercostal space along the right sternal border.
◆ Then move to the pulmonic area, located in the second intercostal space at the left sternal border.
◆ Next, listen to the tricuspid area, which lies in the fifth intercostal space along the left sternal border.
◆ Finally, listen in the mitral area, located in the fifth intercostal space near the midclavicular line.
◆ *Note:* If the patient's heart is enlarged, the mitral area may be closer to the anterior axillary line.

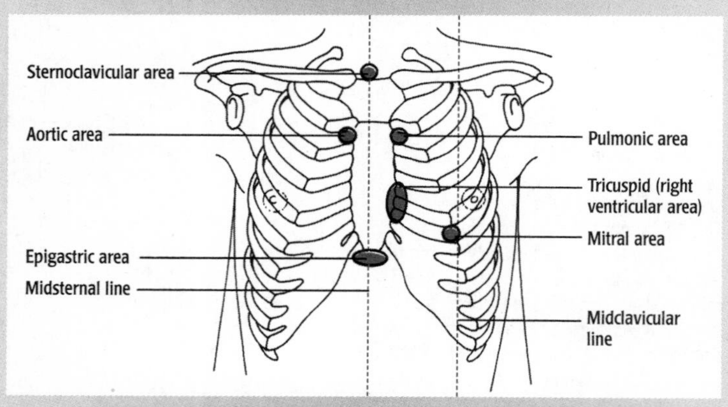

◆ Locate and palpate the patient's arterial pulses. (See *Palpating arterial pulses*.)
◆ If the patient has edema, determine its severity. (See *Evaluating edema,* page 90.)

Checking the neurologic system

Initial questions

◆ Ask the patient to state his full name and the date, time, and place where he is now.

Palpating arterial pulses

To palpate the arterial pulses, you'll apply pressure with your index and middle fingers positioned as shown here.

Carotid pulse

Lightly place your fingers just medial to the trachea and below the angle of the jaw.

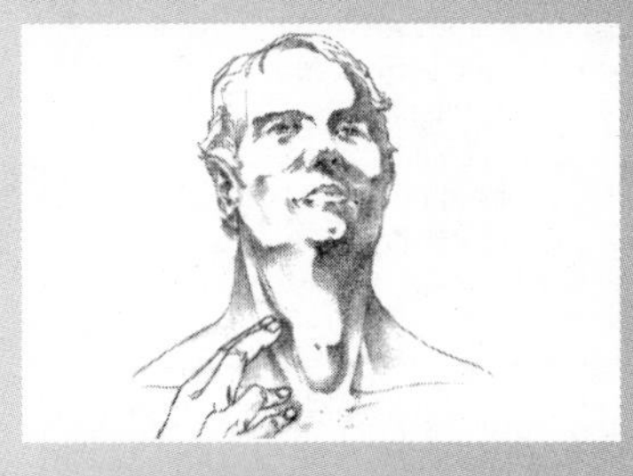

Brachial pulse

Position your fingers medial to the biceps tendon.

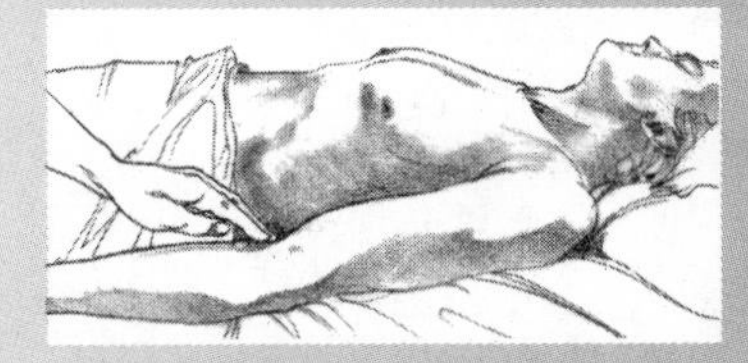

Radial pulse

Apply gentle pressure to the medial and ventral side of the wrist, just below the thumb.

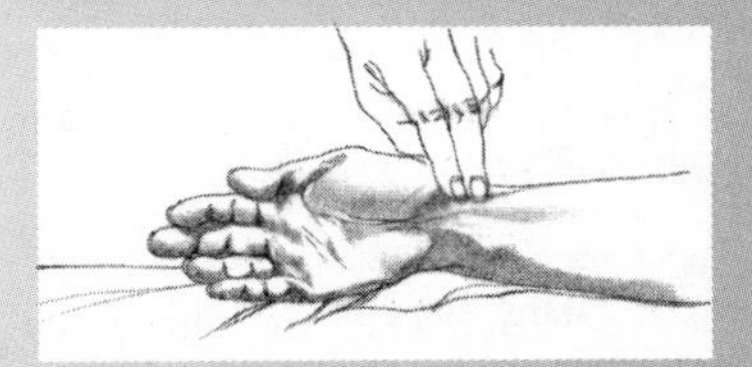

Femoral pulse

Press relatively hard at a point inferior to the inguinal ligament. For an obese patient, palpate in the crease of the groin, halfway between the pubic bone and the hip bone.

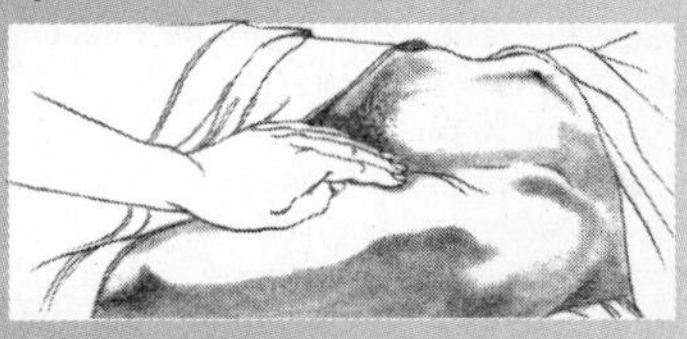

Popliteal pulse

Press firmly against the popliteal fossa at the back of the knee.

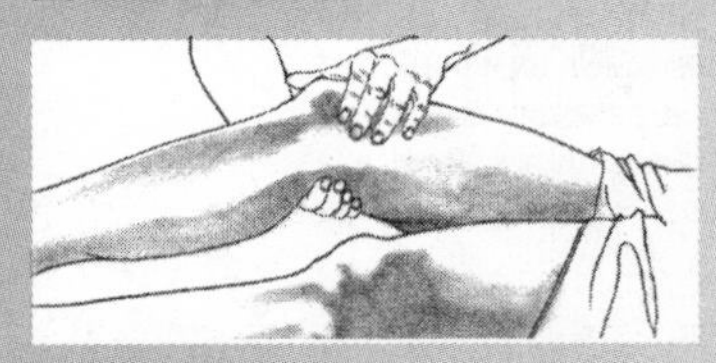

Posterior tibial pulse

Curve your fingers around the medial malleolus, and feel the pulse in the groove between the Achilles' tendon and the malleolus.

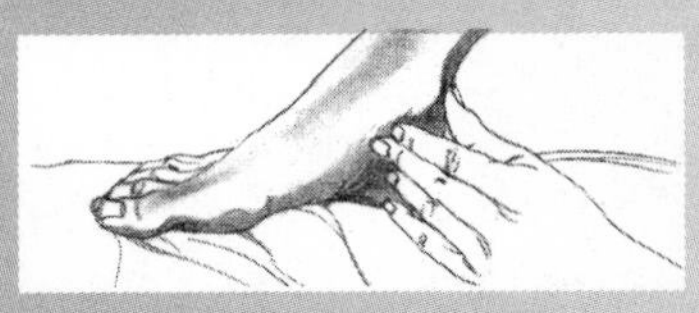

Dorsalis pedis pulse

Lightly touch the medial dorsum of the foot while the patient points his toes down. In this site, the pulse is difficult to palpate and may seem to be absent in some healthy patients.

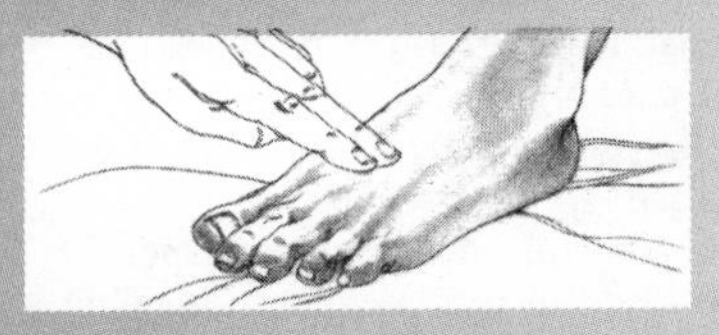

Evaluating edema

To check for pitting edema, press firmly for 5 to 10 seconds over a bony surface, such as the tibia, fibula, sacrum, or sternum. Then remove your finger and note how long the depression remains. Document your observation on a scale of +1 (barely detectable depression) to +4 (persistent pit as deep as 1″ [2.5 cm]).

In severe edema, tissue swells so much that fluid can't be displaced, making pitting impossible. The surface feels rock-hard, and subcutaneous tissue becomes fibrotic. Brawny edema may develop eventually.

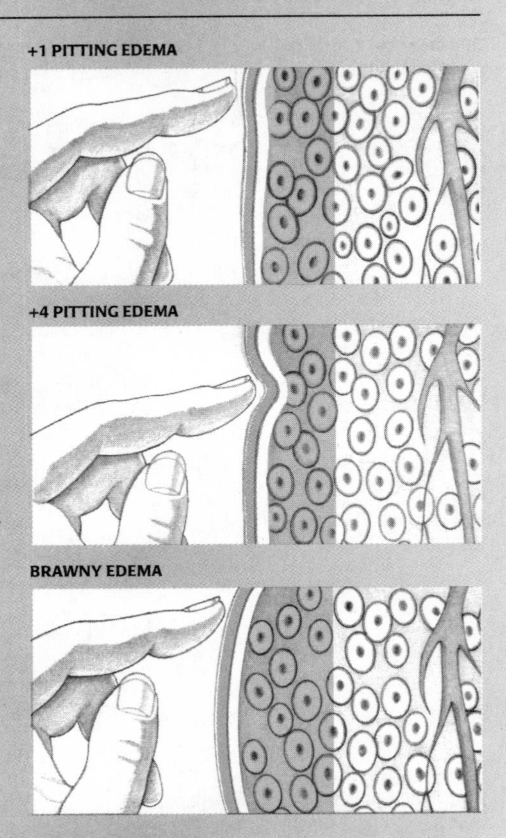

◆ Investigate the character of any headaches (frequency, intensity, location, and duration).

◆ Determine whether your patient has vertigo or syncope.

◆ Ask if he has a history of seizures or use of anticonvulsants.

◆ Explore cognitive disturbances, including recent or remote memory loss, hallucinations, disorientation, speech and language dysfunction, or inability to concentrate. (See *Comparing delirium, dementia, and depression.*)

◆ Ask if the patient has a history of sensory disturbances, including tingling, numbness, and sensory loss.

◆ Explore motor problems, including problems with gait, balance, coordination, tremor, spasm, or paralysis.

◆ Ask the patient if cognitive, sensory, or motor symptoms have interfered with his activities of daily living.

Comparing delirium, dementia, and depression

This table highlights the distinguishing characteristics of delirium, dementia, and depression.

CLINICAL FEATURE	DELIRIUM	DEMENTIA	DEPRESSION
Onset	Acute, sudden	Gradual	Sudden or brief
Course	Short, with diurnal fluctuations in symptoms; symptoms worse at night, in darkness, and on awakening	Lifelong; symptoms progressive and irreversible	Diurnal effects, with symptoms typically worse in the morning; situational fluctuations, but less than with acute confusion
Progression	Abrupt	Slow but uneven	Variable, rapid, or slow, but even
Duration	Hours to less than 1 month; seldom longer	Months to years	At least 2 weeks, but can be several months to years (*Note: Diagnostic and Statistical Manual of Mental Disorders,* Fourth Edition, Text Revision, specifies duration of at least 2 weeks for diagnosis.)
Awareness	Reduced	Clear	Clear
Alertness	Fluctuates; lethargic or hypervigilant	Generally normal	Normal
Attention	Decreased	Generally normal	May decrease temporarily
Orientation	Generally impaired, but reversible	May be impaired as disease progresses	May be disoriented
Memory	Recent and immediate memory impaired	Recent and remote memory impaired	Selective or patchy impairment
Thinking	Disorganized, distorted, and fragmented; incoherent speech, either slow or accelerated	Difficulty with abstraction; impoverished thoughts and impaired judgment; words difficult to find	Intact, with themes of hopelessness, helplessness, or self-deprecation

(continued)

Comparing delirium, dementia, and depression *(continued)*

CLINICAL FEATURE	DELIRIUM	DEMENTIA	DEPRESSION
Perception	Distorted, with illusions, delusions, and hallucinations; difficulty distinguishing between reality and misperceptions	Misperceptions usually absent	Intact, without delusions or hallucinations, except in severe cases
Speech	Incoherent	Dysphasia as disease progresses; aphasia	Normal, slow, or rapid
Psychomotor behavior	Variable; hypokinetic, hyperkinetic, and mixed	Normal; may have apraxia	Variable, with psychomotor retardation or agitation
Sleep and wake cycle	Altered	Fragmented	Insomnia or somnolence
Affect	Variable affective anxiety, restlessness, and irritability; reversible	Superficial, inappropriate, and labile; attempts to conceal deficits in intellect; may show personality changes, aphasia, and agnosia; lacks insight	Depressed, dysphoric mood, with exaggerated and detailed symptoms; preoccupied with personal thoughts; insight present; verbal elaboration
Findings on mental status testing	Distracted from task; numerous errors	Failings highlighted by family; struggles with test, with frequent "near miss" answers; exerts great effort to find an appropriate reply; commonly requests feedback on performance	Failings highlighted by patient; commonly responds, "don't know"; exerts little effort; commonly gives up; appears indifferent toward examination and doesn't care or attempt to find answer

Checking neurologic vital signs

◆ A supplement to routine measurement of temperature, pulse, and respirations, neurologic vital signs are used to evaluate the patient's level of consciousness (LOC), pupillary activity, and level of orientation to time, place, and person.

◆ LOC reflects brain stem function and usually provides the first sign of

Checking mental status

To screen patients for disordered thought processes, ask these questions. An incorrect answer to any question may indicate the need for a complete mental status examination.

QUESTION	FUNCTION SCREENED
What's your name?	Orientation to person
What's your mother's name?	Orientation to other people
What year is it?	Orientation to time
Where are you now?	Orientation to place
How old are you?	Memory
Where were you born?	Remote memory
What did you have for breakfast?	Recent memory
Who is the U.S. president?	General knowledge
Can you count backward from 20 to 1?	Attention span and calculation skills

central nervous system deterioration. (See *Checking mental status*.)

◆ Level of orientation evaluates higher cerebral functions. (See *The cerebrum and its functions,* page 94.)

◆ Changes in LOC, pupillary activity, motor response, and vital signs may signal increased intracranial pressure (ICP). (See *Detecting increased intracranial pressure,* page 95.)

◆ Evaluating muscle strength and tone, reflexes, and posture may also help to identify nervous system damage.

◆ Finally, evaluating the respiratory rate and pattern can help to locate brain lesions and determine their size.

Equipment

Penlight ◆ thermometer ◆ stethoscope ◆ sphygmomanometer ◆ pupil size chart

Implementation tips

◆ Explain the procedure to the patient, even if he's unresponsive.

◆ Check the patient's LOC.

◆ Ask the patient to state his full name. If he responds appropriately, determine his orientation to time, place, and person. Determine the quality of his replies.

◆ Check the patient's ability to understand and follow one-step commands that require a motor response. For example, ask him to open and close his eyes. Note whether he can maintain his LOC.

◆ If the patient doesn't respond to commands, squeeze the nail beds on his fingers and toes with moderate pressure and note his response. Alternately, rub the upper portion of his sternum between the second and third intercostal spaces with your knuckles.

The cerebrum and its functions

The cerebrum is divided into four lobes, based on anatomic landmarks and functional differences. The lobes – parietal, occipital, temporal, and frontal – are named for the cranial bones that lie over them.

This illustration shows the locations of the cerebral lobes and explains their functions. It also shows the location of the cerebellum.

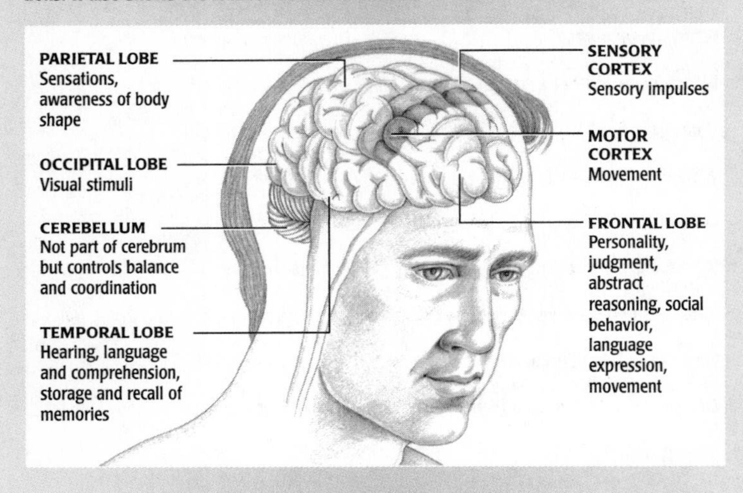

◆ Check the motor responses bilaterally to rule out monoplegia and hemiplegia.

Examine pupils and eye movement

◆ Ask the patient to open his eyes. If he's unresponsive, lift his upper eyelids. Inspect the pupils for size and shape, and compare them for equality. To evaluate them more precisely, use a chart showing the various pupil sizes. (See *Checking the pupils,* page 96.)

◆ Test the patient's direct light response. First, darken the room. Hold each eyelid open in turn, keeping the other eye covered. Swing the penlight from the patient's ear toward the midline of the face. Shine the light directly into the eye. Normally, the pupil constricts immediately when exposed to light and then dilates immediately when the light is removed. Wait 20 seconds before testing the other pupil to allow it to recover from reflex stimulation.

◆ Test consensual light response. Hold both eyelids open, but shine the light into one eye. Watch for constriction in the other pupil, which indicates proper nerve function.

◆ Brighten the room, and ask the conscious patient to open his eyes. Check the eyelids for ptosis or drooping. Then check the extraocular movements. Hold up one finger and ask the patient to follow it with his eyes as you move your finger up, down, laterally, and obliquely. See if the patient's eyes track together to follow your finger (conjugate gaze). Watch for involuntary jerking or oscillating movements (nystagmus).

Detecting increased intracranial pressure

The earlier you recognize the signs of increased intracranial pressure (ICP), the more quickly you can intervene and improve the patient's chance of recovery. By the time late signs appear, interventions may be useless.

CLINICAL FEATURE	EARLY SIGNS	LATE SIGNS
Level of consciousness	◆ Requires increased stimulation ◆ Subtle orientation loss ◆ Restlessness and anxiety ◆ Sudden quietness	◆ Unarousable
Pupils	◆ Pupil changes on side of lesion ◆ One pupil constricts but then dilates (unilateral hippus) ◆ Sluggish reaction of both pupils ◆ Unequal pupils	◆ Pupils fixed and dilated or "blown"
Motor response	◆ Sudden weakness ◆ Motor changes on side opposite the lesion ◆ Positive pronator drift; with palms up, one hand pronates	◆ Profound weakness
Vital signs	◆ Intermittent increases in blood pressure	◆ Increased systolic pressure, profound bradycardia, abnormal respirations (Cushing's syndrome)

◆ Check accommodation. Hold up one finger midline to the patient's face and several feet away. Ask the patient to focus on your finger as you move it toward his nose. His eyes should converge, and his pupils should constrict equally.

◆ If the patient is unconscious, test the oculocephalic (doll's eye) reflex. Hold the patient's eyelids open. Quickly but gently turn the patient's head to one side and then to the other. If the patient's eyes move in the opposite direction from the side to which you turn the head, the reflex is intact.

Alert Never test this reflex if you know or suspect that the patient has a cervical spine injury.

Evaluate motor function

◆ If the patient is conscious, test his grip strength in both hands at the same time. Extend your hands; ask the patient to squeeze your fingers as hard as he can, and compare the strength of each hand. Grip strength is usually slightly stronger in the dominant hand.

◆ Test arm strength by having the patient close his eyes and hold his arms straight out in front of him, palms up. See if either arm drifts downward or pronates, which indicates weakness.

◆ Test leg strength by having the patient raise his legs, one at a time, against gentle downward pressure from your hand.

Checking the pupils

Pupillary changes can signal different conditions. Use these illustrations and lists of causes to help you detect problems.

Bilaterally equal and reactive

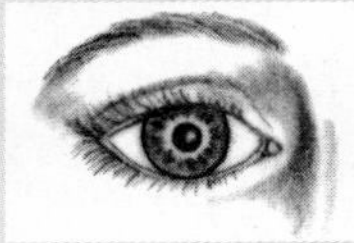
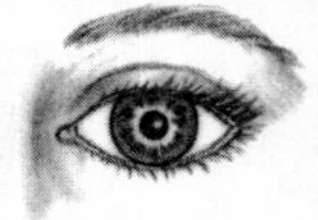

- Normal

Unilateral, dilated (4 mm), fixed, and nonreactive

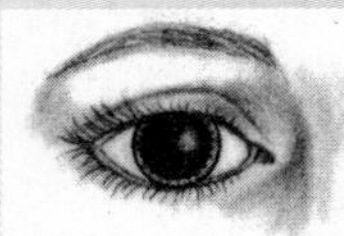
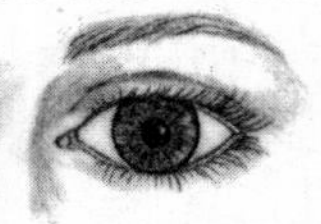

- Uncal herniation with oculomotor nerve damage
- Brain stem compression by an expanding lesion or an aneurysm
- Increased intracranial pressure
- Tentorial herniation
- Head trauma with subsequent subdural or epidural hematoma
- Normal in some people

Bilateral, dilated (4 mm), fixed, and nonreactive

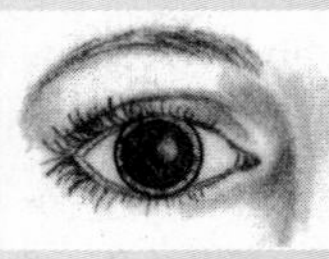
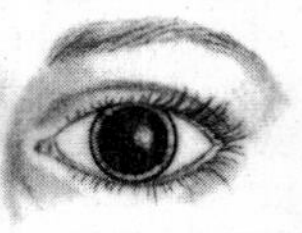

- Severe midbrain damage
- Cardiopulmonary arrest (hypoxia)
- Anticholinergic poisoning
- Deep anesthesia
- Dilating drops

Bilateral, midsized (2 mm), fixed, and nonreactive

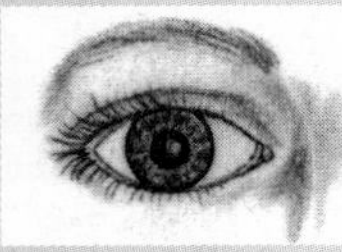
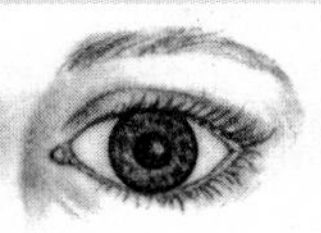

- Midbrain involvement caused by edema, hemorrhage, infarction, laceration, or contusion

Unilateral, small (1.5 mm), and nonreactive

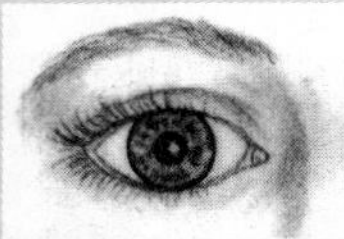
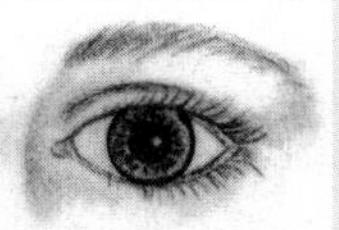

- Disruption of the sympathetic nerve supply to the head caused by a spinal cord lesion above T1

Bilateral, pinpoint (less than 1 mm), and usually nonreactive

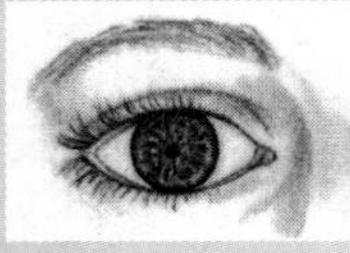
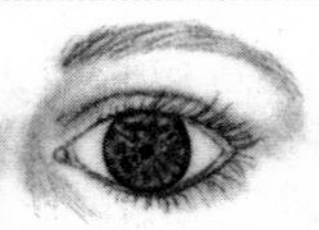

- Lesion of the pons, usually after hemorrhage, leading to blocked sympathetic impulses
- Opiates such as morphine (Pupils may be reactive.)
- Iritis
- Pilocarpine drugs

- If the patient is unconscious, exert pressure on each fingernail bed. If the patient withdraws, compare the strength of each limb.

Alert If decorticate or decerebrate posturing develops in response to painful stimuli, notify the physician immediately. (See *Compar-*

Comparing decerebrate and decorticate postures

Decerebrate posture results from damage to the upper brain stem. In this posture, the arms are adducted and extended, with the wrists pronated and the fingers flexed. The teeth are clenched. The legs are stiffly extended, with plantar flexion of the feet.

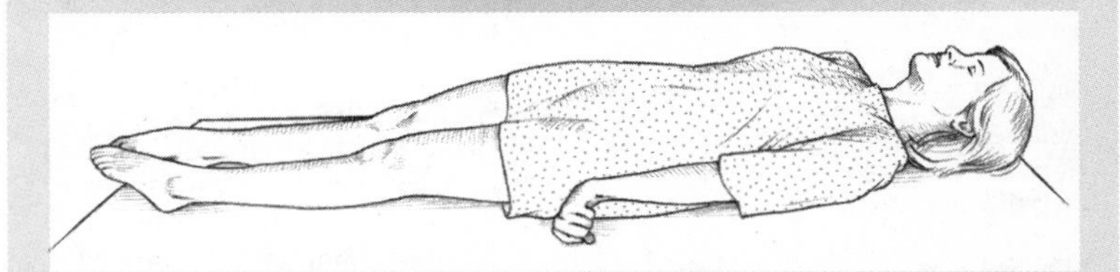

Decorticate posture results from damage to one or both corticospinal tracts. In this posture, the arms are adducted and flexed, with the wrists and fingers flexed on the chest. The legs are stiffly extended and rotated internally, with plantar flexion of the feet.

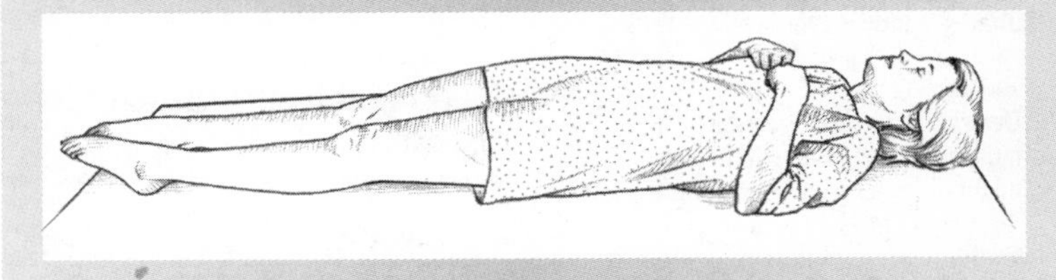

ing decerebrate and decorticate postures.)

◆ Flex and extend the extremities on both sides to evaluate muscle tone.
◆ Test the plantar reflex in all patients. Stroke the lateral aspect of the sole of the patient's foot with your thumbnail. Normally, this elicits flexion of all toes. Watch for a positive Babinski's sign — dorsiflexion of the great toe with fanning of the other toes — that indicates an upper motor neuron lesion.

Complete the neurologic examination
◆ Take the patient's temperature, pulse rate, respiration rate, and blood pressure. Especially check pulse pressure — the difference between systolic and diastolic pressure — because widening pulse pressure can indicate increasing ICP.

Special considerations

Alert If a patient's status was previously stable and he has a sudden change in neurologic or routine vital signs, check his condition further and notify the physician immediately.

Using the Glasgow Coma Scale

◆ The Glasgow Coma Scale provides an objective way to evaluate a patient's LOC and to detect changes from the baseline.
◆ To use this scale, evaluate and score your patient's best eye-opening response, verbal response, and motor response.

The 5 P's of musculoskeletal injury

To swiftly check for musculoskeletal injury, remember the 5 P's: pain, paresthesia, paralysis, pallor, and pulse.

Pain
Ask the patient whether he feels pain. If he does, examine the location, severity, and quality of the pain.

Paresthesia
Check the patient for loss of sensation by touching the injured area with the tip of an open safety pin. Abnormal sensation or loss of sensation indicates neurovascular involvement.

Paralysis
Determine whether the patient can move the affected area. If he can't, he might have nerve or tendon damage.

Pallor
Paleness, discoloration, and coolness on the injured side may indicate neurovascular compromise.

Pulse
Check all pulses distal to the injury site. If a pulse is decreased or absent, blood supply to the area is reduced.

◆ A total score of 15 indicates that the patient is alert; oriented to time, place, and person; and can follow simple commands. A comatose patient will score 7 points or less. A score of 3 indicates a deep coma and a poor prognosis.

Eye-opening response
◆ Open spontaneously (Score: 4)
◆ Open to verbal command (Score: 3)
◆ Open to pain (Score: 2)
◆ No response (Score: 1)

Verbal response
◆ Oriented and converses (Score: 5)
◆ Disoriented and converses (Score: 4)
◆ Uses inappropriate words (Score: 3)
◆ Makes incomprehensible sounds (Score: 2)
◆ No response (Score: 1)

Motor response
◆ Obeys verbal command (Score: 6)
◆ Localizes painful stimulus (Score: 5)
◆ Flexion, withdrawal (Score: 4)
◆ Flexion, abnormal — decorticate rigidity (Score: 3)
◆ Extension — decerebrate rigidity (Score: 2)
◆ No response (Score: 1)

Checking the musculoskeletal system

Initial questions

◆ Ask if the patient has muscle pain, joint pain, swelling, tenderness, or trouble with balance or gait. Does he have joint stiffness? If so, find out when it occurs and how long it lasts. (See *The 5 P's of musculoskeletal injury*.)
◆ Ask whether the patient has noticed noise with joint movement.
◆ Find out if he has arthritis or gout.
◆ Ask about a history of fractures, injuries, back problems, or deformities. Also ask about weakness and paralysis.
◆ Explore limitations on walking, running, or participation in sports. Do muscle or joint problems interfere with activities of daily living?

Age alert If the patient is an infant or a toddler, ask the parents if the patient has achieved developmental milestones — such as sitting up, crawling, and walking.

Determining range of motion

- Observe the patient's posture, gait, and stance.
- Check the patient's joint range of motion (ROM) to test joint function. To determine joint ROM, ask the patient to move specific joints through the normal ROM. If he can't make the movements, move the joints through passive ROM.
- The following pages show each joint and illustrate the tests for ROM, including the expected degree of motion for each joint.

Shoulders

- To determine forward flexion and backward extension, have the patient bring his straightened arm forward and up and then behind him (as shown below).

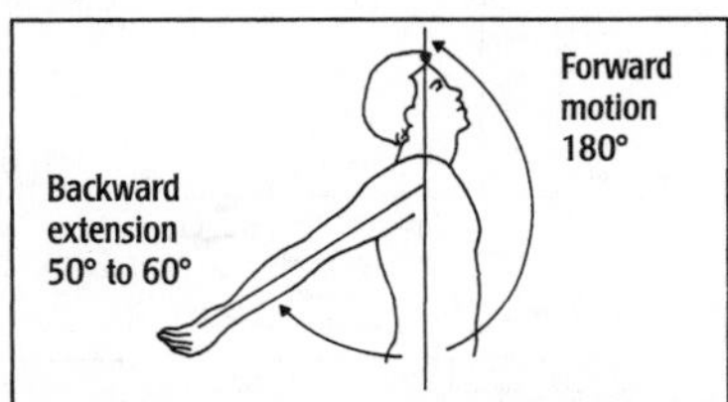

- Check abduction and adduction by asking the patient to bring his straightened arm to the side and up and then in front of him (as shown below).

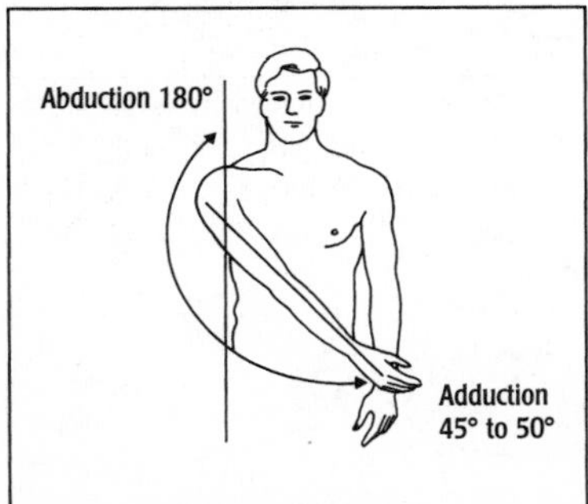

- To determine external and internal rotation, have the patient abduct his arm with his elbow bent. Then ask him to place his hand first behind his head and then behind the small of his back (as shown below).

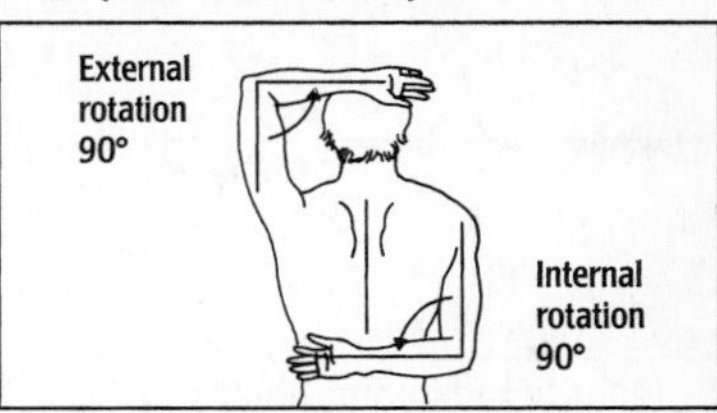

Elbows

- Check flexion by having the patient bend his arm and attempt to touch his shoulder. Check extension by having him straighten his arm (as shown below).

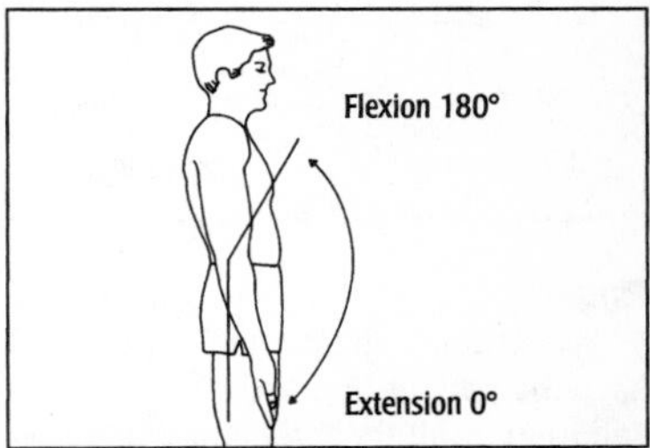

- To determine pronation and supination, hold the patient's elbow in a flexed position, and ask him to rotate his arm until his palm faces the floor. Then rotate his hand back until his palm faces upward (as shown below).

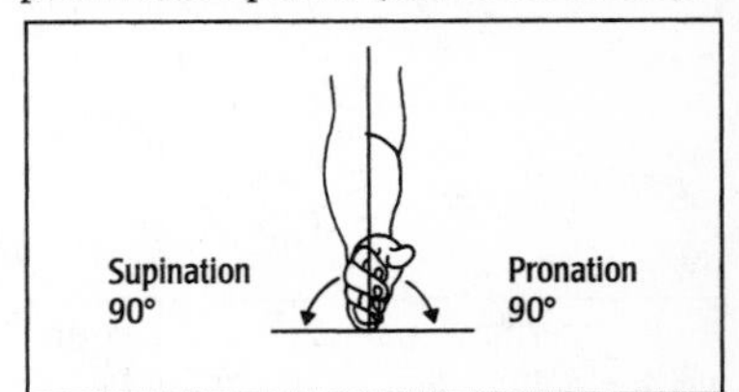

Wrists

- To determine flexion, ask the patient to bend his wrist downward; check extension by having him straighten his wrist. To check for hyperextension, ask him to bend his wrist upward (as shown below).

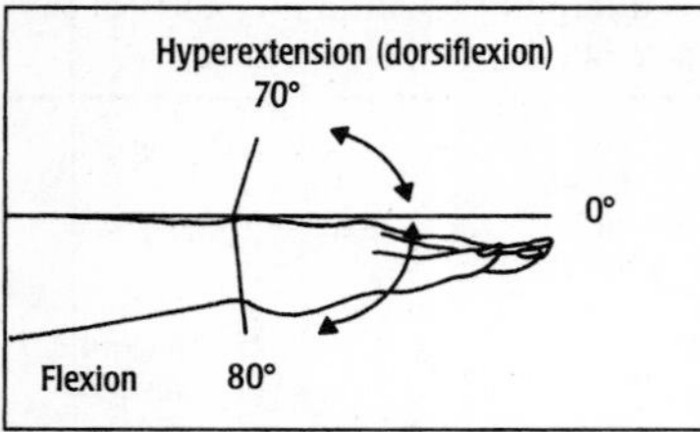

◆ Identify radial and ulnar deviation by asking the patient to move his hand first toward the radial side and then toward the ulnar side (as shown below).

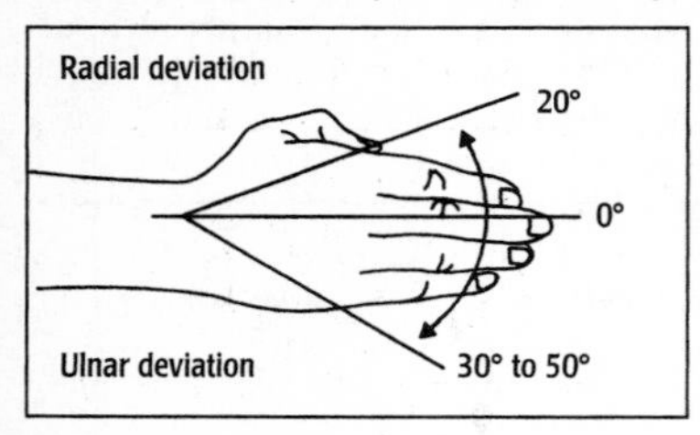

Fingers

◆ To check abduction and adduction, have the patient first spread his fingers and then bring them together. In abduction, there should be 20 degrees between the fingers (as shown below); in adduction, the fingers should touch .

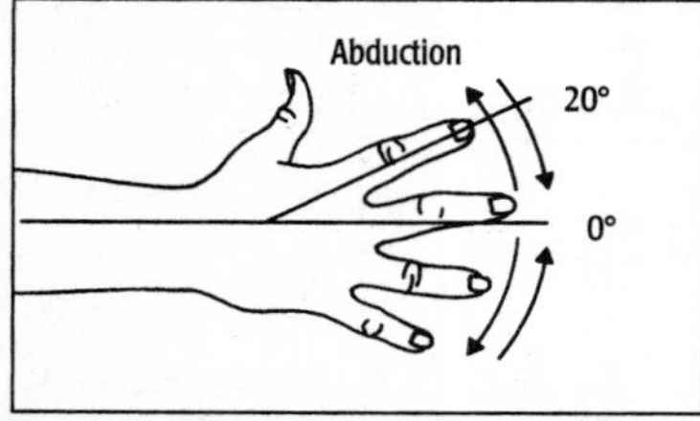

◆ To determine extension and flexion, ask the patient first to straighten his fingers and then to make a fist with his thumb remaining straight (as shown at top of next column).

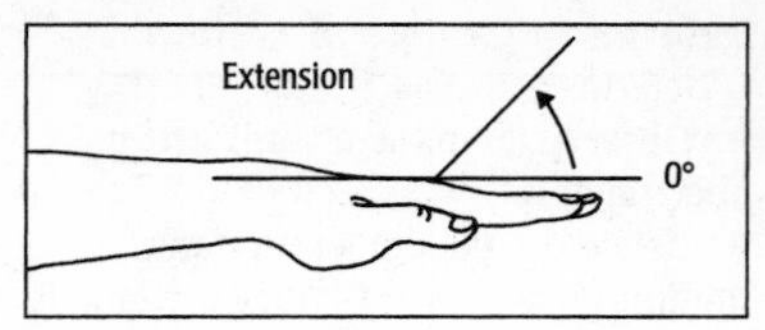

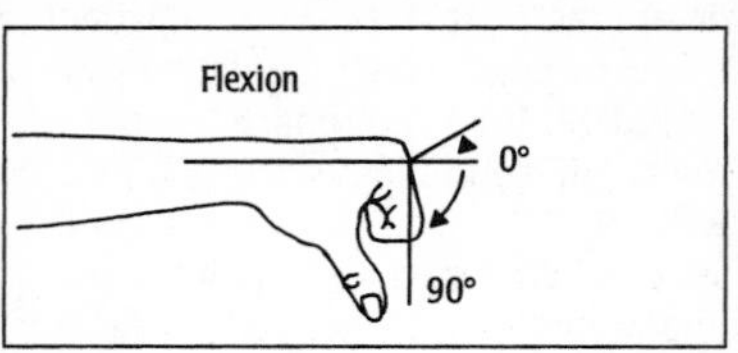

Thumbs

◆ Check extension by having the patient straighten his thumb. To determine flexion, have him bend his thumb at the top joint and then at the bottom (as shown below).

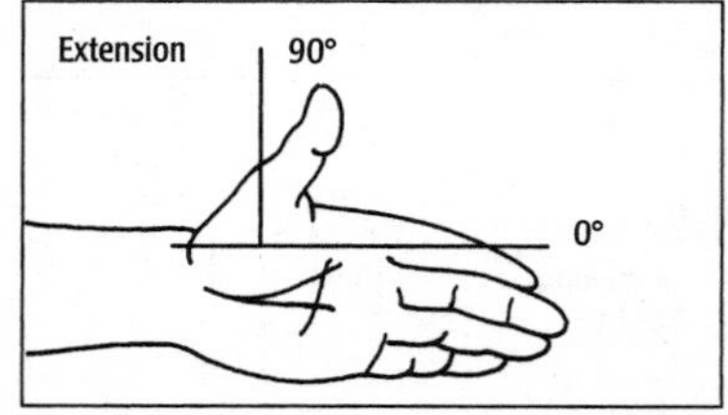

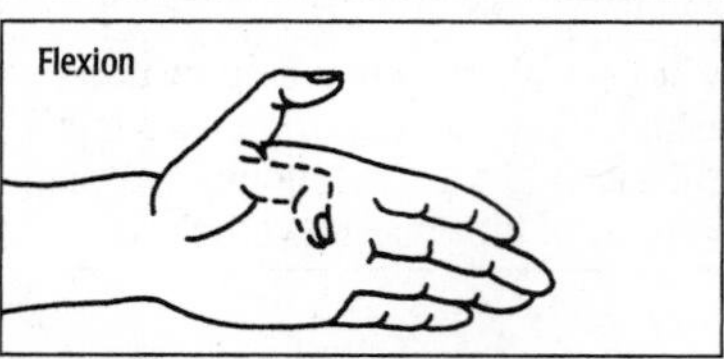

◆ Determine adduction by having the patient extend his hand, bringing his thumb first to the index finger and then to the little finger (as shown below).

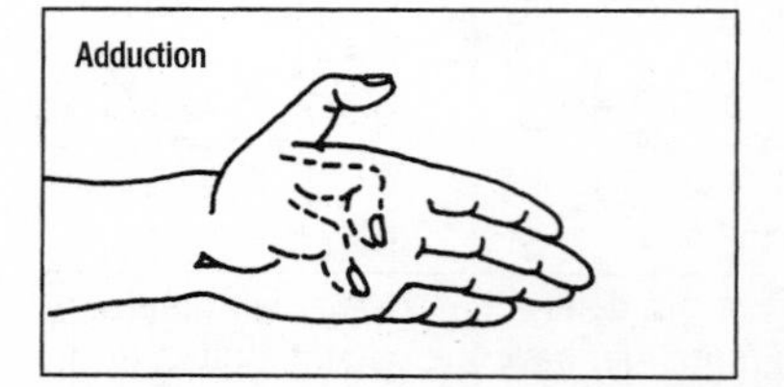

Hips

◆ Determine flexion by asking the patient to bend his knee to his chest while keeping his back straight. If he has undergone total hip replacement, don't perform this movement without the surgeon's permission; motion can dislocate the prosthesis (as shown below).

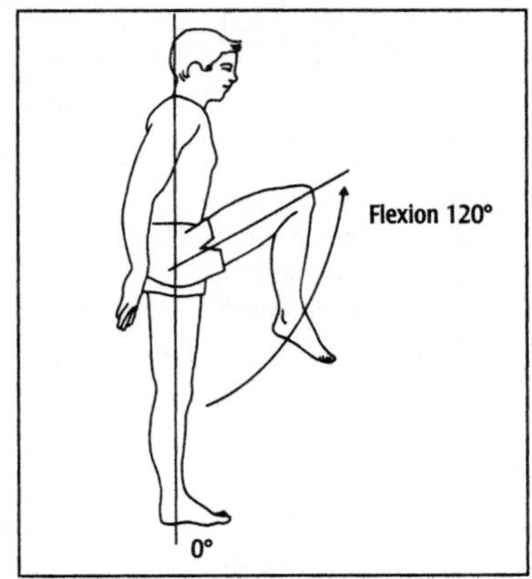

◆ Check extension by having the patient straighten his knee. To determine hyperextension, ask him to extend his leg straight back. This motion can be performed with the patient in the prone or standing position (as shown below).

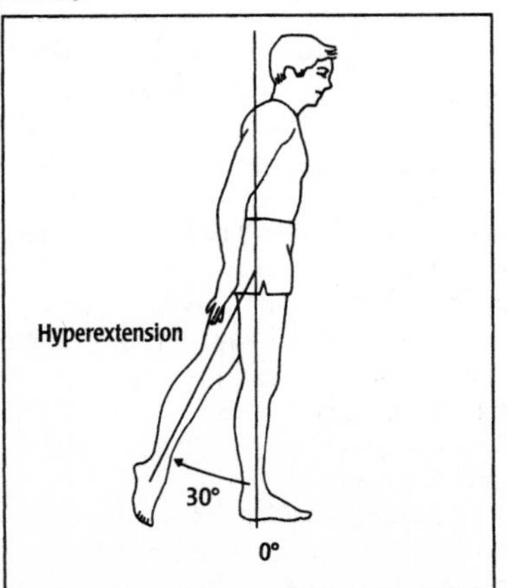

◆ To check abduction, have the patient move his straightened leg away from the midline.

◆ To determine adduction, instruct the patient to move his straightened leg from the midline toward the opposite leg (as shown below).

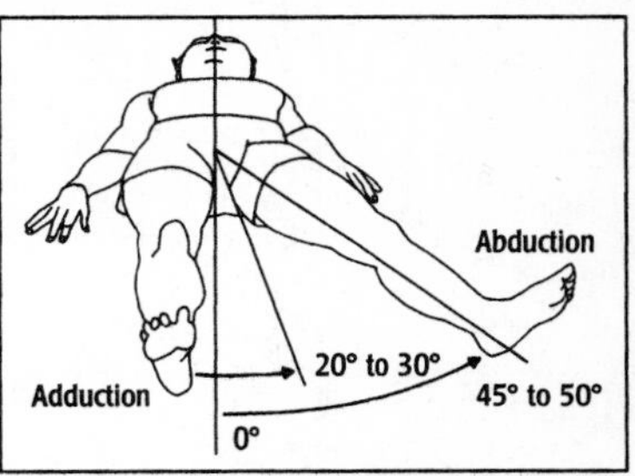

◆ To determine internal and external rotation, ask the patient to bend his knee and turn his leg inward. Then have him turn his leg outward (as shown below).

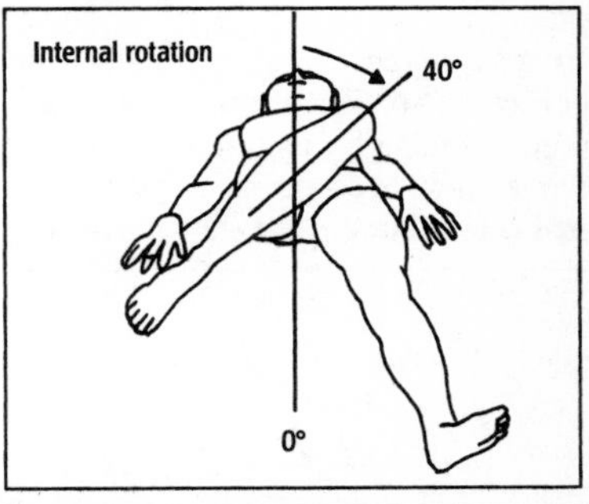

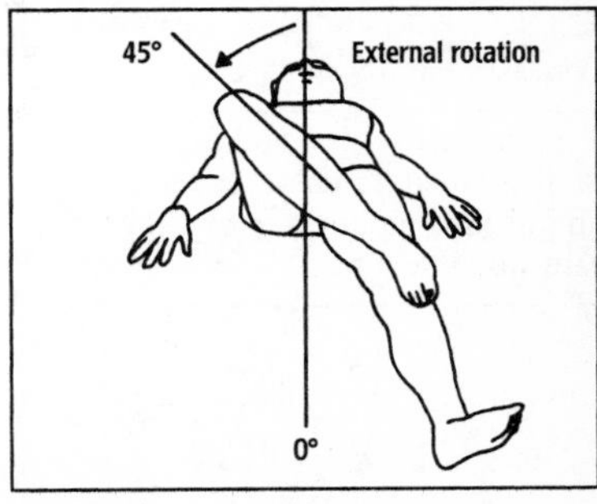

Knees

◆ Ask the patient to straighten his leg at the knee to show extension; ask him to bend his knee and bring his foot up to touch his buttock to show flexion (as shown below).

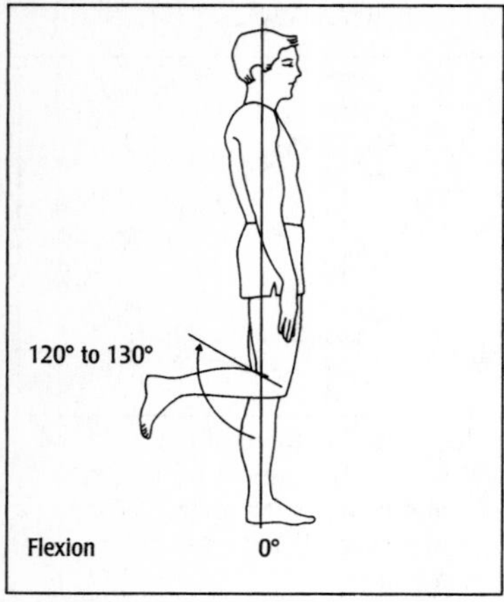

Ankles and feet

◆ Have the patient show plantar flexion by bending his foot downward. Ask him to show hyperextension by bending his foot upward (as shown below).

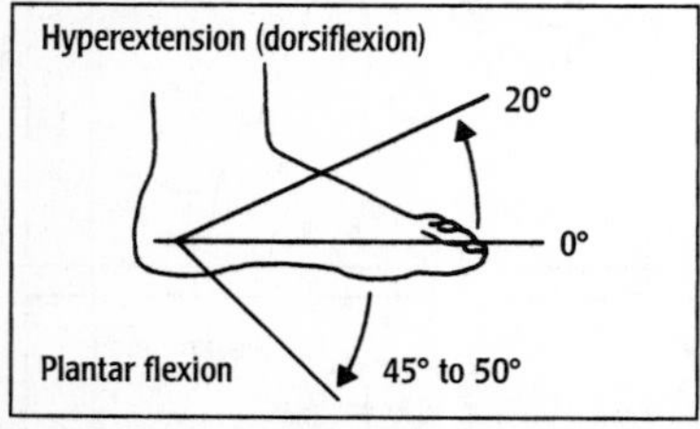

◆ To check eversion and inversion, ask the patient to point his toes. Have him turn his foot inward and then outward (as shown below).

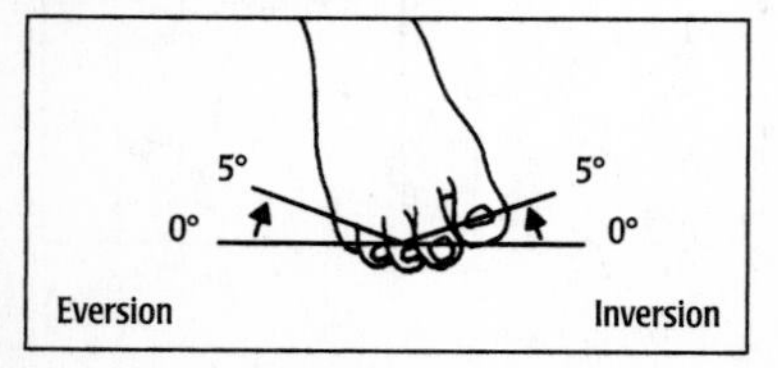

◆ To determine forefoot adduction and abduction, stabilize the patient's heel while he turns his foot first inward and then outward (as shown below).

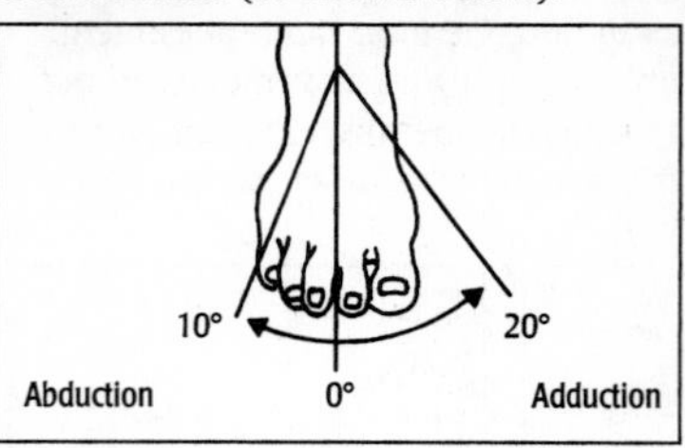

Toes

◆ Check extension and flexion by asking the patient to straighten and then curl his toes. Then check hyperextension by asking him to straighten his toes and point them upward (as shown below).

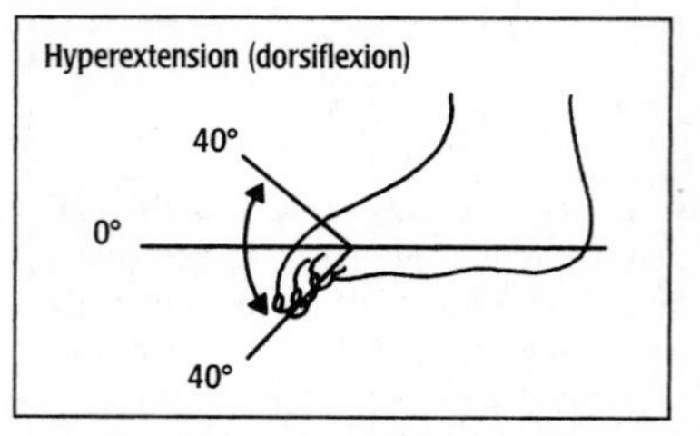

Testing muscle strength

◆ Determine motor function by testing the patient's strength in the affected limb.

◆ Before you begin the muscle strength tests, find out whether the patient is right- or left-handed. The dominant arm is usually stronger.

◆ Have him attempt normal ROM movements against your resistance. Note the strength that the patient exerts. If the muscle group is weak, lessen your resistance to permit accurate observation.

◆ If needed, position the patient so that his limb doesn't have to resist gravity, and repeat the test.

◆ To minimize subjective interpretations of the test findings, rate muscle strength on a scale of 0 to 5, as follows:

0 = No visible or palpable contraction felt; paralysis
1 = Slight palpable contraction felt
2 = Passive ROM maneuvers when gravity is removed
3 = Active ROM against gravity
4 = Active ROM against gravity and light resistance
5 = Active ROM against full resistance; normal strength

Deltoid

◆ With your patient's arm fully extended, place one hand over his deltoid muscle and the other hand on his wrist. Have him abduct his arm to a horizontal position against your resistance; as he does, palpate for deltoid contraction (as shown below).

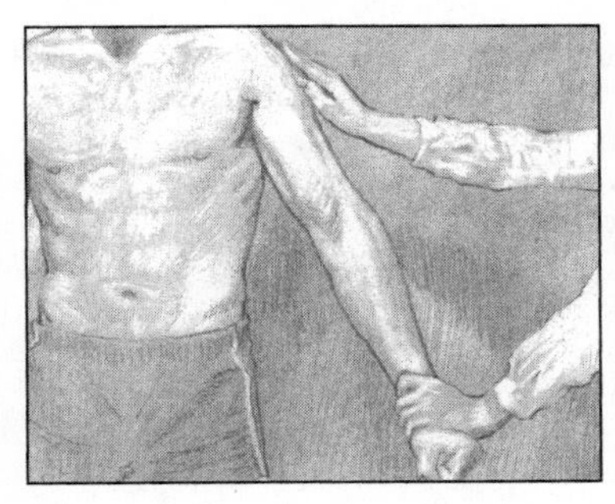

Biceps

◆ With your hand on the patient's fist, have him flex his forearm against your resistance; observe for biceps contraction (as shown below).

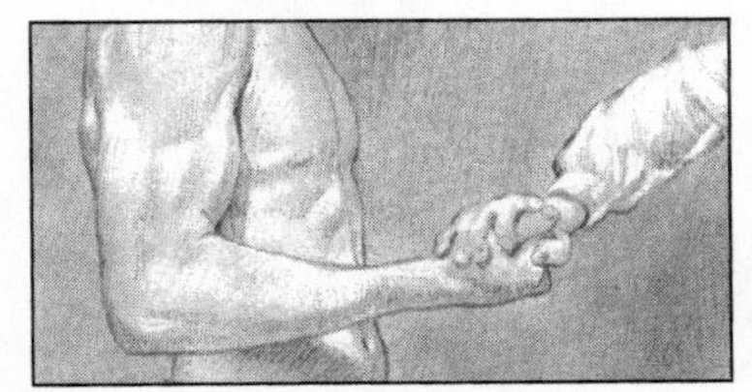

Triceps

◆ Have the patient abduct and hold his arm midway between flexion and extension. Hold and support his arm at the wrist, and ask him to extend it against your resistance. Observe for triceps contraction (as shown below).

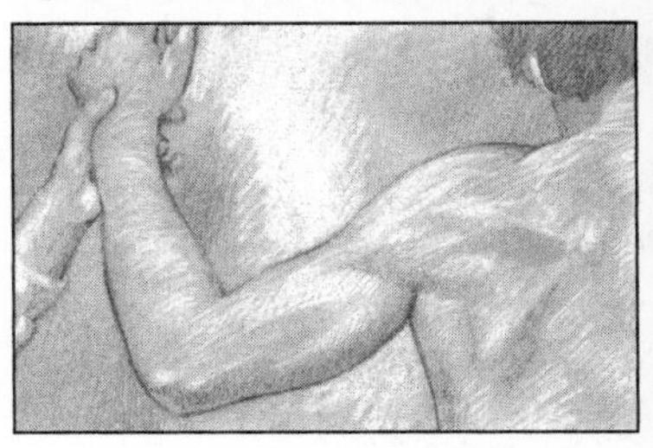

Dorsal interosseous

◆ Have him extend and spread his fingers and resist your attempt to squeeze them together (as shown below).

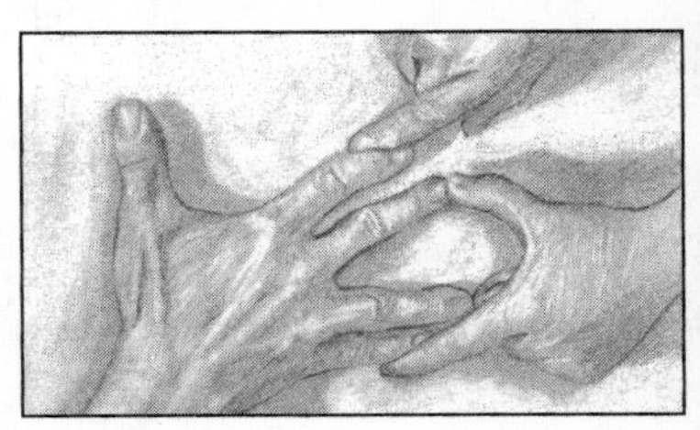

Forearm and hand (grip)

◆ Have the patient grasp your middle and index fingers and squeeze them as hard as he can (as shown below).

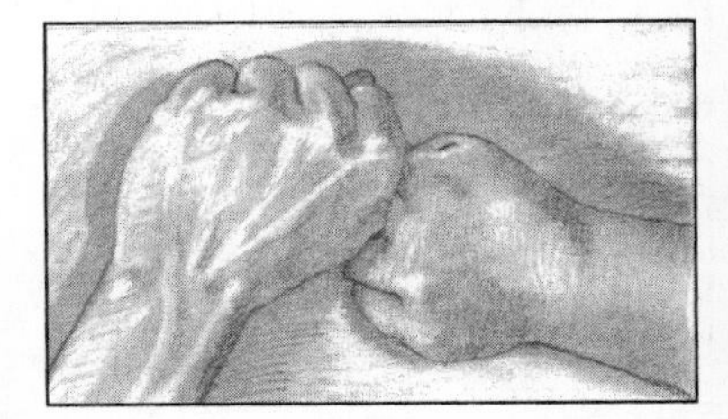

Psoas

◆ Support the patient's leg and have him raise his knee and flex his hip against your resistance (as shown below). Observe for psoas contraction.

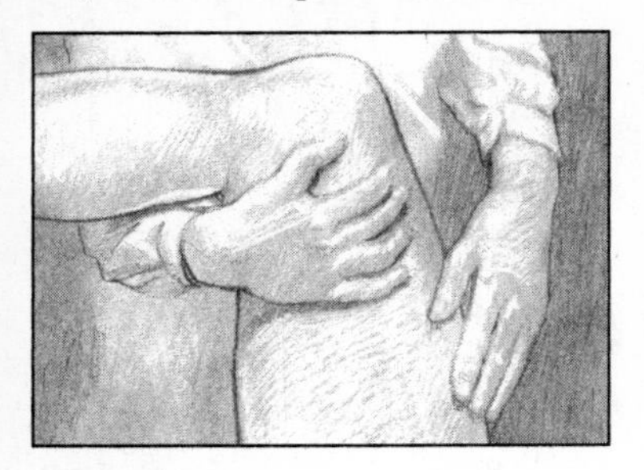

Quadriceps

◆ Have the patient bend his knee slightly while you support his lower leg. Then ask him to extend his knee against your resistance; as he's doing so, palpate for quadriceps contraction (as shown below).

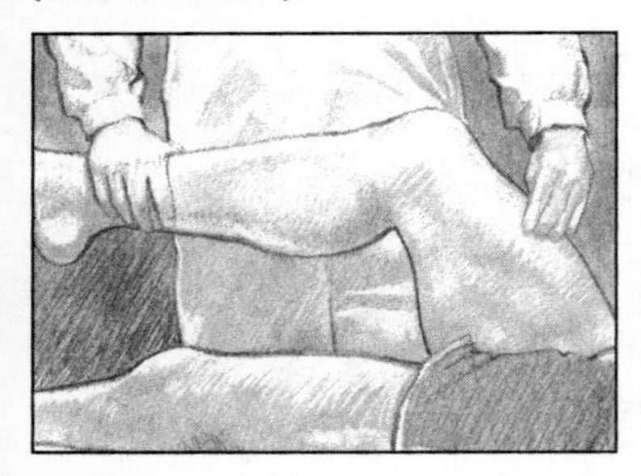

Gastrocnemius

◆ With the patient in the prone position, support his foot and ask him to plantarflex his ankle against your resistance. Palpate for gastrocnemius contraction (as shown below).

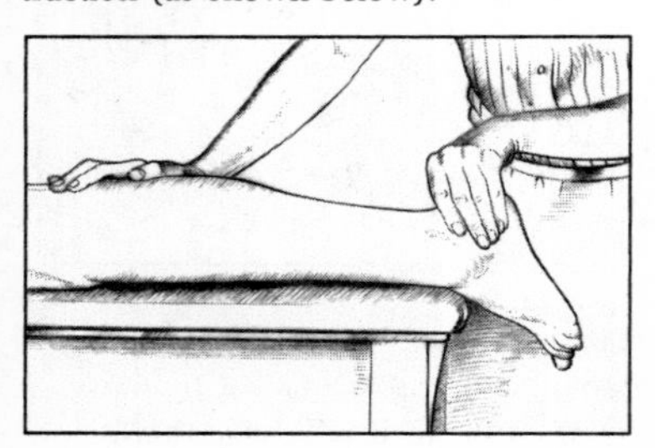

Anterior tibialis

◆ With the patient sitting on the side of the examination table with his legs dangling, place your hand on his foot and ask him to dorsiflex his ankle against your resistance (as shown below).

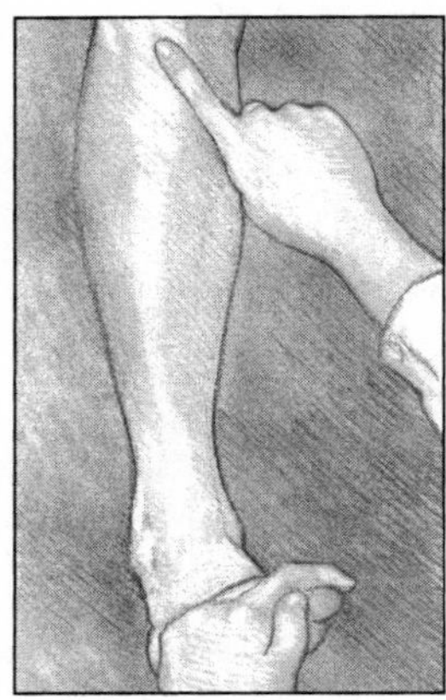

Extensor hallucis longus

◆ With your fingers on his great toe, have him dorsiflex the toe against your resistance. Palpate for extensor hallucis contraction (as shown below).

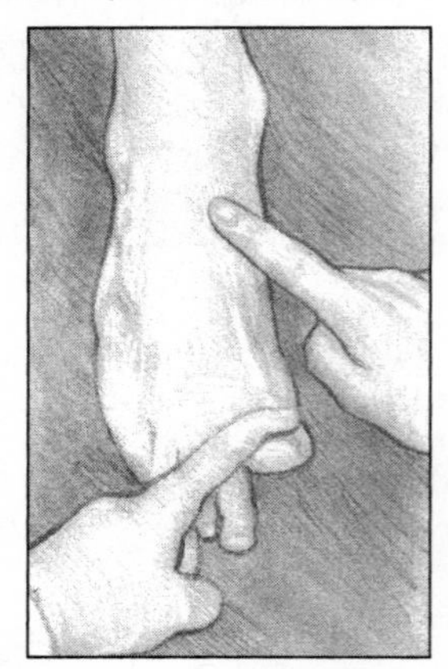

Anatomic structures of the gastrointestinal system

This illustration shows the gastrointestinal system's major anatomic structures. Knowing these structures will help you conduct an accurate physical examination.

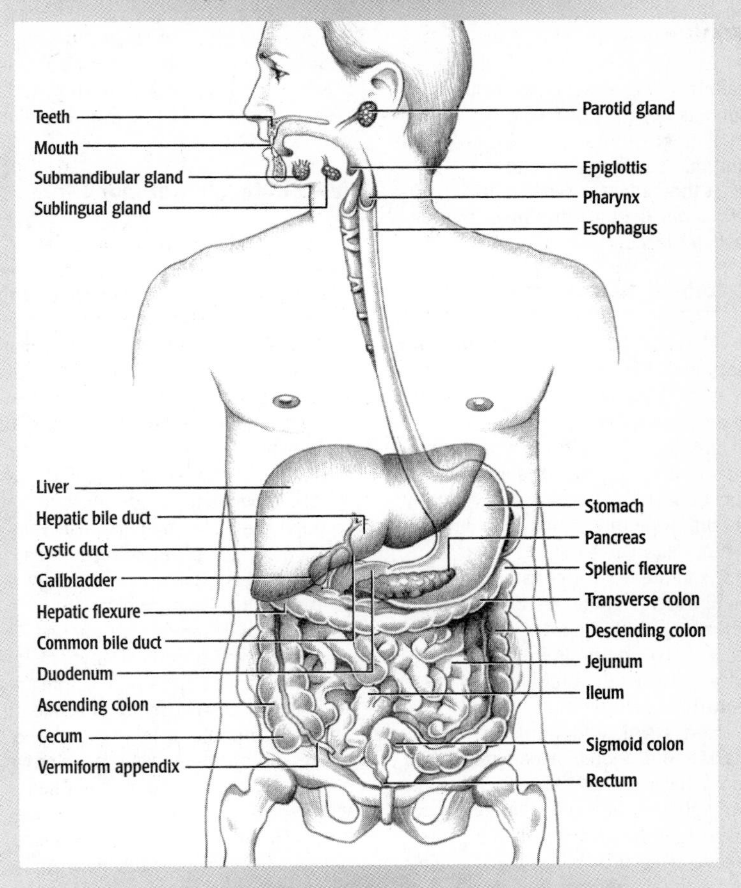

Checking the gastrointestinal system

Initial questions

◆ Explore signs and symptoms, such as appetite and weight changes, dysphagia, nausea, vomiting, heartburn, stomach or abdominal pain, frequent belching or flatulence, hematemesis, and jaundice. (See *Anatomic structures of the gastrointestinal system.*)

◆ Determine how often the patient uses laxatives. Ask about hemorrhoids, rectal bleeding, the character of stools (color, odor, and consistency), and changes in bowel habits. Does the patient have a history of diarrhea, constipation, irritable bowel syndrome, Crohn's disease, colitis, diverticulitis, or cancer?

◆ Has the patient had ulcers?

◆ Ask if the patient has had hernias, gallbladder disease, or liver disease, such as hepatitis or cirrhosis.

◆ Find out if the patient has had abdominal swelling or ascites.

◆ If the patient is older than age 50, ask about the date and results of his last Hemoccult test.

Examining the abdomen

◆ Place the patient in the supine position, with his arms at his sides and his head on a pillow to help relax the abdominal muscles.

◆ Mentally divide the abdomen into quadrants or regions. Systematically inspect all areas, if time and the patient's condition permit, concluding with the symptomatic area.

◆ Examine the patient's entire abdomen, observing the overall contour, color, and skin integrity. Look for rashes, scars, or incisions from past surgeries. Observe the umbilicus for protrusions or discoloration.

◆ Note visible abdominal asymmetry, masses, pulsations, or peristalsis. You can detect masses — especially hepatic and splenic masses — more easily by inspecting the areas while the patient takes a deep breath and holds it. This forces the diaphragm downward, increasing intra-abdominal pressure and reducing the size of the abdominal cavity.

◆ Finally, examine the anal area for redness, irritation, or hemorrhoids.

Alert If the patient is pregnant, vary the position used for examination depending on the stage of pregnancy. For example, if the patient is in her final weeks, avoid the supine position because it may impair respiratory excursion and blood flow. To enhance comfort, have the patient lie on her side or in semi-Fowler's position. Also, during the examination, remember the normal variations of pregnancy: increased pigmentation of the abdominal midline, purplish striae, and upward displacement of the abdominal organs and umbilicus.

Auscultating bowel sounds

◆ Auscultate the abdomen to detect sounds that provide information about bowel motility and the condition of the abdominal vessels and organs.

◆ Bowel sounds result from the movement of air and fluid through the bowel. To auscultate them, press the diaphragm of the stethoscope against the abdomen and listen carefully. Auscultate the four quadrants systematically.

◆ The movement of air and fluid through the bowel by peristalsis normally creates soft, bubbling sounds with no regular pattern, commonly with soft clicks and gurgles interspersed. Loud, rapid, high-pitched, gurgling bowel sounds are hyperactive and may occur normally in a hungry patient. Sounds occurring at a rate of one every minute or longer are hypoactive and normally occur after bowel surgery or after the colon has filled with feces.

◆ When describing bowel sounds, be specific — for example, indicate whether they're quiet or loud gurgles, occasional gurgles, fine tinkles, or loud tinkles.

◆ In a routine complete examination, auscultate for a full 5 minutes before determining that bowel sounds are absent. However, if you're pressed for time, perform a rapid check. If you can't hear bowel sounds within 2 minutes, suspect a serious problem. Even if subsequent palpation stimulates peristalsis, still report a long silence in that quadrant.

◆ Before you report absent bowel sounds, however, make sure that the patient's bladder is empty. A full bladder may obscure the sounds. Gently pressing on the abdominal surface may initiate peristalsis and audible bowel sounds, as will having the patient eat or drink something.

Palpating the abdomen

◆ Abdominal palpation provides useful clues about the character of the abdominal wall; the size, condition, and consistency of the abdominal organs; the presence and nature of abdominal masses; and the presence, degree, and location of abdominal pain.

◆ For a rapid check, palpate mainly to detect areas of pain and tenderness, guarding, rebound tenderness, and costovertebral angle tenderness.

Age alert **An abdominal mass in a child may be a nephroblastoma. To avoid spreading tumor cells, don't palpate it.**

Light palpation

◆ Use light palpation to detect tenderness, areas of muscle spasm or rigidity, and superficial masses.

◆ To palpate for superficial masses in the abdominal wall, have the patient raise his head and shoulders to tighten the abdominal muscles. Tension obscures a deep mass, but a wall mass remains palpable.

◆ Palpate using the finger pads or palmar surface of three to four fingers. Depress ½″ to 1″ (1 to 2.5 cm) using circular motions.

◆ This technique may also help you to determine whether pain originates from the abdominal muscles or from deeper structures.

◆ If you detect tenderness, check for involuntary guarding or abdominal rigidity.

◆ As the patient exhales, palpate the abdominal rectus muscles. Normally, they soften and relax on exhalation; note abnormal muscle tension or inflexibility. Involuntary guarding points to peritoneal irritation. In generalized peritonitis, rigidity is severe and diffuse, commonly described as a "boardlike" abdomen.

◆ A tense or ticklish patient may exhibit voluntary guarding. Help him to relax with deep breathing. He should inhale through his nose and exhale through his mouth.

Checking the genitourinary system

Initial questions

◆ Ask about urine color, oliguria, and nocturia. (See *Evaluating urine color,* page 108.)

◆ Does your patient experience incontinence, dysuria, frequency, urgency, or difficulty with the urinary stream (such as reduced flow or dribbling)?

◆ Ask about pyuria, urine retention, and passage of calculi.

◆ Ask the patient if he has a history of bladder, kidney, or urinary tract infections.

Age alert **If your patient is a child, ask his parents if they've had problems with his toilet training or with bed-wetting.**

Questions for male patients

◆ Ask a male patient about infestations, penile discharge or lesions, and testicular pain or lumps.

◆ Ask if the patient performs testicular self-examinations. Has he had a vasectomy?

Evaluating urine color

For important clues about your patient's health, ask about changes in urine color. Such changes can result from fluid intake, medications, and dietary factors as well as from various disorders.

APPEARANCE	INDICATION
Amber or straw color	Normal
Cloudy	Infection, inflammation, glomerulonephritis, vegetarian diet
Colorless or pale straw color (dilute urine)	Excess fluid intake, anxiety, chronic renal disease, diabetes insipidus, diuretic therapy
Dark brown or black	Acute glomerulonephritis, drugs (such as nitrofurantoin, chlorpromazine, and antimalarials)
Dark yellow or amber (concentrated urine)	Low fluid intake, acute febrile disease, vomiting or diarrhea causing fluid loss
Green-brown	Bile duct obstruction
Orange-red to orange-brown	Urobilinuria, drugs (such as phenazopyridine and rifampin), obstructive jaundice (tea-colored urine)
Red or red-brown	Porphyria, hemorrhage, drugs (such as doxorubicin)

◆ Ask about the patient's sexual history, including sexual orientation, type of activity, frequency, number of partners, safer sex practices, and condom use.
◆ Ask about sexually transmitted diseases (STDs) and other infections. Determine the patient's knowledge of how to prevent STDs, including acquired immunodeficiency syndrome (AIDS).
◆ Find out if the patient has a history of prostate problems.
◆ Ask if he's satisfied with his sexual function. Does he have any concerns about impotence or sterility? Also inquire about his contraceptive practices.

Questions for female patients

◆ Ask your patient about her age at menarche and the character of her menses (frequency, regularity, and duration). What was the date of her last period? Does she have a history of menorrhagia, metrorrhagia, or amenorrhea? If she's postmenopausal, find out her age at menopause.
◆ Ask if she has irregular or painful vaginal bleeding, dyspareunia, or frequent vaginal infections.
◆ Ask about her sexual orientation, type of sexual activity, frequency, number of partners, safe sex practices, and condom use.
◆ Ask about her obstetric history, including the total number of pregnancies (G), number of births (P), number

of premature births, number of abortions, and number of living children. Has she had any problems with fertility?
◆ Has she experienced sexual assault or abuse?
◆ Find out what birth control method she uses.
◆ Determine the dates of her last gynecologic examination and Papanicolaou (Pap) test.
◆ Ask about STDs and other infections. Determine her knowledge of how to prevent STDs, including AIDS.
◆ Ask the patient about her satisfaction with her sexual function.

Inspecting and palpating male genitalia

◆ First, ask the patient to disrobe from the waist down and to cover himself with a drape.
◆ Then put on gloves and examine his penis, scrotum, and testicles, inguinal and femoral areas, and prostate gland.

Penis
◆ Observe the penis. Its size will depend on the patient's age and overall development.
◆ The penile skin should be slightly wrinkled and pink to light brown in a white patient, light brown to dark brown in a black patient.
◆ Check the penile shaft and glans for lesions, nodules, inflammation, and swelling. Also check the glans for smegma, a cheese-like secretion.
◆ Using your thumb and forefinger, palpate the entire penile shaft. It should be somewhat firm, and the skin should be smooth and movable. Note swelling, nodules, or indurations.

Urethral meatus
◆ Put on gloves before examining the urethral meatus.
◆ To inspect a male patient's urethral meatus, have him lie in the supine position and drape him, exposing only his penis.
◆ Gently compress the glans and inspect the urethral meatus for swelling, discharge, inflammation, signs of urethral infection, ulcerations, and lesions, which may indicate an STD.
◆ If you note a discharge, obtain a culture specimen for gonorrhea and chlamydia.

Scrotum and testicles
◆ Have the patient hold his penis away from his scrotum so that you can observe the general size and appearance of the scrotum. The skin will be darker than the rest of the body.
◆ Spread the surface of the scrotum, and examine the skin for swelling, nodules, redness, ulceration, and distended veins.
◆ You'll probably see some sebaceous cysts — firm, white-to-yellow, nontender cutaneous lesions. Also check for pitting edema, a sign of cardiovascular disease.
◆ Spread the pubic hair and check the skin for lesions and parasites.
◆ Gently palpate both testicles between your thumb and first two fingers. Check their size, shape, and response to pressure (typically, deep visceral pain). The testicles should be equal in size. They should feel firm, smooth, and rubbery, and they should move freely in the scrotal sac.

Palpating female breasts and axillae

◆ Have the patient put on a gown. Determine her breast history, including tumors, cancer, cysts, trauma, surgery, galactorrhea, and implants. Ask about mammograms. Ask about lumps, pain, breast changes, and discharge.

- Begin the breast examination with the patient sitting with her arms at her sides.
- Inspect the breasts with the patient's arms over her head and then when she's leaning forward with her hands pressed into her hips. Visually note any abnormalities.
- Palpate each breast using the pads of your fingers. Use a specific pattern, such as spiraling outward, a circular motion, or moving vertically across the breast. Include the tail of Spence and axilla.
- Then examine the breasts with the patient in a supine position. Place a pillow under the side you are examining, and have the patient raise her arm above her head and place her hand behind her head. Palpate each breast as described earlier.
- Note the consistency of the breast tissue. Check for nodules or unusual tenderness. Nodularity may increase before menstruation, and tenderness may result from premenstrual fullness, cysts, or cancer.
- Any lump or mass that feels different from the rest of the breast may represent a pathologic change.
- Palpate the areola and nipple, and gently compress the nipple between your thumb and index finger to detect discharge. If you see discharge, note the color, consistency, and quantity.
- With the patient seated, palpate the axillae. Palpate the right axilla with the middle three fingers of one hand while supporting the patient's arm with your other hand.
- You can usually palpate one or more soft, small, nontender central nodes. If the nodes feel large or hard or are tender, or if the patient has a suspicious-looking lesion, palpate the other groups of lymph nodes.

Inspecting female genitalia

- Before you start the examination, ask the patient to urinate.
- Next, help her into the dorsal lithotomy position, drape her, and put on gloves.
- Observe the skin and hair distribution of the mons pubis. Spread the hair with your fingers to check for lesions and parasites.
- Next, inspect the skin of the labia majora, spreading the hair to look for lesions, parasites, and genital warts. The skin should be slightly darker than the rest of the body, and the labia majora should be round and full.
- Examine the labia minora, which should be dark pink and moist. In nulliparous women, the labia majora and minora lie close together; after vaginal delivery, they may gape open.
- Closely observe each vulvar structure for syphilitic chancres and cancerous lesions.
- Examine the area of Bartholin's and Skene's glands and ducts for swelling, erythema, enlargement, or discharge.
- Next, inspect the urethral opening. It should be a pink, irregular, slitlike opening located at the midline, just above the vagina. It should be the same color as the mucous membranes. Look for erythema, swelling, polyps, discharge, and signs of urethral infection, cystocele, and ulcerations, which may indicate an STD.

4 Data collection findings

Normal findings

To distinguish between health and disease, you must be able to recognize normal data collection findings in each part of the body. When you perform a physical examination, use this head-to-toe roster of normal findings as a reference. It's designed to help you quickly zero in on physical abnormalities and evaluate your patient's overall condition.

Head

Inspection

- A symmetrical, lesion-free skull
- Symmetrical facial structures with normal variations in skin texture and pigmentation
- An ability to shrug the shoulders, a sign that cranial nerve XI (accessory nerve) is functioning normally

Palpation

- No lumps or tenderness on the head
- Symmetrical strength in the facial muscles, a sign that cranial nerves V and VII (trigeminal and facial nerves) are functioning normally
- Symmetrical sensation when you stroke a wisp of cotton on each cheek

Auscultation

- No bruits audible when auscultating the temporal artery

Neck

Inspection

- Unrestricted range of motion in the neck
- No bulging of the thyroid
- Symmetrical lymph nodes with no swelling
- Flat jugular veins

Palpation

- Mobile, soft lymph nodes less than ½″ (1 cm) in diameter with no tenderness
- Symmetrical pulses in the carotid arteries
- A palpable, symmetrical, lump-free thyroid with no tenderness
- Trachea that follows the midline of the neck and isn't tender
- No crepitus, tenderness, or displacement in the cervical spine
- Symmetrical muscle strength in the neck

Auscultation

- No audible carotid bruits

Eyes

Inspection

- No edema, scaling, or lesions on eyelids
- Eyelids that cover corneas completely when closed
- Eyelid color the same as surrounding skin color
- Palpebral fissures of equal height
- Margin of the upper lid falling between the superior pupil margin and the superior limbus
- Symmetrical, lesion-free upper eyelids that don't sag or droop when the eyes are open
- Evenly distributed eyelashes that curve outward
- Globe of the eye neither protruding from nor sunken into the orbit
- Eyebrows with equal size, color, and distribution
- Absence of nystagmus
- Clear conjunctiva with visible small blood vessels and no signs of drainage
- White sclera visible through the conjunctiva
- A transparent anterior chamber that contains no visible material when you shine a penlight into the side of the eye

- Transparent, smooth, and bright cornea with no visible irregularities or lesions
- Round, equal-sized pupils that react to light and accommodation
- Constriction of both pupils when you shine a light on one
- Lacrimal structures free from exudate, swelling, and excessive tearing
- Proper eye alignment
- Parallel eye movement in each of the six cardinal fields of gaze

Palpation

- No eyelid swelling or tenderness
- Globes that feel equally firm, but not overly hard or spongy
- Lacrimal sacs that don't regurgitate fluid

Ears

Inspection

- Bilaterally symmetrical, proportionately sized auricles with a vertical measurement of 1½"to 4"(4 to 10 cm)
- Ear tips that cross the eye-occiput line (an imaginary line extending from the lateral aspect of the eye to the occipital protuberance)
- Long axis of the ear no more than 10 degrees from perpendicular to the eye-occiput line
- Color of ear and facial skin match
- No signs of inflammation, lesions, or nodules
- No cracking, thickening, scaling, or lesions behind the ear when you bend the auricle forward
- No visible discharge from the auditory canal
- A patent external meatus
- Skin color on mastoid process and surrounding area matches
- No redness or swelling
- Normal drum landmarks, a bright reflex, and no canal inflammation or drainage, seen on otoscopic examination

Palpation

- No masses or tenderness on the auricle
- No tenderness on the auricle or tragus during manipulation
- Either small, nonpalpable lymph nodes on the auricle or discrete, mobile lymph nodes that aren't tender
- Well-defined, bony edges on the mastoid process that aren't tender

Nose

Inspection

- Symmetrical, lesion-free nose with no discharge or septal deviation
- Little or no nasal flaring
- Nonedematous frontal and maxillary sinuses
- Pink-red nasal mucosa with no visible lesions and no purulent drainage
- No evidence of foreign bodies or dried blood in the nostrils
- Ability to identify familiar odors

Palpation

- No structural deviation, tenderness, or swelling of the external nose
- No tenderness or edema of the frontal or maxillary sinuses

Mouth

Inspection

- Pink lips with no dryness, cracking, lesions, or cyanosis
- Symmetrical facial structures
- Ability to purse the lips and puff out the cheeks, a sign that cranial nerve VII (facial nerve) is functioning normally
- Ability to open and close the mouth easily
- Light pink, moist oral mucosa with no ulcers or lesions
- Visible salivary ducts with no inflammation
- White, hard palate
- Pink, soft palate

- Pink gums with no tartar, inflammation, hemorrhage, or leukoplakia
- All teeth intact, with no signs of occlusion, caries, or breakage
- Pink tongue that protrudes symmetrically and has no swelling, coating, ulcers, or lesions
- Ability to move the tongue easily and without tremor, a sign that cranial nerve XII (hypoglossal nerve) is functioning normally
- No swelling or inflammation on the anterior and posterior arches
- No lesions or inflammation on the posterior pharynx
- Lesion-free tonsils of appropriate size for the patient's age
- A uvula that moves upward when the patient says "ah" and a gag reflex that can be triggered by touching a tongue blade to the posterior pharynx, both signs that cranial nerves IX and X are functioning normally

Palpation

- Lips free from pain and induration
- No tenderness on the posterior and lateral surfaces of the tongue
- No tenderness or nodules on the floor of the mouth

Lungs

Inspection

- Symmetrical side-to-side configuration of the chest
- Anteroposterior diameter less than the transverse diameter, with a 1:2 ratio in an adult
- Normal chest shape, with no deformities, such as a barrel chest, kyphosis, retraction, sternal protrusion, or depressed sternum
- Costal angle less than 90 degrees, with the ribs joining the spine at a 45-degree angle
- Symmetrical expansion of chest wall during respirations
- Quiet, unlabored respirations with no use of accessory neck, shoulder, or abdominal muscles
- No intercostal, substernal, or supraclavicular retractions
- Normal adult respiratory rate of 12 to 20 breaths/minute, with some variation depending on the patient's age and disease processes
- Regular respiratory rhythm, with expiration taking about twice as long as inspiration
- Diaphragmatic breathing in men and children and thoracic breathing in women

Palpation

- Warm, dry skin
- No tender spots or bulges in the chest
- No asymmetrical expansion, fremitus, or subcutaneous crepitation

Auscultation

- Loud, high-pitched bronchial breath sounds over the trachea
- Intense, medium-pitched bronchovesicular breath sounds over the mainstem bronchi, between the scapulae, and below the clavicles
- Soft, breezy, low-pitched vesicular breath sounds over most of the peripheral lung fields

Heart

Inspection

- No visible pulsations, except at the point of maximum impulse (PMI)
- No lifts (heaves) or retractions in the four valve areas of the chest wall

Palpation

- No detectable vibrations or thrills
- No lifts (heaves)
- No pulsations except at PMI and epigastric area

◆ At the PMI, a localized (less than 1/2″[1 cm] in diameter) tapping pulse possible at the start of systole
◆ In the epigastric area, possible pulsation from the abdominal aorta

Auscultation

S_1

◆ First heart sound (*lub*)
◆ Heard best with the diaphragm of the stethoscope held over the mitral area with the patient in a left-lateral position
◆ In this position, sounds longer, lower, and louder than second heart sound
◆ May be split in the tricuspid area

S_2

◆ Second heart sound (*dub*)
◆ Heard best with the diaphragm of the stethoscope held over the aortic area with the patient sitting and leaning forward
◆ In this position, sounds shorter, sharper, higher, and louder than S_1
◆ May be split in the pulmonic area on inspiration

S_3

◆ Third heart sound
◆ Normal in children and slender, young adults with no cardiovascular disease
◆ Usually disappears by age 25 to 35
◆ In an older adult, may signify ventricular failure
◆ Heard best with the bell of the stethoscope held over the mitral area with the patient in a supine position and exhaling
◆ Sounds short, dull, soft, and low

Murmur

◆ May be functional in children and young adults
◆ Abnormal in older adults
◆ Soft and short, varying with respirations and patient position when harmless (innocent)
◆ Occurs in early systole
◆ Heard best in the pulmonic or mitral area with the patient in a supine position

Abdomen

Inspection

◆ No vascular lesions, jaundice, surgical scars, or rashes
◆ Faint venous patterns (more prominent in slender patients)
◆ Flat, round, or scaphoid abdominal contour
◆ Symmetrical abdomen
◆ Umbilicus midway between the xiphoid process and the symphysis pubis, with a flat or concave shape
◆ No variations in skin color
◆ No apparent bulges
◆ Abdominal movement apparent with respirations
◆ Pink or silver-white striae from pregnancy or weight loss

Light palpation

◆ No tenderness or masses
◆ Abdominal muscles neither tender nor rigid
◆ No guarding, distention, or ascites

Auscultation

◆ High-pitched, gurgling bowel sounds heard every 5 to 15 seconds through the diaphragm of the stethoscope in all four quadrants of the abdomen
◆ Vascular sounds heard through the bell of the stethoscope
◆ Venous hum over the inferior vena cava
◆ No bruits, murmurs, friction rubs, or other venous hums

Arms and legs

Inspection

◆ No gross deformities
◆ Symmetrical body parts

◆ Good body alignment
◆ No involuntary movements
◆ Smooth gait
◆ Full range of motion (ROM) in all muscles and joints
◆ No pain with full ROM
◆ No visible swelling or inflammation of joints or muscles
◆ Equal bilateral limb length and symmetrical muscle mass

Palpation

◆ Normal shape with no swelling or tenderness
◆ Equal bilateral muscle tone, texture, and strength
◆ No involuntary contractions or twitching
◆ Equally strong bilateral pulses

Common chief complaints

A patient's chief complaint is the starting point for almost every initial examination. You may be the patient's first contact, so you'll need a good working knowledge of common chief complaints, what might cause them, which examination steps to pursue, and whether the patient needs medical or nursing intervention.

This alphabetical list examines the most common chief complaints encountered in nursing practice. For each one, you'll find a concise description, detailed questions to ask during the history, areas to focus on during the physical examination, and common causes to consider.

Anxiety

◆ Subjective reaction to a real or imagined threat
◆ Nonspecific feeling of uneasiness or dread
◆ Prompts the body to purposeful action by stimulating the sympathetic nervous system
◆ Normal response to danger and to the physical and emotional stress of illness
◆ May be caused or worsened by many nonpathologic factors, including lack of sleep, poor diet, and excessive intake of caffeine or other stimulants
◆ If mild to moderate, may cause slight physical or psychological discomfort
◆ If severe, may be incapacitating or even life-threatening
◆ If excessive or unwarranted, may indicate an underlying psychological problem

Health history

◆ What are you anxious about? When did the anxiety first occur? What were the circumstances? What do you think caused it? Has this occurred before?
◆ Is the anxiety constant or sporadic? Do you notice any precipitating factors?
◆ How intense is the anxiety on a scale of 0 to 10, with 10 being the worst? What decreases it? What has helped in the past?
◆ Do you smoke? Do you ingest caffeine? Alcohol? Drugs? What medications do you take?

Physical examination

◆ Perform a complete physical examination.
◆ Focus on problems that may be caused or worsened by anxiety.

Causes

Asthma

◆ In an acute asthma attack, sudden anxiety with dyspnea, wheezing, productive cough, accessory muscle use, hyperresonant lung fields, diminished breath sounds, coarse crackles, cyanosis, tachycardia, and diaphoresis

Conversion disorder
- Chronic anxiety expressed through somatic complaints that have no physiologic basis
- Commonly sensorimotor deficits such as blindness and paralysis, but possibly dizziness, chest pain, palpitations, a lump in the throat, or choking

Mood disorders
- Chronic anxiety of varying severity
- Hallmark: Depression on awakening that abates during the day
- Other findings: Dysphoria; anger; insomnia or hypersomnia; decreased libido, interest, energy, and concentration; appetite disturbance; multiple somatic complaints; suicidal thoughts

Hyperthyroidism
- Acute anxiety a possible early sign
- Classic signs: Heat intolerance, weight loss despite increased appetite, nervousness, tremor, palpitations, sweating, an enlarged thyroid, diarrhea and, possibly, exophthalmos

Hyperventilation syndrome
- Acute anxiety, pallor, circumoral and peripheral paresthesia, occasionally carpopedal spasms

Mitral valve prolapse
- May cause panic
- Hallmark: Midsystolic click followed by an apical systolic murmur (click-murmur syndrome)
- May also cause paroxysmal palpitations with sharp, stabbing, or aching precordial pain

Obsessive-compulsive disorder
- Chronic anxiety with recurrent, unshakable thoughts or impulses to perform ritualistic acts that patient recognizes are irrational but can't control
- Anxiety that builds if patient can't perform these acts and diminishes after the action

Phobias
- Chronic anxiety with persistent fear of an object, activity, or situation
- Result is a compelling desire for avoidance that the patient recognizes as irrational but can't suppress

Postconcussion syndrome
- Possible chronic anxiety or periodic attacks of acute anxiety
- Anxiety that's usually most pronounced in situations that demand attention, judgment, or comprehension
- Associated symptoms: irritability, insomnia, dizziness, mild headache

Posttraumatic stress disorder
- Chronic anxiety of varying severity
- Intrusive, vivid memories and thoughts of the traumatic event
- Reliving of the event in dreams and nightmares
- May include insomnia, depression, and feelings of numbness and detachment

Somatoform disorder
- Chronic anxiety and various somatic complaints that have no physiologic basis
- Anxiety and depression that may be prominent or hidden by dramatic, flamboyant, or seductive behavior
- Most common in adolescents and young adults

Other causes
- Angina pectoris
- Antidepressants (may cause paradoxical anxiety)
- Central nervous system stimulants
- Chronic obstructive pulmonary disease
- Heart failure
- Hypochondrial neurosis
- Hypoglycemia
- Myocardial infarction
- Pheochromocytoma
- Pneumothorax

◆ Pulmonary embolism
◆ Sympathomimetic drugs

Cough, nonproductive

◆ Noisy, forceful expulsion of air that doesn't yield sputum or blood
◆ One of the most common signs of a respiratory disorder
◆ Sudden onset
◆ May be self-limiting
◆ If persists beyond 1 month, considered chronic
◆ Commonly results from cigarette smoking
◆ May cause damage, such as airway collapse, rupture of the alveoli, or blebs
◆ If eventually productive, a classic sign of progressive respiratory disease

Health history

◆ When did your cough start? Does a certain body position or a specific activity cause or relieve it? Does it get better or worse at certain times of the day? How does the cough sound? Is it constant or intermittent? Is it annoying or tiring? Does it keep you awake?
◆ Do you have pain with the cough?
◆ Have you noticed recent changes in appetite, energy level, exercise tolerance, or weight? Have you had surgery recently? Do you have allergies? Do you smoke? Have you been recently exposed to fumes or chemicals?
◆ What medications are you taking?

Physical examination

◆ Note whether the patient appears agitated, anxious, confused, diaphoretic, flushed, lethargic, nervous, pale, or restless. Is his skin cold or warm, clammy or dry?
◆ Observe the rate and depth of respirations, noting abnormal patterns. Then examine the patient's chest configuration and chest wall motion.
◆ Check the nose and mouth for congestion, drainage, inflammation, and signs of infection. Then inspect the neck for jugular vein distention and tracheal deviation.
◆ As you palpate the patient's neck, note enlarged lymph nodes or masses.
◆ Finally, auscultate the lungs for crackles, decreased or absent breath sounds, pleural friction rubs, rhonchi, and wheezes.

Causes

Asthma

◆ Attack that typically occurs at night, starts with a nonproductive cough and mild wheezing, and progresses to audible wheezing, chest tightness, a cough that produces thick mucus, and severe dyspnea
◆ Other signs: Accessory muscle use, cyanosis, diaphoresis, flaring nostrils, flushing, intercostal and supraclavicular retractions on inspiration, prolonged expirations, tachycardia, tachypnea

Interstitial lung disease

◆ Nonproductive cough and progressive dyspnea
◆ May also include cyanosis, fatigue, fine crackles, finger clubbing, chest pain, and recent weight loss

Other causes

◆ Airway occlusion
◆ Atelectasis
◆ Common cold
◆ Hypersensitivity pneumonitis
◆ Incentive spirometry
◆ Intermittent positive-pressure breathing
◆ Pericardial effusion
◆ Pleural effusion
◆ Pulmonary embolism
◆ *Hantavirus* infection
◆ Sinusitis
◆ Suctioning

Age alert Acute otitis media, which is common in infants and young children because of their short eustachian tubes, also produces nonproductive coughing.

Cough, productive

- Sudden, forceful, noisy expulsion of air that contains sputum, blood, or both
- Clears airways of secretions that normal mucociliary action doesn't remove
- Most common cause: Cigarette smoking
- Commonly caused by a cardiopulmonary disorder, such as an acute or a chronic infection that causes inflammation, edema, and increased mucus production in the airways
- Also caused by inhalation of antigenic or irritating substances

Health history

- When did your cough start? How much sputum do you cough up daily? Have you ever had a productive cough before?
- How does your cough sound and feel? Does it tend to produce more sputum at certain times of day, with certain meals or activities, in certain environments?
- What are the color, odor, and consistency of the sputum you cough up? Has the amount increased over time?
- Have you noticed recent changes in your appetite or weight?
- Do you have a recent history of surgery or allergies? Do you smoke, or drink alcohol? If so, how much? Do you work around chemicals or respiratory irritants?
- What medications are you taking?
- Do you live or have you lived with anyone diagnosed with tuberculosis?

Physical examination

- Examine the patient's mouth and nose for congestion, drainage, and inflammation. Note his breath odor.
- Inspect the patient's neck for jugular vein distention.
- As he breathes, observe the chest for accessory muscle use, intercostal and supraclavicular retractions, and uneven expansion.
- Palpate the patient's neck for enlarged lymph nodes, masses, and tenderness.
- Finally, auscultate for abnormal breath sounds, crackles, pleural friction rubs, rhonchi, and wheezes.

Causes

Bacterial pneumonia

- Initial dry cough that becomes productive
- Rust-colored sputum in pneumococcal pneumonia; brick-red or currant-jelly sputum in *Klebsiella* pneumonia; salmon-colored sputum in staphylococcal pneumonia; mucopurulent sputum, in streptococcal pneumonia

Lung abscess

- Cardinal sign: Coughing with copious amounts of purulent, foul-smelling, possibly blood-tinged sputum
- Ruptured abscess: May cause anorexia, diaphoresis, dyspnea, fatigue, fever with chills, halitosis, headache, inspiratory crackles, pleuritic chest pain, tubular or amphoric breath sounds, and weight loss

Other causes

- Acute bronchiolitis
- Aspiration and chemical pneumonitis
- Bronchiectasis
- Common cold
- Cystic fibrosis
- Expectorants
- Incentive spirometry
- Intermittent positive-pressure breathing

- ◆ Lung cancer
- ◆ Pertussis
- ◆ Pulmonary embolism
- ◆ Pulmonary edema
- ◆ Tracheobronchitis

Diarrhea

◆ Usually a chief sign of an intestinal disorder
◆ Increased volume of stool compared with usual bowel habits
◆ Varies in severity, and may be acute or chronic
◆ Acute diarrhea: May result from acute infection, stress, fecal impaction, or drug effect
◆ Chronic diarrhea: May result from chronic infection, obstructive and inflammatory bowel disease, malabsorption syndrome, an endocrine disorder, or GI surgery
◆ Periodic diarrhea: May result from food intolerance or from ingestion of caffeine or spicy or high-fiber foods

Health history

◆ Do you have abdominal pain and cramps?
◆ Describe your stool's color, consistency, and frequency. Describe your normal bowel pattern.
◆ Are you weak or fatigued?
◆ What medications do you take?
◆ Have you had GI surgery or radiation therapy recently?
◆ Describe your diet.
◆ Do you have known food allergies?
◆ Have you been experiencing any unusual stress?

Physical examination

◆ If the patient isn't in shock, proceed with a brief physical examination.
◆ Evaluate hydration, check skin turgor and mucous membranes, and take blood pressure with the patient lying, sitting, and standing.
◆ Take the patient's temperature and note chills or rash.
◆ Auscultate bowel sounds.
◆ Inspect the abdomen for distention, and palpate for tenderness.

Causes

Anthrax, GI

◆ Caused by eating contaminated meat from an animal infected with *Bacillus anthracis*
◆ Early signs and symptoms: Decreased appetite, nausea, vomiting, fever
◆ Later signs and symptoms: Severe bloody diarrhea, abdominal pain, hematemesis

Carcinoid syndrome

◆ Severe diarrhea with flushing — usually of the head and neck — commonly caused by emotional stimuli or ingestion of food, hot water, or alcohol
◆ Other signs and symptoms: Abdominal cramps, dyspnea, weight loss, anorexia, weakness, palpitations, valvular heart disease, depression

Cholera

◆ Caused by ingesting water or food contaminated by the bacterium *Vibrio cholerae*
◆ Abrupt watery diarrhea and vomiting
◆ Other signs and symptoms: Thirst (from severe water and electrolyte loss), weakness, muscle cramps, decreased skin turgor, oliguria, tachycardia, hypotension
◆ Without treatment, may be fatal within hours

Clostridium difficile *infection*

◆ May cause no symptoms
◆ May cause soft, unformed stools; watery diarrhea that may be foul-smelling or grossly bloody; abdominal pain, cramping, and tenderness; fever; and a white blood cell count as high as 20,000/μl.

◆ Severe infection: May cause toxic megacolon, colon perforation, or peritonitis

Crohn's disease

◆ Recurring inflammatory disorder that produces diarrhea and abdominal pain with guarding, tenderness, and nausea

◆ May also cause fever, chills, weakness, anorexia, weight loss

Escherichia coli *0157:H7 infection*

◆ Watery or bloody diarrhea, nausea, vomiting, fever, and abdominal cramps after eating undercooked beef or other foods contaminated with this strain of bacteria

◆ May be complicated by hemolytic uremic syndrome, which causes red blood cell destruction and eventually acute renal failure, in children age 5 and younger and in elderly people

Acute viral, bacterial, and protozoal infections (such as cryptosporidiosis)

◆ Sudden onset of watery diarrhea, abdominal pain, cramps, nausea, vomiting, and fever

◆ If significant fluid and electrolyte loss, may cause dehydration and shock

Chronic tuberculosis and fungal and parasitic infections

◆ Less severe but more persistent diarrhea

◆ Accompanied by epigastric distress, vomiting, weight loss and, possibly, passage of blood and mucus

Intestinal obstruction

◆ Partial obstruction: Increased intestinal motility, resulting in thin-stooled diarrhea, abdominal pain with tenderness and guarding, nausea and, possibly, distention

Irritable bowel syndrome

◆ Diarrhea alternating with constipation or normal bowel function

◆ May cause abdominal pain, tenderness, and distention; dyspepsia; and nausea

Ischemic bowel disease

◆ A life-threatening disorder that causes bloody diarrhea with abdominal pain

◆ If severe, may cause shock and require surgery

Lactose intolerance

◆ Diarrhea within several hours of ingesting milk or milk products

◆ Accompanied by cramps, abdominal pain, loud gurgling bowel sounds, bloating, nausea, and flatus

Large-bowel cancer

◆ Bloody diarrhea with partial obstruction

◆ Other signs and symptoms: Abdominal pain, anorexia, weight loss, weakness, fatigue, exertional dyspnea, and depression

Ulcerative colitis

◆ Hallmark: Recurrent bloody diarrhea with pus or mucus

◆ Other signs and symptoms: Tenesmus, hyperactive bowel sounds, cramping lower abdominal pain, low-grade fever, anorexia and, at times, nausea and vomiting

◆ Late findings: Weight loss, anemia, and weakness

Other causes

◆ Foods containing oils that inhibit food absorption, causing acute, uncontrollable diarrhea and rectal leakage

◆ Gastrectomy, gastroenterostomy, pyloroplasty

◆ High-dose radiation therapy (enteritis and diarrhea)

◆ Laxative abuse (acute or chronic diarrhea)
◆ Many antibiotics, such as ampicillin, cephalosporins, tetracyclines, and clindamycin
◆ Other drugs, such as magnesium-containing antacids, colchicine, guanethidine, lactulose, dantrolene, ethacrynic acid, mefenamic acid, methotrexate, metyrosine and, in high doses, cardiac glycosides and quinidine

Age alert Diarrhea in children commonly results from infection, although chronic diarrhea may result from malabsorption syndrome, an anatomic defect, or allergies. Because dehydration and electrolyte imbalance occur rapidly in children, diarrhea can be life-threatening. Diligently monitor all episodes of diarrhea, and immediately replace lost fluids.

Dizziness

◆ Sensation of imbalance or faintness that may include blurred or double vision, confusion, and weakness
◆ May start abruptly or gradually, and may be worsened by standing up quickly and eased by lying down
◆ May be mild or severe, with usually brief episodes
◆ Typically results from inadequate blood flow and oxygen supply to the cerebrum and spinal cord
◆ May occur with anxiety, respiratory and cardiovascular disorders, and postconcussion syndrome
◆ May be a key symptom of certain serious disorders, such as hypertension and vertebrobasilar artery insufficiency

Health history

◆ When did the dizziness start? How severe is it? How often does it occur, and how long does each episode last?
◆ Does the dizziness abate spontaneously? Is it triggered by standing up suddenly or bending over?
◆ Do you have blurred vision, chest pain, a chronic cough, diaphoresis, a headache, or shortness of breath?
◆ Have you ever had hypertension or another cardiovascular disorder? What about diabetes mellitus, anemia, respiratory or anxiety disorders, or head injury?
◆ Which medications are you taking?
◆ For family members: How would you describe the patient's usual level of consciousness (LOC)?

Age alert Many children have trouble describing dizziness and instead complain of tiredness, stomachache, and feeling sick.

Physical examination

◆ Check the patient's current LOC, respirations, and body temperature. As you watch his breathing, look for accessory muscle use or barrel chest. Also look for finger clubbing, cyanosis, dry mucous membranes, and poor skin turgor.
◆ Evaluate the patient's motor and sensory functions and reflexes.
◆ Palpate the extremities for peripheral edema and capillary refill.
◆ Auscultate the patient's heart rate and rhythm and his breath sounds.
◆ Take the patient's blood pressure while he's lying down, sitting, and standing. If the diastolic pressure exceeds 100 mm Hg, notify the physician immediately, and instruct the patient to lie down. A drop of more than 20 mm Hg of systolic pressure or 10 mm Hg of diastolic pressure with position change may indicate orthostatic hypotension.

Causes

Cardiac arrhythmias

◆ Dizziness lasting for several minutes or longer that may precede fainting
◆ Other signs and symptoms: Blurred vision, confusion, hypotension, palpita-

tions, paresthesia, weakness, and an irregular, rapid, or thready pulse

Hypertension

◆ Dizziness that may precede fainting and may be relieved by rest
◆ Other findings: Blurred vision, elevated blood pressure, headache, and retinal changes, such as hemorrhage and papilledema

Transient ischemic attack

◆ Dizziness of varying severity, lasting from a few seconds to 24 hours
◆ May include blindness or visual field deficits, diplopia, hearing loss, numbness, paresis, ptosis, and tinnitus
◆ May be triggered by turning the head to the side
◆ Typically signals an impending stroke

Other causes

◆ Anemia
◆ Certain drugs, such as antihistamines, antihypertensives, anxiolytics, central nervous system depressants, decongestants, opioid analgesics, or vasodilators
◆ Generalized anxiety disorder
◆ Orthostatic hypotension
◆ Panic disorder
◆ Postconcussion syndrome
◆ Some herbal supplements such as St. John's wort

Dysphagia

◆ Difficulty swallowing
◆ The most common — and sometimes the only — symptom of an esophageal disorder
◆ May also result from oropharyngeal, respiratory, and neurologic disorders, thyroid enlargement, anxiety, or from exposure to toxins
◆ Increased risk of aspiration, choking, malnutrition, and dehydration

Health history

◆ When did you start having trouble swallowing? Can you point to the spot where you have the most trouble swallowing?
◆ Is swallowing painful? If so, is the pain constant, or does it come and go?
◆ Does eating make the problem better or worse? Do you have more trouble swallowing solids or liquids? Does the problem go away after you try to swallow a few times? Is swallowing easier if you change position?
◆ Have you or anyone in your family ever had an esophageal, oropharyngeal, respiratory, or neurologic disorder? Have you recently had a tracheotomy or been exposed to a toxin?

Physical examination

◆ Evaluate the patient's swallowing and his cough and gag reflexes.
◆ Listen to his speech, noting signs of muscle, tongue, or facial weakness; aphasia; or dysarthria.
◆ Is the patient's voice nasal or hoarse?
◆ Check his mouth for dry mucous membranes and thick secretions.
◆ Check thyroid size and for presence of masses.

Causes

Airway obstruction

◆ A life-threatening condition
◆ Marked by mild to severe wheezing, respiratory distress, and dysphagia with gagging and dysphonia

Esophageal cancer

◆ Painless dysphagia, usually with rapid weight loss
◆ Dysphagia that becomes painful and constant as cancer advances
◆ Also a cough with hemoptysis, hoarseness, sore throat, and steady chest pain

Age alert For patients older than age 50 with head or neck

cancer, dysphagia is commonly the initial chief complaint.

Esophagitis

- Corrosive esophagitis: Dysphagia with excessive salivation, fever, hematemesis, intense pain in the mouth and anterior chest, and tachypnea
- *Candida* esophagitis: Dysphagia and sore throat
- Reflux esophagitis: A late symptom that usually accompanies stricture

Hiatal hernia

- May cause belching, dysphagia, dyspepsia, flatulence, heartburn, regurgitation, and retrosternal or substernal chest pain that's aggravated by lying down or bending over

Other causes

- Botulism
- Esophageal diverticula
- External esophageal compression
- Hypocalcemia
- Laryngeal nerve damage
- Parkinson's disease
- Radiation therapy
- Tracheotomy

Dyspnea

- Typically described as shortness of breath
- Also includes difficult or uncomfortable breathing
- May vary greatly in severity, which usually isn't related to seriousness of underlying cause
- May arise suddenly or slowly and may subside rapidly or persist for years

Health history

- When did the dyspnea first occur? Did it begin suddenly or gradually? Is it constant or intermittent? Does it occur during activity, while you're resting, or when you're lying flat? Does anything seem to trigger, worsen, or relieve it? Have you ever had dyspnea before?
- Do you have chest pain? A productive or nonproductive cough?
- Have you recently had an upper respiratory tract infection or a traumatic injury? Do you smoke? If so, how much and for how long? Have you been exposed to any allergens? Do you have known allergies?
- Which medications are you taking?

Physical examination

- Observe the patient's respirations, noting their rate and depth as well as breathing difficulties or abnormal respiratory patterns. Check for flaring nostrils, grunting respirations, inspiratory stridor, intercostal retractions during inspirations, and pursed-lip expirations.
- Examine the patient for barrel chest, diaphoresis, jugular vein distention, finger clubbing, and peripheral edema. Note the color, consistency, and odor of sputum.
- Palpate the patient's chest for asymmetrical expansion, decreased diaphragmatic excursion, tactile fremitus, and subcutaneous crepitation. Also check the rate, rhythm, and intensity of the peripheral pulses.
- Auscultate the lungs for bronchophony; crackles; decreased, absent, or unilateral breath sounds; egophony; pleural friction rubs; rhonchi; whispered pectoriloquy; and wheezing.
- Auscultate the heart for abnormal sounds or rhythms and for pericardial friction rubs and tachycardia. Also monitor the patient's blood and pulse pressures.

Causes

Acute respiratory distress syndrome

- Acute dyspnea followed by accessory muscle use, crackles, grunting respirations, progressive respiratory distress, rhonchi, and wheezes

◆ Late stages: Anxiety, cyanosis, decreased mental acuity, and tachycardia
◆ Severe acute respiratory distress syndrome: Signs of shock, such as cool, clammy skin and hypotension
◆ Typically, no history of underlying cardiac or pulmonary disease but a recent pulmonary or systemic insult

Airway obstruction, partial
◆ Inspiratory stridor and sudden shortness of breath
◆ Related findings: Accessory muscle use, anxiety, asymmetrical chest expansion, cyanosis, decreased or absent breath sounds, diaphoresis, hypotension, tachypnea
◆ Possibly caused by aspirated vomitus, a foreign body, or exposure to an allergen

Asthma
◆ Acute dyspneic attacks with accessory muscle use, apprehension, dry cough, flushing or cyanosis, intercostal retractions, tachypnea, tachycardia
◆ Palpation: Decreased tactile fremitus
◆ Auscultation: Wheezing and rhonchi or, during a severe episode, decreased breath sounds

Heart failure
◆ Dyspnea that usually develops gradually or occurs as chronic paroxysmal nocturnal dyspnea
◆ In ventricular failure: Dyspnea with basilar crackles, dependent peripheral edema, distended jugular veins, fatigue, orthopnea, tachycardia, ventricular or atrial gallop, and weight gain
◆ Possible history of cardiovascular disease
◆ May result from a drug that can cause heart failure, such as amiodarone (Cordarone), a beta-adrenergic blocker, or a corticosteroid

Myocardial infarction
◆ Sudden dyspnea with crushing substernal chest pain that may radiate to the back, neck, jaw, and arms
◆ Possible history of heart disease, hypertension, hypercholesterolemia, or use of a drug that may cause heart attack, such as cocaine, dextrothyroxine sodium (Choloxin), estramustine phosphate sodium (Emcyt), or aldesleukin (Proleukin)

Pneumonia
◆ Dyspnea that occurs suddenly, usually with fever, pleuritic chest pain that worsens with deep inspiration, and shaking chills
◆ Dry or productive cough depending on the stage and type of pneumonia
◆ Possible discolored, foul-smelling sputum
◆ Possible crackles, decreased breath sounds, and rhonchi
◆ Possible history of exposure to a contagious organism, hazardous fumes, or air pollution

Pulmonary edema
◆ Severe dyspnea, commonly preceded by signs of heart failure, such as crackles in both lung fields, cyanosis, tachycardia, tachypnea, and marked anxiety
◆ Possible dry cough or one that produces copious amounts of pink, frothy sputum
◆ Possible history of cardiovascular disease, cyanosis, fatigue, and pallor

Pulmonary embolism
◆ Severe dyspnea with intense, angina-like or pleuritic pain aggravated by deep breathing and thoracic movement
◆ Other findings: Crackles, cyanosis, diffuse wheezing, low-grade fever, nonproductive cough, pleural friction rub, restlessness, tachypnea, tachycardia

◆ Possible history of acute myocardial infarction, heart failure, hip or leg fracture, hormonal contraceptive use, pregnancy, thrombophlebitis, or varicose veins

Other causes
◆ Anemia
◆ Anxiety
◆ Cardiac arrhythmias
◆ Cor pulmonale
◆ Inhalation injury
◆ Lung cancer
◆ Pleural effusion
◆ Sepsis

Eye pain

◆ Also known as ophthalmalgia
◆ May be described as burning, throbbing, aching, or stabbing sensation in or around the eye
◆ May also be characterized as a foreign-body sensation
◆ Varies from mild to severe, with duration and exact location providing clues to the cause
◆ Usually results from corneal abrasion, but may also be caused by an eye disorder (such as glaucoma), trauma, or neurologic or systemic disorder — any of which may stimulate nerve endings in the cornea or external eye, producing pain

Health history
◆ Can you describe your eye pain? Is it an ache or a sharp pain? How long does it last? Do you have burning, itching, or discharge?
◆ When did the pain begin? Is it worse in the morning or in the evening?
◆ Have you had recent trauma or surgery?
◆ Do you have headaches? If yes, how often and at what time of day do they occur?

Physical examination
◆ Don't manipulate the eye if you suspect trauma.
◆ Carefully check the lids and conjunctiva for redness, inflammation, and swelling.
◆ Examine the eyes for ptosis or exophthalmos.
◆ Test visual acuity with and without correction, and check extraocular movements.
◆ Characterize discharge.

Causes
Blepharitis
◆ Burning pain in both eyelids accompanied by itching, a sticky discharge, and conjunctival injection
◆ Related findings: Foreign-body sensation, lid ulcerations, and loss of eyelashes

Burns
◆ Chemical burns: Sudden, severe eye pain with erythema and blistering of the face and lids, photophobia, miosis, conjunctival injection, blurring, and inability to keep the eyelids open
◆ Ultraviolet radiation burns: Moderate to severe pain about 12 hours after exposure along with photophobia and vision changes

Chalazion
◆ Localized tenderness and swelling of the upper or lower eyelid
◆ With eversion of the lid, conjunctival injection and a small red lump

Conjunctivitis
◆ Some degree of eye pain and excessive tearing occurs with four types of conjunctivitis.
◆ Allergic conjunctivitis: Bilateral, mild burning pain with itching, conjunctival injection, and a characteristic ropy discharge
◆ Bacterial conjunctivitis: Painful only with corneal involvement; otherwise,

burning, foreign-body sensation, purulent discharge, and conjunctival injection
◆ Fungal conjunctivitis: Pain and photophobia with corneal involvement; also itching, burning, conjunctival injection, and thick, purulent discharge
◆ Viral conjunctivitis: Itching, redness, foreign-body sensation, visible conjunctival follicles, and eyelid edema

Corneal abrasions
◆ Eye pain with foreign-body sensation
◆ Also excessive tearing, photophobia, and conjunctival injection

Corneal ulcers
◆ Severe eye pain with both bacterial and fungal corneal ulcers
◆ Also purulent discharge, sticky eyelids, photophobia, and impaired visual acuity
◆ Bacterial corneal ulcer: Gray-white, irregularly shaped ulcer on the cornea, unilateral pupil constriction, and conjunctival injection
◆ Fungal corneal ulcer: Conjunctival injection, eyelid edema and erythema, and a dense, cloudy, central ulcer surrounded by progressively clearer rings

Foreign body in the cornea or conjunctiva
◆ Sudden, severe pain, usually with intact vision
◆ May include excessive tearing, photophobia, miosis, foreign-body sensation, dark speck on the cornea, and dramatic conjunctival injection

Glaucoma, angle-closure
◆ Pain and pressure over the eye, blurred vision, halo vision, decreased visual acuity, and nausea and vomiting
◆ In acute attack, blurred vision and sudden, excruciating pain in and around the eye, possibly severe enough to cause nausea, vomiting, and abdominal pain
◆ Other findings: Halo vision, rapidly decreasing visual acuity, and a fixed, nonreactive, moderately dilated pupil

Glaucoma, open-angle
◆ Mild aching in the eyes, loss of peripheral vision, halo vision, and reduced visual acuity not corrected by glasses

Age alert Glaucoma, which can cause eye pain, is usually a disease of older patients, becoming clinically significant after age 40. It usually occurs bilaterally and leads to slowly progressive vision loss, especially in the peripheral visual fields.

Iritis, acute
◆ Moderate to severe eye pain with severe photophobia, dramatic conjunctival injection, and blurred vision
◆ Constricted pupil that may respond poorly to light

Migraine headache
◆ Aching eyes and head pain, possibly with nausea, vomiting, blurred vision, and sensitivity to light and noise

Ocular laceration and intraocular foreign bodies
◆ Usually mild to severe unilateral eye pain and impaired visual acuity
◆ May include eyelid edema, conjunctival injection, and an abnormal pupillary response

Optic neuritis
◆ Possible pain in and around the eye
◆ Severe vision loss and tunnel vision that improve in 2 to 3 weeks
◆ Pupils that respond sluggishly to direct light and normally to consensual light

Other causes
◆ Contact lenses
◆ Ocular surgery

Fatigue

- A feeling of excessive tiredness, lack of energy, or exhaustion, accompanied by a strong desire to rest or sleep
- May include weakness, which involves the muscles
- A normal response to physical overexertion, emotional stress, and sleep deprivation
- May also result from psychological and physiologic disorders, especially viral infections and endocrine, cardiovascular, or neurologic disorders

Health history

- When did the fatigue begin? Is it constant or intermittent? If it's intermittent, when does it occur? Does the fatigue worsen with activity and improve with rest, or vice versa? (The former usually signals a physiologic disorder; the latter, a psychological disorder.)
- Have you had any stressful changes at home or at work recently?
- Have you changed your eating habits? Have you recently lost or gained weight?
- Have you or anyone in your family been diagnosed with any cardiovascular, endocrine, or neurologic disorders? What about viral infections or psychological disorders?
- Which medications are you taking?

Age alert Always ask older patients about fatigue because this symptom may be insidious and mask a more serious underlying condition.

Physical examination

- Observe the patient's general appearance for signs of depression or organic illness. Is he unkempt? Expressionless? Tired or unhealthy looking? Is he slumped over?
- Determine his mental status, noting especially agitation, attention deficits, mental clouding, or psychomotor impairment.

Causes

Anemia

- Common first symptom: Fatigue after mild activity
- Other signs and symptoms: Dyspnea, pallor, and tachycardia

Cancer

- Common first symptom: Unexplained fatigue
- Related signs and symptoms that reflect the type, location, and stage of the cancer
- Related signs and symptoms commonly include abnormal bleeding, anorexia, nausea, pain, a palpable mass, vomiting, and weight loss

Chronic infection

- Fatigue: Usually the most prominent — and sometimes the only — symptom

Depression, chronic

- Usually accompanied by persistent fatigue unrelated to exertion
- May also include anorexia, constipation, headache, and sexual dysfunction

Diabetes mellitus

- Fatigue: The most common symptom, which may begin insidiously or abruptly
- Related findings: Polydipsia, polyphagia, polyuria, and weight loss

Heart failure

- Characteristic symptoms: Persistent fatigue and lethargy
- Left-sided heart failure: Exertional and paroxysmal nocturnal dyspnea, orthopnea, and tachycardia
- Right-sided heart failure: Jugular vein distention and, sometimes, a

slight but persistent nonproductive cough

Hypothyroidism

◆ Fatigue early in the course of hypothyroidism, along with forgetfulness, cold intolerance, weight gain, metrorrhagia, and constipation

Myasthenia gravis

◆ Cardinal symptoms: Easy fatigability and muscle weakness that worsen with exertion and abate with rest
◆ Symptoms specific to affected muscle groups

Other causes

◆ Anxiety
◆ Certain drugs, notably antihypertensives and sedatives
◆ Malnutrition
◆ Myocardial infarction
◆ Rheumatoid arthritis
◆ Surgery of most types
◆ Systemic lupus erythematosus

Fever

◆ Abnormal elevation of body temperature above 98.6° F (37° C)
◆ Also known as pyrexia
◆ A common sign arising from disorders that affect virtually every body system, which gives it little diagnostic value when considered alone
◆ Low fever: Oral reading of 99° to 100.4° F [37.2° to 38° C]
◆ Moderate fever: 100.5° to 104° F [38° to 40° C]
◆ High fever: Higher than 104° F [40° C])
◆ A medical emergency if persistently high
◆ If higher than 108° F (42.2° C) causes unconsciousness and, if prolonged, brain damage

Age alert Infants and young children experience higher and more prolonged fevers, more rapid temperature increases, and greater temperature fluctuations than do older children or adults. Older adults don't exhibit temperature changes as readily as younger adults, and usually have a baseline normal temperature reading of less than 98.6° F (37° C).

Health history

◆ What's your normal temperature? When did the fever start? How high did it go? Is the fever constant, or does it disappear and then reappear later?
◆ Do you also have chills, fatigue, or pain?
◆ Have you had any immunodeficiency disorders, infections, recent trauma or surgery, or diagnostic tests?
◆ Have you traveled out of the country recently?
◆ Which medications are you taking? Have you recently had anesthesia?

Causes

Drugs

◆ Hypersensitivity (fever and rash) to such drugs as anti-infectives, barbiturates, iodides, methyldopa (Aldomet), procainamide (Pronestyl), phenytoin (Dilantin), quinidine, and some antitoxins
◆ May also result from chemotherapy drugs, drugs that decrease sweating—such as anticholinergics—and toxic doses of salicylates, amphetamines, and tricyclic antidepressants

Infectious and inflammatory disorders

◆ May cause low fever, as in Crohn's disease and ulcerative colitis, or extremely high fever, as in bacterial pneumonia
◆ May cause remitting fever, as in infectious mononucleosis; sustained fever, as in meningitis; or relapsing fever, as in malaria
◆ May arise abruptly, as in Rocky Mountain spotted fever, or insidiously, as in mycoplasmal pneumonia

◆ Typically accompanies a self-limiting disorder, such as the common cold

Other causes
◆ Blood transfusion reactions
◆ Exercise
◆ Heatstroke
◆ Hypothalamic disease or trauma
◆ Injection of contrast media used in diagnostic tests
◆ Malignant hypothermia
◆ Neuroleptic malignant syndrome
◆ Surgery

Headache

◆ Most common neurologic symptom
◆ May be mild to severe, localized or generalized, and constant or intermittent
◆ Can be vascular, or related to muscle contraction, or a combination
◆ Benign about 90% of the time; occasionally indicates a severe neurologic disorder
◆ May result from disorders associated with intracranial inflammation, increased intracranial pressure (ICP), meningeal irritation, or vascular disturbance
◆ May also result from disorders of the eye or sinus and from the effects of drugs, tests, and treatments

Health history
◆ When did your headache first occur?
◆ Describe your pain on a scale of 0 to 10, with 10 being the worst pain you can imagine. Would you call the pain mild, moderate, or severe?
◆ Is it localized or generalized? If it's localized, where does it occur? Is it constant or intermittent? If it's intermittent, what's the duration?
◆ How would you describe the pain; for example, is it stabbing, dull, throbbing, or viselike?
◆ Does anything seem to trigger it, worsen it, or relieve it? Have you had this kind of headache before?
◆ Have you also had confusion, dizziness, drowsiness, eye pain, fever, muscle twitching, nausea, photophobia, seizures, trouble speaking or walking, neck stiffness, vision disturbances, vomiting, or weakness?
◆ Have you been under unusual stress at home or at work? For family members: Have you noticed changes in the patient's behavior or personality?
◆ Do you have a history of blood disorders, cardiovascular disease, glaucoma, bleeding disorders, hypertension, poor vision, seizures, migraine headaches, or smoking? Have you had a recent traumatic injury, dental work, or a sinus, ear, or systemic infection?
◆ Which medications are you taking?

Physical examination
◆ Observe the rate and depth of the patient's respirations, noting breathing difficulty or abnormal patterns.
◆ Inspect the patient's head for bruising, swelling, and sinus bleeding. Also check for Battle's sign, neck stiffness, otorrhea, and rhinorrhea.
◆ Check the patient's level of consciousness (LOC). Is he drowsy, lethargic, or comatose? Examine his eyes, noting pupil size, equality, and response to light. With the patient both at rest and active, note tremors.
◆ Gently palpate the skull and sinuses for tenderness. Unless head trauma has occurred, slowly move the neck to check for nuchal rigidity or pain. Then check the patient's motor strength. Palpate his peripheral pulses, noting their rate, rhythm, and intensity.
◆ Auscultate over the temporal arteries, listening for bruits.
◆ Also monitor the patient's blood and pulse pressures.

Causes

Brain abscess

◆ Headache that typically intensifies over a few days, localizes to a particular spot, and is aggravated by straining
◆ May be accompanied by decreased LOC (drowsiness to deep stupor), focal or generalized seizures, nausea, and vomiting
◆ Depending on the site, may also cause aphasia, ataxia, impaired visual acuity, hemiparesis, personality changes, or tremors
◆ May include signs of infection
◆ May include a history of systemic, chronic middle ear, mastoid, or sinus infection; osteomyelitis of the skull; a compound fracture; or a penetrating head wound

Brain tumor

◆ Headache that develops near the tumor site and becomes generalized as the tumor grows
◆ Usually pain that's intermittent, deep-seated, dull, and most intense in the morning
◆ Pain that's worsened by coughing, stooping, Valsalva's maneuver, and changes in head position

Cerebral aneurysm, ruptured

◆ A sudden, excruciating headache that may be unilateral and usually peaks within minutes of the rupture
◆ May be accompanied by nausea, vomiting, signs of meningeal irritation, and loss of consciousness
◆ History that may include hypertension or other cardiovascular disorders, a stressful lifestyle, or smoking

Encephalitis

◆ Severe, generalized headache with LOC declining over a 48-hour period
◆ May include fever, focal neurologic deficits, irritability, nausea, nuchal rigidity, photophobia, seizures, and vomiting
◆ May be a history of exposure to viruses that commonly cause encephalitis, such as mumps or herpes simplex

Epidural hemorrhage, acute

◆ Progressively severe headache immediately after a brief loss of consciousness
◆ LOC that declines rapidly and steadily
◆ May include increasing ICP, ipsilateral pupil dilation, nausea, and vomiting
◆ Usually a history of head trauma during previous 24 hours

Glaucoma, acute angle-closure

◆ An ophthalmic emergency that may cause an excruciating headache
◆ May also cause blurred vision, a cloudy cornea, halo vision, a moderately dilated and fixed pupil, photophobia, nausea, and vomiting

Hematoma, subdural

◆ Severe, localized headache, often arising after head trauma; causes a latent period of drowsiness, confusion or personality changes, agitation, and eventual loss of consciousness
◆ Possible later signs of increased ICP
◆ Acute hematoma: When head trauma occurred within 3 days of presenting signs and symptoms
◆ Subacute hematoma: When head trauma occurred within 3 to 20 days before presenting signs and symptoms
◆ Chronic hematoma: When precipitating event occurred more than 3 weeks before signs and symptoms
◆ No history of head trauma in about 50% of patients with chronic subdural hematoma

Hemorrhage, subarachnoid

◆ Sudden, violent headache and dizziness, hypertension, ipsilateral pupil dilation, nausea, nuchal rigidity, sei-

zures, vomiting, and an altered LOC that may progress rapidly to coma
- History that may include congenital vascular defects, arteriovenous malformation, cardiovascular disease, smoking, hypertension, or excessive stress

Hypertension
- Slightly throbbing occipital headache on awakening, possibly decreasing during the day
- A medical emergency if diastolic blood pressure exceeds 120 mm Hg and the headache remains constant, because of the risk of stroke

Meningitis
- Severe, constant, generalized headache that starts suddenly and worsens with movement
- May also cause chills, fever, hyperreflexia, nuchal rigidity, and positive Kernig's and Brudzinski's signs
- Possible recent systemic or sinus infection, dental work, or exposure to bacteria or viruses that commonly cause meningitis, such as *Haemophilus influenzae, Streptococcus pneumoniae,* enteroviruses, and mumps

Migraine
- Severe, throbbing headache that may follow a 5- to 15-minute prodrome of dizziness; tingling of the face, lips, or hands; unsteady gait; and vision disturbances
- May also cause anorexia, nausea, photophobia, drowsiness, and vomiting

Sinusitis, acute
- Dull, periorbital headache that's typically aggravated by bending over or touching the face
- May also cause fever, malaise, nasal discharge, nasal turbinate edema, sinus tenderness, and sore throat
- Relieved by sinus drainage

Other causes
- Cervical traction
- Drugs, such as digoxin (Lanoxin), indomethacin (Indocin), isosorbide (Isordil), nitroglycerin (Nitrostat), or another vasodilator
- Herbal supplements, such as ephedra, ginseng, and St. John's wort
- Lumbar puncture
- Myelography
- Withdrawal from a vasopressor or sympathomimetic

Heartburn

- Substernal burning sensation that rises in the chest and may radiate to the neck or throat
- Also known as pyrosis
- Results from reflux of gastric contents into the esophagus
- Usually accompanied by regurgitation
- Common with pregnancy, ascites, and obesity; may also result from GI disorders, connective tissue disease, and certain drugs
- Usually develops after meals or when a person lies down, bends over, lifts heavy objects, or exercises vigorously
- Usually worsens with swallowing and improves when the person sits upright or takes antacids
- Can be mistaken for a myocardial infarction (MI), but MI usually includes additional symptoms

Health history
- When did the heartburn start? Do certain foods or beverages seem to trigger it? Does stress or fatigue seem to aggravate it? Do movement, certain body positions, or very hot or cold liquids worsen or relieve it?
- Where exactly is the burning sensation? Does it radiate to other areas? Does it cause you to regurgitate sour or bitter fluids?
- Have you ever had heartburn before? If so, what relieved it?

◆ Do you have a history of GI problems or connective tissue disease? *For women of childbearing age:* Are you pregnant?
◆ Which medications are you taking?

Physical examination

◆ Auscultate the heart and lungs to rule out a heart or lung disorder.
◆ Palpate the abdomen for abdominal pain.

Causes

Esophageal cancer

◆ Usually starts with painless dysphagia that progressively worsens
◆ Eventually causes partial obstruction and rapid weight loss
◆ May cause a feeling of substernal fullness, hoarseness, nausea, sore throat, steady pain in the anterior and posterior chest, and vomiting

Gastroesophageal reflux

◆ Most common symptom: Severe, chronic heartburn
◆ Usually occurs within 1 hour after eating and may be triggered by certain foods or beverages
◆ Worsens when the person lies down or bends over and abates when he sits, stands, or takes antacids
◆ Other findings: Dull retrosternal pain that may radiate, hypersalivation, odynophagia, dysphagia, flatulent dyspepsia, and postural regurgitation

Peptic ulcer

◆ Peptic ulcer attack: Usually starts with heartburn and indigestion
◆ Usually a gnawing, burning pain in the left epigastrium; sometimes sharp pain
◆ Pain that typically occurs when the stomach is empty and is relieved by antacids
◆ Pain that may be aggravated by coffee, alcohol, or aspirin ingestion

Scleroderma

◆ A connective tissue disease that may cause esophageal dysfunction, resulting in heartburn, bloating after meals, odynophagia, the sensation of food sticking behind the sternum, and weight loss
◆ Other GI effects: Abdominal distention, constipation or diarrhea, and malodorous, floating stools

Other causes

◆ Certain drugs, such as anticholinergics, aspirin, inhaled beta-adrenergic blockers, inhaled corticosteroids, nonsteroidal anti-inflammatory drugs
◆ Esophageal diverticula
◆ Obesity

Hematuria

◆ Blood in the urine
◆ Cardinal sign of renal and urinary tract disorders
◆ May be visible or occult, which needs confirmation by a urine test
◆ Dark or brownish blood: Renal or upper urinary tract bleeding
◆ Bright red blood: Lower urinary tract bleeding
◆ May reflect continuous or intermittent bleeding
◆ Commonly accompanied by pain
◆ May be aggravated by prolonged standing or walking

Health history

◆ When did you first notice blood in your urine? Does it appear every time you urinate? Are you passing any clots? Does your urine have a foul odor? Have you ever had this problem before?
◆ Do you have any pain? If so, does the pain occur only when you urinate, or is it continuous? On a scale of 0 to 10, with 0 being no pain and 10 being the worst pain imaginable, rate the pain.

◆ Do you have bleeding hemorrhoids? Have you had recent trauma or performed strenuous exercise? Do you have a history of renal, urinary, prostatic, or coagulation disorders? *For female patients:* Are you menstruating?
◆ Which medications are you taking?

Physical examination
◆ Check the urinary meatus for bleeding or abnormalities.
◆ Palpate the abdomen and flanks, noting pain or tenderness.

Causes
Bladder cancer
◆ Primary cause of gross hematuria in men
◆ May produce pain in the bladder, rectum, pelvis, flank, back, or legs
◆ May cause signs of urinary tract infection

Calculi, bladder and renal
◆ Bladder calculi: Usually gross hematuria, pain referred to the penile or vulvar areas and, in some patients, bladder distention
◆ Renal calculi: Either microscopic or gross hematuria
◆ Possible signs and symptoms of urinary tract infection

Glomerulonephritis
◆ Acute form: Typically starts with gross hematuria, and may cause anuria or oliguria, flank and abdominal pain, and increased blood pressure
◆ Chronic form: Typically causes microscopic hematuria, generalized edema, increased blood pressure, and proteinuria

Nephritis
◆ Acute nephritis: Causes fever, a maculopapular rash, and microscopic hematuria
◆ Chronic interstitial nephritis: May cause dilute, almost colorless urine with polyuria and microscopic hematuria

Pyelonephritis, acute
◆ Typically microscopic or gross hematuria that progresses to grossly bloody hematuria
◆ Microscopic hematuria that may persist for a few months after the infection resolves
◆ Other findings: Flank pain, high fever, signs and symptoms of urinary tract infection

Renal infarction
◆ Usually gross hematuria
◆ Other symptoms: anorexia, costovertebral angle tenderness, and constant, severe flank and upper abdominal pain

Other causes
◆ Anticoagulant combined with certain herbal supplements, such as garlic and ginkgo biloba
◆ Benign prostatic hyperplasia
◆ Bladder trauma
◆ Certain drugs, such as anticoagulants; chemotherapy drugs, such as aldesleukin (Proleukin), bacillus Calmette-Guérin intravesical (TheraCys), ifosfamide (Ifex), or leuprolide (Lupron); etretinate (Tegison); and thiabendazole (Mintezol)
◆ Cystoscopy
◆ Obstructive nephropathy
◆ Polycystic kidney disease
◆ Renal biopsy
◆ Renal trauma
◆ Urethral trauma

Hemoptysis

◆ Expectoration of blood or bloody sputum from the lungs or tracheobronchial tree
◆ Usually caused by an abnormality of the tracheobronchial tree
◆ Associated with inflammatory conditions or lesions that cause erosion

and necrosis of the bronchial tissues and blood vessels
- Sometimes confused with bleeding from the mouth, throat, nasopharynx, or GI tract
- When severe, requires emergency endotracheal intubation and suctioning

Health history
- When did you begin coughing blood? How much blood or sputum are you coughing? How often?
- Did you recently have a flulike syndrome? Have you had any recent invasive pulmonary procedures or chest trauma?
- Do you smoke? Did you ever smoke? If so, how much? Have you ever been diagnosed with a cardiac, respiratory, or bleeding disorder?
- Which medications are you taking? Are you taking an anticoagulant?

Physical examination
- After checking the patient's level of consciousness, examine his nose, mouth, and pharynx for sources of bleeding.
- Observe the rate and depth of his respirations, noting breathing difficulty or abnormal breathing patterns. Also, look for abnormal chest movement, accessory muscle use, and retractions.
- Inspect the skin for central and peripheral cyanosis, diaphoresis, lesions, and pallor.
- Palpate the rate, rhythm, and intensity of the peripheral pulses. Then feel the chest, noting abnormal pulsations, diaphragmatic tenderness, and fremitus. Check for respiratory excursion.
- If the patient has a history of trauma, carefully check the position of the trachea, and note edema.
- Auscultate the lungs for crackles, rhonchi, and wheezes and the heart for bruits, gallops, murmurs, and pleural friction rubs.
- Also, monitor the patient's blood pressure and pulse pressure.

Causes
Bronchitis, chronic
- Usually a productive cough that lasts at least 3 months and leads to expectoration of blood-streaked sputum
- Other respiratory signs: Dyspnea, prolonged expiration, scattered rhonchi, wheezing

Lung abscess
- Expectoration of copious amounts of bloody, purulent, foul-smelling sputum
- Also anorexia, chills, diaphoresis, fever, headache, and pleuritic or dull chest pain
- Tubular breath sounds or crackles on auscultation
- Possible recent history of pulmonary infection or evidence of poor oral hygiene, with dental or gingival disease

Lung cancer
- Recurring hemoptysis (an early sign), varying from blood-streaked sputum to blood, caused by ulceration of the bronchus
- Related findings: Anorexia, chest pain, dyspnea, fever, productive cough, weight loss, wheezing

Pulmonary edema
- Expectoration of copious amounts of frothy, blood-tinged, pink sputum
- May also cause dyspnea and orthopnea
- Possible diffuse crackles in both lung fields and a ventricular gallop (S_3)

Tracheal trauma
- Bleeding that seems to come from the back of the throat
- Accompanying signs and symptoms: Airway occlusion, dysphagia, hoarseness, neck pain, respiratory distress

Other causes
- Bronchiectasis
- Coagulation disorders
- Cystic fibrosis
- Lung or airway injuries from diagnostic procedures
- Primary pulmonary hypertension
- Pulmonary emboli

Hoarseness

- Rough or harsh-sounding voice; may be acute or chronic
- May result from laryngeal infections or inflammatory lesions, laryngeal edema, compression or disruption of the vocal cords, recurrent laryngeal nerve damage, or polyps on the vocal cords
- May also occur with aging because laryngeal muscles and mucosa atrophy, reducing control of the vocal cords
- May be worsened by excessive alcohol intake, smoking, inhalation of noxious fumes, excessive talking, and shouting

Health history

- When did the hoarseness start? Is it constant or intermittent? Does anything relieve or worsen it? Have you been overusing your voice?
- Have you also had a cough, a dry mouth, trouble swallowing dry food, shortness of breath, or a sore throat?
- Have you ever had cancer or other disorders? Do you regularly drink alcohol or smoke? If so, how much?

Physical examination

- Inspect the patient's mouth and throat for redness or exudate, which may indicate an upper respiratory tract infection. Ask him to stick out his tongue: If he can't, the hypoglossal nerve (cranial nerve XII) may be impaired.
- As the patient breathes, look for asymmetrical chest expansion, intercostal retractions, nasal flaring, stridor, and other signs of respiratory distress.
- Palpate the patient's neck for masses and the cervical lymph nodes and thyroid gland for enlargement. Then palpate the trachea to check for deviation.
- Auscultate the lungs for crackles, rhonchi, tubular sounds, or wheezes. To detect bradycardia, auscultate the heart.

Causes

Inhalation injury
- Exposure to a fire or an explosion, which may produce coughing, hoarseness, orofacial burns, singed nasal hair, and soot-stained sputum
- Later signs and symptoms: Crackles, rhonchi, wheezes, respiratory distress

Laryngitis
- Acute laryngitis: Sudden hoarseness or complete loss of voice
- Chronic laryngitis: Persistent hoarseness
- Related findings: Cough, fever, pain (especially during swallowing or speaking), profuse diaphoresis, rhinorrhea, sore throat

Vocal cord polyps
- Raspy hoarseness
- Possible chronic cough and crackling voice

Other causes
- Hypothyroidism
- Laryngeal cancer (most common in men ages 50 to 70)
- Prolonged intubation
- Pulmonary tuberculosis
- Rheumatoid arthritis
- Surgical severing of the recurrent laryngeal nerve
- Tracheostomy

Age alert In infants and young children, hoarseness commonly stems from acute laryngotracheobronchitis (croup).

Nausea

- Profound feeling of revulsion to food or a signal of impending vomiting
- Usually accompanied by anorexia, diaphoresis, hypersalivation, pallor, tachycardia, tachypnea, and vomiting
- Common symptom of GI disorder
- May also result from electrolyte imbalances; infections; metabolic, endocrine, and cardiac disorders; early pregnancy; drug therapy; surgery; and radiation therapy
- May be triggered by severe pain, anxiety, alcohol intoxication, overeating, and ingestion of something distasteful

Health history

- When did the nausea begin? Is it intermittent or constant? How severe is it?
- Do you have other signs and symptoms, such as abdominal pain, loss of appetite, changes in bowel habits, excessive belching or gas, weight loss, or vomiting?
- Have you ever had a GI, endocrine, or metabolic disorder? Have you had any recent infections? Have you ever had cancer, radiation therapy, or chemotherapy? *For female patients:* Are you or could you be pregnant?
- Which medications are you taking? Do you drink alcohol and, if so, how much?

Physical examination

- Examine the patient's skin for bruises, jaundice, poor turgor, and spider angiomas. Inspect his abdomen for distention.
- Because palpation can affect the frequency and intensity of bowel sounds, you should auscultate the abdomen first. Listen for bowel sounds in each quadrant. Then using the bell of the stethoscope, listen for abdominal bruits.
- As you palpate the abdomen, note rigidity or tenderness.

Causes

Appendicitis
- Possible nausea and vomiting
- Vague epigastric or periumbilical discomfort that localizes to the right lower quadrant

Cholecystitis, acute
- Commonly, nausea that follows severe right upper quadrant pain that may radiate to the back or shoulders
- Associated findings: Abdominal tenderness, vomiting, possibly abdominal rigidity and distention, diaphoresis, and fever with chills

Gastritis
- Usually, nausea that follows ingestion of alcohol, aspirin, spicy foods, or caffeine
- Possible belching, epigastric pain, fever, malaise, and vomiting of mucus or blood

Other causes
- Certain drugs, such as anesthetics, antibiotics, antineoplastics, ferrous sulfate, potassium (oral), quinidine, or an overdose of a cardiac glycoside or theophylline
- Certain herbal supplements, such as ginkgo biloba and St. John's wort
- Cirrhosis
- Electrolyte imbalance
- Labyrinthitis
- Metabolic acidosis
- Myocardial infarction
- Radiation therapy
- Renal or urologic disorder
- Surgery, especially abdominal
- Ulcerative colitis

Pain, abdominal

◆ May be acute or chronic, diffuse or localized
◆ May originate in the abdominopelvic viscera, the parietal peritoneum, or the capsules of the liver, kidneys, or spleen
◆ Commonly caused by a GI disorder
◆ May stem from a reproductive, genitourinary, musculoskeletal, or vascular disorder; from drug use; or from the effect of a toxin

Health history

◆ When did your pain start? What does it feel like? How long does it last?
◆ Where exactly is it? Does it radiate to other areas, such as your chest or back? Does it get better or worse when you change position, move, exert yourself, cough, eat, or have a bowel movement?
◆ Do you have a fever during episodes of pain? Do you have appetite changes, constipation, diarrhea, nausea, pain with urination, pink or cloudy urine, vomiting, or urinary frequency or urgency?
◆ Do you have a history of adrenal disease, heart disease, recent infection, or recent blunt trauma to the abdomen, flank, or chest? Have you had any condition that could predispose you to emboli? Have you recently had a urinary tract procedure or surgery? Have you traveled to a foreign country recently?
◆ *For women of childbearing age:* What was the date of your last menses? Has your menstrual pattern changed? Could you be pregnant?
◆ Have you ever used I.V. drugs? Do you drink alcohol? If so, how much and how often? Which prescription drugs do you take?

Physical examination

◆ After checking the patient's level of consciousness, check the skin for diaphoresis, jaundice, and turgor. Then check for coolness, discoloration, and edema of the arms and legs.
◆ Inspect the abdomen and chest for signs of trauma: A bluish discoloration around the umbilicus (Cullen's sign) and around the flank area (Turner's sign) can indicate blunt trauma. Obtain and record a baseline measurement of abdominal girth at the umbilicus.
◆ After inspecting for jugular vein distention, observe the rate and depth of respirations, noting abnormal patterns. Observe the color and odor of the patient's urine.
◆ Because palpation can affect the frequency and intensity of bowel sounds, you should auscultate the abdomen first. Listen for bowel sounds in each quadrant, noting whether the sounds are high-pitched and tinkling, hyperactive, or absent.
◆ Listen to the patient's heart and breath sounds for abnormalities. Also, monitor blood and pulse pressures.
◆ As you systematically palpate the abdominal, pelvic, and epigastric areas, note masses, rigidity, tenderness, or tenderness with guarding. *Note:* Don't palpate if you suspect a dissecting abdominal aortic aneurysm.
◆ Check the patient's peripheral pulses for rate, rhythm, and intensity.

Causes

Abdominal aortic aneurysm, dissecting

◆ Constant, dull upper-abdominal pain radiating to the lower back caused by rapid enlargement of the aneurysm and possible rupture
◆ Before rupture, a palpable, pulsating epigastric mass
◆ Systolic bruit that can be auscultated over the aneurysm

- Possible abdominal rigidity, increasing abdominal girth, and signs of hypovolemic shock

Abdominal trauma
- Generalized or localized abdominal pain with abdominal ecchymosis, abdominal tenderness, or vomiting
- If patient is hemorrhaging into the peritoneal cavity, possible abdominal rigidity and increasing abdominal girth
- If an abdominal organ has been perforated, possible hollow bowel sounds or absent bowel sounds
- Probable diaphragmatic tear if bowel sounds can be heard in the chest cavity

Appendicitis
- Sudden pain in the epigastric or umbilical region that increases over a few hours or days, along with flulike symptoms
- Pain (dull or severe) preceded by anorexia, constipation or diarrhea, nausea, and vomiting
- Pain that localizes at McBurney's point in the lower right quadrant
- Possible abdominal rigidity and rebound tenderness

Ectopic pregnancy
- Lower abdominal pain that may be sharp, dull, or cramping, and either constant or intermittent
- May be accompanied by breast tenderness, nausea, vaginal bleeding, vomiting, urinary frequency
- Typically a 1- to 2-month history of amenorrhea
- If the fallopian tube ruptures, sharp lower-abdominal pain that may radiate to the shoulders and neck and become extreme on cervical or adnexal palpation

Hepatitis
- Discomfort or dull pain and tenderness in the right upper quadrant from liver enlargement

Intestinal obstruction
- Short episodes of intense, colicky, cramping pain alternating with pain-free periods

Pancreatitis
- Fulminating, continuous, upper abdominal pain that may radiate to both flanks and to the back

Renal calculi
- Classic symptom: Colicky pain that travels from the costovertebral angle to the flank, suprapubic region, and external genitalia
- Depending on location of calculi, severe abdominal or back pain

Other causes
- Adrenal crisis
- Cholecystitis
- Diabetic ketoacidosis
- Diverticulitis
- Heart failure
- Hepatic abscess
- Mesenteric artery ischemia
- Myocardial infarction
- Nonsteroidal anti-inflammatory drugs
- Ovarian cyst
- Perforated ulcer
- Peritonitis
- Pneumonia
- Pneumothorax
- Pyelonephritis
- Renal infarction
- Salicylate use
- Splenic infarction

Pain, back

- May be acute, chronic, constant, or intermittent

- May remain localized in the back or may radiate along the spine or down one or both legs
- May be worsened by activity (most commonly, stooping or lifting), eased by rest, or unaffected by either
- May be referred from the abdomen, possibly signaling a life-threatening disorder
- Intrinsic back pain: Usually from muscle spasm, nerve root irritation, fracture, or a combination; usually occurs in the lower back or lumbosacral area

Health history

- When did the pain start? What does it feel like? Is it mild, moderate, or severe? Is it constant or intermittent?
- Where exactly is the pain? Is it associated with activity? What relieves or worsens it? *For women of childbearing age:* Does the pain occur before or during your menses?
- Have you had recent episodes of abdominal tenderness or rigidity, fever, nausea, or vomiting? Do you feel unusual sensations in your legs? Have you had urinary frequency or urgency or painful urination?
- Do you have a history of trauma, back surgery, or urinary tract surgery, procedures, obstructions, or infections?
- Which medications are you taking?

Physical examination

- Observe the rate and depth of respirations, noting breathing difficulty or abnormal breathing patterns.
- Check the skin for diaphoresis, discoloration, edema, mottling, and pallor. Then inspect the back, legs, and abdomen for signs of trauma.
- After you check for abdominal distention, measure baseline abdominal girth.
- Because palpation can affect the frequency and intensity of bowel sounds, you should auscultate the abdomen first. Listen for bowel sounds in each quadrant. Then listen over the abdominal aorta for bruits and over the lungs for crackles.
- Palpate the abdominal, epigastric, and pelvic areas for abdominal rigidity, masses, and tenderness. Don't palpate deeply.
- Check the patient's blood and pulse pressures.
- Check the peripheral pulses for rate, rhythm, and intensity.
- Gently palpate the painful area, noting contractions, excessive muscle tone, or spasm. *Note:* Don't palpate if you suspect a dissecting abdominal aortic aneurysm.

Causes

Abdominal aortic aneurysm, dissecting

- Lower back pain and dull upper abdominal pain from a rapidly enlarging aneurysm and early stages of rupture
- Possible tenderness over the area of the aneurysm as well as a pulsating epigastric mass
- Other signs: Absent femoral and pedal pulses, mottled skin below the waist, signs of hypovolemic shock

Pancreatitis

- Fulminating, continuous abdominal pain that may radiate to the back and both flanks
- Possible abdominal tenderness, rigidity, and distention; fever; hypoactive bowel sounds; pallor; tachycardia; and vomiting
- History: Possible alcohol abuse, use of a thiazide diuretic, gallbladder disease, or trauma

Pyelonephritis, acute

- Progressive back pain or flank tenderness with costovertebral angle pain and abdominal pain in one or two quadrants

◆ Also dysuria, high fever, hematuria, nocturia, shaking chills, vomiting, urinary frequency and urgency
◆ May follow a recent urinary tract procedure, urinary tract infection or obstruction, compromised renal function, or neurogenic bladder

Other causes
◆ Appendicitis
◆ Cholecystitis
◆ Herniated disk
◆ Lumbosacral sprain
◆ Osteoporosis
◆ Perforated ulcer
◆ Renal calculi
◆ Tumor
◆ Vertebral osteomyelitis

Pain, chest

◆ Variable description: Dull ache, sensation of heaviness or fullness, feeling of indigestion, or sharp, shooting pain
◆ May be constant or intermittent, may radiate to other body parts, and may arise suddenly or gradually
◆ May indicate several acute and life-threatening cardiopulmonary and GI conditions
◆ May be triggered by stress, anxiety, exertion, deep breathing, or certain foods
◆ May result from musculoskeletal disorders, hematologic disorders, anxiety, and use of certain drugs

Health history
◆ When did the chest pain begin? Did it develop suddenly or gradually? Is the pain localized or diffuse? Does it radiate to your neck, jaw, arms, or back?
◆ Is the pain sharp and stabbing or dull and aching? Is it constant or intermittent? Does breathing, changing positions, or eating certain foods worsen or relieve it? Have you recently taken any medication to relieve chest pain?
◆ Do you have other signs and symptoms, such as coughing, shortness of breath, sweating, headache, nausea, palpitations, vomiting, or weakness?
◆ Have you ever had cardiac or respiratory disease, cardiac surgery, chest trauma, or intestinal disease? Do you have a family history of cardiac disease?
◆ Do you drink alcohol or use illicit drugs? Which medications are you taking?

Physical examination
◆ Check the patient's skin temperature, color, and general appearance, noting coolness, cyanosis, diaphoresis, mottling below the waist, pallor, peripheral edema, and prolonged capillary refill time. Look for facial edema, jugular vein distention, and tracheal deviation. Note signs of altered LOC, anxiety, dizziness, and restlessness.
◆ Observe the rate and depth of the patient's respirations, noting abnormal patterns or trouble breathing. If the patient has a productive cough, examine the sputum.
◆ Palpate the patient's neck, chest, and abdomen. Note asymmetrical chest expansion, masses, subcutaneous crepitation, tender areas, tracheal deviation, and tactile fremitus. Also palpate his peripheral pulses, and record their rate, rhythm, and intensity.
◆ Auscultate the lungs to identify crackles, diminished or absent breath sounds, pleural friction rubs, rhonchi, or wheezes. Auscultate the heart for clicks, gallops, murmurs, and a pericardial friction rub. To check for abdominal bruits, apply the bell of the stethoscope over the abdominal aorta.
◆ Monitor the patient's blood pressure closely.

Causes
Angina
◆ Usually starts gradually, builds to a peak, and subsides slowly

- May occur at rest, or may be provoked by exertion, emotional stress, or a heavy meal
- Typically lasts 2 to 10 minutes
- Usually occurs in the retrosternal region and may radiate to the neck, jaw, and arms
- Associated signs and symptoms: Diaphoresis, dyspnea, nausea, vomiting, palpitations, tachycardia
- Possible atrial gallop (S_4) or murmur

Aortic aneurysm, dissecting
- Sudden, excruciating, tearing pain in the chest and neck, radiating to the upper back, lower back, and abdomen
- Other signs and symptoms: Abdominal tenderness, heart murmur, jugular vein distention, systolic bruits, tachycardia, weak or absent femoral or pedal pulses, and pale, cool, diaphoretic, mottled skin below the waist

Cholecystitis
- Sudden epigastric or right upper quadrant pain
- May be steady or intermittent, may radiate to the back, and may be sharp or intense
- Other signs and symptoms: Chills, diaphoresis, nausea, vomiting
- Possible distention, rigidity, tenderness, and a mass on palpation of the right upper quadrant

Myocardial infarction
- Usually severe, crushing substernal pain that may radiate to the left arm, jaw, or neck
- May be accompanied by anxiety, clammy skin, diaphoresis, dyspnea, a feeling of impending doom, nausea, vomiting, pallor, restlessness
- Possible atrial gallop (S_4), crackles, hypotension, hypertension, murmur, pericardial friction rub
- Commonly a history of heart disease, hypertension, hypercholesterolemia, or cocaine abuse

Peptic ulcer
- A sharp, burning pain arising in the epigastric region, usually hours after eating
- Other signs and symptoms: Epigastric tenderness, nausea, vomiting
- Usually relieved by food or antacids

Pneumothorax
- Sudden, sharp, severe chest pain, usually unilateral, that increases with chest movement
- Possible decreased breath sounds and subcutaneous crepitation
- Other signs and symptoms: Accessory muscle use, anxiety, asymmetrical chest expansion, nonproductive cough, tachycardia, tachypnea
- History that may include chronic obstructive pulmonary disease, lung cancer, diagnostic or therapeutic procedures involving the thorax, or thoracic trauma

Pulmonary embolism
- Typically, sudden dyspnea with intense angina-like or pleuritic ischemic pain that's aggravated by deep breathing and thoracic movement
- Other findings: Anxiety, cough with blood-tinged sputum, crackles, restlessness, tachycardia
- With a large embolism, possible compromise in cardiovascular, pulmonary, and neurologic systems
- History that may include thrombophlebitis, hip or leg fracture, acute myocardial infarction, heart failure, pregnancy, or use of hormonal contraceptives

Other causes
- Abrupt withdrawal of beta-adrenergic blockers
- Acute bronchitis
- Anxiety
- Esophageal reflux
- Esophageal spasm
- Lung abscess

◆ Muscle strain
◆ Pancreatitis
◆ Pneumonia
◆ Rib fracture
◆ Tuberculosis

Palpitations

◆ Conscious awareness of one's own heartbeat
◆ Usually felt over the precordium or in the throat or neck
◆ May feel like pounding, jumping, turning, fluttering, flopping, missing, or skipping heartbeats
◆ May be regular or irregular, fast or slow, and paroxysmal or sustained
◆ Besides cardiac causes, may stem from anxiety, drug reactions, hypertension, thyroid hormone deficiency, or other causes

Health history

◆ When did the palpitations start? Where do you feel them? How would you describe them? What were you doing when they started? How long did they last? Have you ever had palpitations before?
◆ Do you have chest pain, dizziness, or weakness with the palpitations?
◆ Are you under unusual stress at home or at work? Have you recently had multiple blood transfusions or an infusion of phosphate?
◆ Have you ever had thyroid disease, calcium or vitamin D deficiency, malabsorption syndrome, bone cancer, renal disease, hypoglycemia, or cardiovascular or pulmonary disorders that may produce arrhythmias or hypertension?
◆ Which medications are you taking? Are you taking an over-the-counter drug that contains caffeine or a sympathomimetic, such as a cough, cold, or allergy medication? Do you smoke or drink alcohol? If so, how much?

Physical examination

◆ Check the patient's level of consciousness, noting anxiety, confusion, or irrational behavior.
◆ Check the skin for pallor and diaphoresis, and observe the patient's eyes for exophthalmos.
◆ Note the rate and depth of respirations, checking for abnormal patterns and trouble breathing. Also inspect the fingertips for capillary nail bed pulsations.
◆ To check for thyroid gland enlargement, gently palpate the patient's neck. Then palpate the muscles for weakness and twitching.
◆ Evaluate the patient's peripheral pulses, noting the rate, rhythm, and intensity. Check the reflexes for hyperreflexia.
◆ Auscultate the heart for gallops and murmurs and the lungs for abnormal breath sounds. Also monitor blood and pulse pressures.

Causes

Acute anxiety attack

◆ Palpitations typically accompanied by diaphoresis, facial flushing, and trembling
◆ Usually includes hyperventilation, which may lead to dizziness, syncope, and weakness

Cardiac arrhythmias

◆ Paroxysmal or sustained palpitations with dizziness, fatigue, and weakness
◆ Other signs and symptoms: Chest pain, confusion, decreased blood pressure, diaphoresis, pallor, and an irregular, rapid, or slow pulse rate
◆ Possible history of taking a drug that can cause cardiac arrhythmias — such as an antihypertensive, a sympathomimetic, a ganglionic blocker, an anticholinergic, or a methylxanthine

Thyrotoxicosis

- Sustained palpitations that may accompany diaphoresis, diarrhea, dyspnea, heat intolerance, nervousness, tachycardia, tremors, and weight loss despite increased appetite
- Possible exophthalmos and enlarged thyroid gland

Other causes

- Anemia
- Aortic insufficiency
- Certain herbal supplements, such as ginseng and ephedra
- Hypertension
- Hypocalcemia
- Hypoglycemia
- Mitral valve stenosis or prolapse
- Pheochromocytoma

Paresthesia

- An abnormal sensation — commonly described as numbness, prickling, or tingling — felt along the peripheral nerve pathways
- May develop suddenly or gradually, and may be transient or permanent
- A common symptom of many neurologic disorders
- May also occur in certain systemic disorders and with use of certain drugs

Health history

- When did the paresthesia begin? What does it feel like? Where does it occur? Does it come and go, or is it constant?
- Have you had recent trauma, surgery, or an invasive procedure that may have injured the peripheral nerves?
- Have you been exposed to industrial solvents or heavy metals? Have you had long-term radiation therapy?
- Do you have a neurologic, cardiovascular, metabolic, renal, or chronic inflammatory disorder, such as arthritis or lupus erythematosus?
- Which medications are you taking?

Physical examination

- Focus on the patient's neurologic status, checking level of consciousness. Also note the patient's skin color and temperature.
- Test muscle strength and deep tendon reflexes in extremities affected by paresthesia.
- Systematically evaluate light touch, pain, temperature, vibration, and position sensation. Then palpate the pulses.

Causes

Arterial occlusion, acute

- Typically, sudden paresthesia and coldness in one or both legs, aching pain at rest, intermittent claudication, and paresis
- Line of temperature and color demarcation at the level of the occlusion, and a mottled leg below
- Absent pulses below the occlusion, with slow capillary refill time

Brain tumor

- Tumor that affects the parietal lobe: Progressive contralateral paresthesia accompanied by agnosia, anomia, agraphia, apraxia, homonymous hemianopsia, and loss of proprioception

Herniated cervical or lumbar disk

- Acute or gradual paresthesia in the dermatome of the affected spinal nerves
- Other neuromuscular effects: Muscle spasms, severe pain, weakness

Herpes zoster

- Early symptom: Paresthesia in the dermatome supplied by the affected spinal nerve
- Within several days, pruritic, erythematous, vesicular rash with sharp, shooting pain

Spinal cord injury

- In partial spinal cord transection, paresthesia after spinal shock resolves

- May be unilateral or bilateral
- May occur at or below the level of the lesion

Other causes
- Arthritis
- Certain drugs, such as chemotherapy drugs, guanadrel (Hylorel), interferons, and isoniazid (Laniazid)
- Hypocalcemia
- Migraine headache
- Multiple sclerosis
- Parenteral gold therapy
- Peripheral neuropathies
- Poisoning by heavy metal or solvent
- Radiation therapy (long-term)
- Stroke
- Vitamin B_{12} deficiency

Rash, papular

- Small, raised, circumscribed, possibly discolored lesions
- May occur anywhere on the body and in various configurations
- Characteristic sign of many cutaneous disorders
- May also result from allergies or from infectious, neoplastic, or systemic disorders

Age alert In bedridden elderly patients, an erythematous area, sometimes with firm papules, may be the first sign of a developing pressure ulcer.

Health history
- When and where did the rash start? What did it look like? Has it spread or changed in any way? If so, when and how did it spread? Have you recently changed soaps, lotions, or detergents?
- Does the rash itch or burn? Is it painful or tender?
- Have you had a fever, GI distress, or headache? Do you have allergies? Have you had skin disorders, infections, sexually transmitted diseases, or tumors? What childhood diseases have you had?
- Have you recently been bitten by an insect or a rodent? Have you been exposed to anyone with an infectious disease?
- Which medications are you taking? Have you applied topical medications to the rash and, if so, when was the last application?

Physical examination
- Observe the color, configuration, and location of the rash.

Causes
Acne vulgaris
- Inflamed and possibly painful pruritic papules, pustules, nodules, or cysts from rupture of enlarged comedones
- May appear on the face, shoulders, chest, or back

Insect bites
- Allergic reaction to insect venom — especially of ticks, lice, flies, and mosquitoes — that causes a papular, macular, or petechial rash
- Associated findings: Fever, headache, lymphadenopathy, myalgia, nausea, vomiting

Kaposi's sarcoma
- A neoplastic disorder most common among patients with acquired immunodeficiency syndrome
- Produces purple or blue papules or macules on the extremities, ears, and nose
- Lesions that decrease in size with firm pressure but that return to original size in 10 to 15 seconds
- Lesions that may become scaly, ulcerate, and bleed

Psoriasis
- Small, erythematous, pruritic papules on scalp, chest, elbows, knees, back, buttocks, and genitalia that may be painful

◆ Papules that enlarge and coalesce, forming red, elevated plaques covered by silver scales, except in moist areas such as the genitalia
◆ Scales that may flake off easily or may thicken, covering the plaque
◆ Other common findings: Pitted fingernails and arthralgia

Other causes
◆ Adverse effect of succimer (Chemet) treatment for lead poisoning
◆ Infectious mononucleosis
◆ Interferons
◆ Nonsteroidal anti-inflammatory drugs
◆ Sarcoidosis

Rash, pustular

◆ Crops of pustules (small, elevated, circumscribed lesions), vesicles (small blisters), and bullae (large blisters) filled with purulent exudate
◆ Lesions that vary in size and shape and may be generalized or localized (limited to hair follicles or sweat glands)
◆ Caused by skin disorders, systemic disorders, ingestion of certain drugs, and exposure to skin irritants
◆ Although commonly sterile, usually indicates infection

Health history
◆ When and where did the rash erupt? Did another type of skin lesion precede the pustules? Have you recently changed soaps, lotions, or detergents?
◆ What does the rash look like? Has it spread or changed in any way? If so, how and where did it spread?
◆ Have you or has a family member ever had a skin disorder or allergies?
◆ Which medications are you taking? Have you applied topical medication to the rash and, if so, when did you last apply it?

Physical examination
◆ Examine the entire skin surface, noting if it's dry, oily, moist, or greasy.
◆ Record the exact location, distribution, color, shape, and size of the lesions.

Causes
Folliculitis
◆ Bacterial infection of hair follicles
◆ Produces individual pustules, each pierced by a hair, possibly pruritic
◆ Hot-tub folliculitis: Pustules on areas normally covered by a bathing suit

Scabies
◆ Threadlike channels or burrows under the skin, possibly with pustules, vesicles, and excoriation
◆ Lesions that are 1 to 10 cm long with a swollen nodule or red papule containing the itch mite
◆ Common sites: Wrists, elbows, axillae, and waist
◆ *Men:* Commonly crusted lesions on the glans and shaft of the penis and on the scrotum
◆ *Women:* Possible lesions on nipples

Other causes
◆ Acne vulgaris
◆ Blastomycosis
◆ Certain drugs, such as bromides, corticosteroids, corticotropin, iodides, hormonal contraceptives, isoniazid (Laniazid), lithium (Eskalith), phenobarbital (Luminal), and phenytoin (Dilantin)
◆ Furunculosis
◆ Pustular psoriasis

Rash, vesicular

◆ Scattered lesions or linear vesicles that are sharply circumscribed and usually less than 0.5 cm in diameter
◆ Bullae: Lesions larger than 0.5 cm in diameter
◆ May be filled with clear, cloudy, or bloody fluid

◆ May be mild or severe, transient or permanent

Health history

◆ When and where did the rash erupt? Did other skin lesions precede the vesicles?
◆ What does the rash look like? Has it spread or changed in any way? If so, how and where did it spread?
◆ Do you or anyone in your family have a history of allergies or skin disorders?
◆ Have you recently had an infection or been bitten by an insect?

Physical examination

◆ Examine the patient's skin and note the location, general distribution, color, shape, and size of the lesions. Check for crusts, macules, papules, scales, scars, and wheals.
◆ Note whether the outer layer of epidermis separates easily from the basal layer.
◆ Palpate the vesicles or bullae to determine whether they're flaccid or tense.

Causes

Burns

◆ Common in thermal burns that affect the epidermis and part of the dermis
◆ Typically produce vesicles and bullae with erythema, moistness, pain, and swelling

Herpes zoster

◆ Fever and malaise followed by development of vesicular rash along a dermatome
◆ Rash accompanied by pruritus, deep pain, and paresthesia or hyperesthesia, usually of the trunk and sometimes of the arms and legs
◆ Vesicles that erupt, dry up, and form scabs in about 10 days
◆ Occasionally involves the cranial nerves, which produces dizziness, eye pain, facial palsy, hearing loss, impaired vision, and loss of taste

Other causes

◆ Dermatitis
◆ Herpes simplex
◆ Insect bites
◆ Pemphigus
◆ Scabies
◆ Tinea pedis
◆ Toxic epidermal necrolysis

Vision loss

◆ May range from slight impairment to total blindness
◆ May be sudden or gradual, temporary or permanent
◆ May result from eye, neurologic, and systemic disorders as well as from trauma and reactions to certain drugs

Health history

◆ When did your vision loss first occur? Was it sudden or gradual? Does it affect one eye or both eyes? Does it affect all or part of the visual field?
◆ Do you have blurred vision, halo vision, nausea, pain, photosensitivity, or vomiting with the vision loss?
◆ Have you had a recent injury to your face or eyes?
◆ Have you ever had a cardiovascular or endocrine disorder, an infection, or allergies? Does anyone in your family have a history of vision loss or other eye problems?
◆ Which medications are you taking?

Physical examination

◆ Examine the patient's eyes for conjunctival or scleral redness, drainage, edema, foreign bodies, and signs of trauma
◆ With a flashlight, examine the cornea and iris. Observe the size, shape, and color of the pupils.

◆ Test direct and consensual light reflexes, visual accommodation, extraocular muscle function, and visual acuity.
◆ Gently palpate each eye, noting hardness. Auscultate over the neck and temple for carotid bruits.

Causes

Eye trauma

◆ Sudden unilateral or bilateral vision loss
◆ May be total or partial, permanent or temporary
◆ May cause reddened, edematous, lacerated eyelids

Glaucoma

◆ Acute angle-closure glaucoma: Halo vision, nonreactive pupillary response, photophobia, rapid onset of unilateral inflammation and pain, and reduced visual acuity; may cause blindness rapidly
◆ Chronic open-angle glaucoma: Usually bilateral aching eyes, halo vision, peripheral vision loss, and reduced visual acuity; progresses slowly

Other causes

◆ Certain drugs, such as cardiac glycosides, ethambutol (Myambutol), indomethacin (Indocin), and methanol
◆ Congenital rubella or syphilis
◆ Herpes zoster
◆ Marfan's syndrome
◆ Pituitary tumor
◆ Retrolental fibroplasia

Visual floaters

◆ Particles of blood or cellular debris that move about in the vitreous humor and appear as spots or dots when they enter the visual field
◆ Prevalent among elderly and myopic patients
◆ May reflect retinal detachment, an ocular emergency, if sudden or prominent

Health history

◆ When did the floaters first appear? What do they look like? Did they appear suddenly or gradually? If they appeared suddenly, did you also see flashing lights and have a curtainlike loss of vision?
◆ Are you nearsighted, and do you wear corrective lenses?
◆ Do you have a history of eye trauma or other eye disorders, allergies, granulomatous disease, diabetes mellitus, or hypertension?
◆ Which medications are you taking?

Physical examination

◆ Inspect the eyes for signs of injury, such as bruising or edema.
◆ Determine the patient's visual acuity using a Snellen chart or an E chart.

Causes

Retinal detachment

◆ Sudden floaters and flashing lights in the portion of the visual field where the retina has detached
◆ Sensation (painless) of a dark curtain falling in front of the vision
◆ Ophthalmoscopic examination: Gray, opaque, detached retina with an indefinite margin and retinal vessels that appear almost black

Vitreous hemorrhage

◆ Rupture of the retinal vessels
◆ Shower of red or black dots or a red haze across the visual field
◆ Sudden blurred vision in affected eye, possibly with greatly reduced acuity

Other causes

◆ Posterior uveitis

Weight gain

◆ Increased adipose tissue from ingestion of more calories than body needs for energy expenditure

- Commonly related to emotional factors — most commonly anxiety, guilt, and depression — and social factors
- May reflect fluid retention and resulting edema
- Among elderly people, typically reflects sustained food intake despite normal, progressive decline in basal metabolic rate
- Among women, may reflect pregnancy (progressive weight gain) or menstrual cycle (cyclic weight gain)
- Primary sign of many endocrine disorders
- Also occurs with conditions that limit activity, especially cardiovascular and pulmonary disorders
- May result from drug therapy that increases appetite or causes fluid retention or from cardiovascular, hepatic, and renal disorders that cause edema

Health history

- Do you have past patterns of weight gain and loss?
- Do you have a family history of obesity, thyroid disease, or diabetes mellitus?
- Describe your eating habits. Has your appetite increased?
- Do you exercise regularly or at all?
- Have you experienced vision disturbances, hoarseness, paresthesia, or increased urination and thirst?
- Have you had any episodes of impotence?
- *For women:* Have you had menstrual irregularities or experienced weight gain during menstruation? Are you pregnant?
- Have you felt anxious or depressed?
- Are you having trouble with your memory?
- Which medications are you taking?

Physical examination

- Measure skin-fold thickness to estimate fat reserves.
- Note fat distribution, localized or generalized edema, and overall nutritional status.
- Look for other abnormalities, such as abnormal body hair distribution or hair loss and dry skin.
- Take and record the patient's vital signs.

Causes

Acromegaly

- Moderate weight gain
- Other findings: Coarsened facial features, prognathism, enlarged hands and feet, increased sweating, oily skin, deep voice, back and joint pain, lethargy, sleepiness, heat intolerance, occasionally hirsutism

Diabetes mellitus

- Increased appetite
- Other findings: Fatigue, polydipsia, polyuria, nocturia, weakness, polyphagia, somnolence

Heart failure

- Edema despite anorexia
- Other typical findings: Paroxysmal nocturnal dyspnea, orthopnea, fatigue

Hypercortisolism

- Excessive weight gain, usually over the trunk and the back of the neck (buffalo hump)
- Other cushingoid features: Slender limbs, moon face, weakness, purple striae, emotional lability, increased susceptibility to infection.
- *Men:* Possible gynecomastia
- *Women:* Possible hirsutism, acne, menstrual irregularities

Hyperinsulinism

- Increased appetite
- Possible emotional lability, indigestion, weakness, diaphoresis, tachycardia, vision disturbances, syncope

Hypogonadism

◆ Prepubertal: Eunuchoid body proportions with relatively sparse facial and body hair and a high-pitched voice

◆ Postpubertal: Loss of libido, impotence, infertility

Hypothalamic dysfunction

◆ Conditions such as Laurence-Moon-Biedl syndrome

◆ Voracious appetite with subsequent weight gain, altered body temperature and sleep rhythms

Hypothyroidism

◆ Weight gain despite anorexia

◆ Related signs and symptoms: Fatigue; cold intolerance; constipation; menorrhagia; slowed intellectual and motor activity; dry, pale, cool skin; dry, sparse hair; thick, brittle nails

◆ Possible myalgia, hoarseness, hypoactive deep tendon reflexes, bradycardia, and abdominal distention

◆ Eventually, a dull facial expression with periorbital edema

Nephrotic syndrome

◆ Weight gain from edema

◆ Severe cases: Anasarca, which increases body weight up to 50% and may include abdominal distention, orthostatic hypotension, lethargy

Pancreatic islet cell tumor

◆ Excessive hunger that leads to weight gain

◆ Other findings: Emotional lability, weakness, malaise, fatigue, restlessness, diaphoresis, palpitations, tachycardia, vision disturbances, syncope

Preeclampsia

◆ Rapid weight gain that exceeds the normal weight gain of pregnancy

◆ May cause nausea, vomiting, epigastric pain, elevated blood pressure, blurred vision, double vision

Sheehan's syndrome

◆ Possible weight gain

◆ Most common in women with severe obstetric hemorrhage

Other causes

◆ Drugs that cause fluid retention and increased appetite, such as corticosteroids, phenothiazines, and tricyclic antidepressants

◆ Other drugs, such as cyproheptadine, which increases appetite; hormonal contraceptives, which cause fluid retention; and lithium, which can induce hypothyroidism

◆ Nonpathologic causes: Poor eating habits, sedentary recreation, and emotional problems, especially among adolescents

Age alert Weight gain in children can result from an endocrine disorder such as hypercortisolism. Other causes include inactivity caused by Prader-Willi syndrome, Down syndrome, Werdnig-Hoffmann disease, late stages of muscular dystrophy, and severe cerebral palsy.

Weight loss

◆ May reflect decreased food intake, increased metabolic requirements, or a combination of the two

◆ May result from endocrine, neoplastic, GI, and psychological disorders; nutritional deficiency; infection; and neurologic lesions that cause paralysis and dysphagia

◆ May accompany conditions that prevent sufficient food intake, such as painful oral lesions, ill-fitting dentures, and tooth loss

◆ May stem from poverty, adherence to fad diets, excessive exercise, or drug use

Health history

◆ When did you first notice that you were losing weight? How much weight

have you lost? Was the loss intentional? If not, can you think of any reason for it?
- What do you usually eat in a day? Have your eating habits changed recently? Why?
- Have your stools changed recently? For instance, have you noticed bulky, floating stools, or have you had diarrhea? What about abdominal pain, excessive thirst, excessive urination, heat intolerance, nausea, or vomiting?
- Have you felt anxious or depressed? If so, why?
- Which medications are you taking? Do you take diet pills or laxatives to lose weight?

Physical examination

- Record the patient's height and weight. As you take vital signs, note the patient's general appearance. Does he appear well-nourished? Do his clothes fit? Is muscle wasting evident?
- Next, examine the skin for turgor and abnormal pigmentation, especially around the joints. Do you see jaundice or pallor?
- Examine the patient's mouth, including the condition of teeth or dentures. Also, check the eyes for exophthalmos and the neck for swelling.
- Finally, palpate the patient's abdomen for liver enlargement, masses, and tenderness.

Causes

Anorexia nervosa
- A psychogenic disorder most common in young women
- Characterized by severe, self-imposed weight loss
- May include amenorrhea, blotchy or sallow skin, cold intolerance, constipation, frequent infections, loss of fatty tissue, loss of scalp hair, and skeletal muscle atrophy

Cancer
- Commonly causes weight loss
- Associated signs and symptoms based on type, location, and stage of tumor
- Typically causes abnormal bleeding, anorexia, fatigue, nausea, pain, a palpable mass, and vomiting

Crohn's disease
- Weight loss accompanied by abdominal pain, anorexia, and chronic intestinal cramping
- Other findings: Abdominal distention, tenderness, and guarding; diarrhea; hyperactive bowel sounds; pain; tachycardia

Depression
- Possible weight loss, anorexia, apathy, fatigue, feelings of worthlessness, and insomnia or hypersomnia
- Other signs and symptoms: Incoherence, indecisiveness, suicidal thoughts or behavior

Leukemia
- Acute leukemia: Progressive weight loss with bleeding tendencies, high fever, and severe prostration
- Chronic leukemia: Progressive weight loss with anemia, anorexia, bleeding, enlarged spleen, fatigue, fever, pallor, and skin eruptions

Other causes
- Adrenal insufficiency
- Certain drugs, such as amphetamines, chemotherapy drugs, laxatives, and thyroid treatments
- Cryptosporidiosis
- Diabetes mellitus
- Gastroenteritis
- Lymphoma
- Thyrotoxicosis
- Ulcerative colitis

5 Common disorders

Alzheimer's disease

Overview

- Degenerative disorder of the cerebral cortex, especially the frontal lobe
- Accounts for more than 50% of all cases of dementia
- Poor prognosis
- No cure or definitive treatment

Causes
- Unknown

Risk factors
Neurochemical
- Neurotransmitter deficiency

Environmental
- Aluminum and manganese
- Trauma
- Genetic abnormality on chromosome 21
- Slow-growing central nervous system viruses

Data collection

History
- History obtained from a family member or caregiver
- Insidious onset
- Almost imperceptible initial changes
- Forgetfulness and subtle memory loss
- Recent memory loss
- Difficulty learning and remembering new information
- Decline in personal hygiene
- Inability to concentrate
- Tendency toward repetitive actions and restlessness
- Negative personality changes (irritability, depression, paranoia, hostility)
- Nocturnal awakening
- Disorientation
- Suspicion and fear of imaginary people and situations
- Misperception of environment
- Misidentification of objects and people
- Complaints of stolen or misplaced objects
- Labile emotions
- Mood swings, sudden angry outbursts, and sleep disturbances

Physical findings
- Impaired sense of smell (usually an early symptom)
- Impaired stereognosis
- Gait disorders
- Tremors
- Loss of recent memory
- Positive snout reflex
- Organic brain disease in adults
- Urinary or fecal incontinence
- Seizures

Diagnostic tests
- Diagnosis of exclusion
- Tests to rule out other diseases
- Positive diagnosis only with autopsy

Imaging
- Position emission tomography shows metabolic activity of the cerebral cortex.
- Computed tomography scan shows excessive and progressive brain atrophy.
- Magnetic resonance imaging rules out intracranial lesions.
- Cerebral blood flow studies show abnormalities in blood flow to the brain.

Diagnostic procedures
- Cerebrospinal fluid analysis shows chronic neurologic infection.
- EEG evaluates the brain's electrical activity and may show slowing of brain waves in the late stages of the disease.

Other

◆ Neuropsychologic tests may show impaired cognitive ability and reasoning.

Treatment

General

◆ Behavioral interventions (patient-centered or caregiver training) focused on managing cognitive and behavioral changes
◆ Well-balanced diet (may need to be monitored)
◆ Safe activities, as tolerated (may need to be monitored)

Medications

◆ Anticholinesterase agents
◆ Anticonvulsants (experimental)
◆ Antidepressants
◆ Anti-inflammatories (experimental)
◆ Anxiolytics
◆ Cerebral vasodilators
◆ Neurolytics
◆ N-methyl-D-aspartate antagonist
◆ Psychostimulators
◆ Vitamin E

Nursing interventions

◆ Provide an effective communication system.
◆ Use soft tones and a slow, calm manner when speaking to the patient.
◆ Allow the patient enough time to answer questions.
◆ Protect the patient from injury.
◆ Provide rest periods.
◆ Provide an exercise program.
◆ Encourage independence.
◆ Offer frequent toileting.
◆ Assist with hygiene and dressing.
◆ Give prescribed drugs.
◆ Provide familiar objects to help with orientation and behavior control.
◆ Monitor fluid intake, nutritional status, and safety.

Patient teaching

◆ Be sure to cover:
- the disease process
- the exercise regimen
- the importance of cutting food and providing finger foods, if indicated
- the need to use plates with rim guards, built-up utensils, and cups with lids
- promotion of independence.

◆ Refer the patient (and his family or caregivers) to the Alzheimer's Association.
◆ Refer the patient (and his family or caregivers) to a local support group.
◆ Refer the patient (and his family or caregivers) to social services for additional support.

Arterial occlusive disease

Overview

◆ Obstruction or narrowing of the lumen of the aorta and its major branches
◆ May affect the carotid, vertebral, innominate, subclavian, femoral, iliac, renal, mesenteric, and celiac arteries
◆ Prognosis depends on the location of the occlusion and the development of collateral circulation

Causes

◆ Atheromatous debris (plaques)
◆ Atherosclerosis
◆ Direct blunt or penetrating trauma
◆ Embolism
◆ Fibromuscular disease
◆ Immune arteritis
◆ Indwelling arterial catheter
◆ Raynaud's disease
◆ Thromboangiitis obliterans
◆ Thrombosis

Risk factors

- Advanced age
- Diabetes mellitus
- Dyslipidemia
- Hypertension
- Smoking

Data collection

History

- One or more risk factors
- Family history of vascular disease
- Intermittent claudication
- Pain on resting
- Poor healing of wounds or ulcers
- Impotence
- Dizziness or near syncope
- Symptoms of transient ischemic attack

Physical findings

- Trophic changes of the affected arm or leg
- Diminished or absent pulses in the affected arm or leg
- Ischemic ulcers
- Pallor with elevation of the affected arm or leg
- Dependent rubor
- Arterial bruit
- Hypertension
- Pain
- Pulselessness distal to the occlusion
- Paralysis and paresthesia in the affected arm or leg
- Poikilothermy (temperature of affected area matches surrounding environmental temperature)

Diagnostic tests

Imaging

- Arteriography shows the type, location, and degree of obstruction and any collateral circulation.
- Ultrasonography and plethysmography show decreased blood flow distal to the occlusion.
- Doppler ultrasonography has a relatively low-pitched sound and shows a monophasic waveform.
- EEG and computed tomography scan may show brain lesions.

Other tests

- Segmental limb pressures and pulse volume measurements show the location and extent of the occlusion.
- Ophthalmodynamometry shows the degree of obstruction in the internal carotid artery.
- Electrocardiogram may show cardiovascular disease.

Treatment

General

- Control of hypertension, diabetes, and dyslipidemia
- Foot and leg care
- Low-fat, low-cholesterol, high-fiber diet
- Regular walking program
- Smoking cessation
- Weight control

Medications

- Anticoagulants
- Antidiabetic drugs
- Antihypertensives
- Antiplatelet drugs
- Lipid-lowering drugs
- Niacin or vitamin B complex
- Thrombolytics

Surgery

- Amputation
- Atherectomy
- Bowel resection
- Bypass graft
- Embolectomy
- Endarterectomy
- Endovascular stent placement
- Laser angioplasty
- Laser surgery
- Lumbar sympathectomy
- Patch grafting

◆ Percutaneous transluminal angioplasty

Nursing interventions

For chronic arterial occlusive disease

◆ Use preventive measures, such as minimal pressure mattresses, heel protectors, a foot cradle, or a footboard.
◆ Avoid restrictive clothing, including antiembolism stockings.
◆ Give prescribed drugs.
◆ Allow the patient to express fears and concerns.

For preoperative care during an acute episode

◆ Determine the patient's circulatory status.
◆ Give prescribed analgesics.
◆ Give prescribed heparin or thrombolytics.
◆ Wrap the patient's affected foot in soft cotton batting, and reposition it frequently to prevent pressure on any one area.
◆ Strictly avoid elevating or applying heat to the affected leg.

For postoperative care

◆ Watch the patient closely for signs of hemorrhage.
◆ If the patient has mesenteric artery occlusion, connect a nasogastric tube to low intermittent suction.
◆ Give prescribed analgesics.
◆ Assist with early ambulation, but don't let the patient sit for a long period.
◆ After amputation, check the residual limb carefully for drainage, and note and record the color and amount of drainage as well as the time.
◆ Elevate the residual limb, as ordered.
◆ Monitor distal pulses.

Patient teaching

◆ Be sure to cover:
– the disorder, diagnosis, and treatment
– medications and potential adverse reactions
– when to notify the physician
– diet restrictions
– the regular exercise program
– foot care
– signs and symptoms of graft occlusion
– signs and symptoms of arterial insufficiency and occlusion
– the need to avoid crossing the legs and wearing constrictive clothing or garters
– modification of risk factors
– the need to avoid temperature extremes.
◆ Refer the patient to a physical and occupational therapist, as indicated.
◆ Refer the patient to a podiatrist for foot care, as needed.
◆ Refer the patient to an endocrinologist for glucose control, as indicated.
◆ Refer the patient to a smoking-cessation program, as indicated.

Asthma

Overview

◆ A chronic reactive airway disorder that involves episodic, reversible airway obstruction caused by bronchospasm, increased mucus secretion, and mucosal edema
◆ Signs and symptoms that range from mild wheezing and dyspnea to life-threatening respiratory failure
◆ Signs and symptoms of bronchial airway obstruction that may persist between acute episodes

Causes

◆ Sensitivity to specific external allergens
◆ Internal, hypoallergenic factors

Extrinsic asthma (atopic asthma)
- ◆ Animal dander
- ◆ Food additives that contain sulfites or other sensitizing substances
- ◆ House dust or mold
- ◆ Kapok or feather pillows
- ◆ Pollen

Intrinsic asthma (nonatopic asthma)
- ◆ Emotional stress
- ◆ Genetic factors

Bronchoconstriction
- ◆ Cold air
- ◆ Drugs, such as aspirin, beta-adrenergic blockers, and nonsteroidal anti-inflammatories
- ◆ Exercise
- ◆ Hereditary predisposition
- ◆ Psychological stress
- ◆ Sensitivity to allergens or irritants such as pollutants
- ◆ Tartrazine
- ◆ Viral infections

Data collection

History
- ◆ Development of symptoms after a severe respiratory tract infection, especially in adults (intrinsic asthma)
- ◆ Symptoms aggravated by irritants, emotional stress, fatigue, endocrine changes, temperature and humidity variations, and exposure to noxious fumes (intrinsic asthma)
- ◆ Simultaneous onset of severe, multiple asthma symptoms or insidious onset with gradually increasing respiratory distress
- ◆ Exposure to a particular allergen followed by sudden onset of dyspnea, wheezing, and tightness in the chest and a cough that produces thick, clear, or yellow sputum

Physical findings
- ◆ Ability to speak only a few words before pausing for breath
- ◆ Diaphoresis
- ◆ Diminished breath sounds
- ◆ Hyperresonance
- ◆ Increased anteroposterior thoracic diameter
- ◆ Inspiratory and expiratory wheezes
- ◆ Prolonged expiratory phase of respiration
- ◆ Tachycardia, tachypnea, and mild systolic hypertension
- ◆ Use of accessory respiratory muscles
- ◆ Visible dyspnea
- ◆ Cyanosis, confusion, and lethargy, which indicate onset of life-threatening status asthmaticus and respiratory failure

Diagnostic tests
Laboratory
- ◆ Arterial blood gas (ABG) analysis shows hypoxemia.
- ◆ Increased serum immunoglobulin E levels are caused by an allergic reaction.
- ◆ A complete blood count with differential shows an increased eosinophil count.

Imaging
- ◆ Chest X-rays may show hyperinflation and areas of focal atelectasis.

Diagnostic procedures
- ◆ Pulmonary function tests may show decreased peak flow and forced expiratory volume in 1 second, low-normal or decreased vital capacity, and increased total lung and residual capacities.
- ◆ Skin testing may identify specific allergens.
- ◆ Bronchial challenge testing shows the clinical significance of allergens that are identified by skin testing.

Other tests
- ◆ Pulse oximetry measurements may show decreased oxygen saturation.

Treatment

General
◆ Identification and avoidance of precipitating factors
◆ Desensitization to specific antigens
◆ Establishment and maintenance of a patent airway
◆ Fluid replacement
◆ Activity as tolerated
◆ In patients unresponsive to drug therapy, possible admission for further treatment, which may include intubation or mechanical ventilation

Medications
◆ Antibiotics (if coexistant infection)
◆ Anticholinergic bronchodilators
◆ Bronchodilators
◆ Corticosteroids
◆ Histamine antagonists
◆ I.V. magnesium sulfate (controversial)
◆ Leukotriene antagonists
◆ Low-flow oxygen
◆ Trial of heliox (helium-oxygen mixture) before intubation

Nursing interventions
◆ Give prescribed drugs.
◆ Place the patient in high Fowler's position.
◆ Encourage pursed-lip and diaphragmatic breathing.
◆ Give prescribed humidified oxygen.
◆ Adjust oxygen according to the patient's vital signs and ABG values.
◆ Assist with intubation and mechanical ventilation, if appropriate.
◆ Perform postural drainage and chest percussion, if tolerated.
◆ Suction the intubated patient, as needed.
◆ Treat the patient's dehydration with I.V. or oral fluids, as tolerated.
◆ Anticipate bronchoscopy or bronchial lavage.
◆ Keep the room temperature comfortable.
◆ Use an air conditioner or a fan in hot, humid weather.

Patient teaching

◆ Be sure to cover:
- the disorder, diagnosis, and treatment
- medications and potential adverse reactions
- when to notify the physician
- the importance of avoiding known allergens and irritants
- the use of a metered-dose inhaler or dry powder inhaler
- pursed-lip and diaphragmatic breathing
- the use of a peak flow meter
- effective coughing techniques
- the importance of maintaining adequate hydration.

◆ Refer the patient to a local asthma support group.

Bronchitis, chronic

Overview

◆ Inflammation of the lining of the bronchial tubes
◆ A form of chronic obstructive pulmonary disease
◆ Characterized by excessive production of tracheobronchial mucus with a cough for at least 3 months each year for 2 consecutive years
◆ Severity linked to the amount of cigarette smoke or other pollutants inhaled and the duration of inhalation
◆ Worsening of cough and related symptoms by respiratory tract infections
◆ Development of significant airway obstruction in a few patients with chronic bronchitis

Causes
- Cigarette smoking
- Environmental pollution
- Exposure to organic or inorganic dusts and noxious gas
- Possible genetic predisposition

Data collection

History
- Cough, initially prevalent in winter, but gradually becoming year-round
- Exertional dyspnea
- Frequent upper respiratory tract infections
- Increasingly severe coughing episodes
- Longtime smoker
- Productive cough
- Worsening dyspnea

Physical findings
- Cough that produces copious gray, white, or yellow sputum
- Cyanosis (patient sometimes referred to as a "blue bloater")
- Jugular vein distention
- Pedal edema
- Prolonged expiratory time
- Rhonchi
- Substantial weight gain
- Tachypnea
- Use of accessory respiratory muscles
- Wheezing

Diagnostic tests
Laboratory
- Arterial blood gas analysis shows decreased partial pressure of oxygen and normal or increased partial pressure of carbon dioxide.
- Sputum culture shows many microorganisms and neutrophils.

Imaging
- Chest X-ray may show hyperinflation and increased bronchovascular markings.

Diagnostic procedures
- Pulmonary function test results show increased residual volume, decreased vital capacity and forced expiratory flow, and normal static compliance and diffusing capacity.

Other tests
- Electrocardiography may show atrial arrhythmias; peaked P waves in leads II, III, and aV_F; and right ventricular hypertrophy.

Treatment

General
- Activity, as tolerated, with frequent rest periods
- Adequate fluid intake
- Avoidance of air pollutants
- Chest physiotherapy
- High-calorie, protein-rich diet
- Smoking cessation
- Ultrasonic or mechanical nebulizer treatments

Medications
- Antibiotics
- Bronchodilators
- Corticosteroids
- Diuretics
- Oxygen

Surgery
- Tracheostomy in advanced disease

Nursing interventions
- Give prescribed drugs.
- Encourage the patient to express fears and concerns.
- Include the patient and family in care decisions.
- Perform chest physiotherapy.
- Provide a high-calorie, protein-rich diet.
- Offer small, frequent meals.
- Encourage energy-conservation techniques.
- Ensure adequate oral fluid intake.

- Provide frequent mouth care.
- Encourage daily activity.
- Provide diversional activities, as appropriate.
- Provide frequent rest periods.

Patient teaching

- Be sure to cover:
  - the disorder, diagnosis, and treatment
  - medications and possible adverse reactions
  - when to notify the physician
  - infection control practices
  - the importance of influenza and pneumococcus vaccines
  - the importance of home oxygen therapy, if needed, including a demonstration, if needed
  - postural drainage and chest percussion
  - coughing and deep-breathing exercises
  - inhaler use
  - high-calorie, protein-rich meals
  - adequate hydration
  - avoidance of inhaled irritants
  - prevention of bronchospasm.
- Refer the patient to a smoking-cessation program, if indicated.
- Refer the patient to the American Lung Association for information and support.

Cancer, breast

Overview

- Malignant proliferation of the epithelial cells that line the ducts or lobules of the breast
- Prognosis considerably affected by early detection and treatment

Causes

- Unknown

Risk factors

- Alcohol or tobacco use
- Antihypertensive therapy
- Early onset of menses, late menopause
- Estrogen therapy
- Family history of breast cancer, particularly in first-degree relatives, including the patient's parents and siblings
- Fibrocystic disease
- High-fat diet
- History of endometrial or ovarian cancer
- History of unilateral breast cancer
- Long menstrual cycles
- Nulliparous patient or first pregnancy after age 30
- Positive results on tests for genetic mutations (BRCA 1)
- Older than age 45 and premenopausal
- Radiation exposure

Data collection

History

- Detection of a painless lump or mass in the breast
- Change in breast tissue
- History of risk factors

Physical findings

- Clear, milky, or bloody nipple discharge, nipple retraction, scaly skin around the nipple, and skin changes, such as dimpling or inflammation
- Edema of the arm
- Hard lump, mass, or thickening of breast tissue
- Lymphadenopathy

Diagnostic tests

Laboratory

- Alkaline phosphatase levels and liver function test results show distant metastasis.
- A hormonal receptor assay determines whether the tumor is estrogen- or progesterone-dependent and guides

decisions about therapy that blocks the action of estrogen, which may support tumor growth.

Imaging

- Mammography can show a tumor that's too small to palpate.
- Ultrasonography can distinguish between a fluid-filled cyst and a solid mass.
- Chest X-rays can pinpoint metastasis in the chest.
- Scans of the bone, brain, liver, and other organs can detect distant metastasis.

Diagnostic procedures

- Fine-needle aspiration and excisional biopsy provide cells for histologic examination that may confirm the diagnosis.

Treatment

General

- Usually depends on stage and type of disease, the patient's age and menopausal status, and the disfiguring effects of surgery
- May include any combination of surgery, radiation therapy, chemotherapy, and hormone therapy
- May be improved by preoperative breast irradiation
- May include arm-stretching exercises after surgery
- May involve primary radiation therapy

Medications

- Antiestrogen therapies
- Aromatase inhibitors
- Chemotherapy drugs
- Hormonal therapies
- Monoclonal antibody therapy (for metastatic disease)
- Selective estrogen receptor modulators

Surgery

- Lumpectomy
- Partial, total, or modified radical mastectomy

Nursing interventions

- Provide information about the disease process, diagnostic tests, and treatment.
- Give prescribed drugs.
- Provide emotional support.

Patient teaching

- Be sure to cover:
  - all procedures and treatments
  - activities or exercises that promote healing
  - breast self-examination (now considered optional by the American Cancer Society)
  - the risks and the signs and symptoms of recurrence
  - the need to avoid venipuncture and blood pressure monitoring using the affected arm.
- Refer the patient to local and national support groups.

Cancer, colorectal

Overview

- Almost always adenocarcinoma (about half sessile lesions of rectosigmoid area, the rest polypoid lesions)
- Slow progression
- Five-year survival rate of 50%
- Curable in 75% of patients if early diagnosis allows resection before involvement of nodes
- Second most common visceral neoplasm in United States and Europe

Causes

- Unknown

Risk factors

- Age older than 40
- Digestive tract disease
- Excessive intake of saturated animal fat
- Family history of colon cancer
- High-protein, low-fiber diet
- History of familial polyposis
- History of ulcerative colitis

Data collection

History

- Abdominal aching, pressure, or dull cramps
- Black, tarry stools
- Diarrhea, anorexia, obstipation, weight loss, and vomiting
- Intermittent abdominal fullness
- Rectal bleeding
- Rectal pressure
- Tumors of the right side of the colon: No signs and symptoms in the early stages because stool is liquid in that part of the colon
- Urgent need to defecate on arising
- Weakness

Physical findings

- Abdominal distention or visible masses
- Enlarged abdominal veins
- Enlarged inguinal and supraclavicular nodes
- Abnormal bowel sounds
- Abdominal masses (bulky for right-side tumors, easier detection of transverse-section tumors)
- Generalized abdominal tenderness

Diagnostic tests

Laboratory

- A fecal occult blood test may show blood in the stools, a warning sign of rectal cancer.
- The carcinoembryonic antigen test permits patient monitoring before and after treatment to detect metastasis or recurrence.

Imaging

- Excretory urography verifies bilateral renal function and allows inspection to detect displacement of the kidneys, ureters, or bladder by a tumor pressing against these structures.
- Barium enema studies use dual contrast of barium and air to show the location of lesions that aren't detectable manually or visually. This test shouldn't precede colonoscopy or excretory urography because barium sulfate interferes with these tests.
- A computed tomography scan allows better visualization if a barium enema test yields inconclusive results or if metastasis to the pelvic lymph nodes is suspected.

Diagnostic procedures

- Proctoscopy or sigmoidoscopy permits visualization of the lower GI tract. It can detect up to 66% of colorectal cancers.
- Colonoscopy permits visual inspection and photography of the colon up to the ileocecal valve and provides access for polypectomy and biopsy of suspected lesions.

Other tests

- Digital rectal examination can be used to detect almost 15% of colorectal cancers; specifically, it can be used to detect suspicious rectal and perianal lesions.

Treatment

General

- Radiation preoperatively and postoperatively to induce tumor regression
- High-fiber diet
- After surgery, avoidance of heavy lifting and contact sports

Medications

- Analgesics

- Chemotherapy for metastasis, residual disease, or recurrent inoperable tumor

Surgery

- Resection or right hemicolectomy for advanced disease (Surgery may include resection of the terminal segment of the ileum, cecum, ascending colon, and right half of the transverse colon with corresponding mesentery.)
- Right colectomy that includes the transverse colon and mesentery corresponding to the midcolic vessels, or segmental resection of the transverse colon and associated midcolic vessels
- Resection usually limited to the sigmoid colon and mesentery
- Anterior or low anterior resection (A newer method that uses a stapler allows for much lower resections than were possible in the past.)
- Abdominoperineal resection and permanent sigmoid colostomy required

Nursing interventions

- Provide support, and encourage the patient to express his concerns.
- Give prescribed drugs.

Postoperative

- Bowel function
- Complications
- Electrolyte levels
- Hydration and nutritional status
- Intake and output
- Pain control
- Psychological status
- Vital signs
- Wound site

Patient teaching

- Be sure to cover:
  - the disease process, treatment, and postoperative course
  - stoma care
  - the need to avoid heavy lifting
  - the need to keep follow-up appointments
  - risk factors and signs of reoccurrence.
- Refer the patient to resource and support services.

Cancer, prostate

Overview

- Proliferation of cancer cells that usually takes the form of adenocarcinomas and typically originates in the posterior prostate gland
- May progress to widespread bone metastasis and death

Causes

- Unknown

Risk factors

- Age older than 40
- Exposure to heavy metals
- Family history
- Infection
- Vasectomy

Data collection

History

- Symptoms rare in early stages of disease
- Later, urinary problems, such as difficulty starting a urine stream, dribbling, and retention of urine

Physical findings

- In early stages: A flat, firm, nodular mass with a sharp edge
- In advanced disease: Edema of the scrotum or leg, with a hard lump in the prostate region

Diagnostic tests

Laboratory

- Serum prostate-specific antigen (PSA) level is elevated. (An elevated PSA level may indicate cancer with or without metastases.)

Imaging

- Transrectal prostatic ultrasonography shows the size of the prostate and the presence of abnormal growths.
- Bone scan and excretory urography determine the extent of disease.
- Magnetic resonance imaging and computed tomography scan define the extent of the tumor.

Other tests

- The standard screening tests are digital rectal examination and PSA test. Positive results on these tests identify cancer. The American Cancer Society recommends yearly screening for men older than age 40.

Treatment

General

- Radiation therapy or internal beam radiation
- Varies with stage of cancer
- Well-balanced diet

Medications

- Chemotherapy
- Hormonal therapy

Surgery

- Cryosurgical ablation
- Orchiectomy
- Prostatectomy
- Radical prostatectomy
- Transurethral resection of the prostate

Nursing interventions

- Give medications as ordered.
- Encourage the patient to express his feelings.
- Provide emotional support.

Patient teaching

- Be sure to cover:
  - the disorder, diagnosis, and treatment
  - perineal exercises that decrease incontinence
  - the importance of follow-up care
  - medications, dosages, and possible adverse reactions.
- Refer the patient to appropriate resources and support services, as needed.

Coronary artery disease

Overview

- Heart disease that results from narrowing of the coronary arteries over time as a result of atherosclerosis
- Primary effect: Loss of oxygen and nutrients to myocardial tissue because of decreased coronary blood flow

Causes

- Atherosclerosis
- Congenital defects
- Coronary artery spasm
- Dissecting aneurysm
- Infectious vasculitis
- Syphilis

Risk factors

- Diabetes
- Family history
- High cholesterol level
- Hormonal contraceptives
- Increased homocysteine levels
- Obesity
- Sedentary lifestyle
- Smoking
- Stress

Data collection

History

- Angina that may radiate to the left arm, neck, jaw, or shoulder blade
- Angina that commonly occurs after physical exertion but may also follow emotional excitement, exposure to cold, or a large meal
- May develop during sleep and wake the patient
- Nausea
- Vomiting
- Fainting
- Sweating
- Stable angina (predictable and relieved by rest or nitrates)
- Unstable angina (increased frequency and duration, more easily induced, generally indicates extensive or worsening disease and, untreated, may progress to myocardial infarction)
- Crescendo angina (effort-induced pain that occurs with increasing frequency and with decreasing provocation)
- Prinzmetal's or variant angina pectoris (severe pain that occurs at rest without provocation or effort)

Physical findings

- Arteriovenous nicking of the retina
- Cool extremities
- Decreased or absent peripheral pulses
- Hypertension
- Obesity
- Positive Levine sign (holding the fist to the chest)
- Xanthoma

Diagnostic tests

Imaging

- Myocardial perfusion imaging with thallium 201 during treadmill exercise shows ischemic areas of the myocardium. These are visualized as "cold spots."
- Pharmacologic myocardial perfusion imaging in arteries with stenosis shows a decrease in blood flow that's proportional to the percentage of occlusion.
- Multiple-gated acquisition scanning shows cardiac wall motion and reflects injury to cardiac tissue.

Diagnostic procedures

- Electrocardiographic findings may be normal between anginal episodes. During angina, the findings may show ischemic changes.
- Exercise testing may be performed to detect ST-segment changes during exercise, which indicate ischemia, and to determine a safe exercise prescription.
- Coronary angiography shows the location and degree of coronary artery stenosis or obstruction, the collateral circulation, and the condition of the artery beyond the narrowing.
- Stress echocardiography may show abnormal wall motion.

Treatment

General

- Lifestyle changes, such as smoking cessation and maintaining ideal body weight
- Low-fat, low-sodium diet
- Possible activity restrictions
- Regular exercise
- Stress reduction techniques, especially if known stressors cause pain

Medications

- Antihypertensives
- Antilipemics
- Antiplatelets
- Aspirin
- Estrogen replacement therapy
- Nitrates
- Beta-adrenergic blockers
- Calcium channel blockers

Surgery
- ◆ Angioplasty
- ◆ Atherectomy
- ◆ Coronary artery bypass graft
- ◆ "Keyhole" or minimally invasive surgery
- ◆ Laser angioplasty
- ◆ Placement of an endovascular stent

Nursing interventions
- ◆ Ask the patient to grade the severity of his pain on a scale of 0 to 10, with 10 being the most severe.
- ◆ Keep nitroglycerin available for immediate use. Instruct the patient to call immediately, before taking nitroglycerin, if pain occurs.
- ◆ Observe the patient for signs and symptoms that may signify worsening of his condition.
- ◆ Perform vigorous chest physiotherapy and guide the patient in pulmonary self-care.
- ◆ Monitor abnormal bleeding and distal pulses after interventions or procedures.
- ◆ Monitor drainage of the chest tube after surgery.

Patient teaching
- ◆ Be sure to cover:
  - coronary artery disease risk factors
  - the need to avoid activities that precipitate episodes of pain
  - effective coping mechanisms for dealing with stress
  - the need to follow the prescribed drug regimen
  - the importance of following a low-sodium, low-calorie diet
  - the importance of regular, moderate exercise.
- ◆ Refer the patient to a weight-loss program, if needed.
- ◆ Refer the patient to a smoking-cessation program, if needed.
- ◆ Refer the patient to a cardiac rehabilitation program, if indicated.

Diabetes mellitus

Overview
- ◆ Chronic disease of absolute or relative insulin deficiency or resistance
- ◆ Characterized by disturbances in the metabolism of carbohydrates, proteins, and fats
- ◆ Two primary forms:
  - Type 1, characterized by absolute insulin insufficiency
  - Type 2, characterized by insulin resistance with varying degrees of insulin secretory defects
- ◆ Pre-diabetes: Fasting glucose is $\geq$ 100 mg/dl and $<$ 126 mg/dl

Causes
- ◆ Autoimmune disease (type 1)
- ◆ Genetic factors

Risk factors
- ◆ Family history of diabetes
- ◆ Viral infections (type 1)

Type 2
- ◆ Race
- ◆ Obesity: BMI $\geq$ 27 kg/m^2
- ◆ History of gestational diabetes, previous glucose intolerance, or delivery of an infant weighing $>$ 9 lb (4.1 kg)
- ◆ HDL $\leq$ 35 mg/dl or triglyceride level $\geq$ 250 mg/dl
- ◆ Hypertension: $\geq$ 140/90 mm Hg
- ◆ Age $\geq$ 45
- ◆ Sedentary lifestyle

Alert Unless a diabetic woman's glucose levels are well controlled before conception and during pregnancy, her neonate has two to three times the risk of congenital malformations and fetal distress.

Data collection

History
- ◆ Dehydration

- Dry, itchy skin
- Dry mucous membranes
- Frequent skin and urinary tract infections
- Nocturnal diarrhea
- Numbness or pain in hands or feet
- Polydipsia
- Polyuria, nocturia
- Poor skin turgor
- Postprandial feeling of nausea or fullness
- Sexual problems
- Vision changes
- Weakness and fatigue
- Weight loss and hunger

Type 1
- Rapidly developing symptoms

Type 2
- Family history of diabetes mellitus
- Other endocrine diseases
- Pregnancy
- Recent stress or trauma
- Severe viral infection
- Use of drugs that increase blood glucose levels
- Vague, long-standing symptoms that develop gradually

Physical findings
- Cool skin temperature
- Decreased peripheral pulses
- Diminished deep tendon reflexes
- Dry mucous membranes
- "Fruity" breath odor in ketoacidosis
- Muscle wasting and loss of subcutaneous fat (type 1)
- Obesity, particularly in the abdominal area (type 2)
- Orthostatic hypotension
- Poor skin turgor
- Possible hypovolemia and shock in ketoacidosis and hyperosmolar hyperglycemic state
- Retinopathy or cataract formation
- Skin changes, especially on the legs and feet

Diagnostic tests
Laboratory
- Fasting plasma glucose level is 126 mg/dl or greater on at least two occasions.
- Random blood glucose level is 200 mg/dl or greater.
- Two-hour postprandial blood glucose level is 200 mg/dl or greater.
- Glycosylated hemoglobin value is increased.
- Urinalysis may show acetone or glucose.

Diagnostic procedures
- Ophthalmologic examination may show diabetic retinopathy.

Treatment

General
- Exercise and diet control
- Strict glycemic control for prevention of complications
- Modest calorie restriction for weight loss or maintenance
- American Diabetes Association recommendations to reach target glucose, hemoglobin A_{1c}, lipid, and blood pressure levels
- Regular aerobic exercise

Medications
- Exogenous insulin (type 1, possibly type 2)
- Oral antidiabetic drugs (type 2)

Surgery
- Pancreas transplantation

Nursing interventions
- Give prescribed drugs.
- Give rapidly absorbed carbohydrates for hypoglycemia or, if the patient is unconscious, give glucagon or I.V. dextrose, as ordered.
- Give I.V. fluids and insulin replacement for hyperglycemic crisis, as ordered.

◆ Provide meticulous skin care, especially to the feet and legs.
◆ Treat all injuries, cuts, and blisters immediately.
◆ Avoid constricting hose, slippers, or bed linens.
◆ Encourage adequate fluid intake.
◆ Encourage the patient to express feelings and concerns.
◆ Offer emotional support.
◆ Help the patient to develop effective coping strategies.

Patient teaching

◆ Be sure to cover:
- the disorder, diagnosis, and treatment
- medications and potential adverse reactions
- when to notify the physician
- the prescribed meal plan
- the prescribed exercise program
- signs and symptoms of infection, hypoglycemia, hyperglycemia, and diabetic neuropathy
- self-monitoring of blood glucose level
- complications of hyperglycemia
- foot care
- the importance of annual regular ophthalmologic examinations
- safety precautions
- management of diabetes during illness.

◆ Refer the patient to a dietitian.
◆ Refer the patient to a podiatrist if indicated.
◆ Refer the patient to an ophthalmologist.
◆ Refer adult diabetic patients who are planning families for preconception counseling.
◆ Refer the patient to the Juvenile Diabetes Research Foundation, the American Association of Diabetes Educators, and the American Diabetes Association, as appropriate, to obtain additional information.

Emphysema

Overview

◆ Chronic lung disease characterized by permanent enlargement of air spaces distal to the terminal bronchioles and by exertional dyspnea
◆ One of several diseases usually labeled collectively as chronic obstructive pulmonary disease or chronic obstructive lung disease

Causes
◆ Cigarette smoking
◆ Genetic deficiency of alpha$_1$-antitrypsin

Data collection

History
◆ Anorexia and weight loss
◆ Chronic cough
◆ Malaise
◆ Shortness of breath
◆ Smoking

Physical findings
◆ Barrel chest
◆ Clubbed fingers and toes
◆ Crackles
◆ Cyanosis
◆ Decreased breath sounds
◆ Decreased chest expansion
◆ Decreased tactile fremitus
◆ Distant heart sounds
◆ Hyperresonance
◆ Inspiratory wheeze
◆ Prolonged expiratory phase with grunting respirations
◆ Pursed-lip breathing
◆ Tachypnea
◆ Use of accessory muscles

Diagnostic tests
Laboratory
◆ Arterial blood gas analysis shows decreased partial pressure of oxygen;

partial pressure of carbon dioxide is normal until late in the disease.
◆ Red blood cell count shows an increased hemoglobin level late in the disease.

Imaging
◆ Chest X-ray may show:
- a flattened diaphragm
- reduced vascular markings at the lung periphery
- overaeration of the lungs
- a vertical heart
- enlarged anteroposterior chest diameter
- a large retrosternal air space.

Diagnostic procedures
◆ Pulmonary function tests typically show:
- increased residual volume and total lung capacity
- reduced diffusing capacity
- increased inspiratory flow.
◆ Electrocardiography may show tall, symmetrical P waves in leads II, III, and aV_F; a vertical QRS axis; and signs of right ventricular hypertrophy late in the disease.

Treatment

General
◆ Activity, as tolerated
◆ Adequate hydration
◆ Chest physiotherapy
◆ High-protein, high-calorie diet
◆ Possible transtracheal catheterization and home oxygen therapy

Medications
◆ Antibiotics
◆ Anticholinergics
◆ Bronchodilators
◆ Corticosteroids
◆ Mucolytics
◆ Oxygen

Surgery
◆ Insertion of a chest tube for pneumothorax

Nursing interventions
◆ Give prescribed drugs.
◆ Provide supportive care.
◆ Help the patient adjust to lifestyle changes demanded by a chronic illness.
◆ Encourage the patient to express fears and concerns.
◆ Perform chest physiotherapy.
◆ Provide a high-calorie, protein-rich diet.
◆ Give small, frequent meals.
◆ Encourage daily activity and diversional activities.
◆ Provide frequent rest periods.

Patient teaching

◆ Be sure to cover:
- the disorder, diagnosis, and treatment
- medications and potential adverse reactions
- when to notify the physician
- the importance of avoiding smoking and areas where smoking is permitted
- the need to avoid crowds and people with infections
- home oxygen therapy, if indicated
- transtracheal catheter care, if needed
- coughing and deep-breathing exercises
- the proper use of handheld inhalers
- the importance of a high-calorie, protein-rich diet
- adequate oral fluid intake
- avoidance of respiratory irritants
- signs and symptoms of pneumothorax.

Alert Urge the patient to notify the physician about sudden worsening of dyspnea or sharp pleuritic chest pain that's worsened by chest movement, breathing, or coughing.

◆ Refer the patient to a smoking-cessation program if indicated.
◆ Refer the patient for influenza and pneumococcal pneumonia immunizations as needed.
◆ Refer the family of a patient with familial emphysema for screening for alpha$_1$-antitrypsin deficiency.

Gastroenteritis

Overview

◆ Self-limiting inflammation of the stomach and small intestine
◆ Intestinal flu, traveler's diarrhea, viral enteritis, and food poisoning

Causes
◆ Amoebae, especially *Entamoeba histolytica*
◆ Bacteria, such as *Staphylococcus aureus, Salmonella, Shigella, Clostridium botulinum, Clostridium perfringens,* and *Escherichia coli*
◆ Drug reactions to antibiotics
◆ Food allergens
◆ Enzyme deficiencies
◆ Ingestion of toxins, such as poisonous plants and toadstools
◆ Parasites, such as *Ascaris, Enterobius,* and *Trichinella spiralis*
◆ Viruses, such as adenoviruses, echoviruses, and coxsackieviruses

Data collection

History
◆ Abdominal pain and discomfort
◆ Acute onset of diarrhea
◆ Exposure to contaminated food
◆ Malaise and fatigue
◆ Nausea and vomiting
◆ Recent travel

Physical findings
◆ Decreased blood pressure
◆ Hyperactive bowel sounds
◆ Slight abdominal distention
◆ Poor skin turgor (with dehydration)

Diagnostic tests
Laboratory
◆ Gram stain, stool culture (by direct rectal swab), or blood culture shows the causative agent.

Treatment

General
◆ Activity, as tolerated (Encourage mobilization.)
◆ Avoidance of milk products
◆ Electrolyte solutions
◆ Initially, clear liquids as tolerated
◆ Rehydration
◆ Supportive treatment for nausea, vomiting, and diarrhea

Medications
◆ Antibiotics
◆ Antidiarrheal therapy
◆ Antiemetics
◆ I.V. fluids

Nursing interventions
◆ Allow uninterrupted rest periods.
◆ Replace lost fluids and electrolytes through diet or I.V. fluids.
◆ Give prescribed drugs.

Patient teaching

◆ Be sure to cover:
- the disorder, diagnosis, and treatment
- diet modifications
- prescribed drugs, including administration and possible adverse effects
- preventive measures
- how to perform warm sitz baths three times daily to relieve anal irritation.

Gastroesophageal reflux disease

Overview

◆ Persistent reflux of gastric or duodenal contents, or both, into the esophagus, causing acute epigastric pain, usually after a meal without associated belching or vomiting
◆ Also called GERD

Causes
◆ Any condition or position that increases intra-abdominal pressure
◆ Hiatal hernia with an incompetent sphincter
◆ Idiopathic
◆ Pyloric surgery (alteration or removal of the pylorus), which allows reflux of bile or pancreatic juice

Risk factors
◆ Any agent that lowers pressure in the lower esophageal sphincter (LES): acidic and fatty food, alcohol, cigarettes, anticholinergics (atropine, belladonna, propantheline) or other drugs (morphine, diazepam, calcium channel blockers, meperidine)
◆ Nasogastric intubation for more than 4 days

Data collection

History
◆ Minimal or no symptoms in one-third of patients
◆ Heartburn that typically occurs 1½ to 2 hours after eating
◆ Heartburn that worsens with vigorous exercise, bending, lying down, wearing tight clothing, coughing, constipation, or obesity
◆ Relief obtained by using antacids or sitting upright
◆ Regurgitation without associated nausea or belching
◆ Sensation of accumulation of fluid in the throat without a sour or bitter taste
◆ Chronic pain radiating to the neck, jaws, and arms that may mimic angina pectoris
◆ Nocturnal hypersalivation and wheezing

Physical findings
◆ Bright red or dark brown blood in the vomitus
◆ Chronic cough
◆ Odynophagia (sharp substernal pain on swallowing), possibly followed by a dull substernal ache
◆ Laryngitis and morning hoarseness

Diagnostic tests
Imaging
◆ Barium swallow with fluoroscopy shows evidence of recurrent reflux.

Diagnostic procedures
◆ Ambulatory 24-hour pH monitoring shows the degree of gastroesophageal reflux and is the gold standard for diagnosis when endoscopy is negative.
◆ Gastroesophageal scintillation testing shows reflux.
◆ Esophageal manometry shows abnormal LES pressure and sphincter incompetence.
◆ The result of an acid perfusion (Bernstein) test confirms esophagitis.
◆ The results of esophagoscopy (endoscopy) and biopsy confirm pathologic changes in the mucosa in some patients.

Treatment

General
◆ Avoidance of dietary causes

Diet and lifestyle choices that alter LES pressure

Diet and lifestyle choices can increase or decrease lower esophageal sphincter (LES) pressure. Consider these factors when you plan the patient's treatment.

Choices that increase LES pressure
- Carbohydrates
- Low-dose ethanol
- Nonfat milk
- Protein

Choices that decrease LES pressure
- Antiflatulents (simethicone)
- Chocolate
- Cigarette smoking
- High-dose ethanol
- Fat
- Lying on the right or left side
- Orange juice
- Sitting
- Tomatoes
- Whole milk

- Avoidance of eating 3 hours before sleep (see *Diet and lifestyle choices that alter LES pressure*)
- Lifestyle changes
- Lifting restrictions for surgical treatment
- Parenteral nutrition or tube feedings
- Positional therapy
- No activity restrictions for medical treatment
- Removal of the cause
- Weight reduction, if appropriate

Medications
- Antacids
- Cholinergics (rarely)
- Histamine-2 receptor antagonists
- Proton pump inhibitors

Surgery
- Esophagectomy
- Hiatal hernia repair
- Vagotomy or pyloroplasty

Nursing interventions
- Offer emotional and psychological support.
- Assist with diet modification.
- Perform chest physiotherapy and give oxygen after surgery, if needed.
- Place the patient in semi-Fowler's position if he has a nasogastric tube.

Patient teaching

- Be sure to cover:
  - the disorder, diagnosis, and treatment
  - the causes of gastroesophageal reflux disease
  - the prescribed antireflux regimen of medication, diet, and positional therapy
  - development of a diet plan
  - the need to identify situations or activities that increase intra-abdominal pressure
  - the need to avoid substances that reduce sphincter control
  - signs and symptoms to watch for and report.

Heart failure

Overview

- Myocardial dysfunction that leads to impaired heart pumping performance or to an abnormal circulatory congestion
- May cause peripheral edema from congested systemic venous circulation or pulmonary edema from congested pulmonary circulation
- Usually occurs in a damaged left ventricle, but may occur mainly in the

right ventricle or secondary to left-sided heart failure

Causes

- Anemia
- Arrhythmias
- Atherosclerosis with myocardial infarction
- Constrictive pericarditis
- Emotional stress
- Hypertension
- Increased intake of salt or water
- Infections
- Mitral stenosis secondary to rheumatic heart disease, constrictive pericarditis, or atrial fibrillation
- Mitral or aortic insufficiency
- Myocarditis
- Pregnancy
- Pulmonary embolism
- Thyrotoxicosis
- Ventricular and atrial septal defects

Data collection

History

- Anorexia
- Disorder or condition that can cause heart failure
- Dyspnea or paroxysmal nocturnal dyspnea
- Fatigue
- Insomnia
- Nausea
- Peripheral edema
- Sense of abdominal fullness (particularly in right-sided heart failure)
- Substance abuse (alcohol, drugs, tobacco)
- Weakness

Physical findings

- Ascites
- Cough that produces pink, frothy sputum
- Cyanosis of the lips and nail beds
- Decreased pulse oximetry
- Decreased pulse pressure
- Decreased urinary output
- Diaphoresis
- Hepatomegaly and, possibly, splenomegaly
- Jugular vein distention
- Moist, bibasilar crackles, rhonchi, and expiratory wheezing
- Pale, cool, clammy skin
- Peripheral edema
- Pulsus alternans
- S_3 and S_4 heart sounds
- Tachycardia

Diagnostic tests

Laboratory

- B-type natriuretic peptide immunoassay value is elevated.

Imaging

- Chest X-rays show increased pulmonary vascular markings, interstitial edema, or pleural effusion, and cardiomegaly.
- Echocardiography shows decreased ejection fraction, or abnormal heart size, shape, or movement.

Diagnostic procedures

- Electrocardiography shows enlargement, or ischemia and may show atrial fibrillation, tachycardia, or extrasystole.
- Pulmonary artery pressure monitoring shows elevated pulmonary artery and pulmonary artery wedge pressures in left-sided heart failure, and elevated right atrial or central venous pressure in right-sided heart failure.

Treatment

General

- Activity, as tolerated
- Antiembolism stockings
- Elevation of legs
- Fluid restriction
- Low-fat diet, if indicated
- Sodium-restricted diet
- Walking program

Medications

- Angiotensin-converting enzyme inhibitors

- ◆ Angiotensin receptor blockers
- ◆ Anticoagulants
- ◆ Beta-adrenergic blockers
- ◆ Cardiac glycosides
- ◆ Diuretics
- ◆ Inotropic drugs
- ◆ Oxygen
- ◆ Potassium supplements
- ◆ Vasodilators

Surgery

◆ For valvular dysfunction with recurrent acute heart failure, surgical replacement
◆ Heart transplantation
◆ Placement of a stent
◆ Placement of a ventricular assist device

Nursing interventions

◆ Place the patient in Fowler's position, and give supplemental oxygen.
◆ Provide continuous cardiac monitoring during the acute and advanced stages of disease.
◆ Help the patient with range-of-motion exercises.
◆ Apply antiembolism stockings, and check for calf pain and tenderness.
◆ Monitor the patient's weight daily to detect peripheral edema and other signs and symptoms of fluid overload.

Patient teaching

◆ Be sure to cover:
- the disorder, diagnosis, and treatment
- signs and symptoms of worsening heart failure
- when to notify the physician
- the importance of follow-up care
- the need to avoid high-sodium foods
- the need to avoid fatigue
- instructions about fluid restrictions
- the need for the patient to weigh himself every morning at the same time, before eating and after urinating; to keep a record of his weight; and to report a weight gain of 3 to 5 lb (1.5 to 2.5 kg) in 1 week
- the importance of smoking cessation, if appropriate
- weight reduction, as needed
- medication dosage, administration, potential adverse effects, and monitoring needs.

◆ Encourage follow-up care.
◆ Refer the patient to a smoking-cessation program, if appropriate.

Hepatitis, viral

Overview

◆ Infection and inflammation of the liver by a virus
◆ Six types now recognized (A, B, C, D, E, and G), and a seventh suspected
◆ Marked by hepatic cell destruction, necrosis, and autolysis, leading to anorexia, jaundice, and hepatomegaly
◆ In most patients, eventual regeneration of hepatic cells, with little or no residual damage, allowing recovery
◆ Complications more likely with advanced age and serious underlying disorders
◆ Poor prognosis if edema and hepatic encephalopathy develop

Causes

◆ Infection with one of the six major forms of the virus

Type A

◆ Transmission by the fecal-oral or parenteral route
◆ Ingestion of contaminated food, milk, or water

Type B

◆ Transmission by contact with contaminated human blood, secretions, and stools

Type C

◆ Transmission mainly via sharing of needles by I.V. drug users, blood transfusions, and tattoo needles

Type D

◆ Found only in patients with an acute or a chronic episode of hepatitis B

Type E

◆ Transmission by the parenteral route and often water-borne

Type G

◆ Believed to be blood-borne, with routes of transmission similar to those of hepatitis B and C

Data collection

History

◆ No signs or symptoms of disease in 50% to 60% of people with hepatitis B
◆ No signs or symptoms of disease in 80% of people with hepatitis C
◆ Revelation of a source of transmission

Prodromal stage

◆ Anorexia and mild weight loss
◆ Arthralgia and myalgia (hepatitis B)
◆ Changes in senses of taste and smell
◆ Depression
◆ Fatigue and generalized malaise
◆ Headache and photophobia
◆ Nausea and vomiting
◆ Weakness

Clinical jaundice stage

◆ Abdominal pain or tenderness
◆ Anorexia
◆ Indigestion
◆ Possible jaundice of the sclerae, mucous membranes, and skin
◆ Pruritus

Posticteric stage

◆ Decrease in most symptoms

Physical findings

Prodromal stage

◆ Clay-colored stools
◆ Dark urine
◆ Fever (100° to 102° F [37.8° to 38.9° C])

Clinical jaundice stage

◆ Abdominal tenderness in the right upper quadrant
◆ Cervical adenopathy
◆ Rash, erythematous patches, or hives
◆ Splenomegaly
◆ Tender, enlarged liver

Posticteric stage

◆ Decrease in liver enlargement

Diagnostic tests

Laboratory

◆ In patients with suspected viral hepatitis, a hepatitis profile is routinely performed. The result identifies antibodies specific to the causative virus and establishes the type of hepatitis.
- Type A: An antibody to hepatitis A confirms the diagnosis.
- Type B: Hepatitis B surface antigens and hepatitis B antibodies confirm the diagnosis.
- Type C: The diagnosis depends on serologic testing for the specific antibody 1 or more months after the onset of acute illness. Until then, the diagnosis is established principally by obtaining negative test results for hepatitis A, B, and D.
- Type D: Intrahepatic delta antigens or immunoglobulin (Ig) M antidelta antigens are detected in acute disease (or, in chronic disease, IgM and IgG), establishing the diagnosis.
- Type E: The detection of hepatitis E antigens supports the diagnosis and may rule out hepatitis C.

- Type G: The detection of hepatitis G ribonucleic acid supports the diagnosis. (Serologic assays are being developed.)
◆ Additional findings from liver function studies support the diagnosis.
- Serum aspartate aminotransferase and serum alanine aminotransferase levels are increased in the prodromal stage of acute viral hepatitis.
- Serum alkaline phosphatase levels are slightly increased.
- Serum bilirubin levels are elevated and may remain elevated late in the course of disease, especially in patients with severe disease.
- Prothrombin time is prolonged (more than 3 seconds longer than normal, indicating severe liver damage).
- White blood cell counts commonly show transient neutropenia and lymphopenia, followed by lymphocytosis.

Diagnostic procedures
◆ Liver biopsy shows chronic hepatitis.

Treatment

General

For hepatitis C
◆ Aimed at clearing hepatitis C virus from the body, stopping or slowing hepatic damage, and providing symptomatic relief
◆ Alcohol cessation
◆ Avoidance of contact sports and strenuous activity
◆ Frequent rest periods, as needed
◆ Parenteral feeding, if appropriate
◆ Small, high-calorie, high-protein meals (Protein intake is reduced if signs of precoma — lethargy, confusion, and mental changes — develop.)
◆ Symptomatic care

Medications
◆ Alfa-2b interferon (hepatitis B and C)
◆ Antiemetics
◆ Cholestyramine
◆ Lamivudine (hepatitis B)
◆ Ribavirin (hepatitis C)
◆ Standard Ig
◆ Vaccine

Surgery
◆ Possible liver transplantation (hepatitis C)

Nursing interventions
◆ Observe standard precautions to prevent disease transmission.
◆ Provide rest periods throughout the day.
◆ Give prescribed drugs.
◆ Encourage oral fluid intake.

Patient teaching

◆ Be sure to cover:
- the disorder, diagnosis, and treatment
- measures to prevent spread of the disease
- the importance of rest and a proper diet that includes a variety of healthy foods
- the need to avoid alcohol
- medications, dosages, and possible adverse effects
- the need to avoid over-the-counter medications unless approved by the physician
- the need for follow-up care.

◆ Refer the patient to Alcoholics Anonymous, if indicated.

Human immunodeficiency virus and acquired immunodeficiency syndrome

Overview

◆ Infection with human immunodeficiency virus (HIV) type 1, the retrovirus that causes acquired immunodeficiency syndrome (AIDS)

- Increased susceptibility to opportunistic infections, unusual cancers, and other abnormalities
- Progressive failure of the immune system
- Transmission by contact with infected blood or body fluids, usually through identifiable high-risk behaviors

Causes

- Infection with HIV, a retrovirus

Risk factors

- Contact with infected blood or body fluids, such as semen, breast milk, and saliva
- History of sexually transmitted disease
- Placental transmission
- Sharing of needles or syringes by I.V. drug users
- Unprotected sexual intercourse, particularly anal intercourse

Data collection

History

- A mononucleosis-like syndrome after a high-risk exposure, possibly followed by an asymptomatic period that may last years
- A latent stage in which the only sign of HIV infection is laboratory evidence of seroconversion

Physical findings

- Persistent generalized adenopathy
- Neurologic symptoms resulting from HIV encephalopathy
- Nonspecific symptoms (weight loss, fatigue, night sweats, fevers)
- Opportunistic infection or cancer (Kaposi's sarcoma)

Age alert Bacterial infections occur more commonly in children with AIDS.

Diagnostic tests

Laboratory

- A screening test (enzyme-linked immunosorbent assay) and a confirmatory test (Western blot) show HIV antibodies, which indicate HIV infection.
- A $CD4^+$ T-cell count of less than 200 cells/µl in a patient with HIV confirms AIDS diagnosis

Treatment

General

- Disease-specific therapy for a variety of neoplastic diseases, premalignant diseases, and organ-specific syndromes
- Regular exercise, as tolerated, with adequate rest periods
- Symptom management (fatigue and anemia)
- Variety of therapeutic options for opportunistic infections (the leading cause of illness and death in HIV-infected patients)
- Well-balanced diet

Medications

- Anti-infective drugs
- Antineoplastic drugs
- Highly active antiretroviral therapy
- Immunomodulatory drugs

Primary therapy

- Nonnucleoside reverse transcriptase inhibitors
- Nucleoside reverse transcriptase inhibitors
- Protease inhibitors

Nursing interventions

- Help the patient cope with an altered body image, the emotional burden of serious illness, and the threat of death.
- Avoid using glycerin swabs on the mucous membranes. Use normal saline or bicarbonate mouthwash for daily oral rinsing.

◆ Ensure adequate fluid intake during episodes of diarrhea.
◆ Provide meticulous skin care, especially in the debilitated patient.
◆ Encourage the patient to maintain as much physical activity as he can tolerate. Make sure his schedule includes time for exercise and rest.
◆ Watch for progression of lesions in Kaposi's sarcoma.
◆ Monitor the patient for opportunistic infections or signs of disease progression.

Patient teaching

◆ Be sure to cover:
- medication regimens
- the importance of informing sexual partners, caregivers, and health care workers about HIV infection status
- the signs of infection and the importance of seeking immediate medical attention
- the symptoms of AIDS dementia and its stages and progression.

◆ Refer the patient to a local support group.
◆ Refer the patient to hospice care, as indicated.

Hypertension

Overview

◆ Intermittent or sustained elevation of diastolic or systolic blood pressure
◆ Usually benign initially, progressing slowly to accelerated or malignant state
◆ Two major types:
- Essential (also called primary or idiopathic) hypertension
- Secondary hypertension, which results from renal disease or another identifiable cause

◆ A severe, fulminant form — malignant hypertension — that may arise from either type and that is a medical emergency

Causes
◆ Unknown

Risk factors
◆ Aging
◆ Black race (in the United States)
◆ Diet high in sodium and saturated fat
◆ Excessive alcohol intake
◆ Family history
◆ Hormonal contraceptive use
◆ Obesity
◆ Sedentary lifestyle
◆ Stress
◆ Tobacco use

Data collection

History
◆ In many cases, no symptoms, with disorder detected incidentally during evaluation for another disorder or during routine blood pressure screening
◆ Symptoms that show the effect of hypertension on the organ systems
- Awakening with a headache in the occipital region that subsides spontaneously after a few hours
- Blurred vision
- Dizziness, fatigue, and confusion
- Epistaxis
- Hematuria
- Palpitations, chest pain, and dyspnea

Physical findings
◆ Bounding pulse
◆ Bruits over the abdominal aorta and femoral arteries or the carotids
◆ Elevated blood pressure on at least two consecutive occasions after initial screenings (normal: systolic pressure less than 120 mm Hg and diastolic pressure less than 80 mm Hg)

- Hemorrhages, exudates, and papilledema of the eye in late stages of disease, if patient has hypertensive retinopathy
- Peripheral edema in late stages of disease
- Pulsating abdominal mass suggesting an abdominal aneurysm
- S_4 heart sound

Diagnostic tests

Laboratory

- Urinalysis may show protein, red blood cells, or white blood cells (suggesting renal disease) or glucose (suggesting diabetes mellitus).
- Serum potassium levels are less than 3.5 mEq/L, possibly indicating adrenal dysfunction (primary hyperaldosteronism).
- Blood urea nitrogen levels are normal or elevated to more than 20 mg/dl, and serum creatinine levels are normal or elevated to more than 1.5 mg/dl, suggesting renal disease.

Imaging

- Excretory urography may show renal atrophy, indicating chronic renal disease; one kidney more than 5/8″ (1.6 cm) shorter than the other suggests unilateral renal disease.
- Chest X-rays may show cardiomegaly.
- Renal arteriography may show renal artery stenosis.

Diagnostic procedures

- Electrocardiography may show left ventricular hypertrophy or ischemia.
- An oral captopril challenge may be done to test for renovascular hypertension.
- Ophthalmoscopy shows arteriovenous nicking and, in hypertensive encephalopathy, edema.

Treatment

General

- Adequate calcium, magnesium, and potassium in diet
- Diet low in sodium and saturated fat
- In secondary hypertension, correction of the underlying cause and control of hypertensive effects
- Lifestyle changes, such as weight control, limiting alcohol use, regular exercise, and smoking cessation
- Regular exercise program

Medications

- Aldosterone antagonist
- Alpha-receptor antagonists
- Angiotensin-converting enzyme inhibitors
- Angiotensin receptor blockers
- Beta-adrenergic blockers
- Calcium channel blockers
- Diuretics
- Vasodilators

Nursing interventions

- Give medications, as ordered.
- Encourage diet changes, as appropriate.
- Help the patient identify risk factors and modify his lifestyle, as appropriate.
- Monitor vital signs, especially blood pressure.

Patient teaching

- Be sure to cover:
  - the disorder, diagnosis, and treatment
  - how to use a self-monitoring blood pressure cuff and record the reading in a journal for review by the physician
  - the importance of complying with antihypertensive therapy and establishing a daily routine for taking medications
  - the need to report adverse drug effects

- the need to avoid high-sodium antacids and over-the-counter cold and sinus medications that contain potentially harmful vasoconstrictors
- the need for the patient to examine and modify his lifestyle, including diet
- the need for a routine exercise program, particularly aerobic walking
- dietary restrictions
- the importance of follow-up care.

◆ Refer the patient to stress-reduction therapy or support groups, as needed.

Influenza

Overview

◆ Acute, highly contagious infection of the respiratory tract
◆ Ability to mutate into different strains so that no immunologic resistance is present in those at risk (antigenic variation)
◆ Antigenic variation characterized as antigenic drift (minor changes that occur yearly or every few years) and antigenic shift (major changes that lead to pandemics)
◆ Also called the grippe or the flu

Causes

◆ Type A: Most prevalent; occurs annually, with new serotypes causing epidemics every 3 years
◆ Type B: Also annual, but causes epidemics only every 4 to 6 years
◆ Type C: Endemic and causes only sporadic cases
◆ Infection transmitted by inhaling a respiratory droplet from an infected person or by indirect contact (drinking from a contaminated glass)

Data collection

History

◆ Fatigue, listlessness, and weakness
◆ Headache
◆ Malaise
◆ Myalgia
◆ No influenza vaccine received during the past season
◆ Usually, recent exposure (typically within 48 hours) to a person with influenza

Physical findings

◆ Cervical adenopathy and tenderness
◆ Diminished breath sounds in areas of consolidation
◆ Erythema of the nose and throat without exudate
◆ Fever (usually higher in children)
◆ Red, watery eyes; clear nasal discharge
◆ Signs of croup or dry cough
◆ Tachypnea, shortness of breath, and cyanosis
◆ With bacterial pneumonia, purulent or bloody sputum

Diagnostic tests

◆ After an epidemic is confirmed, diagnosis requires only observation of signs and symptoms.

Laboratory

◆ Inoculation of chicken embryos with nasal secretions from an infected patient shows the influenza virus.
◆ Throat swabs, nasopharyngeal washes, or sputum cultures show isolation of the influenza virus.
◆ Immunodiagnostic techniques show viral antigens in tissue culture or in exfoliated nasopharyngeal cells obtained by washings.
◆ White blood cell (WBC) counts are increased in secondary bacterial infection.
◆ WBC counts are decreased in overwhelming viral or bacterial infection.

Treatment

General

- Fluid and electrolyte replacement
- Increased fluid intake
- Oxygen and assisted ventilation, if indicated
- Rest periods, as needed

Medications

- Acetaminophen or aspirin
- Antibiotics
- Antiviral drugs
- Guaifenesin or an expectorant

Nursing interventions

- Give drugs, as ordered.
- Follow standard precautions.
- Give oxygen therapy, if warranted.
- Monitor patient for signs and symptoms of dehydration.

Patient teaching

- Be sure to cover:
  - the disorder, diagnosis, and treatment
  - use of mouthwash or warm saline gargles to ease sore throat
  - importance of increasing fluid intake to prevent dehydration
  - use of a warm bath or a heating pad to relieve myalgia
  - importance of proper hand-washing technique and tissue disposal to prevent the virus from spreading
  - need for influenza immunization.

Irritable bowel syndrome

Overview

- A common condition marked by chronic or periodic diarrhea alternating with constipation
- Accompanied by straining and abdominal cramps
- Initial episodes occurring early in life and in the late teens to 20s
- Good prognosis
- Also known as spastic colon, spastic colitis, or mucous colitis

Causes

- Unknown

Other possible triggers

- Allergy to certain foods or drugs
- Anxiety and stress
- Dietary factors, such as fiber, raw fruits, coffee, alcohol, and foods that are cold, highly seasoned, or laxative in nature
- Hormones
- Lactose intolerance
- Laxative abuse

Data collection

History

- Abdominal bloating
- Anxiety and fatigue
- Chronic constipation, diarrhea, or both
- Contributing psychological factors (such as a recent stressful life change) that may have triggered or worsened symptoms
- Dyspepsia
- Faintness and weakness
- Heartburn
- Lower abdominal pain (typically in the left lower quadrant) usually relieved by defecation or passage of gas
- Small stools with visible mucus or pasty, pencil-like stools instead of diarrhea

Physical findings

- Normal bowel sounds
- Tympany over a gas-filled bowel

Diagnostic tests

- Testing involves studies to rule out other, more serious disorders.

Laboratory
◆ Examination of stools shows no occult blood, parasites, or pathogenic bacteria.
◆ Results of complete blood count, serologic tests, serum albumin test, and erythrocyte sedimentation rate are normal.

Imaging
◆ Barium enema may show a colonic spasm, and the descending colon may appear tubular. Barium enema is also used to rule out certain other disorders, such as diverticula, tumors, and polyps.

Diagnostic procedures
◆ Sigmoidoscopy may show spastic contractions.

Treatment

General
◆ Avoidance of sorbitol, nonabsorbable carbohydrates, and lactose-containing foods
◆ Diet based on the patient's symptoms
◆ Increased dietary bulk
◆ Increased fluid intake
◆ Initially, an elimination diet
◆ Lifestyle modifications
◆ Regular exercise
◆ Stress management

Medications
◆ Anticholinergic, antispasmodic drugs
◆ Antidiarrheals
◆ Antiemetics
◆ Laxatives
◆ Mild tranquilizers
◆ Simethicone
◆ Tricyclic antidepressants

Nursing interventions
◆ Because the patient with irritable bowel syndrome isn't hospitalized, nursing interventions usually focus on patient teaching.

Patient teaching

◆ Be sure to cover:
- the disorder, diagnosis, and treatment
- dietary plans and implementation
- the need to drink 8 to 10 glasses of water or other compatible fluids daily
- the proper use of prescribed medication, including the desired effects and possible adverse reactions
- the need to implement lifestyle changes that reduce stress
- smoking cessation
- the need for regular physical examinations. (For patients older than age 40, emphasize the need for colorectal cancer screening, including annual proctosigmoidoscopy and rectal examinations.)

Lyme disease

Overview

◆ A multisystem disorder caused by a spirochete

Causes
◆ The spirochete *Borrelia burgdorferi,* which is carried by the minute tick *Ixodes dammini* (also called *I. scapularis*) or another tick in the Ixodidae family

Data collection

History
◆ Fever (up to 104° F [40° C]) and chills
◆ Onset of symptoms in warmer months
◆ Recent exposure to ticks

◆ Severe headache and stiff neck, with eruption of rash

Physical findings

◆ Regional lymphadenopathy
◆ Tenderness at the site of skin lesions or in the posterior cervical area

Early stage

◆ Arthralgia
◆ Erythema migrans
◆ Headache
◆ Mild dyspnea
◆ Myalgia
◆ Tachycardia or irregular heartbeat

Later stage

◆ Bell's palsy
◆ Cardiac symptoms, such as heart failure, pericarditis, and dyspnea
◆ Fibromyalgia
◆ Intermittent arthritis
◆ Neurologic signs, such as memory impairment
◆ Neurologic symptoms such as memory impairment and myelitis
◆ Ocular signs such as conjunctivitis

Diagnostic tests

Laboratory

◆ Assays for anti-*B. burgdorferi* show evidence of previous or current infection.
◆ Enzyme-linked immunosorbent technology or indirect immunofluorescence microscopy shows immunoglobulin (Ig) M levels that peak 3 to 6 weeks after infection. IgG antibodies are detected several weeks after infection, may continue to develop for several months, and usually persist for years.
◆ Positive Western blot assay shows serologic evidence of past or current infection with *B. burgdorferi.*
◆ Polymerase chain reaction is used in patients who have joint and cerebrospinal fluid (CSF) involvement.
◆ Serologic testing isn't useful early in the course of Lyme disease because of its low sensitivity. However, it may be more useful in later stages of disease, when the sensitivity and specificity of the test are improved.

Diagnostic procedures

◆ Lumbar puncture with analysis of the CSF may show antibodies to *B. burgdorferi.*
◆ Skin biopsy may be used to detect *B. burgdorferi.*

Treatment

General

◆ Prompt tick removal using proper technique
◆ Rest periods when needed

Medications

◆ I.V. or oral antibiotics (started as soon as possible after infection occurs)

Nursing interventions

◆ Plan care to provide adequate rest.
◆ Give prescribed drugs.
◆ Help with range-of-motion and strengthening exercises (with arthritis).
◆ Encourage verbalization, and provide support.

Patient teaching

◆ Be sure to cover:
- the disorder, diagnosis, and treatment
- medications, dosages, and possible adverse effects
- the importance of follow-up care and the need to report recurrent or new symptoms to the physician
- prevention of Lyme disease, such as avoiding tick-infested areas, covering the skin with clothing, using insect repellants, inspecting exposed skin for attached ticks at least every 4 hours, and removing ticks

- information about the vaccine for persons at risk for contracting Lyme disease.
- ◆ If the patient is in the late stages of disease, refer him to a dermatologist, neurologist, cardiologist, or infectious disease specialist, as indicated.

Multiple sclerosis

Overview

- ◆ Progressive demyelination of the white matter of the brain and spinal cord
- ◆ Characterized by exacerbations and remissions
- ◆ In some cases, rapid progression, with death occurring within months
- ◆ Variable prognosis (Most patients with multiple sclerosis [70%] lead active lives with prolonged remissions.)
- ◆ Also known as MS

Causes

- ◆ Allergic response
- ◆ Autoimmune response of the nervous system
- ◆ Events that precede the onset of disease:
  - Emotional stress
  - Overwork
  - Fatigue
  - Pregnancy
  - Acute respiratory tract infections
- ◆ Exact cause unknown
- ◆ Genetic factors possibly also involved
- ◆ Slow-acting viral infection

Risk factors

- ◆ Anorexia nervosa
- ◆ Anoxia
- ◆ Nutritional deficiencies
- ◆ Toxins
- ◆ Trauma
- ◆ Vascular lesions

Data collection

History

- ◆ Blurred vision or diplopia
- ◆ Bowel disturbances (involuntary evacuation or constipation)
- ◆ Dysphagia
- ◆ Emotional lability
- ◆ Fatigue (typically the most disabling symptom)
- ◆ Symptoms related to the extent and site of myelin destruction, the extent of remyelination, and the adequacy of subsequent restored synaptic transmission
- ◆ Symptoms transient or lasting for hours or weeks
- ◆ Symptoms unpredictable and difficult to describe
- ◆ Urinary problems
- ◆ Vision problems and sensory impairment (the first signs)

Physical findings

- ◆ Gait ataxia
- ◆ Intention tremor
- ◆ Muscle weakness of the involved area
- ◆ Nystagmus and scotoma
- ◆ Ophthalmoplegia
- ◆ Optic neuritis
- ◆ Paralysis, ranging from monoplegia to quadriplegia
- ◆ Poor articulation
- ◆ Spasticity and hyperreflexia

Diagnostic tests

- ◆ Diagnosis may require years of testing and observation.

Laboratory

- ◆ Cerebrospinal fluid analysis shows mononuclear cell pleocytosis, an elevated level of total immunoglobulin (Ig) G, and the presence of oligoclonal Ig.

Imaging

◆ Magnetic resonance imaging is the most sensitive method for detecting focal lesions associated with multiple sclerosis.

Other tests

◆ EEG abnormalities occur in one-third of patients with multiple sclerosis.

◆ Evoked potential studies show slowed conduction of nerve impulses.

Treatment

General

◆ Symptomatic treatment for acute exacerbations and related signs and symptoms

◆ Diet high in fluid and fiber in case of constipation

◆ Frequent rest periods

Medications

◆ Alkylating drugs

◆ Antimetabolites

◆ Biologic response modifiers

◆ Immunosuppressants

◆ I.V. steroids followed by oral corticosteroids

Nursing interventions

◆ Provide emotional and psychological support.

◆ Help with the physical therapy program.

◆ Provide adequate rest periods.

◆ Promote emotional stability.

◆ Keep the bedpan or urinal readily available because the need to void is immediate.

◆ Provide bowel and bladder training, if indicated.

◆ Give prescribed drugs.

◆ Monitor functional changes, including speech, vision, energy, sensory impairment, and muscle dysfunction.

Understanding types of multiple sclerosis

Various terms are used to describe different types of multiple sclerosis.

◆ *Relapsing remitting:* clear relapses (or acute attacks or exacerbations), with full recovery and no lasting disability. Between attacks, the disease doesn't worsen.

◆ *Primary progressive:* steadily progressing or worsening, with minor recovery or plateaus. This form is uncommon and may involve different brain and spinal cord damage from other forms.

◆ *Secondary progressive:* beginning as a pattern of clear relapses and recovery, but becoming steadily progressive and worsening between acute attacks.

◆ *Progressive-relapsing:* steadily progressing from the onset but with clear, acute attacks. This form is rare.

In addition, the differential diagnosis must rule out spinal cord compression, foramen magnum tumor (which may mimic the exacerbations and remissions of multiple sclerosis), multiple small strokes, syphilis or another infection, thyroid disease, and chronic fatigue syndrome.

Patient teaching

◆ Be sure to cover:

- the disease process (see *Understanding types of multiple sclerosis*)
- medication and adverse effects
- the importance of avoiding stress, infections, and fatigue
- the importance of maintaining independence
- the need to avoid exposure to bacterial and viral infections
- nutritional management

– the importance of adequate fluid intake and regular urination.
◆ Refer the patient to the National Multiple Sclerosis Society.
◆ Refer the patient to physical and occupational rehabilitation programs, as indicated.

Myocardial infarction

Overview

◆ Reduced blood flow through one or more coronary arteries, causing myocardial ischemia and necrosis
◆ Site of infarction depends on the vessels involved
◆ Also called MI and heart attack

Causes
◆ Atherosclerosis
◆ Coronary artery stenosis or spasm
◆ Platelet aggregation
◆ Thrombosis

Risk factors
◆ Diabetes mellitus
◆ Elevated serum triglyceride, low-density lipoprotein, and cholesterol levels, and decreased serum high-density lipoprotein levels
◆ Excessive intake of saturated fats, carbohydrates, or salt
◆ Family history of coronary artery disease (CAD)
◆ Hypertension
◆ Middle-age or older (40 to 70)
◆ Obesity
◆ Sedentary lifestyle
◆ Smoking
◆ Stress or type A personality
◆ Use of such drugs as amphetamines or cocaine

Data collection

History
◆ Possible CAD with increasing frequency, severity, or duration of angina
◆ Cardinal symptom: Persistent, crushing substernal pain or pressure that may radiate to the left arm, jaw, neck, and shoulder blades, and may persist for 12 hours or longer
◆ Little or no pain in an elderly patient or a patient with diabetes; pain possibly mild and confused with indigestion in other patients
◆ Fatigue, nausea, vomiting, and shortness of breath, accompanied by a feeling of impending doom
◆ Sudden death (may be the first and only indication of MI)

Physical findings
◆ A systolic murmur of mitral insufficiency
◆ An S_4 heart sound, an S_3 heart sound, and paradoxical splitting of the S_2 heart sound with ventricular dysfunction
◆ Diaphoresis
◆ Dyspnea
◆ Extreme anxiety and restlessness
◆ Hypertension
◆ In inferior MI, bradycardia and hypotension
◆ Low-grade fever for the next few days
◆ Pericardial friction rub with transmural MI or pericarditis
◆ Tachycardia

Diagnostic tests
Laboratory
◆ Serum creatine kinase (CK) level is elevated, especially CK-MB isoenzyme, which is the cardiac muscle fraction of CK.
◆ Serum lactate dehydrogenase (LD) level is elevated; LD_1 isoenzyme level (found in cardiac tissue) is higher than LD_2 level (in serum).

◆ An elevated white blood cell count usually appears on the second day and lasts for 1 week.
◆ Myoglobin (the hemoprotein found in cardiac and skeletal muscle) is detected. It's released with muscle damage, as soon as 2 hours after an MI.
◆ Troponin I and troponin T levels are elevated only when cardiac muscle damage occurs. Troponin levels are more specific than CK-MB level. (Troponin levels increase within 4 to 6 hours of myocardial injury and may remain elevated for 5 to 11 days.)

Imaging
◆ Nuclear medicine scans performed with I.V. technetium 99m pertechnetate can identify acutely damaged muscle by detecting accumulations of radioactive nucleotide. An area of accumulation appears as a "hot spot" on the film. Myocardial perfusion imaging with thallium 201 shows a "cold spot" (a poorly perfused area of the heart where thallium does not appear) in most patients during the first few hours after a transmural MI.
◆ Echocardiography shows ventricular wall dyskinesia with a transmural MI and helps evaluate the ejection fraction.

Diagnostic procedures
◆ Serial 12-lead electrocardiography (ECG) readings may be normal or inconclusive during the first few hours after an MI. Characteristic abnormalities include serial ST-segment depression in a subendocardial MI and ST-segment elevation and Q waves, representing scarring and necrosis, respectively, in a transmural MI.
◆ Coronary artery catheterization may be performed to detect left- or right-sided heart failure, to identify areas of blockage and necrosis, and to monitor the response to treatment.

Treatment

General
◆ Bed rest, with a commode available at the bedside
◆ Calorie restriction, if indicated
◆ For arrhythmias, a pacemaker or electrical cardioversion
◆ For cardiogenic shock, intra-aortic balloon pump
◆ Gradual increase in activity, as tolerated
◆ Low-fat, low-cholesterol diet

Medications
◆ Angiotensin-converting enzyme inhibitors
◆ Antiarrhythmics and antianginals
◆ Aspirin
◆ Beta-adrenergic blockers
◆ Calcium channel blockers
◆ Inotropic drugs
◆ I.V. heparin
◆ I.V. morphine
◆ I.V. thrombolytic therapy started within 3 hours of the onset of symptoms
◆ Oxygen
◆ Stool softeners

Surgery
◆ Percutaneous revascularization
◆ Surgical revascularization

Nursing interventions
◆ Evaluate pain and give analgesics, as ordered. Record the severity, location, type, and duration of pain. Avoid I.M. injections.
◆ Check the patient's blood pressure before and after giving nitroglycerin.
◆ During episodes of chest pain, obtain ECG.
◆ Organize patient care and activities to provide periods of uninterrupted rest.
◆ Provide a low-cholesterol, low-sodium diet with caffeine-free beverages.

◆ Allow the patient to use a bedside commode.
◆ Assist with range-of-motion exercises.
◆ Provide emotional support, and help reduce stress and anxiety.
◆ A patient who has undergone percutaneous transluminal coronary angioplasty will need sheath care. Watch for bleeding. Keep the leg with the sheath insertion site immobile. Maintain strict bed rest. Check peripheral pulses in the affected leg often.

Patient teaching

◆ Be sure to cover:
- procedures (answering questions for the patient and family members)
- medications, dosages, adverse reactions, and signs of toxicity to watch for and report
- dietary restrictions
- progressive resumption of sexual activity
- appropriate responses to new or recurrent symptoms
- typical and atypical chest pain and the need to report pain to the physician.

◆ Refer the patient to a cardiac rehabilitation program.
◆ Refer the patient to a smoking-cessation program, if needed.
◆ Refer the patient to a weight-reduction program, if needed.

Osteoarthritis

Overview

◆ Chronic degeneration of joint cartilage
◆ Most common form of arthritis
◆ Range of disability, from minor limitation to near immobility
◆ Knees and hips most commonly affected
◆ Varying rates of progression

Causes
◆ Advanced age
◆ Congenital abnormality
◆ Endocrine disorders such as diabetes mellitus
◆ Metabolic disorders such as chondrocalcinosis
◆ Possible hereditary factors
◆ Secondary osteoarthritis
◆ Traumatic injury

Data collection

History
◆ Aching during changes in weather
◆ Deep, aching joint pain
◆ "Grating" feeling when the joint moves
◆ Limited movement
◆ Pain after exercise or weight bearing
◆ Pain that may be relieved by rest
◆ Predisposing traumatic injury
◆ Stiffness in the morning and after exercise

Physical findings
◆ Contractures
◆ Deformity of the involved areas
◆ Gait abnormalities
◆ Hard nodes on the distal and proximal interphalangeal joints that may be red, swollen, and tender
◆ Joint swelling
◆ Loss of finger dexterity
◆ Muscle atrophy
◆ Muscle spasms, limited movement, and joint instability

Diagnostic tests
Laboratory
◆ Synovial fluid analysis rules out inflammatory arthritis.

Imaging
◆ X-rays of the affected joint may show narrowing of the joint space or margins, cystlike bony deposits in the joint space and margins, sclerosis of the subchondral space, joint deformity or articular damage, bony growths at weight-bearing areas, and possible joint fusion.
◆ Radionuclide bone scan may be used to rule out inflammatory arthritis by showing normal uptake of the radionuclide.
◆ Magnetic resonance imaging shows the affected joint, adjacent bones, and progression of disease.

Diagnostic procedures
◆ Neuromuscular tests may show reduced muscle strength.

Other tests
◆ Arthroscopy shows the internal joint structures and identifies soft-tissue swelling.

Treatment

General
◆ Activity, as tolerated
◆ Assistive mobility devices
◆ Pain relief
◆ Physical therapy
◆ Steps to improve mobility
◆ Steps to minimize disability

Medications
◆ Analgesics

Surgery
◆ Arthrodesis
◆ Arthroplasty (partial or total)
◆ Osteoplasty
◆ Osteotomy

Nursing interventions
◆ Allow adequate time for self-care.
◆ Adjust pain medications to allow for maximum rest.
◆ Identify techniques that promote rest and relaxation.
◆ Give anti-inflammatory medications.
◆ If the hand joints are affected, use hot soaks and paraffin dips.
◆ If the lumbosacral spinal joints are affected, provide a firm mattress.
◆ If the cervical spinal joints are affected, apply a cervical collar.
◆ If the hip is affected, apply moist heat pads and administer antispasmodic drugs.
◆ If the knee is affected, help with range-of-motion (ROM) exercises.
◆ Apply elastic supports or braces.
◆ Check the patient's crutches, cane, braces, or walker for proper fit.

Patient teaching

◆ Be sure to cover:
- the disorder, diagnosis, and treatment
- the need for adequate rest during the day, after exertion, and at night
- methods to conserve energy
- the need to take medications exactly as prescribed
- adverse reactions to medications
- the need to wear support shoes that fit well and the importance of repairing worn heels
- the need to install safety devices at home
- the importance of ROM exercises and the need to perform them as gently as possible
- the need to maintain proper body weight
- the use of crutches or other orthopedic devices.

◆ Refer the patient to occupational or physical therapy, as indicated.

Osteoporosis

Overview

◆ Loss of calcium and phosphate from bones, causing increased vulnerability to fractures
◆ Primary or secondary to underlying disease
◆ Types of primary osteoporosis: postmenopausal osteoporosis (type I) and age-associated osteoporosis (type II)
◆ Secondary osteoporosis: Caused by an identifiable agent or disease

Causes
◆ Alcoholism
◆ Bone immobilization
◆ Exact cause unknown
◆ Hyperthyroidism
◆ Lactose intolerance
◆ Liver disease
◆ Malabsorption
◆ Malnutrition
◆ Osteogenesis imperfecta
◆ Prolonged therapy with steroids or heparin
◆ Rheumatoid arthritis
◆ Scurvy
◆ Sudeck's atrophy (localized in the hands and feet, with recurring attacks)

Risk factors
◆ Declining gonadal adrenal function
◆ Faulty protein metabolism (caused by estrogen deficiency)
◆ Mild, prolonged negative calcium balance
◆ Sedentary lifestyle

Data collection

History
◆ Postmenopausal patient
◆ Condition known to cause secondary osteoporosis
◆ Snapping sound or sudden pain in the lower back when bending down to lift something
◆ Possible slow development of pain (over several years)
◆ With vertebral collapse, backache and pain radiating around the trunk
◆ Pain aggravated by movement or jarring

Physical findings
◆ Decreased spinal movement, with flexion more limited than extension
◆ Humped back
◆ Loss of height
◆ Markedly aged appearance
◆ Muscle spasm

Diagnostic tests
Laboratory
◆ Normal serum calcium, phosphorus, and alkaline levels
◆ Elevated parathyroid hormone level

Imaging
◆ X-ray studies show characteristic degeneration in the lower thoracolumbar vertebrae.
◆ Computed tomography scan determines spinal bone loss.
◆ Bone scans show injured or diseased areas.

Diagnostic procedures
◆ Bone biopsy shows thin, porous, but otherwise normal bone.

Other tests
◆ Dual or single photon absorptiometry (measurement of bone mass) shows loss of bone mass.

Treatment

General
◆ Control of bone loss
◆ Control of pain
◆ Diet that's rich in vitamin D, calcium, and protein

◆ Physical therapy program of gentle exercise and activity
◆ Prevention of additional fractures
◆ Reduction and immobilization of fractures
◆ Supportive devices

Medications

◆ Calcitonin
◆ Calcium and vitamin D supplements
◆ Estrogen
◆ Sodium fluoride

Surgery

◆ Open reduction and internal fixation for femur fractures

Nursing interventions

◆ Encourage careful positioning, ambulation, and prescribed exercises.
◆ Promote self-care, and allow adequate time.
◆ Encourage mild exercise.
◆ Assist with walking.
◆ Perform passive range-of-motion exercises.
◆ Promote physical therapy sessions.
◆ Use safety precautions.
◆ Give analgesia, as ordered.
◆ Apply heat.
◆ Monitor the skin for redness, warmth, and new sites of pain.
◆ Monitor exercise tolerance and joint mobility.

Patient teaching

◆ Be sure to cover:
- the disorder, diagnosis, and treatment
- the prescribed drug regimen
- how to recognize significant adverse reactions
- the need to perform monthly breast self-examination while receiving estrogen therapy
- the need to report vaginal bleeding promptly
- the need to report new pain sites immediately
- the importance of sleeping on a firm mattress
- the need to avoid excessive bed rest
- the use of a back brace, if appropriate
- the use of proper body mechanics
- the use of home safety devices
- the importance of a calcium-rich diet.

◆ Refer the patient to physical and occupational therapy, as appropriate.

Otitis media

Overview

◆ Inflammation of the middle ear associated with the accumulation of fluid
◆ Acute, chronic, suppurative, or secretory

Causes

◆ Acute otitis media: Bacterial infection with *Streptococcus pneumoniae, Haemophilus influenzae,* or *Moraxella catarrhalis*
◆ Suppurative otitis media: Bacterial infection with pneumococci, group A beta-hemolytic streptococci, staphylococci, or gram-negative bacteria
◆ Chronic suppurative otitis media: Inadequate treatment of acute episodes of otitis media or infection by resistant strains of bacteria
◆ Secretory otitis media: Viral infection, allergy, or barotrauma
◆ Chronic secretory otitis media: Overgrowth of adenoidal tissue, edema, chronic sinus infection, or inadequate treatment of acute suppurative otitis media

Age alert Acute otitis media is an emergency in an immunocompromised child.

Pediatric patients
- Peak incidence between ages 6 and 24 months
- Decreased incidence after age 3 years
- Most common during the winter months

Data collection

History
- Allergies
- Dizziness
- Nausea, vomiting
- Severe, deep, throbbing ear pain
- Upper respiratory tract infection

Acute secretory otitis media
- Popping, crackling, or clicking sounds on swallowing or moving the jaw
- Sensation of fullness in the ear
- Sensation of hearing an echo when speaking

Tympanic membrane rupture
- Pain that suddenly stops
- Recent air travel or scuba diving

Physical findings
- Blue-black tympanic membrane with hemorrhage into the middle ear
- Clear or amber fluid behind the tympanic membrane
- Conductive hearing loss (varies with the size and type of tympanic membrane perforation and the amount of ossicular destruction)
- Mild to high fever
- Obscured or distorted bony landmarks of the tympanic membrane in acute suppurative otitis media
- Painless, purulent discharge in chronic suppurative otitis media
- Pulsating discharge with tympanic perforation
- Retraction of the tympanic membrane in acute secretory otitis media
- Sneezing and coughing with upper respiratory tract infection

Chronic otitis media
- Cholesteatoma
- Mobility of the tympanic membrane decreased or absent
- Thickening and scarring of the tympanic membrane

Diagnostic tests
Laboratory
- Culture and sensitivity tests of exudate show the causative organism.
- Complete blood count shows leukocytosis.

Imaging
- Radiographic studies show mastoid involvement.

Diagnostic procedures
- Tympanometry detects hearing loss and evaluates the condition of the middle ear.
- Audiometry shows the degree of hearing loss.
- Pneumatic otoscopy may show decreased mobility of the tympanic membrane.

Age alert In adults, unilateral serous otitis media should always be evaluated for a nasopharyngeal-obstructing lesion such as carcinoma.

Treatment

General
- In acute secretory otitis media, Valsalva's maneuver several times daily (may be the only treatment required)
- Treatment of underlying cause
- Elimination of eustachian tube obstruction

Medications
- Analgesics
- Antibiotic

- Aspirin or acetaminophen
- Nasopharyngeal decongestant therapy
- Sedatives (in small children)

Surgery
- Cholesteatoma excision
- Mastoidectomy
- Myringoplasty
- Myringotomy and aspiration of fluid from the middle ear, followed by insertion of a polyethylene tube into the tympanic membrane
- Stapedectomy for otosclerosis
- Tympanoplasty

Nursing interventions
- Answer all questions.
- Encourage discussion of concerns about hearing loss.

With hearing loss
- Offer reassurance, when appropriate, that hearing loss caused by serious otitis media is temporary.
- Provide clear, concise explanations.
- Face the patient when speaking, and enunciate clearly and slowly.
- Allow time for the patient to grasp what was said.
- Provide a pencil and paper.
- Alert the staff to the patient's communication difficulty.

After myringotomy
- Wash hands before and after performing ear care.
- Maintain drainage flow.
- Place sterile cotton loosely in the external ear to absorb drainage and prevent infection. Change the cotton when it becomes damp. Avoid placing cotton or plugs deeply into the ear canal.
- Give analgesics as ordered.
- Give antiemetics after tympanoplasty and reinforce the dressings.
- Monitor the patient for excessive bleeding or discharge.
- Watch for and immediately report pain and fever caused by acute secretory otitis media.

Patient teaching

- Be sure to cover:
  - proper instillation of ointment, drops, and ear wash, as ordered
  - medications and adverse effects
  - the importance of taking antibiotics
  - the need for adequate fluid intake
  - the correct instillation of nasopharyngeal decongestants
  - the use of fitted earplugs for swimming after myringotomy and tympanostomy tube insertion
  - the need to notify the physician if the tube falls out and if ear pain, fever, or pus-filled discharge occurs
  - strategies for preventing recurrence.

Parkinson's disease

Overview

- Brain disorder causing progressive deterioration, with muscle rigidity, akinesia, and involuntary tremors
- Usual cause of death: Aspiration pneumonia
- One of the most common crippling diseases in the United States

Causes
- Exposure to toxins, such as manganese dust and carbon monoxide
- Drug-induced effect (haloperidol [Haldol], methyldopa, reserpine)
- Type A encephalitis
- Usually unknown

Data collection

History
- Akinesia
- Dysarthria

- Dysphagia
- Fatigue with activities of daily living
- Increased perspiration
- Insidious (unilateral pill-roll) tremor, which increases during stress or anxiety and decreases with purposeful movement and sleep
- Insomnia
- Mood changes
- Muscle cramps of the legs, neck, and trunk
- Muscle rigidity
- Oily skin

Physical findings
- Difficulty walking
- Difficulty pivoting
- Drooling
- High-pitched, monotonous voice
- Lack of parallel motion in gait
- Loss of balance
- Loss of posture control with walking
- Masklike facial expression
- Muscle rigidity causing resistance to passive muscle stretching
- Oculogyric crises (eyes fixed upward, with involuntary tonic movements)

Diagnostic tests
Imaging
- Computed tomography scan or magnetic resonance imaging rules out other disorders, such as intracranial tumors.

Treatment

General
- Assistive devices to aid ambulation
- High-bulk foods
- Physical therapy and occupational therapy
- Small, frequent meals

Medications
- Anticholinergics
- Antihistamines
- Antiviral drugs
- Dopamine replacement drugs
- Enzyme-inhibiting drugs
- Tricyclic antidepressants

Surgery
- Used when drug therapy is unsuccessful
- Stereotaxic neurosurgery
- Destruction of the ventrolateral nucleus of the thalamus

Nursing interventions
- Take measures to prevent aspiration.
- Protect the patient from injury.
- Stress the importance of rest periods between activities.
- Ensure adequate nutrition.
- Provide frequent warm baths and massage.
- Encourage the patient to enroll in a physical therapy program.
- Provide emotional and psychological support.
- Encourage the patient to be independent.
- Assist with ambulation and range-of-motion exercises.
- Postoperatively, monitor for signs of hemorrhage and increased intracranial pressure.

Patient teaching

- Be sure to cover:
  - the disorder, diagnosis, and treatment
  - medications, dosages, and adverse reactions
  - measures to prevent pressure ulcers and contractures
  - household safety measures
  - the importance of daily bathing
  - methods to improve communication
  - the importance of a swallowing therapy regimen (aspiration precautions).

◆ Refer the patient to occupational and physical rehabilitation, as indicated.

Peptic ulcer

Overview

◆ Circumscribed lesion in the mucosal membrane of the lower esophagus, stomach, duodenum, or jejunum
◆ Occurs in two major forms: duodenal ulcer and gastric ulcer (both chronic)
◆ Duodenal ulcers: Account for about 80% of peptic ulcers, affect the proximal part of the small intestine, and follow a chronic course characterized by remissions and exacerbations (About 5% to 10% of patients with duodenal ulcers have complications that warrant surgery.)
◆ Gastric ulcers: Occur in the gastric mucosa and have a wide spectrum of clinical presentations, ranging from asymptomatic to vague epigastric pain, nausea, and iron deficiency anemia to acute life-threatening hemorrhage.

Causes

◆ *Helicobacter pylori*
◆ Pathologic hypersecretory states
◆ Use of glucocorticoids or nonsteroidal anti-inflammatory drugs (NSAIDs)

Risk factors

◆ Cigarette smoking
◆ Exposure to irritants
◆ Genetic factors
◆ Normal aging
◆ Psychogenic factors
◆ Trauma
◆ Type A blood (for gastric ulcer)
◆ Type O blood (for duodenal ulcer)

Data collection

History

◆ History of a predisposing factor
◆ Left epigastric pain described as heartburn or indigestion and accompanied by a feeling of fullness or distention
◆ Periods of worsening and remitting symptoms, with remissions lasting longer than exacerbations

Gastric ulcer

◆ Nausea or vomiting
◆ Pain triggered or worsened by eating
◆ Recent loss of weight or appetite

Duodenal ulcer

◆ Pain that awakens the patient from sleep
◆ Pain relieved by eating; may occur 1½ to 3 hours after food intake
◆ Weight gain

Physical findings

◆ Epigastric tenderness
◆ Hyperactive bowel sounds
◆ Pallor

Diagnostic tests

Laboratory

◆ Complete blood count shows anemia.
◆ Testing shows occult blood in the stools.
◆ Venous blood sample shows *H. pylori* antibodies.
◆ White blood cell count is elevated.
◆ Urea breath test shows low levels of exhaled carbon 13.
◆ Fasting serum gastrin level rules out Zollinger-Ellison syndrome.

Imaging

◆ Barium swallow or upper GI and small-bowel series may reveal the ulcer.

- Upper GI tract X-rays show mucosal abnormalities.

Diagnostic procedures

- Upper GI endoscopy or esophagogastroduodenoscopy confirm the ulcer and permit cytologic studies and biopsy to rule out *H. pylori* or cancer.
- Gastric secretory studies show hyperchlorhydria.

Treatment

General

- Avoidance of dietary irritants
- Iced saline lavage, possibly containing norepinephrine
- Laser or cautery during endoscopy
- Nothing by mouth if GI bleeding is evident
- Smoking cessation
- Stress reduction
- Symptomatic care

Medications

For H. pylori

- Amoxicillin, clarithromycin (Biaxin), and omeprazole (Prilosec)

For gastric or duodenal ulcer

- Antacids
- Anticholinergics (for duodenal ulcers; usually contraindicated in gastric ulcers)
- Antisecretory agents if the ulcer resulted from NSAID use, when NSAIDs must be continued
- Coating agents (for duodenal ulcer)
- Histamine-receptor antagonists or gastric acid pump inhibitor
- Prostaglandin analogues
- Proton pump inhibitors
- Sedatives and tranquilizers (for gastric ulcer)

Surgery

- Indicated for perforation, lack of response to conservative treatment, suspected cancer, or other complications
- Type varies with the location and extent of the ulcer; major operations: bilateral vagotomy, pyloroplasty, and gastrectomy

Nursing interventions

- Give medications as ordered.
- Provide six small meals or small hourly meals, as ordered.
- Offer emotional support.
- Monitor the patient for signs and symptoms of bleeding.
- Provide pain control.

After surgery

- Monitor bowel function.
- Maintain nasogastric tube function and drainage.
- Check fluid and nutritional status.
- Care for the wound site.
- Watch for signs and symptoms of metabolic alkalosis or perforation.

Patient teaching

- Be sure to cover:
  - the disorder, diagnosis, and treatment
  - medications, dosages, and possible reactions to medications
  - warnings against using over-the-counter medications, especially aspirin, aspirin-containing products, and NSAIDs, unless the physician approves
  - warnings against using caffeine and alcohol during exacerbations
  - appropriate lifestyle changes
  - dietary modifications.
- Refer the patient to a smoking-cessation program, if indicated.

Pneumonia

Overview

- Acute infection of the lung parenchyma that impairs gas exchange

◆ May be classified by etiology, location, or type

Causes

Bacterial and viral pneumonia

◆ Abdominal and thoracic surgery
◆ Alcoholism
◆ Aspiration
◆ Atelectasis
◆ Bacterial or viral respiratory infection
◆ Cancer
◆ Chronic illness and debilitation
◆ Chronic respiratory disease
◆ Endotracheal intubation or mechanical ventilation
◆ Exposure to noxious gases
◆ Immunosuppressive therapy
◆ Influenza
◆ Malnutrition
◆ Smoking
◆ Sickle cell disease
◆ Tracheostomy

Aspiration pneumonia

◆ Caustic substance entering the airway

Risk factors

◆ Advanced age
◆ Debilitation
◆ Decreased level of consciousness
◆ Impaired gag reflex
◆ Nasogastric (NG) tube feedings
◆ Poor oral hygiene

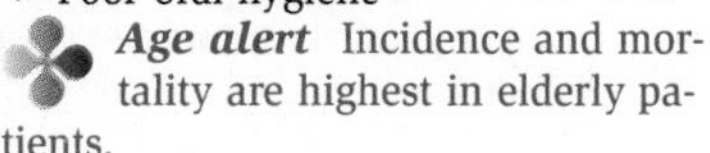
Age alert Incidence and mortality are highest in elderly patients.

Data collection

History

Bacterial pneumonia

◆ Sudden onset of:
- Pleuritic chest pain
- Chills
- Cough
- Production of purulent sputum

Viral pneumonia

◆ Constitutional symptoms
◆ Fever
◆ Nonproductive cough

Aspiration pneumonia

◆ Fever
◆ Malaise
◆ Weight loss

Physical findings

◆ Crackles, wheezing, or rhonchi
◆ Decreased breath sounds
◆ Decreased fremitus
◆ Dullness over the affected area
◆ Fever
◆ Sputum production
◆ Tachypnea
◆ Use of accessory muscles

Diagnostic tests

Laboratory

◆ Complete blood count shows leukocytosis.
◆ Blood culture findings are positive for the causative organism.
◆ Arterial blood gas analysis shows hypoxemia.
◆ Fungal or acid-fast bacilli cultures identify the causative agent.
◆ Assay shows Legionella-soluble antigen in urine.
◆ Sputum culture, Gram stain, and smear show the infecting organism.

Imaging

◆ Chest X-rays usually show patchy or lobar infiltrates.

Diagnostic procedures

◆ Bronchoscopy or transtracheal aspiration specimens identify the causative agent.

Other tests

◆ Pulse oximetry may show decreased oxygen saturation.

Treatment

General
- ◆ Adequate fluids
- ◆ Bed rest initially, with progress as tolerated
- ◆ High-calorie, high-protein diet
- ◆ Mechanical ventilation (positive end-expiratory pressure) for respiratory failure

Medications
- ◆ Analgesics
- ◆ Antibiotics
- ◆ Antitussives
- ◆ Bronchodilators
- ◆ Humidified oxygen

Surgery
- ◆ Drainage of parapneumonic pleural effusion or lung abscess

Nursing interventions
- ◆ Give medications as ordered.
- ◆ Give I.V. fluids and electrolyte replacement as ordered.
- ◆ Maintain a patent airway and adequate oxygenation.
- ◆ Give supplemental oxygen as ordered. Give oxygen cautiously if the patient has chronic lung disease.
- ◆ Suction the patient as needed.
- ◆ Obtain sputum specimens as needed.
- ◆ Provide a high-calorie, high-protein diet of soft foods.
- ◆ Give supplemental oral feedings, NG tube feedings, or parenteral nutrition if needed.
- ◆ Take steps to prevent aspiration during NG feedings.
- ◆ Dispose of secretions properly.
- ◆ Provide a quiet, calm environment with frequent rest periods.
- ◆ Include the patient in care decisions whenever possible.

Patient teaching
- ◆ Be sure to cover:
  - the disorder, diagnosis, and treatment
  - medications and possible adverse reactions
  - the need for adequate fluid intake
  - the importance of getting adequate rest
  - deep-breathing and coughing exercises
  - chest physiotherapy
  - the need to avoid irritants that stimulate secretions
  - when to notify the physician
  - home oxygen therapy, if required
  - ways to prevent pneumonia.
- ◆ Refer the patient to a smoking-cessation program, if indicated.

Pulmonary embolism

Overview
- ◆ Obstruction of the pulmonary arterial bed that occurs when a mass (such as a dislodged thrombus) lodges in the main pulmonary artery or branch, partially or completely obstructing it
- ◆ Usually originates in the deep veins of the leg
- ◆ Can be asymptomatic, but sometimes causes rapid death from pulmonary infarction

Causes
- ◆ Atrial fibrillation
- ◆ Deep vein thrombosis
- ◆ Pelvic, renal, and hepatic vein thrombosis
- ◆ Rarely, other types of emboli, such as bone, air, fat, amniotic fluid, tumor cells, or a foreign body
- ◆ Right heart thrombus
- ◆ Upper-extremity thrombosis
- ◆ Valvular heart disease

Risk factors
- Increased blood coagulability
- Predisposing disorders, such as thromboembolism and thrombophlebitis
- Surgery
- Various treatments
- Venous stasis or injury

Data collection

History
- Pleuritic pain or angina
- Predisposing factor
- Shortness of breath for no apparent reason

Physical findings
- Crackles
- Hypotension
- Large embolus: Cyanosis, syncope, and distended jugular veins
- Low-grade fever
- Productive cough, possibly with blood-tinged sputum
- Restlessness
- S_3 and S_4 gallop, with increased intensity of the pulmonic component of S_2
- Tachycardia
- Transient pleural friction rub
- Warmth, tenderness, and edema of the lower leg
- Weak, rapid pulse

Diagnostic tests
Laboratory
- Arterial blood gas values show hypoxemia.
- D-dimer level is elevated.

Imaging
- Lung ventilation-perfusion scan shows a ventilation-perfusion mismatch.
- Pulmonary angiography shows a pulmonary vessel filling defect or an abrupt vessel ending as well as the location and extent of pulmonary embolism.
- Chest X-rays may show a small infiltrate or effusion.
- Spiral chest computed tomography scan may show central pulmonary emboli.

Diagnostic procedures
- Electrocardiography may show right axis deviation, right bundle-branch block, or atrial fibrillation.

Treatment

General
- Bed rest during the acute phase
- Maintenance of adequate cardiovascular and pulmonary function
- Mechanical ventilation, if indicated
- Possible fluid restriction

Medications
- Antiarrhythmics
- Antibiotics (for septic embolus)
- Anticoagulation
- Corticosteroids (controversial)
- Diuretics
- Oxygen therapy
- Thrombolytics
- Vasopressors (for hypotension)

Surgery
- Pulmonary embolectomy
- Vena caval filter placement
- Vena caval interruption

Nursing interventions
- Give medications as ordered.
- Avoid I.M. injections.
- Encourage active and passive range-of-motion exercises, unless contraindicated.
- Avoid massage of the lower legs.
- Apply antiembolism stockings.
- Provide adequate nutrition.
- Assist with ambulation as soon as the patient is stable.

◆ Encourage the use of incentive spirometry.

Patient teaching

◆ Be sure to cover:
- the disease, diagnosis, and treatment
- medications and possible adverse reactions
- ways to prevent deep vein thrombosis and pulmonary embolism
- signs and symptoms of abnormal bleeding
- how to prevent abnormal bleeding
- how to monitor anticoagulant effects
- dietary sources of vitamin K
- when to notify the physician.

◆ Refer the patient to a weight management program, if indicated.

Renal failure, acute

Overview

◆ Sudden interruption of renal function as a result of obstruction, reduced circulation, or renal parenchymal disease
◆ Classified as prerenal failure, intrarenal failure (also called intrinsic, or parenchymal, failure), or postrenal failure
◆ Usually reversible with treatment
◆ If not treated, may progress to end-stage renal disease, uremia, and death
◆ Normally, three distinct phases: Oliguric, diuretic, and recovery

Oliguric phase

◆ This phase may last a few days or several weeks.
◆ Urine output drops to less than 400 ml/day.
◆ Excess fluid volume, azotemia, and electrolyte imbalance occur.
◆ Local mediators are released, causing intrarenal vasoconstriction.
◆ Medullary hypoxia causes cellular swelling and adherence of neutrophils to capillaries and venules.
◆ Hypoperfusion occurs.
◆ Cellular injury and necrosis occur.
◆ Reperfusion causes reactive oxygen species to form, leading to further cellular injury.

Diuretic phase

◆ Renal function is recovered.
◆ Urine output gradually increases.
◆ Glomerular filtration rate improves, although tubular transport systems remain abnormal.

Recovery phase

◆ The recovery phase may last 3 to 12 months or longer.
◆ Renal function gradually returns to normal or near normal.

Causes

Prerenal failure

◆ Hemorrhagic blood loss
◆ Hypotension or hypoperfusion
◆ Hypovolemia
◆ Loss of plasma volume
◆ Water and electrolyte losses

Intrarenal failure

◆ Acute tubular necrosis
◆ Coagulation defects
◆ Glomerulopathy
◆ Malignant hypertension

Postrenal failure

◆ Bladder neck obstruction
◆ Obstructive uropathy, which is usually bilateral
◆ Ureteral destruction

Data collection

History

◆ Predisposing disorder

◆ Recent fever, chills, or a central nervous system disorder
◆ Recent GI problem

Physical findings

◆ Altered level of consciousness
◆ Bibasilar crackles
◆ Bleeding abnormalities
◆ Dry mucous membranes
◆ Dry, pruritic skin
◆ Irritability, drowsiness, or confusion
◆ Oliguria or anuria, depending on the phase of renal failure
◆ Tachycardia
◆ Uremic breath odor

Diagnostic tests

Laboratory

◆ Blood urea nitrogen, serum creatinine, and potassium levels are elevated.
◆ Hematocrit, blood pH, bicarbonate, and hemoglobin levels are decreased.
◆ Urine casts and cellular debris are present, and the specific gravity is decreased.
◆ In glomerular disease, proteinuria and urine osmolality are near the serum osmolality level.
◆ Urine sodium level is less than 20 mEq/L if oliguria results from decreased perfusion.
◆ Urine sodium level is greater than 40 mEq/L if oliguria results from an intrarenal problem.
◆ Urine creatinine clearance is used to measure the glomerular filtration rate and estimate the number of remaining functioning nephrons.

Imaging

◆ These imaging tests may show the cause of renal failure:
- kidney ultrasonography
- kidney-ureter-bladder radiography
- excretory urography renal scan
- retrograde pyelography
- computed tomography scan
- nephrotomography.

Diagnostic procedures

◆ Electrocardiography shows tall, peaked T waves; a widening QRS complex; and disappearing P waves in hyperkalemia.

Treatment

General

◆ Hemodialysis or peritoneal dialysis (if appropriate)
◆ Fluid restriction
◆ High-calorie, low-protein, low-sodium, and low-potassium diet
◆ Rest periods when fatigued

Medications

◆ Diuretics
◆ In hyperkalemia, hypertonic glucose-and-insulin infusions, sodium bicarbonate, and sodium polystyrene sulfonate
◆ Supplemental vitamins

Surgery

◆ Creation of vascular access for hemodialysis

Nursing interventions

◆ Give medication as ordered.
◆ Encourage the patient to express his feelings and concerns.
◆ Provide emotional support.
◆ Identify patients at risk for acute tubular necrosis, and take preventive steps.
◆ Monitor the patient's weight daily.
◆ Monitor the dialysis access site.

Patient teaching

◆ Be sure to cover:
- the disorder, diagnosis, and treatment
- medications, dosages, and possible adverse reactions
- the recommended fluid allowance
- the importance of complying with the diet and medication regimen

– the importance of monitoring weight daily and reporting changes of 3 lb (1.4 kg) or more immediately
– the signs and symptoms of edema and the importance of reporting them to the physician.

Renal failure, chronic

Overview

◆ End result of a gradually progressive loss of renal function
◆ Few symptoms until more than 75% of glomerular filtration is lost, with symptoms worsening as renal function declines
◆ Fatal unless treated; to sustain life, maintenance dialysis or kidney transplantation may be needed

Causes
◆ Chronic glomerular disease
◆ Chronic infections such as chronic pyelonephritis
◆ Collagen diseases such as systemic lupus erythematosus
◆ Congenital anomalies such as polycystic kidney disease
◆ Endocrine disease
◆ Nephrotoxic agents
◆ Obstructive processes such as calculi
◆ Vascular diseases

Data collection

History
◆ Amenorrhea
◆ Dry mouth
◆ Fasciculations and twitching
◆ Fatigue
◆ Hiccups
◆ Impotence
◆ Infertility and decreased libido
◆ Muscle cramps
◆ Nausea
◆ Pathologic fractures
◆ Predisposing factor

Physical findings
◆ Abdominal pain on palpation
◆ Altered level of consciousness
◆ Bibasilar crackles
◆ Cardiac arrhythmias
◆ Decreased urine output
◆ Growth retardation (in children)
◆ Gum ulceration and bleeding
◆ Hypotension or hypertension
◆ Pale, yellow-bronze skin color
◆ Peripheral edema
◆ Pleural friction rub
◆ Poor skin turgor
◆ Thin, brittle fingernails and dry, brittle hair
◆ Uremic fetor

Diagnostic tests
Laboratory
◆ Blood urea nitrogen, serum creatinine, sodium, and potassium levels are elevated.
◆ Arterial blood gas (ABG) values show decreased arterial pH and bicarbonate levels.
◆ Hematocrit and hemoglobin level are low; red blood cell (RBC) survival time is decreased.
◆ Mild thrombocytopenia and platelet defects appear.
◆ Aldosterone secretion is increased.
◆ Hyperglycemia and hypertriglyceridemia occur.
◆ High-density lipoprotein levels are decreased.
◆ ABG values show metabolic acidosis.
◆ Urine specific gravity is fixed at 1.010.
◆ Proteinuria, glycosuria, and urinary RBCs, leukocytes, casts, and crystals are detected.

Imaging
◆ Kidney-ureter-bladder radiography, excretory urography, nephrotomogra-

phy, renal scan, and renal arteriography show reduced kidney size.

Diagnostic procedures
◆ Renal biopsy allows histologic identification of the underlying pathology.
◆ EEG shows changes that suggest metabolic encephalopathy.

Treatment

General
◆ Fluid restriction
◆ Hemodialysis or peritoneal dialysis
◆ Low-protein (with peritoneal dialysis, high-protein), high-calorie, low-sodium, low-phosphorus, and low-potassium diet
◆ Rest periods when fatigued

Medications
◆ Antiemetics
◆ Antihypertensives
◆ Antipruritics
◆ Cardiac glycosides
◆ Erythropoietin
◆ Iron and folate supplements
◆ Loop diuretics
◆ Supplementary vitamins and essential amino acids

Surgery
◆ Creation of vascular access for dialysis
◆ Possible kidney transplantation

Nursing interventions
◆ Give medication as ordered.
◆ Perform meticulous skin care.
◆ Encourage the patient to express his feelings.
◆ Provide emotional support.
◆ Monitor the patient's weight and signs and symptoms of fluid overload daily.

Patient teaching

◆ Be sure to cover:
- the disorder, diagnosis, and treatment
- dietary changes
- fluid restrictions
- care of the dialysis site, as appropriate
- the importance of wearing or carrying medical identification.

◆ Refer the patient to appropriate resources and support services.

Rheumatoid arthritis

Overview

◆ Chronic, systemic, symmetrical inflammatory disease (see *Identifying rheumatoid arthritis,* page 206)
◆ Peripheral joints and surrounding muscles, tendons, ligaments, and blood vessels primarily affected
◆ Marked by spontaneous remissions and unpredictable exacerbations
◆ Potentially crippling

Causes
◆ Unknown
◆ Possible effect of infection (viral or bacterial), hormonal factors, and lifestyle

Data collection

History
◆ Bilateral, symmetrical symptoms that may extend to the wrists, elbows, knees, and ankles
◆ Insidious onset of nonspecific symptoms including fatigue, malaise, persistent low-grade fever, anorexia, weight loss, and vague articular symptoms
◆ Later, more specific localized articular symptoms, commonly in the fingers
◆ Numbness or tingling in feet, or weakness or loss of sensation in fingers

Identifying rheumatoid arthritis

A patient who meets four of the seven American College of Rheumatology criteria is classified as having rheumatoid arthritis. The patient must experience the first four criteria for at least 6 weeks, and a physician must observe the second through fifth criteria.

Criteria

1. Morning stiffness in and around the joints that lasts for 1 hour before full improvement
2. Arthritis in three or more joint areas, with at least three joint areas (as observed by a physician) showing soft-tissue swelling or joint effusions, not just bony overgrowth (The 14 possible areas involved include the right and left proximal interphalangeal, metacarpophalangeal, wrist, elbow, knee, ankle, and metatarsophalangeal joints.)
3. Arthritis of the hand joints, including the wrist, metacarpophalangeal joint, or proximal interphalangeal joint
4. Arthritis that involves the same joint areas on both sides of the body
5. Subcutaneous rheumatoid nodules over bony prominences
6. The finding of abnormal amounts of serum rheumatoid factor by any method that produces a positive result in fewer than 5% of patients without rheumatoid arthritis
7. Radiographic changes, usually on posteroanterior radiographs of the hand and wrist, that show erosions or unequivocal bony decalcification localized in or most noticeable adjacent to the involved joints

- Pain on inspiration
- Shortness of breath
- Stiff joints
- Stiff, weak, or painful muscles

Physical findings

- Boggy wrists
- Eye redness
- Foreshortened hands
- Joint deformities and contractures
- Joints that are warm to the touch
- Leg ulcers
- Pericardial friction rub
- Positive Babinski's sign
- Red, painful, swollen arms
- Rheumatoid nodules

Diagnostic tests

Laboratory

- Rheumatoid factor test result is positive in 75% to 80% of patients, as indicated by a titer of 1:160 or higher.
- Synovial fluid analysis shows increased volume and turbidity but decreased viscosity and complement (C3 and C4) levels; white blood cell count may exceed 10,000/µl.
- Serum globulin levels are elevated.
- Erythrocyte sedimentation rate is elevated.
- Complete blood count shows moderate anemia and slight leukocytosis.

Imaging

- In early stages of the disease, X-rays show bone demineralization and soft-tissue swelling. Later, they help determine the extent of cartilage and bone destruction, erosion, subluxations, and deformities and show the characteristic pattern of these abnormalities.
- Magnetic resonance imaging and computed tomography scans may provide information about the extent of damage.

Other tests

◆ Synovial tissue biopsy shows inflammation.

Treatment

General

◆ Adequate sleep (8 to 10 hours every night)

◆ Application of moist heat

◆ Frequent rest periods between activities

◆ Range-of-motion (ROM) exercises and carefully individualized therapeutic exercises

◆ Splinting

Medications

◆ Antimalarials (hydroxychloroquine)

◆ Antineoplastic drugs

◆ Corticosteroids

◆ Gold salts

◆ Nonsteroidal anti-inflammatory drugs

◆ Penicillamine

◆ Salicylates

Surgery

◆ Advanced disease: Joint reconstruction or total joint arthroplasty

◆ Arthrodesis (joint fusion)

◆ Metatarsal head and distal ulnar resectional arthroplasty and insertion of a silicone prosthesis between the metacarpophalangeal and proximal interphalangeal joints

◆ Osteotomy

◆ Repair of ruptured tendon

◆ Synovectomy

Nursing interventions

◆ Give analgesics as ordered, and watch for adverse reactions.

◆ Perform meticulous skin care.

◆ Supply adaptive devices, such as a zipper-pull, easy-to-open beverage cartons, lightweight cups, and unpackaged silverware.

After total knee or hip arthroplasty

◆ Give blood replacement products, antibiotics, and analgesics as ordered.

◆ Have the patient perform active dorsiflexion; immediately report inability to do so.

◆ Supervise isometric exercises every 2 hours.

◆ After total hip arthroplasty, check traction for pressure areas and keep the head of the bed raised 30 to 45 degrees.

◆ Change or reinforce dressings, as needed, using sterile technique.

◆ Have the patient turn, cough, and breathe deeply every 2 hours.

◆ After total knee arthroplasty, keep the leg extended and slightly elevated.

◆ After total hip arthroplasty, keep the hip in abduction. Watch for and immediately report inability to rotate the hip or bear weight on it, increased pain, or a leg that appears shorter than the other leg.

◆ Assist the patient in activities, keeping his weight on the unaffected side.

Patient teaching

◆ Be sure to cover:
- the disorder, diagnosis, and treatment
- the chronic nature of rheumatoid arthritis and the possible need for major lifestyle changes
- the importance of a balanced diet and weight control
- the importance of adequate sleep
- sexual concerns.

◆ If the patient requires total knee or hip arthroplasty, be sure to cover:
- preoperative and surgical procedures
- postoperative exercises, with supervision of the patient's practice to ensure that he's performing the exercises correctly

- deep-breathing and coughing exercises to perform after surgery
- the need to perform frequent ROM leg exercises after surgery
- the use of a constant-passive-motion device after total knee arthroplasty or placement of an abduction pillow between the legs after total hip arthroplasty
- how to use a trapeze to move about in bed
- dosages and possible adverse reactions to medications.

◆ Refer the patient to the Arthritis Foundation.

◆ Refer the patient to physical and occupational therapy.

Seizure disorder

Overview

◆ Neurologic condition characterized by recurrent seizures

◆ Intelligence not affected

◆ Good seizure control achieved in about 80% of patients with strict adherence to prescribed treatment

◆ Also known as epilepsy

Causes

◆ Idiopathic in 50% of cases

Nonidiopathic epilepsy

◆ Anoxia

◆ Apparent familial connection in some seizure disorders

◆ Birth trauma

◆ Brain tumors or other space-occupying lesions

◆ Genetic abnormalities (tuberous sclerosis and phenylketonuria)

◆ Ingestion of toxins, such as mercury, lead, or carbon monoxide

◆ Meningitis, encephalitis, or brain abscess

◆ Metabolic abnormalities (hypoglycemia, pyridoxine deficiency, hypoparathyroidism)

◆ Perinatal infection or injury

◆ Stroke

◆ Traumatic injury

Data collection

History

◆ Description of a pungent smell

◆ Description of an aura

◆ Dreamy feeling

◆ GI distress

◆ Headache

◆ Lethargy

◆ Mood changes

◆ Myoclonic jerking

◆ Precipitating factors or events possibly reported

◆ Rising or sinking feeling in the stomach

◆ Seizure occurrence unpredictable and unrelated to activities

◆ Unusual taste in the mouth

◆ Vision disturbance

Physical findings

◆ Findings possibly normal while the patient isn't having a seizure and when the cause is idiopathic

◆ Findings related to the underlying cause of the seizure

Diagnostic tests

Laboratory

◆ Serum glucose and calcium test results rule out other diagnoses.

Imaging

◆ Computed tomography scan and magnetic resonance imaging may indicate abnormalities in internal structures.

◆ Skull radiography may show skull fractures or certain neoplasms within the brain.

◆ Brain scan may show malignant lesions when the X-ray findings are normal or questionable.
◆ Cerebral angiography may show cerebrovascular abnormalities, such as aneurysm or tumor.

Other tests
◆ EEG shows paroxysmal abnormalities. (A negative finding doesn't rule out epilepsy because paroxysmal abnormalities occur intermittently.)

Treatment

General
◆ Activity as tolerated
◆ Detailed presurgical evaluation to characterize the seizure type, frequency, and site of onset and the patient's psychological functioning and degree of disability to select candidates for surgery when medical treatment is unsuccessful
◆ No dietary restrictions
◆ Protection of the airway during seizures
◆ Safety measures
◆ Stimulation of the vagal nerve by a pacemaker

Medications
◆ Anticonvulsants

Surgery
◆ Correction of the underlying problem
◆ Removal of a demonstrated focal lesion

Nursing interventions
◆ Institute seizure precautions.
◆ Prepare the patient for surgery if indicated.
◆ Give prescribed anticonvulsants.
◆ Monitor seizure activity.

Patient teaching

◆ Be sure to cover:
- the disorder, diagnosis, and treatment
- the importance of maintaining a normal lifestyle
- the importance of complying with the prescribed drug schedule
- adverse drug effects
- care during a seizure
- the importance of regular meals and checking with the physician before dieting
- the importance of carrying a medical identification card or wearing medical identification jewelry.

◆ Refer the patient to the Epilepsy Foundation of America.
◆ Refer the patient to his state's motor vehicle department for information about obtaining a driver's license.

Stroke

Overview

◆ Sudden impairment of blood circulation to the brain
◆ Most common cause of neurologic disability
◆ About 50% of stroke survivors permanently disabled
◆ Recurrence possible within weeks, months, or years
◆ Formerly known as cerebrovascular accident (CVA) or brain attack

Causes
Cerebral thrombosis
◆ Most common cause of stroke
◆ Obstruction of a blood vessel in the extracerebral vessels
◆ Site possibly intracerebral

Cerebral embolism

- Second most common cause of stroke
- Cardiac arrhythmias
- Endocarditis
- History of rheumatic heart disease
- Posttraumatic valvular disease
- After open-heart surgery

Cerebral hemorrhage

- Third most common cause of stroke
- Arteriovenous malformation
- Cerebral aneurysms
- Chronic hypertension

Risk factors

- Alcohol use
- Cardiac arrhythmias
- Diabetes mellitus
- Elevated cholesterol and triglyceride levels
- Familial history of cerebrovascular disease
- Gout
- Heart disease
- High red blood cell count
- High serum triglyceride levels
- History of transient ischemic attack
- Obesity
- Smoking
- Use of hormonal contraceptives in conjunction with smoking and hypertension

Data collection

History

- Gradual onset of dizziness, mental disturbances, or seizures
- Loss of consciousness or sudden aphasia
- One or more risk factors
- Sudden onset of hemiparesis or hemiplegia
- Varying clinical features, depending on:
  - Artery affected
  - Severity of damage
  - Extent of collateral circulation

Physical findings

- With stroke in the left hemisphere, signs and symptoms on the right side
- With stroke in the right hemisphere, signs and symptoms on the left side
- With stroke that causes cranial nerve damage, signs and symptoms on the same side
- Change in level of consciousness
- With a conscious patient, anxiety along with communication and mobility difficulties
- Urinary incontinence
- Loss of voluntary muscle control
- Hemiparesis or hemiplegia
- Decreased deep tendon reflexes
- Hemianopsia on the affected side of the body
- With left-sided hemiplegia, problems with visuospatial relations
- Sensory losses

Diagnostic tests

Laboratory

- Laboratory tests — including levels of anticardiolipin antibodies, antiphospholipid, factor V (Leiden) mutation, antithrombin III, protein S, and protein C — may show increased risk of thrombosis.

Imaging

- Magnetic resonance imaging and magnetic resonance angiography allow the size and location of the lesion to be evaluated.
- Cerebral angiography details the disruption of cerebral circulation and is the test of choice for examining the entire cerebral blood flow.
- Computed tomography scan detects structural abnormalities.
- Positron emission tomography provides data on cerebral metabolism and changes in cerebral blood flow.

Other tests

- Transcranial Doppler studies are used to evaluate the velocity of blood flow.

◆ Carotid Doppler is used to measure flow through the carotid arteries.
◆ Two-dimensional echocardiogram is used to evaluate the heart for dysfunction.
◆ Cerebral blood flow studies are used to measure blood flow to the brain.
◆ Electrocardiogram shows reduced electrical activity in an area of cortical infarction.

Treatment

General
◆ Care measures to help the patient adapt to specific deficits
◆ Varies, depending on the cause and clinical manifestations
◆ Careful management of blood pressure
◆ Physical, speech, and occupational rehabilitation
◆ Puréed dysphagia diet or tube feedings, if indicated

Medications
◆ Analgesics
◆ Anticoagulants
◆ Anticonvulsants
◆ Antidepressants
◆ Antihypertensives
◆ Antiplatelets
◆ Lipid-lowering drugs
◆ Stool softeners
◆ Tissue plasminogen activator when the cause isn't hemorrhagic (emergency care within 3 hours of onset of the symptoms)

Surgery
◆ Craniotomy
◆ Endarterectomy
◆ Extracranial-intracranial bypass
◆ Ventricular shunts

Nursing interventions
◆ Maintain a patent airway and oxygenation.
◆ Offer the urinal or bedpan every 2 hours.
◆ Insert an indwelling urinary catheter if needed.
◆ Ensure adequate nutrition.
◆ Provide careful mouth care.
◆ Provide meticulous eye care.
◆ Follow the physical therapy program, and help the patient with exercise.
◆ Maintain communication with the patient.
◆ Provide psychological support.
◆ Set realistic short-term goals.
◆ Protect the patient from injury.
◆ Provide careful positioning to prevent aspiration and contractures.
◆ Take steps to prevent complications.
◆ Give medications as ordered.
◆ Monitor the patient for the development of deep vein thrombosis and pulmonary embolus.

Patient teaching

◆ Be sure to cover:
- the disorder, diagnosis, and treatment
- occupational and speech therapy programs
- dietary regimen
- medication regimen
- adverse drug reactions
- stroke prevention.

◆ Refer the patient to home care services.
◆ Refer the patient to outpatient services, speech, and occupational rehabilitation programs, as indicated.

Thrombophlebitis

Overview

◆ Development of a thrombus that may cause vessel occlusion or embolization
◆ Acute condition characterized by inflammation and thrombus formation

◆ May occur in deep or superficial veins
◆ Typically occurs at the valve cusps because venous stasis encourages accumulation and adherence of platelet and fibrin

Causes

◆ Fracture of the spine, pelvis, femur, or tibia
◆ Hormonal contraceptives such as estrogens
◆ May be idiopathic
◆ Neoplasms
◆ Pregnancy and childbirth
◆ Prolonged bed rest
◆ Surgery
◆ Trauma
◆ Venous stasis
◆ Venulitis

Data collection

History

◆ Asymptomatic in up to 50% of patients with deep vein thrombophlebitis
◆ Possible tenderness, aching, or severe pain in the affected leg or arm; fever, chills, and malaise

Physical findings

◆ Lymphadenitis in patients with extensive vein involvement
◆ Positive cuff sign
◆ Possible positive Homans' sign
◆ Possible sensation of warmth in the affected leg or arm
◆ Redness, swelling, and tenderness of the affected leg or arm

Diagnostic tests

◆ Doppler ultrasonography shows reduced blood flow to a specific area and obstruction to venous flow, particularly in iliofemoral deep vein thrombophlebitis.
◆ Plethysmography shows decreased circulation distal to the affected area and is more sensitive than ultrasonography in detecting deep vein thrombophlebitis.
◆ Phlebography confirms the diagnosis and shows filling defects and diverted blood flow.

Treatment

General

◆ Antiembolism stockings
◆ Application of warm, moist compresses to the affected area
◆ Bed rest, with elevation of the affected extremity

Medications

◆ Analgesics
◆ Anticoagulants
◆ Thrombolytics

Surgery

◆ Caval interruption with transvenous placement of a vena cava filter
◆ Embolectomy
◆ Simple ligation to vein plication, or clipping

Nursing interventions

◆ Enforce bed rest as ordered and elevate the patient's affected arm or leg, but avoid compressing the popliteal space.
◆ Apply warm compresses or a covered aquathermia pad.
◆ Give analgesics, as ordered.
◆ Mark, measure, and record the circumference of the affected arm or leg daily, and compare this measurement with that of the other arm or leg.
◆ Give anticoagulants, as ordered.
◆ Perform or encourage range-of-motion exercises.
◆ Use pneumatic compression devices.
◆ Apply antiembolism stockings.
◆ Encourage early ambulation.
◆ Monitor the results of laboratory tests.

◆ Monitor the patient for signs and symptoms of pulmonary embolism.

Patient teaching

◆ Be sure to cover:
- the disorder, diagnosis, and treatment
- the importance of follow-up blood studies to monitor anticoagulant therapy
- how to give injections (if the patient requires subcutaneous anticoagulation therapy after discharge)
- the need to avoid prolonged sitting or standing to help prevent a recurrence
- the proper application and use of antiembolism stockings
- the importance of adequate hydration
- the need to use an electric razor and to avoid products that contain aspirin.

Tuberculosis

Overview

◆ Acute or chronic lung infection characterized by pulmonary infiltrates and the formation of granulomas with caseation, fibrosis, and cavitation
◆ Excellent prognosis with proper treatment and compliance
◆ Also known as TB

Causes

◆ Exposure to *Mycobacterium tuberculosis*
◆ In some cases, exposure to other strains of mycobacteria

Risk factors

◆ Close contact with a patient newly diagnosed with tuberculosis
◆ Drug and alcohol abuse
◆ Gastrectomy
◆ History of previous exposure to tuberculosis
◆ History of silicosis, diabetes, malnutrition, cancer, Hodgkin's disease, or leukemia
◆ Homelessness
◆ Immunosuppression and use of corticosteroids
◆ Multiple sexual partners
◆ Recent immigration from Africa, Asia, Mexico, or South America
◆ Residence in a nursing home, mental health facility, or prison

Data collection

History

In primary infection
◆ Anorexia and weight loss
◆ Low-grade fever
◆ May be asymptomatic after a 4- to 8-week incubation period
◆ Night sweats
◆ Weakness and fatigue

In reactivated infection
◆ Chest pain
◆ Low-grade fever
◆ Productive cough (blood or mucopurulent or blood-tinged sputum)

Physical findings

◆ Bronchial breath sounds
◆ Crepitant crackles
◆ Dullness over the affected area
◆ Wheezes
◆ Whispered pectoriloquy

Diagnostic tests

Laboratory
◆ Tuberculin skin test result is positive in both active and inactive tuberculosis.
◆ Stains and cultures of sputum, cerebrospinal fluid, urine, abscess drainage, or pleural fluid show heat-sensitive, nonmotile, aerobic, acid-fast bacilli.

Preventing the spread of tuberculosis

Explain respiratory and standard precautions to a hospitalized patient who has tuberculosis. Before discharge, tell him that he must take precautions to keep from spreading the disease, such as wearing a mask around others, until his physician tells him that he's no longer contagious. He should tell all health care providers he sees, including his dentist and optometrist, that he has tuberculosis so that they can take infection-control precautions.

Teach the patient other specific precautions to avoid spreading the infection. For example, tell him to cough and sneeze into tissues and to dispose of the tissues properly. Stress the importance of washing his hands thoroughly in hot, soapy water after handling his own secretions. Also, instruct him to wash his eating utensils separately in hot, soapy water.

Imaging

◆ Chest X-rays show nodular lesions, patchy infiltrates, cavity formation, scar tissue, and calcium deposits.
◆ Computed tomography or magnetic resonance imaging shows the presence and extent of lung damage.

Diagnostic procedures

◆ Bronchoscopy specimens show heat-sensitive, nonmotile, aerobic, acid-fast bacilli.

Treatment

General

◆ Rest initially, with resumption of activity as tolerated
◆ After 2 to 4 weeks, when the disease is no longer infectious, resumption of normal activities while continuing to take medication
◆ Well-balanced, high-calorie diet

Medications

◆ Antitubercular therapy for at least 6 months with daily oral doses of:
- isoniazid
- pyrazinamide
- rifampin
- ethambutol added in some cases.

◆ Second-line drugs include:
- aminosalicylic acid (para-aminosalicylic acid)
- capreomycin
- cycloserine
- pyrazinamide
- streptomycin.

Surgery

◆ For complications that require invasive or surgical intervention

Nursing interventions

◆ Give therapy.
◆ Isolate the patient in a quiet, properly ventilated room, and maintain tuberculosis precautions.
◆ Provide diversional activities.
◆ Dispose of secretions properly.
◆ Provide adequate rest periods.
◆ Provide a well-balanced, high-calorie diet.
◆ Provide small, frequent meals.
◆ Consult with a dietitian if oral supplements are needed.
◆ Perform chest physiotherapy.
◆ Provide supportive care.
◆ Include the patient in care decisions.
◆ Monitor visual acuity if the patient is taking ethambutol.

Patient teaching

◆ Be sure to cover:
- the disorder, diagnosis, and treatment

- medications and potential adverse reactions
- when to notify the physician
- the need for isolation
- the importance of postural drainage and chest percussion
- the importance of coughing and deep-breathing exercises, including a demonstration, if needed
- the importance of regular follow-up examinations
- the signs and symptoms of recurring tuberculosis
- the possibility that rifampin may decrease the effectiveness of hormonal contraceptives
- the need for a balanced, high-calorie, high-protein diet
- measures to prevent tuberculosis. (See *Preventing the spread of tuberculosis*.)

◆ Refer anyone exposed to an infected patient for testing and follow-up.
◆ Refer the patient to a support group such as the American Lung Association.
◆ Refer the patient to a smoking-cessation program, if indicated.

Urinary tract infection, lower

Overview

◆ Bacterial infection of the lower urinary tract system
◆ Two forms:
- Cystitis (infection of the bladder)
- Urethritis (infection of the urethra)

◆ Nearly 10 times more common in females than in males
◆ Usually responds readily to treatment
◆ Possible recurring and resistant bacterial flare-ups during therapy
◆ Also known as lower UTI

Age alert In men and children, lower UTIs are typically linked to anatomic or physiologic abnormalities. These patients need close evaluation.

Causes

◆ Ascending infection by a single gram-negative, enteric bacterium, such as *Escherichia coli, Klebsiella, Proteus, Enterobacter, Pseudomonas,* or *Serratia*
◆ Simultaneous infection with multiple pathogens
◆ Recurrence from persistent infection (usually from renal calculi, chronic bacterial prostatitis, or a structural anomaly that causes infection)

Risk factors

◆ Bowel incontinence
◆ Diabetes
◆ Immobility
◆ Inadequate fluid consumption
◆ Natural anatomical variations
◆ Trauma or invasive procedures
◆ Urinary catheter
◆ Urinary stasis
◆ Urinary tract obstruction
◆ Vesicourethral reflux

Data collection

History

◆ Bladder cramps or spasms
◆ Feeling of warmth during urination
◆ Lower back or flank pain
◆ Malaise and chills
◆ Nausea and vomiting
◆ Nocturia or dysuria
◆ Pruritus
◆ Urethral discharge (in men)
◆ Urinary urgency and frequency

Physical findings

◆ Cloudy, foul-smelling urine
◆ Fever
◆ Hematuria
◆ Pain or tenderness over the bladder

Diagnostic tests

Laboratory

◆ Microscopic urinalysis shows red blood cell and white blood cell counts greater than 10 per high-power field, suggesting lower UTI.

◆ Clean-catch urinalysis shows bacterial count of more than 100,000/ml, confirming UTI.

◆ Sensitivity testing determines appropriate antimicrobial drug.

◆ If the patient's history and physical examination warrant, a blood test or a stained smear of urethral discharge rules out sexually transmitted disease.

Imaging

◆ Voiding cystourethrography or excretory urography may disclose congenital anomalies that predispose the patient to recurrent UTI.

Treatment

General

◆ Increased fluid intake

◆ Increased fruit juice intake, especially cranberry

◆ Sitz baths or warm compresses

Medications

◆ Antimicrobials

Surgery

◆ In case of recurrent infections from infected renal calculi, chronic prostatitis, or structural abnormalities

Nursing interventions

◆ Collect all urine specimens appropriately.

◆ Encourage oral fluid intake unless contraindicated.

◆ Give drugs as prescribed.

◆ Use sitz baths or warm compresses, as needed.

Patient teaching

◆ Be sure to cover:

- the disorder, diagnosis, and treatment
- the proper technique for providing an uncontaminated urine specimen
- the importance of completing the prescribed course of antimicrobial therapy
- medications, dosages, and possible adverse effects
- warm sitz baths to relieve perineal discomfort
- proper cleaning after toileting.

6 Common procedures

Bladder irrigation, continuous

◆ Continuous bladder irrigation is used to flush small blood clots that form after prostate or bladder surgery, and it may be used to treat an irritated, inflamed, or infected bladder lining.
◆ The continuous flow of irrigating solution through the bladder also creates a mild tamponade that may help prevent venous hemorrhage.
◆ The catheter may be inserted in the operating room after surgery, or it may be inserted at the bedside in nonsurgical patients.
◆ The procedure requires placement of a triple-lumen catheter.
◆ One lumen controls balloon inflation, one allows irrigant inflow, and one allows irrigant outflow.

Equipment

One 4,000-ml container or two 2,000-ml containers of irrigating solution (usually normal saline solution) or the prescribed amount of medicated solution ◆ Y-type tubing made specifically for bladder irrigation ◆ alcohol or povidone-iodine pad ◆ I.V. pole or bedside pole attachment ◆ drainage bag and tubing

Implementation

◆ Double-check the irrigating solution against the physician's order. Usually, normal saline solution is prescribed for bladder irrigation after prostate or bladder surgery. The patient will need large volumes of solution for the first 24 to 48 hours after surgery. Make sure the solution is at room temperature or slightly warmed for patient comfort.
◆ If the patient had surgery, make sure you're using Y-type tubing because it allows immediate irrigation with reserve solution.
◆ If the solution contains an antibiotic, check the patient's chart to make sure he isn't allergic to the drug.
◆ Wash your hands. Assemble all equipment at the patient's bedside. Explain the procedure and provide privacy.
◆ Insert the spike of the Y-type tubing into the container of irrigating solution. (If you have a two-container system, insert one spike into each container.) (See *Setup for continuous bladder irrigation.*)
◆ Squeeze the drip chamber on the spike of the tubing.
◆ Open the flow clamp and flush the tubing to remove air, which could cause bladder distention. Then close the clamp.
◆ Hang the irrigating solution on the I.V. pole.
◆ Clean the opening to the inflow lumen of the catheter with the alcohol or povidone-iodine pad.
◆ Insert the distal end of the Y-type tubing securely into the inflow lumen (third port) of the catheter.
◆ Make sure that the outflow lumen is securely attached to the tubing of the drainage bag.
◆ Open the flow clamp under the container of irrigating solution, and set the drip rate as ordered.
◆ To prevent air from entering the system, replace the primary container before it empties completely.
◆ If you have a two-container system, simultaneously close the flow clamp under the nearly empty container and open the flow clamp under the reserve container. This prevents reflux of irrigating solution from the reserve container into the nearly empty one. Hang a new reserve container on the I.V. pole and insert the tubing, maintaining asepsis.
◆ Empty the drainage bag about every 4 hours or as often as needed. Use

Setup for continuous bladder irrigation

During continuous bladder irrigation, a triple-lumen catheter allows irrigating solution to flow into the bladder through one lumen and to flow out through another, as shown in the inset. The third lumen is used to inflate the balloon that holds the catheter in place.

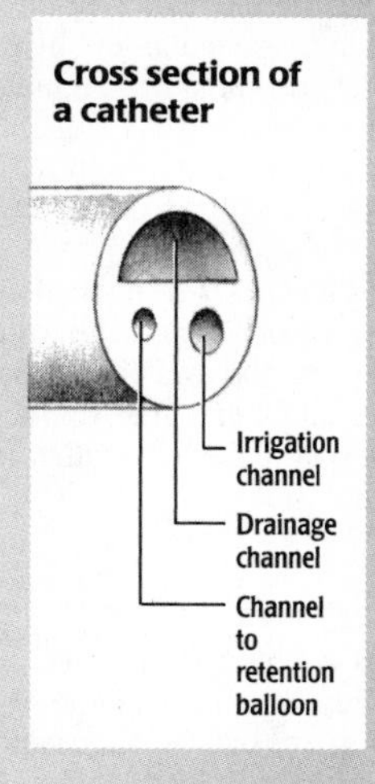

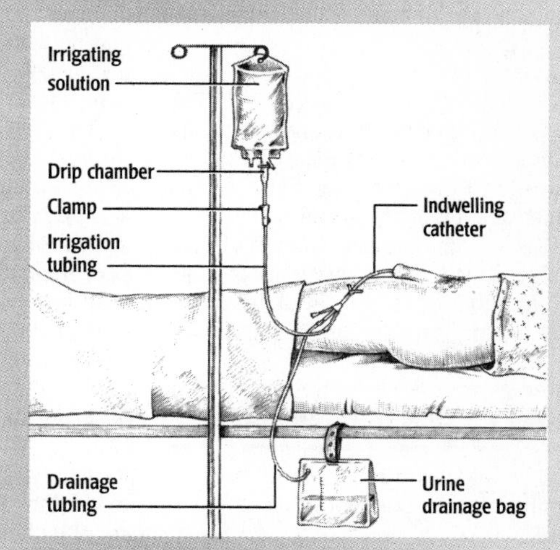

sterile technique to avoid the risk of contamination.

◆ Monitor the patient's vital signs at least every 4 hours during irrigation. Increase the frequency of monitoring if the patient's condition becomes unstable.

Special considerations

◆ Unless specified otherwise, the patient should remain on bed rest while receiving continuous bladder irrigation.

◆ Check the inflow and outflow lines periodically for kinks to make sure the solution is running freely. If the solution flows rapidly, check the lines often.

◆ Measure the outflow volume accurately. It should, allowing for urine production, exceed inflow volume.

Alert If the inflow volume exceeds the outflow volume postoperatively, suspect bladder rupture at the suture lines or renal damage, and notify the physician immediately.

◆ Check outflow for changes in appearance and for blood clots, especially if irrigation is being performed postoperatively to control bleeding.

– If the drainage is bright red, irrigating solution is usually infused rapidly, with the clamp wide open, until the drainage clears. Notify the physician at once if you suspect hemorrhage.

– If the drainage is clear, the solution is usually given at a rate of 40 to 60 gtt/minute. The physician typically specifies the rate for antibiotic solutions.

◆ Encourage oral fluid intake of 2 to 3 qt/day (2 to 3 L/day), unless con-

traindicated by another medical condition.
◆ Watch for interruptions in the continuous irrigation system; these can predispose the patient to infection.
◆ Check often for obstruction in the outflow lumen of the catheter. Obstruction can lead to bladder distention.

Documentation

◆ Record the date, time, and amount of fluid given (on the intake and output record) each time you finish a container of solution.
◆ Record the time and amount of fluid each time you empty the drainage bag.
◆ Note the appearance of drainage.
◆ Note any patient complaints.

Blood glucose monitoring

◆ Two major processes permit nonlaboratory measurement of blood glucose.
– In color reflectance photometry, a reagent patch on the tip of a handheld plastic strip (such as Glucostix or Chemstrip bG) changes color in response to the amount of glucose in the blood sample. Comparing the color change with a standardized color chart provides a semiquantitative measurement of blood glucose levels. The strip may also be inserted in a portable blood glucose meter (such as Glucometer or Accu-Chek) to provide quantitative measurements that compare in accuracy with laboratory tests.
– In biosensor or electrochemical testing, an electrical charge that is proportional to the blood glucose content is created. A plastic strip containing a small blood sample on a marked membrane is inserted into the meter and read in 5 to 45 seconds.
◆ Both metering systems provide accurate results when used as directed. Capillary blood samples can be obtained from a fingerstick, heelstick or earlobe, and some newer models also accept samples from the palm, forearm, or thigh.
◆ These tests can monitor abnormal blood glucose levels in patients with diabetes, screen for diabetes mellitus and neonatal hypoglycemia, and help distinguish diabetic coma from nondiabetic coma.
◆ The tests can be performed in the hospital, physician's office, or the patient's home.
◆ Specialized machines have been designed for low vision users, users with poor manual dexterity, and users who wish to record and store large amounts of related information, such as diet, for later retrieval.

Equipment

Reagent strips ◆ gloves ◆ portable blood glucose meter, if available ◆ alcohol pads ◆ gauze pads ◆ disposable lancets or mechanical blood-letting device ◆ small adhesive bandage ◆ watch or clock with a second hand, if meter is unavailable

Implementation

◆ Verify the patient's identity using two patient identifiers. Explain the procedure to the patient. If the patient is a child, explain the procedure to the parents and child. Provide privacy.
◆ Select the puncture site — usually the lateral side of a fingertip.

Age alert Select the heel or great toe for an infant.

◆ Wash your hands and put on gloves.
◆ If needed, dilate the capillaries by applying warm, moist compresses to the area for about 10 minutes or place the limb in a dependent position below the heart.

◆ Wipe the puncture site with an alcohol pad, and dry it thoroughly with a gauze pad.
◆ To collect a sample from the fingertip with a disposable lancet (smaller than 2 mm) or an Autolet (which uses a spring-loaded lancet), position the lancet on the side of the patient's fingertip, perpendicular to the fingerprint lines. Pierce the skin sharply and quickly to minimize the patient's pain and anxiety and to increase blood flow.
◆ After puncturing the fingertip, don't squeeze the puncture site to avoid diluting the sample with tissue fluid.
◆ Touch a drop of blood to the reagent patch or membrane on the strip; make sure you cover the entire area.
◆ After collecting the blood sample, briefly apply pressure to the puncture site to prevent painful extravasation of blood into subcutaneous tissues. Ask an adult patient to hold a gauze pad firmly over the puncture site until bleeding stops.
◆ If reading the test without a meter, leave the blood on the reagent strip for exactly 60 seconds. Compare the color change on the strip with the standardized color chart on the product container.
◆ If you're using a blood glucose meter, follow the manufacturer's instructions and read the result on the digital display.
◆ After bleeding has stopped, you may apply a small adhesive bandage to the puncture site, if needed.

Special considerations

◆ Before using reagent strips, check the expiration date on the package, and replace outdated strips. Check for special instructions related to the specific reagent. The reagent area of a fresh strip should match the color of the "0" block on the color chart. Protect the strips from light, heat, and moisture.
◆ Before using a blood glucose meter, calibrate it and run it with a control sample to ensure accurate test results. Follow the manufacturer's instructions for calibration.
◆ Avoid selecting cold, cyanotic, or swollen puncture sites to ensure an adequate blood sample. If you can't obtain a capillary sample, perform venipuncture and place a large drop of venous blood on the reagent strip. If you want to test blood from a refrigerated sample, allow the blood to return to room temperature before testing it.
◆ To help detect abnormal glucose metabolism and diagnose diabetes mellitus, the physician may order other blood glucose tests.

Documentation

◆ Record the reading from the reagent strip or blood glucose meter (in your notes or on a special flowchart, if available).
◆ Document the time and date of the test.
◆ Record how the patient tolerated the procedure and any teaching done.

Chest physiotherapy

◆ Chest physiotherapy (PT) includes postural drainage, coughing and deep-breathing exercises, and chest percussion and vibration.
◆ Together, these techniques mobilize and eliminate secretions, reexpand lung tissue, and promote efficient use of the respiratory muscles.
◆ Chest PT is critically important for bedridden patients by helping to prevent or treat atelectasis and pneumonia, two potentially serious respiratory complications.
◆ Postural drainage performed with percussion and vibration encourages peripheral pulmonary secretions to

empty by gravity into the major bronchi or trachea and is accomplished by sequential repositioning of the patient.
- Usually, secretions drain best with the patient positioned with the bronchi perpendicular to the floor.
- Lower- and middle-lobe bronchi usually empty best with the patient in the head-down position; upper lobe bronchi, in the head-up position.

◆ Percussing the chest with cupped hands mechanically dislodges thick, tenacious secretions from the bronchial walls.

◆ Vibration can be used with or instead of percussion in a patient who's frail, in pain, or recovering from thoracic surgery or trauma.

◆ Candidates for chest PT include patients who expectorate large amounts of sputum, such as those with bronchiectasis or cystic fibrosis.

◆ The procedure hasn't proved effective in treating patients with status asthmaticus, lobar pneumonia, or acute exacerbations of chronic bronchitis when the patient has scant secretions and is being mechanically ventilated. It also has little value for patients with stable, chronic bronchitis.

◆ Contraindications include active pulmonary bleeding with hemoptysis, the immediate posthemorrhage stage, fractured ribs, an unstable chest wall, lung contusions, pulmonary tuberculosis, untreated pneumothorax, acute asthma or bronchospasm, lung abscess or tumor, bony metastasis, head injury, and recent myocardial infarction.

Equipment

Stethoscope ◆ emesis basin ◆ facial tissues ◆ suction equipment as needed ◆ equipment for oral care ◆ trash bag

Implementation

◆ Gather the equipment at the bedside. Set up suction equipment, if needed, and test its function.

◆ Explain the procedure to the patient, provide privacy, and wash your hands.

◆ Auscultate the patient's lungs with a stethoscope to determine the patient's baseline respiratory status.

◆ Position the patient as needed using pillows.
- For patients with generalized disease, drainage usually starts with the lower lobes, continues with the middle lobes, and ends with the upper lobes.
- For patients with localized disease, drainage starts with the affected lobes and proceeds to the other lobes to avoid spreading the disease to uninvolved areas.

◆ Instruct the patient to remain in each position for 10 to 15 minutes. During this time, perform percussion and vibration as ordered. (See *Performing percussion and vibration*.)

◆ After you perform postural drainage, percussion, or vibration, instruct the patient to cough to remove loosened secretions.
- Tell him to inhale deeply through his nose and then to exhale in three short huffs.
- Instruct him to inhale deeply again and then to cough through a slightly open mouth.
- Three consecutive coughs are highly effective.
- An effective cough sounds deep, low, and hollow; an ineffective one, high-pitched.

◆ Have the patient exercise for about 1 minute, then have him rest for 2 minutes. Gradually progress to 10-minute exercise periods done four times daily.

Performing percussion and vibration

To perform percussion, instruct the patient to breathe slowly and deeply, using the diaphragm, to promote relaxation. Hold your hands in a cupped shape, with your fingers flexed and your thumbs pressed tightly against your index fingers. Percuss each segment for 1 to 2 minutes by alternating your hands against the patient in a rhythmic manner. Listen for a hollow sound on percussion to verify that you're performing the technique correctly.

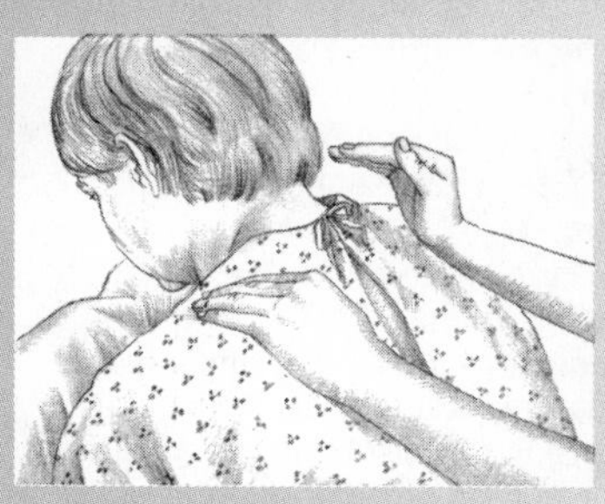

To perform vibration, ask the patient to inhale deeply and then to exhale slowly through pursed lips. While the patient exhales, firmly press your fingers and the palms of your hands against the chest wall. Tense the muscles of your arms and shoulders in an isometric contraction to send fine vibrations through the chest wall. Vibrate during five exhalations over each chest segment.

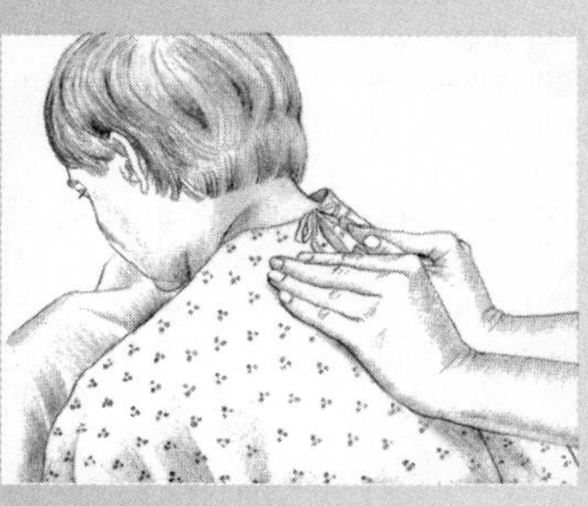

◆ Provide oral hygiene because secretions may have a foul taste or a stale odor.
◆ Dispose of secretions with suction equipment or tissues and a trash bag.
◆ Provide an emesis basin if needed.
◆ Auscultate the patient's lungs to evaluate the effectiveness of therapy.

Special considerations

◆ For optimal effectiveness and safety, modify chest PT according to the patient's condition.
– For example, start or increase the flow of supplemental oxygen, if indicated.
– Also, suction a patient who has an ineffective cough reflex.
– If the patient tires quickly during therapy, shorten the sessions. Fatigue leads to shallow respirations and increased hypoxia.
◆ Chest PT should be limited to 30 minutes or less, as tolerated. Drainage of different lobes may need to be done during separate PT sessions.
◆ If the patient is receiving chest PT to prevent dehydration of mucus and promote easier mobilization, make sure he takes in plenty of fluids.
◆ Avoid performing postural drainage immediately before or within 1½ hours after meals to avoid nausea and aspiration of food or vomitus.
◆ Because chest percussion can induce bronchospasm, adjunct treatment (for example, intermittent positive-pressure breathing, aerosol, or nebulizer therapy) should precede chest PT.
◆ To avoid injuring the spine or internal organs, don't percuss over the spine, liver, kidneys, or spleen. Also,

don't percuss over bare skin or a woman's breasts. Percuss over soft clothing (but not over buttons, snaps, or zippers), or place a thin towel over the chest wall. Remove jewelry that might scratch or bruise the patient.
◆ Observe the patient for complications.
– During postural drainage in head-down positions, pressure on the diaphragm by abdominal contents can impair respiratory excursion and lead to hypoxia or orthostatic hypotension.
– The head-down position may also lead to increased intracranial pressure, which precludes the use of chest PT in a patient with acute neurologic impairment.
– Vigorous percussion or vibration can cause rib fracture, especially if the patient has osteoporosis.
– In a patient with emphysema and blebs, coughing can lead to pneumothorax.

Patient teaching tip Preoperatively, explain coughing and deep-breathing exercises so the patient can practice them when he's pain-free. Postoperatively, splint the patient's incision using your hands or, if possible, teach the patient to splint it himself to minimize pain during coughing.

Documentation

◆ Record the date and time of chest PT.
◆ Note positions used to drain secretions.
◆ Record the length of time each position maintained.
◆ Note the chest segments percussed or vibrated.
◆ Record color, amount, odor, and viscosity of secretions produced.
◆ Note any presence of blood.
◆ Note complications and nursing actions taken.
◆ Note patient's tolerance of treatment.

Colostomy and ileostomy care

◆ A patient with an ascending or transverse colostomy or an ileostomy must wear an external pouch to collect emerging fecal matter, which is typically watery or pasty.
◆ Besides collecting waste matter, the pouch helps to control odor and protect the stoma and peristomal skin.
◆ All pouching systems must be changed immediately if a leak develops, and every pouch must be emptied when it's one-third to one-half full. The patient with an ileostomy may need to empty his pouch four or five times daily.
◆ The best time to change the pouching system is when the bowel is least active, usually 2 to 4 hours after meals.
◆ After a few months, most patients can predict their best changing time.
◆ Most disposable pouching systems can be used for 2 to 7 days; some models last even longer.
◆ The selection of a pouching system should take into consideration which system provides the best adhesive seal and skin protection for the individual patient.
◆ The type of pouch selected also depends on the location and structure of the stoma, the availability of supplies, the wear time, the consistency of effluent, personal preference, and cost.
◆ Pouching systems may be drainable or closed-bottomed, disposable or reusable, adhesive-backed, and one- or two-piece. (See *Comparing ostomy pouching systems*.)

Equipment

Pouching system ◆ stoma measuring guide ◆ stoma paste (if drainage is wa-

Comparing ostomy pouching systems

Manufactured in many shapes and sizes, ostomy pouches are fashioned for comfort, safety, and easy application. For example, a disposable, closed-end pouch may meet the needs of a patient who irrigates, who wants added security, or who wants to discard the pouch after each bowel movement. Another patient may prefer a reusable, drainable pouch. Some commonly available pouches are described here.

Disposable pouches

The patient who must empty his pouch often (because of diarrhea or a new colostomy or ileostomy) may prefer a one-piece, drainable, disposable pouch with a closure clamp attached to a skin barrier (below left).

These transparent or opaque, odor-proof, plastic pouches come with attached adhesive or karaya seals. Some pouches have microporous adhesive or belt tabs. The bottom opening allows for easy draining. This pouch may be used permanently or temporarily, until the stoma size stabilizes.

Also disposable and made of transparent or opaque, odor-proof plastic, a one-piece, disposable, closed-end pouch (below right) may come in a kit with an adhesive seal, belt tabs, a skin barrier, or a carbon filter for gas release. A patient with a regular bowel elimination pattern may choose this style for added security and confidence.

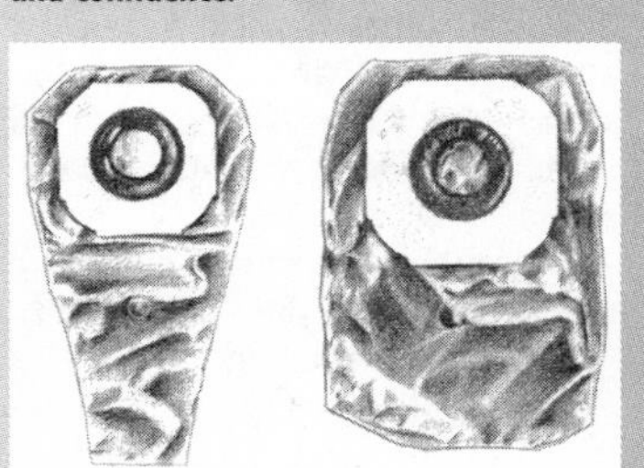

A two-piece, disposable, drainable pouch with a separate skin barrier (shown below) permits frequent changes and minimizes skin breakdown. Also made of transparent or opaque, odor-proof plastic, this style comes with belt tabs and usually snaps to the skin barrier with a flange mechanism.

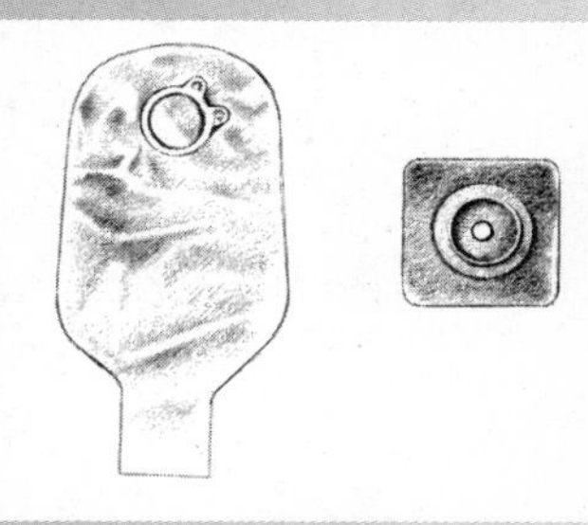

Reusable pouches

Typically manufactured from sturdy, opaque, hypoallergenic plastic, the reusable pouch comes with a separate, custom-made faceplate and O-ring (as shown below). Some pouches have a pressure valve for releasing gas. The device has a 1- to 2-month life span, depending on how frequently the patient empties the pouch.

Reusable equipment may benefit a patient who needs a firm faceplate or who wishes to minimize cost. However, many reusable ostomy pouches aren't odor-proof.

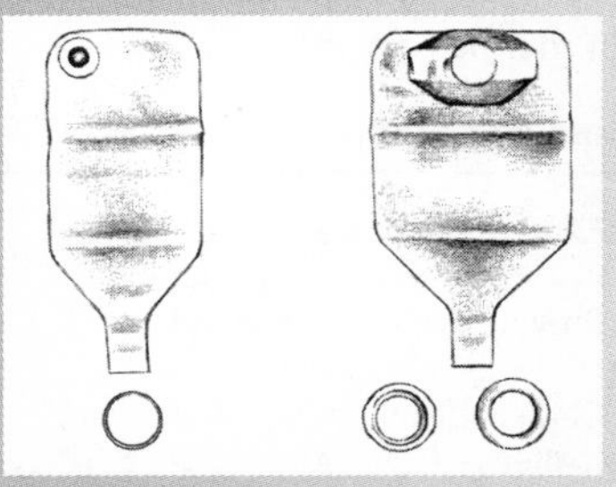

Applying a skin barrier and pouch

Fitting a skin barrier and an ostomy pouch properly can be done in a few steps. The commonly used, two-piece pouching system with flanges is shown here.

1. Measure the stoma using a measuring guide.

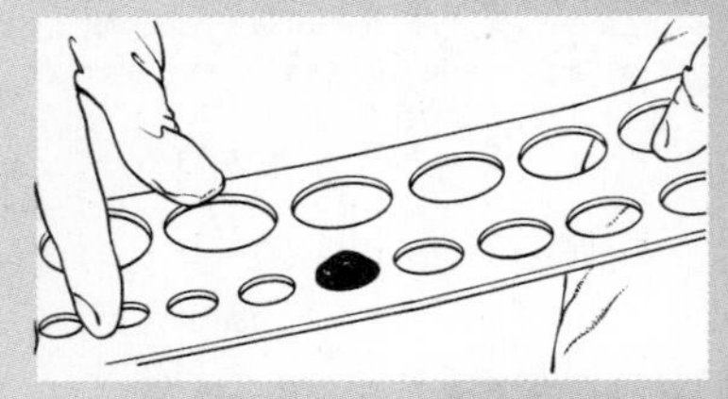

2. Trace the appropriate circle carefully on the back of the skin barrier.

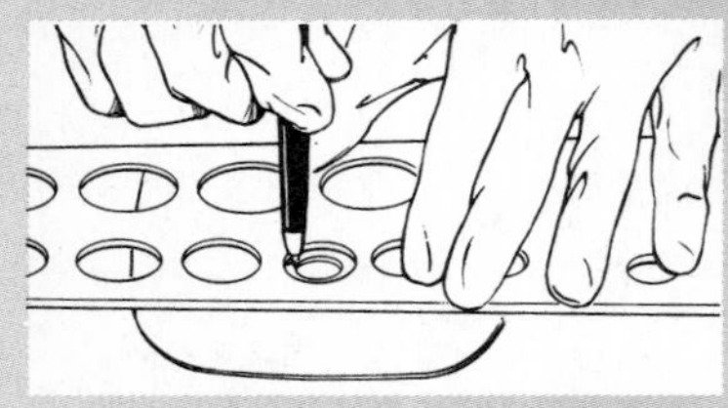

3. Cut the circular opening in the skin barrier. Bevel the edges to prevent them from irritating the patient.

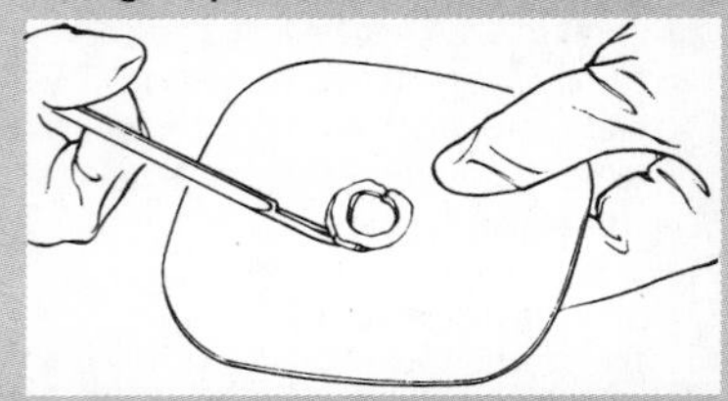

4. Remove the backing from the skin barrier and moisten it or apply barrier paste as needed along the edge of the circular opening.

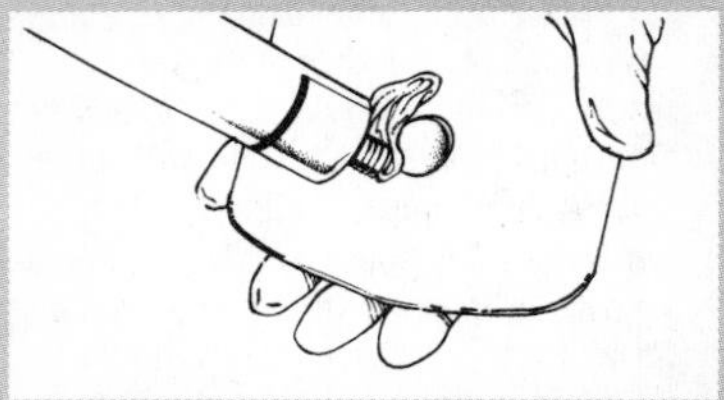

tery to pasty or stoma secretes excess mucus) ◆ scissors ◆ water ◆ closure clamp ◆ toilet or bedpan ◆ gloves ◆ facial tissue ◆ prepared skin barrier ◆ gauze pad ◆ optional: ostomy belt, paper tape, mild nonmoisturizing soap, skin shaving equipment

Implementation

◆ Explain the procedure to the patient.
◆ Provide privacy and emotional support.
◆ Gather the equipment and take it to the patient's bedside.

Fitting the pouch and skin barrier

◆ For a pouch with an attached skin barrier, measure the stoma with the stoma-measuring guide. Select the opening size that matches the stoma.
◆ For an adhesive-backed pouch with a separate skin barrier, measure the stoma with the measuring guide and select the opening that matches the stoma.
– Trace the selected size opening onto the paper back of the skin barrier.
– Cut out the opening.
– If the pouch has precut openings, which can be handy for a round stoma, select an opening that's 1/8″ [3 mm] larger than the stoma. If the

5. Center the skin barrier over the stoma, with the adhesive side down, and gently press it to the skin.

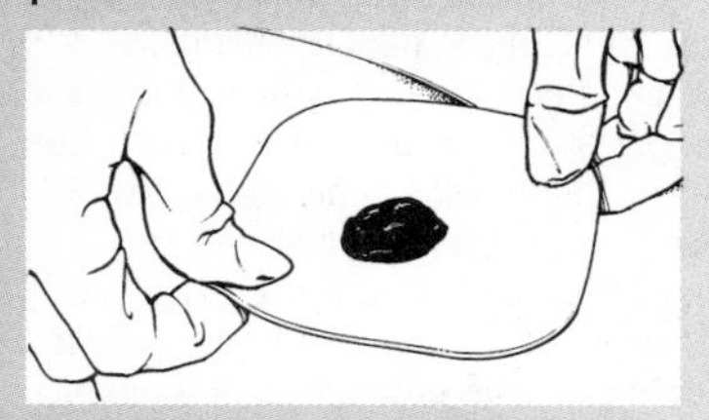

6. Gently press the pouch opening onto the ring until it snaps into place.

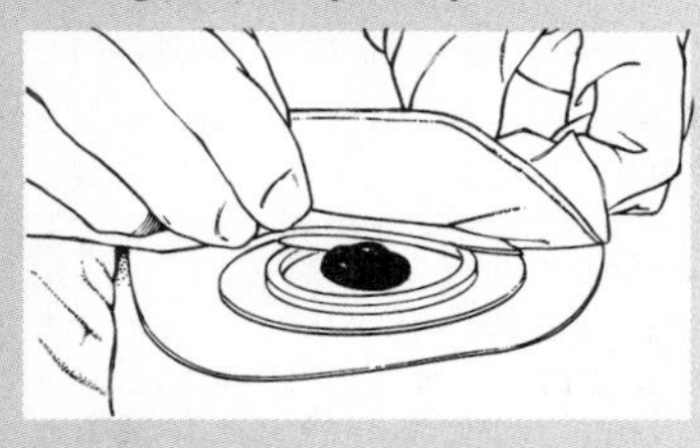

pouch comes without an opening, cut the hole 1/8″ wider than the measured tracing.

– The cut-to-fit system works best for an irregularly shaped stoma.

◆ For a two-piece pouching system with flanges, follow the instructions shown in *Applying a skin barrier and pouch.*

◆ Avoid fitting the pouch too tightly because the stoma has no pain receptors. A constrictive opening could injure the stoma or the skin without the patient feeling discomfort.

◆ Avoid cutting the opening too big because a large opening may expose the skin to fecal matter and moisture.

◆ A patient with a descending or sigmoid colostomy who has formed stools and whose ostomy doesn't secrete much mucus may choose to wear only a pouch. In this case, make sure that the pouch opening closely matches the stoma size.

◆ Between 6 weeks and 1 year after surgery, the stoma will shrink to its permanent size, then pattern-making preparations won't be needed unless the patient gains weight, has additional surgery, or injures the stoma.

Applying or changing the pouch

◆ Collect all equipment. Wash your hands and provide privacy. Explain the procedure to the patient.

◆ Put on gloves.

◆ As you perform each step, explain what you're doing and why because the patient will eventually perform the procedure himself.

◆ Remove and discard the old pouch.

◆ Wipe the stoma and the peristomal skin gently with a facial tissue.

◆ Carefully wash the stoma with mild nonmoisturizing soap and water, and dry the peristomal skin by patting it gently. Let the skin dry thoroughly.

◆ Inspect the peristomal skin and stoma.

◆ If needed, shave the surrounding hair (in a direction away from the stoma) to promote a better seal and avoid skin irritation from hair pulling against the adhesive.

◆ If you're applying a separate skin barrier, peel off the paper backing of the prepared skin barrier, center the barrier over the stoma, and press gently to ensure adhesion.

◆ You may want to outline the stoma on the back of the skin barrier (depending on the product) with a thin ring of stoma paste to provide extra skin protection. Skip this step if the patient has a sigmoid or descending

colostomy, formed stools, and little mucus.
◆ Remove the paper backing from the adhesive side of the pouching system, and center the pouch opening over the stoma. Press gently to secure.
◆ For a pouching system with flanges, align the lip of the pouch flange with the bottom edge of the skin barrier flange. Gently press around the circumference of the pouch flange, beginning at the bottom, until the pouch adheres securely to the barrier flange. (The pouch will click into its secured position.) Hold the barrier against the skin, and gently pull on the pouch to confirm the seal between flanges.
◆ Encourage the patient to stay quietly in position for about 5 minutes to improve adherence. The patient's body warmth also helps to improve adherence and to soften a rigid skin barrier.
◆ Attach an ostomy belt to secure the pouch further, if desired. (Some pouches have belt loops, and others have plastic adapters for belts.)
◆ Leave a small amount of air in the pouch to allow drainage to fall to the bottom.
◆ Apply the closure clamp, if needed.
◆ If desired, apply paper tape in a picture-frame fashion to the pouch edges for additional security.

Emptying the pouch

◆ Explain the procedure to the patient and provide privacy. Wash your hands.
◆ Gather the equipment at bedside or help the patient get to the bathroom.
◆ Put on gloves.
◆ Tilt the bottom of the pouch upward, and remove the closure clamp.
◆ Turn up a cuff on the lower end of the pouch, and allow the pouch to drain into the toilet or bedpan.
◆ Wipe the bottom of the pouch with a gauze pad, and reapply the closure clamp.
◆ The bottom portion of the pouch can be rinsed with cool tap water. Don't aim water up near the top of the pouch because the water may loosen the seal on the skin.
◆ A two-piece flanged system can also be emptied by unsnapping the pouch. Let the drainage flow into the toilet.
◆ Release flatus through the gas release valve, if the pouch has one. Otherwise, release flatus by tilting the bottom of the pouch upward, releasing the clamp, and expelling the flatus. To release flatus from a flanged system, loosen the seal between the flanges.
◆ Never make a pinhole in a pouch to release gas. The hole destroys the odor-proof seal.

Special considerations

◆ After you perform the procedure and explain it to the patient, encourage the patient's increasing involvement in self-care.
◆ Use adhesive solvents and removers only after patch testing the patient's skin. Some products may irritate skin or produce hypersensitivity reactions.
◆ Consider using a liquid skin sealant to give the skin added protection from drainage and adhesive irritants.
◆ Remove the pouching system if the patient reports burning or itching beneath it or purulent drainage around the stoma.
◆ Notify the physician or therapist of skin irritation, breakdown, rash, or unusual appearance of the stoma or peristomal area.
◆ Use commercial pouch deodorants, if desired. However, most pouches are odor-free, and odor should be evident only when you empty the pouch or if it leaks.
◆ Before the patient is discharged, suggest that he avoid odor-causing foods, such as fish, eggs, onions, and garlic.

◆ If the patient wears a reusable pouching system, suggest that he obtain two or more systems so that he can wear one while the other dries after it's cleaned with soap and water or a commercially prepared cleaning solution.
◆ Failure to fit the pouch properly over the stoma or improper use of a belt can injure the stoma.
◆ Be alert for a possible allergic reaction to adhesives or other ostomy products.

Documentation

◆ Record date and time of the pouching system change. Note how the patient tolerated the procedure.
◆ Note character of drainage, including color, amount, type, and consistency.
◆ Note the appearance of the stoma and the peristomal skin.
◆ Document patient teaching content.
◆ Record patient's response to self-care instruction.
◆ Record your evaluation of the patient's learning progress.

Colostomy irrigation

◆ Irrigation of a colostomy serves two purposes:
– It lets a patient with a descending or sigmoid colostomy regulate bowel function.
– It cleans the large bowel before and after tests, surgery, or other procedures.
◆ Colostomy irrigation may begin as soon as bowel function resumes after surgery. However, most clinicians suggest waiting until the patient's bowel movements are more predictable.
◆ Initially, the nurse or the patient irrigates the colostomy at the same time every day, recording the amount of output and any spillage that occurs between irrigations.
◆ About 4 to 6 weeks may pass before colostomy irrigation establishes a predictable pattern of elimination.

Equipment

Colostomy irrigation set (contains an irrigation drain or sleeve, an ostomy belt [if needed] to secure the drain or sleeve, water-soluble lubricant, drainage pouch clamp, and irrigation bag with clamp, tubing, and cone tip) ◆ 1 L of tap water irrigant warmed to about 100° F (37.8° C) ◆ warmed normal saline solution (for cleansing enemas) ◆ I.V. pole or wall hook ◆ washcloth and towel ◆ water ◆ ostomy pouching system ◆ linen-saver pad ◆ gloves ◆ optional: bedpan or chair, mild nonmoisturizing soap, rubber band or clip, and small dressing, bandage, or commercial stoma cap

Implementation

◆ Gather equipment at the bedside or help the patient get to the bathroom. Provide privacy. Wash your hands and put on gloves.
◆ Explain each step of the procedure to the patient because he'll probably be irrigating the colostomy himself.
◆ Depending on the patient's condition, colostomy irrigation may be performed in bed using a bedpan or in the bathroom using the toilet or a chair.
– For irrigation with the patient in bed, place the bedpan beside the bed and elevate the head of the bed to between 45 and 90 degrees, if allowed.
– For irrigation in the bathroom, have the patient sit on the toilet or on a chair facing the toilet, whichever he finds more comfortable.
◆ Set up the irrigation bag with tubing and a cone tip.

◆ Fill the irrigation bag with warmed tap water (or normal saline solution, if the irrigation is to clean the bowel).
◆ Hang the bag on the I.V. pole or a wall hook. The bottom of the bag should be at the patient's shoulder level to prevent fluid from entering the bowel too quickly. Most irrigation sets also have a clamp that regulates the flow rate.
◆ Prime the tubing with irrigant to prevent air from entering the colon and possibly causing cramps and gas pains.
◆ If the patient is in bed, place a linen-saver pad under him to protect the sheets from getting soiled.
◆ If the patient uses an ostomy pouch, remove it.
◆ Place the irrigation sleeve over the stoma. If the sleeve doesn't have an adhesive backing, secure the sleeve with an ostomy belt. If the patient has a two-piece pouching system with flanges, snap off the pouch and save it. Snap on the irrigation sleeve.
◆ Place the open-ended bottom of the irrigation sleeve in the bedpan or toilet to promote drainage by gravity. If needed, cut the sleeve so that it meets the water level inside the bedpan or toilet. Effluent may splash from a short sleeve or may not drain from a long one.
◆ Lubricate your gloved small finger with water-soluble lubricant, and insert the gloved finger into the stoma. If you're teaching the patient, have him do this to determine the bowel angle at which to insert the cone safely. Expect the stoma to tighten when the finger enters the bowel and then to relax in a few seconds.
◆ Lubricate the cone with water-soluble lubricant to prevent it from irritating the mucosa.
◆ Angle the cone to match the bowel angle, and insert it into the top opening of the irrigation sleeve and then into the stoma. Insert the cone gently but snugly; never force it into place.
◆ Unclamp the irrigation tubing, and let the water flow slowly.
- If you don't have a clamp to control the flow rate of the irrigant, pinch the tubing to control the flow.
- The water should enter the colon over a period of 10 to 15 minutes.
- If the patient reports cramping, slow or stop the flow, keep the cone in place, and have the patient take a few deep breaths until the cramping stops.
- Cramping during irrigation may result from a bowel that's ready to empty, water that's too cold, a rapid flow rate, or air in the tubing.
◆ Have the patient remain stationary for 15 to 20 minutes to let the initial effluent drain.
◆ If the patient is ambulatory, he can stay in the bathroom until all effluent empties, or he can clamp the bottom of the drainage sleeve with a rubber band or clip and return to bed. Explain that ambulation and activity stimulate elimination.
◆ Suggest that a nonambulatory patient lean forward or massage his abdomen to stimulate elimination.
◆ Wait about 45 minutes for the bowel to finish eliminating the irrigant and effluent. Then remove the irrigation sleeve.
◆ If the irrigation was intended to clean the bowel, repeat the procedure with warmed normal saline solution until the return solution appears clear.
◆ Using a washcloth, mild nonmoisturizing soap, and water, clean the area around the stoma. Rinse and dry the area thoroughly with a clean towel.
◆ Inspect the skin and stoma for changes in appearance.
- Although it's usually dark pink to red, the color of the stoma may change with the patient's status.
- Notify the physician of marked changes in stoma color.

- A pale hue may result from anemia.
- Substantial darkening suggests a change in blood flow to the stoma.

◆ Apply a clean pouch. If the patient has a regular pattern of bowel elimination, he may prefer a small dressing, bandage, or commercial stoma cap.

◆ If the irrigation sleeve is disposable, discard it. If it's reusable, rinse it and hang it to dry along with the irrigation bag, tubing, and cone.

Special considerations

◆ Irrigating a colostomy to establish a regular bowel elimination pattern isn't successful in all patients.
- Keep a record of results.
- If the bowel continues to move between irrigations, try decreasing the volume of irrigant.
- Increasing the volume of irrigant won't help, because it only stimulates peristalsis.
- Also consider irrigating every other day.

◆ Irrigation may help regulate bowel function in patients with a descending or sigmoid colostomy because this is the bowel's stool storage area. However, a patient with an ascending or transverse colostomy won't benefit from irrigation. A patient with a descending or sigmoid colostomy who's missing part of the ascending or transverse colon may not be able to irrigate successfully, because his ostomy may function as an ascending or transverse colostomy.

◆ If diarrhea develops, stop irrigations until stools form again.

◆ Irrigation alone won't achieve regularity for the patient. He must also observe a complementary diet and exercise regimen.

◆ If the patient has a strictured stoma that prohibits cone insertion, remove the cone from the irrigation tubing and replace it with a soft silicone catheter.
- Angle the catheter gently 2″ to 4″ (5 to 10 cm) into the bowel to instill the irrigant.
- Don't force the catheter into the stoma, and don't insert it farther than the recommended length because you may perforate the bowel.

◆ Observe the patient for complications.
- Bowel perforation may occur if a catheter is incorrectly inserted into the stoma.
- Fluid and electrolyte imbalances may result from using too much irrigant.

Documentation

◆ Record the date and time of irrigation. Note the patient's tolerance of the procedure.

◆ Note type and amount of irrigant used.

◆ Note the color of the stoma.

◆ Note the character of drainage, including color, consistency, and amount.

◆ Record patient teaching content.

◆ Note patient's response to self-care instruction.

◆ Record your evaluation of the patient's learning progress.

Defibrillation

◆ An LPN assists an RN with this procedure.

◆ Defibrillation is the standard treatment for ventricular fibrillation.

◆ It involves using electrode paddles to direct an electric current through the patient's heart.
- The current causes the myocardium to depolarize, which in turn encourages the sinoatrial node to resume control of the electrical activity of the heart.
- The electrode paddles that deliver the current may be placed on the pa-

Understanding the implantable cardioverter-defibrillator

The implantable cardioverter-defibrillator (ICD) has a programmable pulse generator and lead system that monitors the activity of the heart, detects ventricular bradyarrhythmias and tachyarrhythmias, and responds with appropriate therapies. The range of therapies includes antitachycardia and bradycardia pacing, cardioversion, and defibrillation. Newer defibrillators can also pace both the atrium and the ventricle.

Implantation of an ICD is similar to that of a permanent pacemaker. The cardiologist positions the lead (or leads) transvenously in the endocardium of the right ventricle (and the right atrium, if both chambers require pacing). The lead connects to a generator box, which is implanted on the left or right side of the upper chest, near the clavicle.

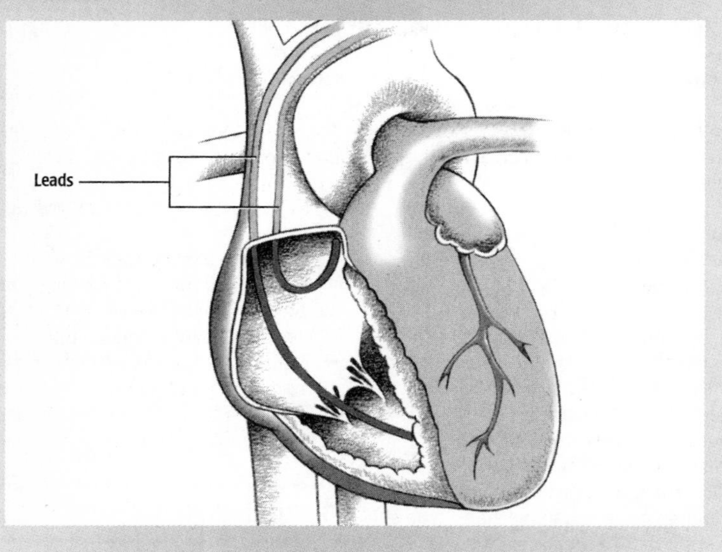

tient's chest or, during cardiac surgery, directly on the myocardium.

◆ Because ventricular fibrillation leads to immediate death if it isn't corrected, the success of defibrillation depends on early recognition and quick treatment of this arrhythmia.

◆ Patients with a history of ventricular fibrillation may be candidates for receiving an implantable cardioverter-defibrillator, a sophisticated device that automatically discharges an electric current when it senses a ventricular tachyarrhythmia. (See *Understanding the implantable cardioverter-defibrillator*.)

◆ In addition to treating ventricular fibrillation, defibrillation may be used to treat ventricular tachycardia that doesn't produce a pulse.

Equipment

Defibrillator ◆ external paddles ◆ conductive medium pads ◆ electrocardiogram (ECG) monitor with recorder ◆

supplemental oxygen therapy equipment ◆ emergency cardiac drugs

Implementation

◆ Check to see if the patient has a pulse. If he doesn't, call for help, and perform cardiopulmonary resuscitation (CPR) until the defibrillator and other emergency equipment arrive.
◆ If the defibrillator has "quick look" capability, place the external paddles on the patient's chest to view his cardiac rhythm quickly. Otherwise, connect the monitoring leads of the ECG monitor with recorder to the patient, and check his cardiac rhythm.
◆ If the patient has ventricular fibrillation or pulseless ventricular tachycardia, prepare to defibrillate.
◆ Expose the patient's chest, and apply conductive medium pads at the paddle placement positions.
- For anterolateral placement, place one paddle to the right of the upper sternum, just below the right clavicle, and the other over the fifth or sixth intercostal space at the left anterior axillary line.
- For anteroposterior placement, place the anterior paddle directly over the heart at the precordium, to the left of the lower sternal border. Place the flat posterior paddle under the patient's body, beneath the heart and immediately below the scapulae, but not under the vertebral column.
◆ Turn on the defibrillator.
◆ For external defibrillation in an adult patient, set the energy level to 200 joules, unless you're using a biphasic defibrillator, which uses lower energy settings. (See *Biphasic defibrillators*.)
◆ Charge the paddles by pressing the charge buttons, which are located either on the machine or on the paddles.
◆ Place the paddles over the conductive pads and press firmly against the patient's chest using 25 lb (11.3 kg) of pressure.
◆ Recheck the patient's cardiac rhythm.
◆ If the patient remains in ventricular fibrillation or pulseless ventricular

Biphasic defibrillators

Most defibrillators are monophasic; they deliver a single current of electricity that travels in one direction between the two pads or paddles on the patient's chest. To work, they require a high amount of electric current.

Recently, biphasic defibrillators have been introduced into facilities. Placement of the pads or paddles is the same as with monophasic defibrillators. The difference is that the electric current discharged from the pads or paddles travels in a positive direction for a specified duration and then reverses and flows in a negative direction for the remaining time of the electrical discharge.

This type of defibrillator delivers two currents of electricity and lowers the defibrillation threshold of the heart muscle, making it possible to defibrillate ventricular fibrillation successfully with smaller amounts of energy. Instead of 200 joules, an initial shock of 150 joules is usually effective. The biphasic defibrillator adjusts for differences in impedance (the resistance of the current through the chest). This helps reduce the number of shocks needed to terminate ventricular fibrillation.

Biphasic technology uses lower energy levels and fewer shocks. Thus, it reduces the damage to the myocardial muscle. Biphasic defibrillators, when used at the clinically appropriate energy level, may be used for defibrillation and – when placed in the synchronized mode – for synchronized cardioversion.

tachycardia, instruct all personnel to stand clear of the patient and the bed.

◆ Discharge the current by pressing both paddle charge buttons at once.

◆ Leaving the paddles in position on the patient's chest, recheck the patient's cardiac rhythm and have someone else check his pulse.

◆ If needed, prepare to defibrillate a second time. Instruct a colleague to reset the energy level on the defibrillator to 200 to 300 joules. Announce that you're preparing to defibrillate, and follow the procedure described earlier.

◆ Recheck the patient. If defibrillation is needed again, instruct a colleague to reset the energy level to 360 joules. Then follow the same procedure as before.

◆ Perform the three countershocks in rapid succession, rechecking the patient's rhythm before each defibrillation.

◆ If the patient still has no pulse after three initial defibrillations, resume CPR, give supplemental oxygen, and begin giving appropriate emergency cardiac drugs. Also, consider possible causes for failure of the patient's rhythm to convert, such as acidosis or hypoxia.

◆ If defibrillation restores a normal rhythm, provide appropriate care.

- Check the patient's central and peripheral pulses, and measure the patient's blood pressure, heart rate, and respiratory rate.
- Check the patient's level of consciousness, cardiac rhythm, breath sounds, skin color, and urine output.
- Obtain baseline arterial blood gas values and a 12-lead ECG.
- Provide supplemental oxygen, ventilation, and drugs as needed.
- Check the patient's chest for electrical burns, and treat them as ordered with corticosteroid or lanolin-based creams.

◆ Prepare the defibrillator for immediate reuse.

Special considerations

◆ Defibrillators vary from one manufacturer to the next, so familiarize yourself with the equipment. Defibrillator operation should be checked at least every 8 hours and after each use.

◆ Defibrillation can be affected by several factors, including the size and placement of the paddles, the condition of the patient's myocardium, the duration of the arrhythmia, chest resistance, and the number of countershocks.

◆ Defibrillation can cause accidental electric shock to those providing care.

◆ Using too little conductive medium can cause skin burns.

Documentation

◆ Record procedures, including the patient's ECG rhythms, before and after defibrillation.

◆ Note the number of times defibrillation was performed.

◆ Record the voltage used during each attempt.

◆ Record whether the patient's pulse returned.

◆ Note the dosage, route, and time of drug administration.

◆ Note whether CPR was used.

◆ Note how the airway was maintained.

◆ Record the patient's outcome.

Defibrillation, automated external

◆ Automated external defibrillators (AEDs) are commonly used to meet the need for early defibrillation, which is considered the most effective treatment for ventricular fibrillation.

◆ Some facilities require an AED in every noncritical care unit. Their use is also becoming common in such public places as shopping malls, sports stadiums, and airplanes.

◆ Instruction in using an AED is required as part of basic life support (BLS) and advanced cardiac life support (ACLS) training.

◆ AEDs are used increasingly to provide early defibrillation, even when no health care provider is present. The device interprets the victim's cardiac rhythm and gives the operator step-by-step directions on how to proceed if the person needs defibrillation. Most AEDs have a "quick look" feature that allows you to see the rhythm with the paddles before the electrodes are connected.

◆ The AED is equipped with a microcomputer that senses and analyzes a patient's heart rhythm at the push of a button. Then it audibly or visually prompts you to deliver a shock.

◆ All models have the same basic function, but they operate differently. For example, all AEDs communicate directions through messages shown on a display screen, by voice commands, or both. Some AEDs display a patient's heart rhythm simultaneously.

◆ All devices record your interactions with the patient during defibrillation, either on a cassette tape or in a solid-state memory module.

◆ Some AEDs have an integral printer that allows immediate documentation of the event.

◆ Facility policy determines who's responsible for reviewing all AED interactions; the patient's physician always has that option.

◆ Local and state regulations govern who's responsible for collecting AED case data for reporting purposes.

Equipment

AED ◆ two prepackaged electrodes ◆ electrode connector cables

Implementation

◆ After you discover that your patient is unresponsive to your questions, pulseless, and apneic, follow BLS and ACLS protocols.

◆ Ask a colleague to bring the AED into the patient's room and set it up before the code team arrives.

◆ Open the foil packets that contain the two electrode pads.

◆ Attach the white electrode cable connector to one pad and the red electrode cable connector to the other. The electrode pads aren't site-specific.

◆ Expose the patient's chest.

◆ Remove the plastic backing film from the electrode pads, and place the electrode pad that's attached to the white cable connector on the right upper portion of the patient's chest, just beneath his clavicle.

◆ Place the pad that's attached to the red cable connector to the left of the apex of the heart. To remember where to place the pads, think "white — right, red — ribs." (Placement for the electrode pads is the same for both manual defibrillation and cardioversion.)

◆ Firmly press the ON button, and wait while the machine performs a brief self-test. Most AEDs indicate their readiness by sounding a computerized voice that says "Stand clear" or by emitting a series of loud beeps.

◆ If the AED isn't functioning properly, it conveys the message "Don't use the AED. Remove and continue cardiopulmonary resuscitation [CPR]."

◆ Remember to report any AED malfunctions according to facility procedure.

◆ Now the machine is ready to analyze the patient's heart rhythm. Ask

everyone to stand clear, and press the ANALYZE button when you are prompted by the machine.
- Be careful not to touch or move the patient while the AED is in analysis mode.
- If you get the message "Check electrodes," make sure that the electrodes are correctly placed and that the patient cable is securely attached; then press the ANALYZE button again.
- In 15 to 30 seconds, the AED will analyze the patient's rhythm.

◆ If a shock isn't needed, the AED displays a "No shock indicated" message and prompts you to "Check patient."

◆ If the patient needs a shock, the AED will display a "Stand clear" message and emit a beep that changes into a steady tone as it's charging.

◆ When an AED is fully charged and ready to deliver a shock, it prompts you to press the SHOCK button. (Some fully automatic AED models automatically deliver a shock within 15 seconds after analyzing the patient's rhythm.)

◆ Make sure that no one is touching the patient or his bed, and call out "Stand clear." Then press the SHOCK button on the AED. Most AEDs are ready to deliver a shock within 15 seconds.

◆ After the first shock, the AED automatically reanalyzes the patient's heart rhythm. If no additional shock is needed, the machine prompts you to check the patient.

◆ If the patient is still in ventricular fibrillation, the AED automatically begins to recharge at a higher joule level to prepare for a second shock. Repeat the steps that you performed before shocking the patient.

◆ According to the AED algorithm, the patient can be shocked up to three times at increasing joule levels (200, 200 to 300, and 360 joules).

◆ If the patient is still in ventricular fibrillation after three shocks, resume CPR for 1 minute.

◆ Then press the ANALYZE button on the AED to identify the heart rhythm. If the patient is still in ventricular fibrillation, continue the algorithm sequence until the code team leader arrives.

◆ After the code, remove and transcribe the computer memory module or tape, or prompt the AED to print a rhythm strip with the code data. Follow facility policy for analyzing and storing the code data.

Special considerations

◆ Defibrillators vary from one manufacturer to another, so familiarize yourself with the equipment at your facility.

◆ The operation of the defibrillator should be checked at least every 8 hours and after each use.

◆ Defibrillation can cause accidental electric shock to those providing care.

Documentation

◆ Record all information required by the appropriate code form.

◆ Record the patient's name, age, medical history, and chief complaint, if available.

◆ Note the time you found the patient in arrest.

◆ Note the time CPR began.

◆ Note the time when the AED was applied.

◆ Record the number of shocks the patient received.

◆ Note the time that the patient's pulse was regained.

◆ Record all postarrest care given.

◆ Note findings of physical examination.

Doppler use

◆ The Doppler ultrasound blood flow detector is more sensitive than palpation for determining a patient's pulse rate; it's especially useful for a pulse that's faint or weak on palpation.
◆ Unlike palpation, which detects expansion and retraction of the arterial walls, this instrument detects the motion of red blood cells (RBCs).

Equipment

Doppler ultrasound blood flow detector ◆ coupling or transmission gel ◆ soft cloth ◆ antiseptic solution or soapy water

Implementation

◆ Apply a small amount of coupling or transmission gel (not water-soluble lubricant) to the ultrasound probe.
◆ Position the probe on the skin directly over the selected artery.
◆ If the device you're using has a speaker, turn the instrument on. Moving counterclockwise, set the volume control to the lowest setting.
◆ If your model doesn't have a speaker, plug in the earphones and slowly raise the volume. This device is basically a stethoscope fitted with an audio unit, a volume control, and a transducer, which amplifies the movement of RBCs.
◆ To obtain the best signals with either device, tilt the probe 45 degrees from the artery and apply gel between the skin and the probe. Slowly move the probe in a circular motion to locate the center of the artery and the Doppler signal — a hissing noise at the heartbeat. If needed for future use, mark the location with a permanent marker.
◆ Avoid moving the probe rapidly because it distorts the signal.
◆ Count the signals for 60 seconds to determine the pulse rate.
◆ After you've measured the pulse rate, clean the probe with a soft cloth soaked in antiseptic solution or soapy water.
◆ Don't immerse the probe in water or bump it against a hard surface.

Documentation

◆ Note the location and quality of the pulse.
◆ Record the patient's pulse rate.
◆ Note the time of measurement.

Electrocardiography

◆ One of the most valuable and frequently used diagnostic tools, electrocardiography measures the heart's electrical activity as waveforms.
◆ Impulses moving through the heart's conduction system create electric currents that can be monitored on the body's surface. Electrodes attached to the skin can detect these electric currents and transmit them to an electrocardiogram (ECG) machine, which records cardiac activity.
◆ An ECG can be used to identify myocardial ischemia and infarction, rhythm and conduction disturbances, chamber enlargement, electrolyte imbalances, and drug toxicity.
◆ The standard 12-lead ECG uses a series of electrodes placed on the limbs and the chest wall to assess the heart from 12 different views (leads). (See *12-lead electrocardiogram electrode placement*, page 238).
- The 12 leads consist of three standard bipolar limb leads (designated I, II, III), three unipolar augmented leads (aV_R, aV_L, aV_F), and six unipolar precordial leads (V_1 to V_6).

12-lead electrocardiogram electrode placement

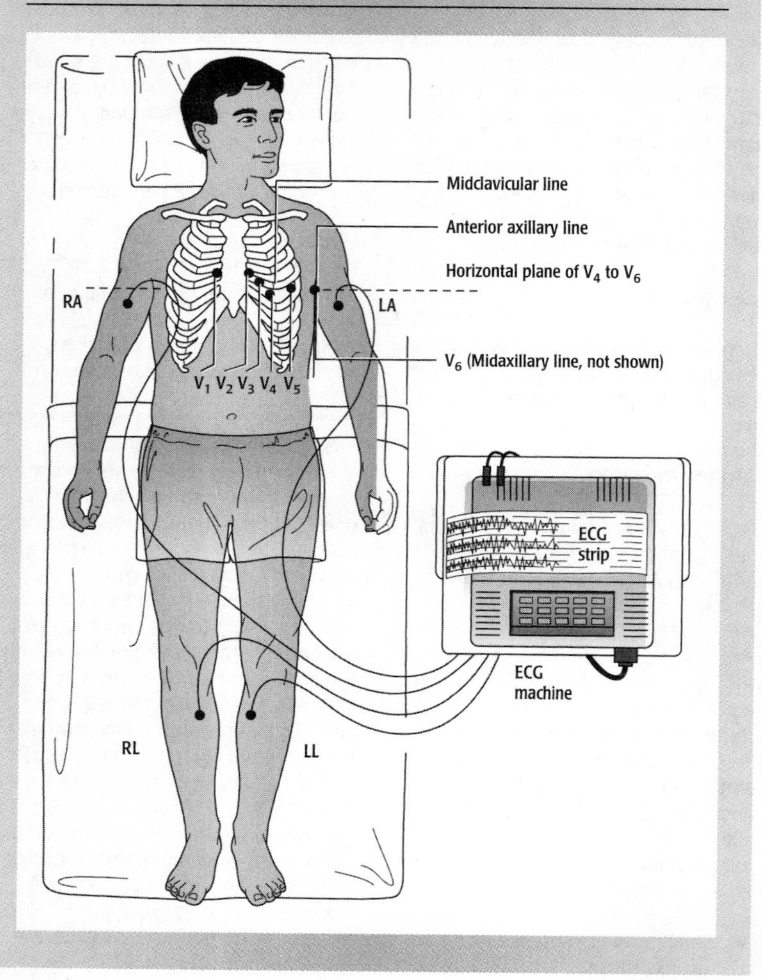

- The limb leads and augmented leads show the heart from the frontal plane.
- The precordial leads show the heart from the horizontal plane.

◆ The ECG device measures and averages the differences between the electrical potential of the electrode sites for each lead and graphs them over time. This creates the standard ECG complex, called PQRST.

- The P wave represents atrial depolarization.
- The QRS complex represents ventricular depolarization.

- The T wave represents ventricular repolarization.

◆ Variations of standard ECG include exercise ECG (stress ECG) and ambulatory ECG (Holter monitoring).
- Exercise ECG monitors heart rate, blood pressure, and ECG waveforms as the patient walks on a treadmill, pedals a stationary bicycle, or pedals an arm exercise machine.
- Patients unable to exercise may be given adenosine (Adenocard) or dipyridamole (Persantine) to mimic the effects of exercise on the heart.
- For thallium or myoview exercise ECGs, radionucleotide drugs are given to enable heart scans to be done in addition to the ECG.
- For ambulatory ECG, the patient wears a portable Holter monitor to record heart activity continually over 24 hours.

◆ Today, ECG is typically accomplished using a multichannel method. All ten electrodes are attached to the patient at once, and the machine prints a simultaneous view of all leads.

Equipment

ECG machine ◆ recording paper ◆ disposable pregelled electrodes ◆ 4″ × 4″ gauze pads ◆ optional: clippers, marking pen

Implementation

◆ Verify the patient's identity using two patient identifiers.

◆ Place the ECG machine close to the patient's bed, and plug the power cord into the wall outlet.

◆ Keep the patient away from objects that might cause electrical interference, such as equipment, fixtures, and power cords.

◆ As you set up the machine to record a 12-lead ECG, explain the procedure to the patient and provide privacy.
- Tell him that the test records the heart's electrical activity and it may be repeated at certain intervals.
- Emphasize that no electrical current will enter his body and that the test is painless.
- Also, tell him that the test typically takes about 5 minutes.

◆ Wash your hands.

◆ Have the patient lie in a supine position in the center of the bed with his arms at his sides. You may raise the head of the bed to promote his comfort.

◆ Expose his arms and legs, and drape him appropriately.
- His arms and legs should be relaxed to minimize muscle trembling, which can cause electrical interference.
- If the bed is too narrow, place the patient's hands under his buttocks to prevent muscle tension.
- Also use this technique if the patient is shivering or trembling.
- Make sure his feet aren't touching the bed board.

◆ Select flat, fleshy areas to place the electrodes. Avoid muscular and bony areas. If the patient has an amputated limb, choose a site on the residual limb.

◆ Clean excess oil or other substances from the skin to enhance electrode contact.

◆ Apply the disposable electrodes. Peel off the contact paper and apply them directly to the prepared site, as recommended by the manufacturer's instructions.

◆ To guarantee the best connection to the leadwire, position disposable electrodes on the legs with the lead connection pointing superiorly.

◆ Connect the limb leadwires to the electrodes.

◆ You'll see that the tip of each leadwire is lettered and color-coded for easy identification.

- The white or RA leadwire goes to the right arm.
- The green or RL leadwire goes to the right leg.
- The red or LL leadwire goes to the left leg.
- The black or LA leadwire goes to the left arm.
- The V_1 to V_6 leadwires go to the chest.

◆ Expose the patient's chest. Apply a disposable electrode at each electrode position.

◆ If your patient is female, place the chest electrodes below the breast tissue. In a large-breasted woman, you may need to displace the breast tissue laterally.

◆ Check to see that the paper speed selector is set to the standard 25 mm/second and that the machine is set to full voltage. The machine will record a normal standardization mark—a square that's the height of two large squares or 10 small squares on the recording paper.

◆ If needed, enter the appropriate patient identification data.

◆ If any part of the waveform extends beyond the paper when you record the ECG, adjust the normal standardization to half-standardization. Note this adjustment on the ECG strip because this will need to be considered in interpreting the results.

◆ Now you're ready to start recording.

- Ask the patient to relax and breathe normally.
- Tell him to lie still and not to talk when you record his ECG.

◆ Then press the AUTO button.

- Observe the tracing quality.
- The machine will record all 12 leads automatically, recording three consecutive leads simultaneously.
- Some machines have a display screen so you can preview waveforms before the machine records them on paper.

◆ When the machine finishes recording the 12-lead ECG, remove the electrodes and clean the patient's skin.

Special considerations

◆ Small areas of hair on the patient's chest or extremities may be clipped, but this usually isn't needed.

◆ If the patient's skin is exceptionally oily, scaly, or diaphoretic, rub the electrode site with a dry 4″ × 4″ gauze or alcohol pad before applying the electrode to help reduce interference in the tracing.

◆ If the patient's respirations distort the recording, ask him to hold his breath briefly to reduce baseline wander in the tracing.

◆ If the patient has a pacemaker, you can perform an ECG with or without a magnet, according to the physician's orders. Be sure to note the presence of a pacemaker and the use of the magnet on the ECG printout.

Documentation

◆ Record the patient's name, identification number, facility name, date, and time on the ECG recording.

◆ Note any appropriate clinical information on the ECG.

◆ Record the date and time of test in your notes.

◆ Note significant responses by the patient in your notes.

Feeding tube maintenance and removal

◆ Inserting a feeding tube nasally or orally into the stomach or duodenum provides nourishment to a patient who can't or won't eat.
◆ The tube also allows supplemental feedings for a patient with very high nutritional requirements, such as an unconscious patient or one with extensive burns.
◆ The preferred route is nasal, but the oral route may be used for patients with such conditions as a deviated septum or an injury of the head or nose.
◆ The physician may order duodenal feeding if the patient can't tolerate gastric feeding or if gastric feeding may cause aspiration.
◆ The absence of bowel sounds or possible intestinal obstruction contraindicates the use of a feeding tube.
◆ Feeding tubes differ somewhat from standard nasogastric tubes.
– Made of silicone, rubber, or polyurethane, feeding tubes have small diameters and great flexibility.
– These qualities reduce oropharyngeal irritation, necrosis resulting from pressure on the tracheoesophageal wall, irritation of the distal esophagus, and discomfort from swallowing.
– To facilitate passage, some feeding tubes are weighted with tungsten.
– Some tubes need a guide wire to keep them from curling in the back of the throat.
– These small-bore tubes usually have radiopaque markings and a water-activated coating that provides a lubricated surface.
◆ Precise placement of the feeding tube is especially important because small-bore feeding tubes may slide into the trachea without causing immediate signs or symptoms of respiratory distress, such as coughing, choking, gasping, or cyanosis.
◆ The patient will usually cough if the tube enters the larynx. Ask the patient to speak. If he can't, the tube is in the larynx and should be withdrawn at once.
◆ The nurse is responsible for rechecking the position of the feeding tube before giving any liquid, medication, or feeding, and for maintaining patency of the tube.

Equipment

For checking position

Linen-saver pad ◆ emesis basin ◆ 60-ml syringe ◆ pH indicator paper

For removal

Linen-saver pad ◆ tube clamp ◆ bulb syringe

Implementation

◆ Explain to the patient that when the feeding tube is inserted he may have some nasal discomfort, and that he may gag and his eyes may water. Tell him that swallowing will make advancement of the tube easier.
◆ Arrange with the patient to have a signal that he can use if he wants the procedure to be stopped briefly during insertion.

Checking position of the tube

◆ Provide privacy and wash your hands.
◆ Determine if the tape or line marking optimal tube placement length is still in position (if available).
◆ Gently try to aspirate gastric secretions.
– If no gastric secretions return, the tube may not be lying near any pooled gastric secretions. Reposition the patient on his left side to move the tube

into pooled gastric secretions, and aspirate again.

– Placement may need to be verified by radiograph.

◆ Check the aspirate for pH using the pH indicator paper.

– A pH of 5 or less with a clear, slightly yellow, or grassy-green color aspirate generally confirms gastric placement.

– A pH of 6 or more with light to golden yellow or brownish-green color aspirate indicates small bowel placement.

– A pH greater than 6 with clear aspirate with white mucus shreds may indicate pulmonary placement.

◆ Patients on stomach acid-reducing medications, those with GI bleeding, and those on continuous feedings may require initial and periodic radiographic placement confirmation as the pH test may not be accurate. Check your facility guidelines.

◆ Report any problems verifying placement to the clinical supervisor at once, and notify the physician as appropriate.

Removing the tube

◆ Protect the patient's chest with a linen-saver pad. Provide privacy.

◆ Flush the tube with air from a bulb syringe, clamp or pinch it to prevent aspiration of fluid during withdrawal, and withdraw the tube gently but quickly.

◆ Promptly cover and discard the used tube.

Special considerations

◆ To maintain patency, flush the feeding tube with up to 60 ml of normal saline solution or water before and after each medication and tube feeding or every 4 hours if on continuous tube feedings, per your facility's guidelines.

◆ Retape the tube at least daily and as needed. Alternate taping the tube toward the inner and the outer side of the nose to avoid constant pressure on the same nasal area.

◆ Inspect the skin for redness and breakdown.

◆ Provide nasal hygiene daily using cotton-tipped applicators and water-soluble lubricant to remove crusted secretions.

◆ Help the patient brush his teeth, gums, and tongue with mouthwash or a mild saline solution at least twice daily.

◆ When aspirating gastric contents to check tube placement, pull gently on the syringe plunger to prevent trauma to the stomach lining or bowel. If you meet resistance during aspiration, stop the procedure because resistance may result simply from the tube lying against the stomach wall. If the tube coils above the stomach, you won't be able to aspirate the stomach contents. To rectify this situation, change the patient's position or withdraw the tube a few inches, readvance it, and try to aspirate again.

◆ If the tube was inserted with a guide wire, don't use the guide wire to reposition the tube. However, the physician may do so, using fluoroscopic guidance.

Patient teaching tip If the patient will use a feeding tube at home, verify that appropriate nursing referrals for home care have been made, and reinforce the teaching on how to use and care for a feeding tube. Assist the patient in getting information on how to obtain equipment, how to check the position of the tube and how to remove it, how to prepare and store feeding formula, and how to solve problems regarding tube position and patency. Reinforce the teaching of the patient on watching for complications related to prolonged intubation, such as skin erosion at the nostril, sinusitis, esophagitis, esophagotracheal fistula, gastric ulceration, and pulmonary and oral infection.

Documentation

Checking tube position

- Record the date and time.
- Note measures taken to verify placement.
- Note a description of the aspirate amount, color, character, and pH.
- Record whether tube placement was verified clinically or by radiograph.
- Note the name of the person performing the procedure.
- Note when the tube is flushed (on the patient's intake and output record).
- Note how the patient tolerated the procedure and any teaching done.

Tube removal

- Record the date and time.
- Note the patient's tolerance of the procedure.

Gastrostomy feeding button care

- A gastrostomy feeding button is an alternative feeding device for an ambulatory patient who's receiving long-term enteral feedings.
- Approved by the Food and Drug Administration for 6-month implantation, feeding buttons can be used to replace gastrostomy tubes, if needed.
- The button can usually be inserted into a stoma in less than 15 minutes.
- The feeding button has a mushroom dome at one end and two wing tabs and a flexible safety plug at the other. When inserted into an established stoma, the button lies almost flush with the skin, with only the top of the safety plug visible.
- In addition to its cosmetic appeal, the device is easily maintained, reduces skin irritation and breakdown, and is less likely to become dislodged or to migrate than an ordinary feeding tube.
- A one-way antireflux valve mounted just inside the mushroom dome prevents accidental leakage of gastric contents.
- The device usually is replaced after 3 to 4 months because the antireflux valve wears out.

Equipment

Gastrostomy feeding button of the correct size (all three sizes, if correct one isn't known) ◆ gloves ◆ feeding accessories, including adapter, feeding catheter, food syringe or bag, and formula ◆ catheter clamp ◆ cleaning equipment, including water, cotton-tipped applicator, pipe cleaner, and mild soap or povidone-iodine solution ◆ optional: pump to provide continuous infusion over several hours

Implementation

- Explain the insertion, reinsertion, and feeding procedure to the patient. Tell him that a physician will perform the initial insertion.
- Wash your hands and put on gloves.
- Attach the adapter and feeding catheter to the food syringe or bag. Clamp the catheter, and fill the syringe or bag and catheter with formula. Refill the syringe before it's empty. These steps prevent air from entering the stomach and distending the abdomen.
- Open the safety plug, and attach the adapter and feeding catheter to the gastrostomy feeding button. Elevate the food syringe or bag above the patient's stomach level, and gravity-feed the formula for 15 to 30 minutes, varying the

How to reinsert a gastrostomy feeding button

If your patient's gastrostomy feeding button pops out (with coughing, for instance), the device will need to be reinserted. Here are some steps to follow.

Prepare the equipment

Collect the feeding button, an obturator, and water-soluble lubricant. If the button will be reinserted, wash it with soap and water and rinse it thoroughly.

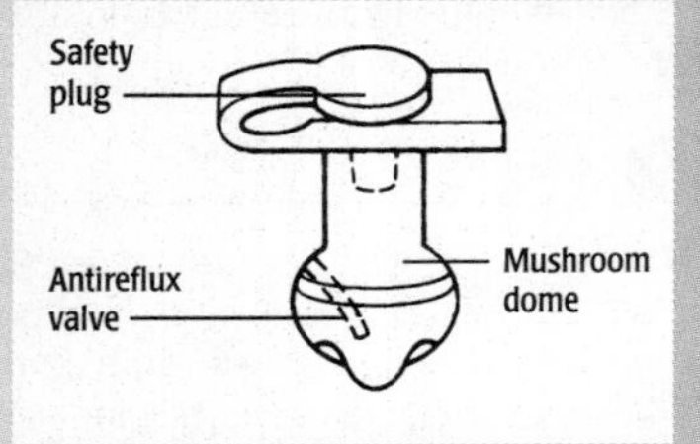

Insert the button

◆ Check the depth of the patient's stoma to make sure that you have a feeding button of the correct size. Then clean around the stoma.

◆ Lubricate the obturator with a water-soluble lubricant, and distend the button several times to ensure the patency of the antireflux valve within the button.

◆ Lubricate the mushroom dome and the stoma. Gently push the button through the stoma into the stomach.

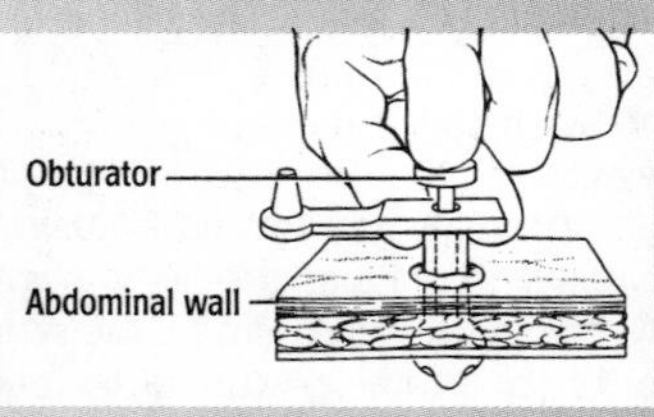

◆ Remove the obturator by gently rotating it as you withdraw it, to keep the antireflux valve from adhering to it. If the valve sticks, gently push the obturator back into the button until the valve closes.

◆ After you remove the obturator, make sure that the valve is closed. Then close the flexible safety plug, which should be relatively flush with the skin surface.

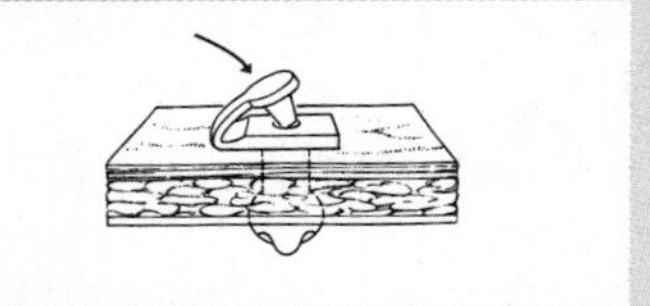

◆ If you need to administer a feeding right away, open the safety plug and attach the feeding adapter and feeding tube. Deliver the feeding as ordered.

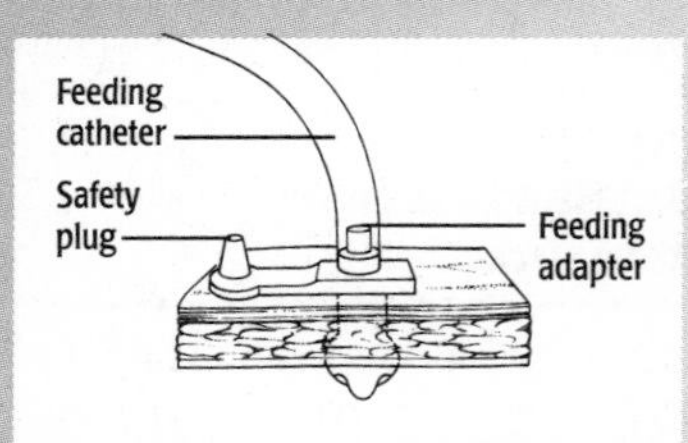

height as needed to alter the flow rate. Use a pump for continuous infusion or for feedings that last several hours.

◆ After the feeding, flush the button with 10 ml of water.

◆ Clean the inside of the feeding catheter with a cotton-tipped applicator and water to preserve its patency and to dislodge formula or food particles.

◆ Lower the food syringe or bag below the patient's stomach level to allow belching.
◆ Remove the adapter and feeding catheter.
– The antireflux valve should prevent gastric reflux.
– Snap the safety plug into place to keep the lumen clean and prevent leakage if the antireflux valve fails.
◆ If the patient feels nauseated or vomits after the feeding, vent the button with the adapter and feeding catheter to help control the vomiting.
◆ Wash the catheter and food syringe or bag in mild soap, and rinse thoroughly.
◆ Clean the catheter and adapter with a pipe cleaner.
◆ Rinse the equipment well before using it for the next feeding.
◆ Soak the equipment once weekly according to manufacturer guidelines.

Special considerations

◆ If the button pops out during feeding, reinsert it, estimate the amount of formula already delivered, and resume feeding. (See *How to reinsert a gastrostomy feeding button.*)
◆ Once daily, clean the peristomal skin with mild soap and water or povidone-iodine solution and let the skin air-dry for 20 minutes to minimize skin irritation.
◆ Also clean the site whenever spillage from the feeding bag occurs.

Patient teaching tip Before discharge, make sure the patient can insert and care for the gastrostomy feeding button. If needed, teach him or a family member or caregiver how to reinsert the button by first practicing on a model. Offer written instructions, and answer the patient's questions about obtaining replacement supplies.

Documentation

◆ Record feeding time and duration.
◆ Note amount and type of feeding formula used.
◆ Note patient tolerance.
◆ Record intake and output, as needed.
◆ Note appearance of the stoma and surrounding skin.
◆ Record patient teaching and patient's response.

Incentive spirometry

◆ Incentive spirometry involves the use of a breathing device to help the patient achieve maximal ventilation.
◆ The device measures respiratory flow or respiratory volume and induces the patient to take a deep breath and hold it for several seconds.
– This deep breath increases lung volume, boosts alveolar inflation, and promotes venous return.
– This exercise also establishes alveolar hyperinflation for a longer time than is possible with a normal deep breath, thus preventing and reversing the alveolar collapse that causes atelectasis and pneumonitis.
◆ Devices used for incentive spirometry provide a visual incentive to breathe deeply.
– Some are activated when the patient inhales a certain volume of air; the device then estimates the amount of air inhaled.
– Others contain plastic floats that rise according to the amount of air that the patient pulls through the device when he inhales.
◆ Patients at low risk for atelectasis may use a flow incentive spirometer. Patients at high risk may need a volume incentive spirometer, which measures lung inflation more precisely.

◆ Incentive spirometry benefits a patient who needs prolonged bed rest, especially a postoperative patient, who may regain his normal respiratory pattern slowly because of abdominal or thoracic surgery, advanced age, inactivity, obesity, smoking, and decreased ability to cough effectively and expel lung secretions.

Equipment

Flow or volume incentive spirometer, as indicated, with sterile disposable tube and mouthpiece (the tube and mouthpiece are sterile on first use and clean on subsequent uses) ◆ stethoscope ◆ warm water

Implementation

◆ Read the manufacturer's instructions for spirometer setup and operation.
◆ Check the patient's condition.
◆ Assemble the ordered equipment at the patient's bedside.
◆ Wash your hands.
◆ Explain the procedure to the patient, making sure he understands the importance of performing incentive spirometry regularly to maintain alveolar inflation.
◆ Remove the sterile disposable tube and mouthpiece from the package, and attach them to the device.
◆ Set the flow rate or volume goal, as determined by the physician or respiratory therapist and based on the patient's preoperative performance.
◆ Turn on the machine, if needed.
◆ Help the patient into a comfortable sitting or semi-Fowler's position to promote optimal lung expansion.
– Tilting a flow incentive spirometer decreases the required patient effort and reduces the effectiveness of the exercise.
– If you're using a flow incentive spirometer and the patient can't assume or maintain this position, he can perform the procedure in any position as long as the device remains upright.
◆ Auscultate the patient's lungs with a stethoscope to provide a baseline for comparison with posttreatment auscultation.
◆ Instruct the patient to place the sterile mouthpiece in his mouth and to close his lips tightly around it. A weak seal may alter flow or volume readings.
◆ Instruct the patient to exhale normally and then to inhale as slowly and deeply as possible. If he has trouble with this step, tell him to suck as he would through a straw, but more slowly.
◆ Ask the patient to retain the entire volume of air that he inhaled for 3 seconds or, if you're using a device with a light indicator, until the light turns off.
◆ This deep breath creates sustained transpulmonary pressure near the end of inspiration and is sometimes called a sustained maximal inspiration.
◆ Tell the patient to remove the mouthpiece and exhale normally. Allow him to relax and take several normal breaths before attempting another breath with the spirometer.
◆ Repeat this sequence 5 to 10 times during every waking hour. Note tidal volumes.
◆ Evaluate the patient's ability to cough effectively.
– Encourage him to cough after each effort because deep lung inflation may loosen secretions and facilitate their removal.
– Examine the expectorated secretions.
◆ Auscultate the patient's lungs, and compare the findings with those of the first auscultation.
◆ Remove the mouthpiece, wash it in warm water, and shake it dry.
◆ Avoid immersing the spirometer itself because this enhances bacterial growth and impairs the effectiveness of

the internal filter in preventing inhalation of extraneous material.

◆ Place the mouthpiece in a plastic storage bag between exercises. Label it and the spirometer, if applicable, with the patient's name so that another patient doesn't inadvertently use the equipment.

◆ If the patient used a flow incentive spirometer, compute the volume by multiplying the setting by the duration that the patient kept the ball (or balls) suspended, as follows. If the patient suspended the ball for 3 seconds at a setting of 500 cc during each of 10 breaths, multiply 500 cc by 3 seconds and then record this total (1,500 cc) and the number of breaths, as follows: 1,500 cc × 10 breaths.

◆ If the patient used a volume incentive spirometer, take the volume reading directly from the spirometer. For example, record 1,000 cc × 5 breaths.

Special considerations

◆ If the patient is scheduled for surgery, check beforehand his respiratory pattern and his ability to meet appropriate postoperative goals.

◆ Teach him how to use the spirometer before surgery so that he can concentrate on your instructions and practice the exercise.

◆ A preoperative evaluation will also help in establishing postoperative therapeutic goals.

◆ Exercise frequency varies with the patient's condition and ability.

◆ Avoid exercising at mealtime, to prevent nausea.

◆ If the patient has trouble breathing only through his mouth, provide a noseclip to measure each breath fully.

◆ Provide paper and a pencil so that the patient can note exercise times.

◆ Immediately after surgery, monitor the patient's exercise often to ensure compliance and evaluate achievement.

Documentation

◆ Record any preoperative teaching.

◆ Record preoperative flow or volume levels.

◆ Note date and time of the procedure.

◆ Note the type of spirometer used.

◆ Record low or volume levels achieved.

◆ Note the number of breaths taken.

◆ Note the patient's condition before and after the procedure.

◆ Note the patient's tolerance of the procedure.

◆ Record results of both auscultations.

◆ Record the volume (by computation if you used a flow incentive spirometer. or directly from the spirometer if you used a volume incentive spirometer).

Latex allergy protocol

◆ Latex, a natural product of the rubber tree, is commonly used in barrier protection products and medical equipment — and more and more nurses and patients are becoming hypersensitive to it.

◆ Those at increased risk for latex allergy include people who have had or will undergo multiple surgical procedures (especially those with a history of spina bifida), health care workers (especially those in the emergency department and operating room), workers who manufacture latex and latex-containing products, and people with a genetic predisposition to latex allergy.

◆ Intraoperative reactions to latex commonly stem from latex contact with mucous membranes or intraperitoneal serosal lining; inhalation of airborne latex particles during anesthesia; and injection of antibiotics and anesthetic agents through latex ports.

◆ People allergic to certain cross-reactive foods — including apricots, cherries, grapes, kiwis, passion fruit,

Latex allergy screening

To determine if your patient has a latex sensitivity or allergy, ask the following screening questions:
- ◆ What is your occupation?
- ◆ Have you had an allergic reaction, local sensitivity, or itching after exposure to any latex products, such as balloons or condoms?
- ◆ Do you have shortness of breath or wheezing after blowing up balloons or after a dental visit? Do you have itching in or around your mouth after eating a banana?

If your patient answers "yes" to any of these questions, proceed with the following questions:
- ◆ Do you have a history of allergies, dermatitis, or asthma? If so, what type of reaction do you have?
- ◆ Do you have any congenital abnormalities? If yes, explain.
- ◆ Do you have any food allergies? If so, what specific allergies do you have? Describe your reaction.
- ◆ If you have shortness of breath or wheezing when blowing up latex balloons, describe your reaction.
- ◆ Have you had any previous surgical procedures? Did you have any complications? If so, describe them.
- ◆ Have you had previous dental procedures? Did you have any complications? If so, describe them.
- ◆ Are you exposed to latex in your occupation? Do you have a reaction to latex products at work? If so, describe your reaction.

bananas, avocados, chestnuts, tomatoes, and peaches — may also be allergic to latex. Exposure to latex elicits an allergic response similar to the response elicited by these foods.

◆ For allergic people, latex becomes a hazard when its protein comes in direct contact with the mucous membranes or is inhaled, as occurs when powdered latex surgical gloves are used. People with asthma are at greater risk for worsening symptoms from airborne latex.

◆ The diagnosis of latex allergy is based on the patient's history and findings on physical examination. Laboratory testing should be performed to confirm or exclude the diagnosis. Skin testing can be done, and a few blood tests are approved by the Food and Drug Administration. Some laboratories may also perform an enzyme-linked immunosorbent assay.

◆ Latex allergy can produce various signs and symptoms, including generalized itching (on the hands and arms, for example); itchy, watery, or burning eyes; sneezing and coughing (hay fever–type signs and symptoms); rash; hives; bronchial asthma, scratchy throat, or trouble breathing; edema of the face, hands, or neck; and anaphylaxis.

◆ To help identify people at risk, ask specific questions about latex allergy during the health history. (See *Latex allergy screening*.)

◆ If the patient's history shows a latex sensitivity, the physician will assign him to one of three categories based on the extent of his sensitization.
- Group 1 patients have a history of anaphylaxis or a systemic reaction when exposed to a natural latex product.
- Group 2 patients have a clear history of a nonsystemic allergic reaction.
- Group 3 patients don't have a history of latex hypersensitivity, but are considered high risk because of a medical condition, occupation, or crossover allergy.

◆ If you determine that the patient is sensitive to latex, make sure he doesn't come in contact with it because he could suffer a life-threatening hypersensitivity reaction.

- Creating a latex-free environment is the only way to safeguard the patient.
- Many facilities now designate latex-free equipment that's usually kept on a cart that can be moved into the patient's room.

Equipment

Latex allergy patient identification wristband ◆ latex-free equipment, including room contents

Implementation

◆ After you've determined that the patient has a latex allergy or is sensitive to latex, arrange for him to be placed in a private room.
◆ If that isn't possible, make the room latex-free, even if his roommate hasn't been designated as hypersensitive to latex, to prevent the spread of airborne particles from latex products used on the other patient.

For all patients in groups 1 and 2

◆ Ask all patients being admitted to the delivery room, or short procedure unit, or having a surgical procedure if they have a latex allergy. If they don't know, determine if they have risk factors for latex allergy.
◆ If the patient has a confirmed latex allergy, bring a cart with latex-free equipment into his room.
◆ If policy requires that the patient wear a latex allergy patient identification wristband, place it on the patient.
◆ If the patient will be receiving anesthesia, make sure that LATEX ALLERGY is clearly visible on the front of his chart. Notify the circulating nurse in the surgical unit, the nurses in the postanesthesia care unit, and all other team members that the patient has a latex allergy.
◆ If the patient must be transported to another area of the facility, make sure that the latex-free cart accompanies him and that all health care workers who come in contact with him are wearing nonlatex gloves. The patient should wear a mask with cloth ties when leaving his room to protect him from inhaling airborne latex particles.
◆ Watch for signs and symptoms of allergic reaction. (See *Signs and symptoms of latex allergy.*)
◆ If the patient will have an I.V. line, make sure that only latex-free products are used to establish I.V. access.
◆ Make sure to use only latex-free I.V. products and supplies.
◆ Use a nonlatex tourniquet. If none are available, use a latex tourniquet over clothing.

Signs and symptoms of latex allergy

Conscious patient
◆ Abnormal cramps
◆ Anxiety
◆ Bronchoconstriction
◆ Diarrhea
◆ Faintness
◆ Generalized pruritus
◆ Itchy eyes
◆ Nausea
◆ Shortness of breath
◆ Swelling of soft tissue (hands, face, and tongue)
◆ Vomiting

Anesthetized patient
◆ Bronchospasm
◆ Cardiopulmonary arrest
◆ Facial edema
◆ Flushing
◆ Hypotension
◆ Laryngeal edema
◆ Tachycardia
◆ Urticaria
◆ Wheezing

Managing a latex allergy reaction

If you determine that your patient is having an allergic reaction to a latex product, act immediately. Make sure that you perform emergency interventions using latex-free equipment. If the latex product that caused the reaction is known, remove it and perform, or assist in performing, the following measures:

◆ If the allergic reaction develops during drug administration or a procedure, stop the drug or procedure immediately.
◆ Assess the patient's airway, breathing, and circulation.
◆ Give 100% oxygen with continuous pulse oximetry.
◆ Start I.V. volume expanders with lactated Ringer's solution or normal saline solution.
◆ Give epinephrine according to the patient's symptoms.
◆ Give famotidine, as ordered.
◆ If the patient has bronchospasm, give nebulized albuterol, as ordered.
◆ Secondary treatment for latex allergy reaction is aimed at the swelling and tissue reaction and at breaking the chain of allergic events. It includes:
- diphenhydramine
- methylprednisolone
- famotidine.
◆ Document the event and the exact cause (if known). If latex particles have entered the I.V. line, insert a new I.V. line with a new catheter, new tubing, and new infusion attachments as soon as possible.

◆ Use latex-free equipment for oxygen administration. Remove the elastic and tie the equipment on with gauze.
◆ Wrap your stethoscope with a nonlatex product to protect the patient from latex contact.
◆ Wrap a transparent semipermeable dressing over the patient's finger before using pulse oximetry.
◆ Use latex-free syringes when giving drugs.
◆ If the patient has an allergic reaction to latex, act immediately. (See *Managing a latex allergy reaction.*)

Special considerations

◆ Signs and symptoms of latex allergy usually occur within 30 minutes after anesthesia is induced. However, the time of onset can range from 10 minutes to 5 hours.
◆ As a health care worker, you're in a position to develop latex hypersensitivity.
- Use latex-free products whenever possible to help reduce your exposure to latex.
- If you suspect that you're sensitive to latex, contact the employee health services department about facility protocol for latex-sensitive employees.
◆ Patients who don't have a history of latex hypersensitivity but have an associated medical condition, occupation, or crossover allergy should be aware of the risk of latex hypersensitivity.

Alert Don't assume that if something doesn't look like rubber it isn't latex. Latex is found in various types of equipment, including electrocardiograph leads, oral and nasal airway tubing, tourniquets, nerve stimulation pads, temperature strips, and blood pressure cuffs.

Documentation

◆ Document in the patient's chart (according to facility policy) that the patient has a latex allergy.

◆ If the patient has a latex hypersensitivity reaction, document the time of each event, symptoms, any known triggers, and response to reaction.

Manual ventilation

◆ Manual ventilation involves using a handheld resuscitation bag, which is an inflatable device that can be attached to a face mask or directly to an endotracheal (ET) or tracheostomy tube to allow manual delivery of oxygen or room air to the lungs of a patient who can't breathe by himself.
◆ Usually used in an emergency, manual ventilation can also be performed while the patient is disconnected temporarily from a mechanical ventilator, such as during a tubing change, during transport, or before suctioning. In these cases, use of the handheld resuscitation bag maintains ventilation.
◆ Giving oxygen with a resuscitation bag can help improve a compromised cardiorespiratory system.

Equipment

Handheld resuscitation bag ◆ mask ◆ oxygen source (wall unit or tank) ◆ oxygen tubing ◆ nipple adapter attached to oxygen flowmeter ◆ optional: oxygen accumulator and positive end-expiratory pressure (PEEP) valve; oropharyngeal airway or nasopharyngeal airway

Implementation

◆ Unless the patient is intubated or has a tracheostomy, select a mask that fits snugly over the patient's mouth and nose.
◆ Attach the mask to the resuscitation bag.
◆ If oxygen is readily available, connect the handheld resuscitation bag to the oxygen source. Attach one end of the oxygen tubing to the bottom of the bag and the other end to the nipple adapter on the flowmeter of the oxygen source.
◆ Turn on the oxygen, and adjust the flow rate according to the patient's condition.
– For example, if the patient has a low partial pressure of arterial oxygen, he'll need a higher fraction of inspired oxygen (FIO_2).
– To increase the concentration of inspired oxygen, you can add an oxygen accumulator (also called an oxygen reservoir). This device, which attaches to an adapter on the bottom of the bag, permits an FIO_2 of up to 100%. If time allows, set up suction equipment.
◆ Before you use the handheld resuscitation bag, remove any objects from the patient's upper airway. (This action alone restores spontaneous respirations in some instances.)
◆ Also, suction the patient to remove secretions that may obstruct the airway, impeding resuscitation efforts.
◆ If the patient has a tracheostomy or an ET tube in place, suction the tube.
◆ If needed, insert an oropharyngeal or nasopharyngeal airway to maintain airway patency.
◆ If appropriate, remove the headboard and stand at the head of the bed to help keep the patient's neck extended and to free space at the side of the bed for other activities, such as cardiopulmonary resuscitation.
◆ Tilt the patient's head backward, if not contraindicated, and pull his jaw forward to move the tongue away from the base of the pharynx and prevent obstruction of the airway. (See *How to apply a handheld resuscitation bag and mask,* pages 252 and 253.)
◆ Keeping your nondominant hand on the patient's mask, exert downward pressure to seal the mask against his face. For an adult patient, use your

How to apply a handheld resuscitation bag and mask

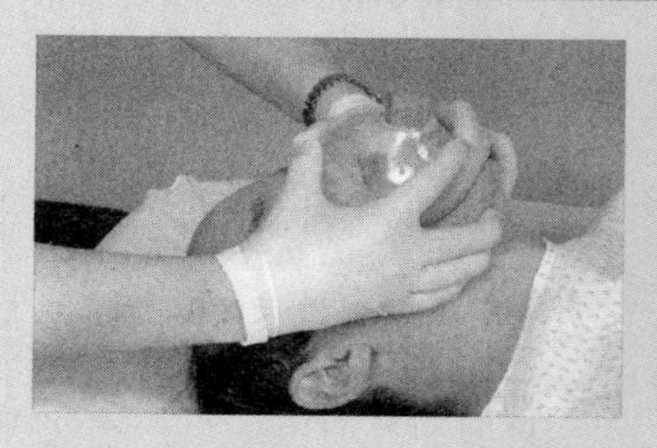

Place the mask over the patient's face so that the apex of the triangle covers the bridge of his nose and the base lies between his lower lip and his chin.

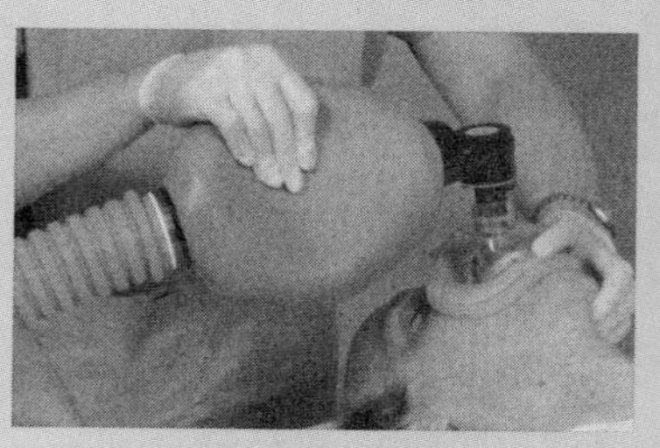

Make sure that the patient's mouth remains open underneath the mask. Attach the bag to the mask and to the tubing that leads to the oxygen source.

dominant hand to compress the bag every 5 seconds to deliver about 1 L (1,000 cc) of air.

Age alert For infants and children, use a pediatric handheld resuscitation bag. For a child, deliver 15 breaths/minute, or one compression of the bag every 4 seconds; for an infant, 20 breaths/minute, or one compression every 3 seconds. Infants and children should receive 250 to 500 cc of air with each compression.

◆ Deliver breaths with the patient's own inspiratory effort, if any is present. Don't try to deliver a breath as the patient exhales.

◆ Watch the patient's chest to make sure it rises and falls with each compression. If it doesn't, check the fit of the mask and the patency of the patient's airway. If needed, reposition the patient's head and ensure patency with an oral airway.

Special considerations

◆ Add PEEP to manual ventilation by attaching a PEEP valve to the resuscitation bag. This may improve oxygenation if the patient hasn't responded to an increased fraction of inspired oxygen levels. Always use a PEEP valve to manually ventilate a patient who has been receiving PEEP on the ventilator.

◆ If the patient has a cervical injury, avoid neck hyperextension; instead, use the jaw-thrust technique to open the airway. If you need both hands to keep the patient's mask in place and maintain hyperextension, use the lower part of your arm to compress the bag against your side.

◆ Observe the patient for vomiting through the clear part of the mask. If vomiting occurs, stop the procedure immediately, lift the mask, wipe and suction the vomitus, and resume resuscitation.

◆ Underventilation commonly occurs because it's difficult to keep the handheld resuscitation bag positioned tightly on the patient's face while ensuring an open airway. In addition, the volume of air delivered to the patient varies with the type of bag used and the hand size of the person who is compressing the bag. An adult with a small or medium hand may not consistently deliver 1 L (1,000 cc) of air with each compression of the bag. For these

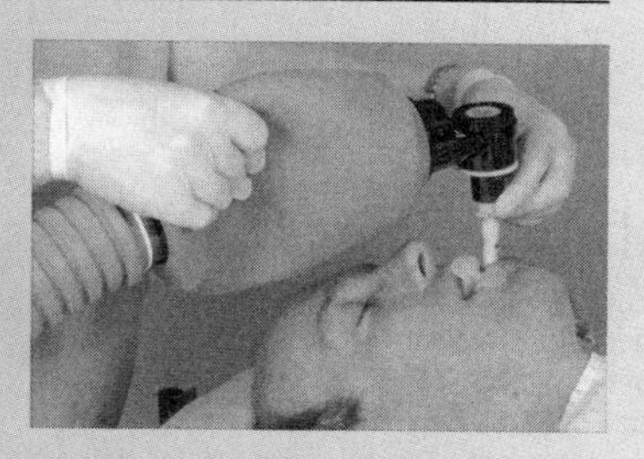

If the patient has a tracheostomy tube or an endotracheal tube in place, remove the mask from the bag and attach the handheld resuscitation bag directly to the tube.

reasons, have someone assist with the procedure, if possible.

◆ Aspiration of vomitus can result in pneumonia, and gastric distention may occur if air is forced into the patient's stomach.

Documentation

Emergency situation

◆ Record the date and time of the procedure.
◆ Record manual ventilation efforts.
◆ Note complications that occurred and nursing action taken.
◆ Note the patient's response to treatment.

Nonemergency situation

◆ Record the date and time of the procedure.
◆ Note the reason for the procedure.
◆ Record the length of time the patient was disconnected from mechanical ventilation and received manual ventilation.
◆ Note complications that occurred and nursing actions taken.
◆ Note the patient's tolerance of the procedure.

Nasogastric tube insertion and removal

◆ An LPN assists an RN with this procedure.
◆ Usually inserted to decompress the stomach, a nasogastric (NG) tube can prevent vomiting after major surgery.
◆ An NG tube is typically in place for 48 to 72 hours after surgery, by which time peristalsis usually resumes. However, the tube may remain in place for shorter or longer periods, depending on its use.
◆ The NG tube has other diagnostic and therapeutic applications, especially in assessing and treating upper GI bleeding, collecting gastric contents for analysis, performing gastric lavage, aspirating gastric secretions, and giving drugs and nutrients.
◆ Inserting an NG tube requires close observation of the patient and verification of proper placement.
◆ An NG tube must be inserted with extra care in pregnant patients and in those with an increased risk of complications. For example, a physician will order an NG tube for a patient with aortic aneurysm, myocardial infarction, gastric hemorrhage, or esophageal varices only if he believes that the benefits outweigh the risks.
◆ Most NG tubes have a radiopaque marker or strip at the distal end to allow the position of the tube to be verified by X-ray. If an X-ray doesn't confirm placement, the physician may order fluoroscopy.
◆ The most common types of NG tubes are the Levin tube, which has one lumen, and the Salem sump tube, which has two lumens, one for suction and drainage and a smaller one for ventilation. Air flows through the vent lumen continuously, protecting the delicate gastric mucosa by preventing a vacuum from forming should the tube adhere to the stomach lining. The

Types of nasogastric tubes

The physician will choose the type and diameter of the nasogastric (NG) tube that best suits the patient's needs, including lavage, aspiration, enteral therapy, or stomach decompression. Choices may include the Levin tube and the Salem sump tube.

Levin tube
The Levin tube is a rubber or plastic tube that has a single lumen, a length of 42″ to 50″ (106.5 to 127 cm), and holes at the tip and along the side.

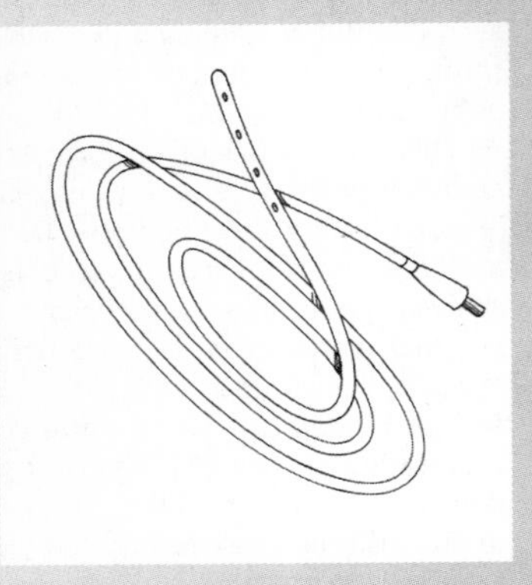

Salem sump tube
The Salem sump tube is a double-lumen tube that's made of clear plastic and has a blue sump port (pigtail) that allows atmospheric air to enter the patient's stomach. Thus, the tube floats freely and doesn't adhere to or damage the gastric mucosa. The larger port of this 48″ (122 cm) tube serves as the main suction conduit. The tube has openings at 45, 55, 65, and 75 cm as well as a radiopaque line to verify placement.

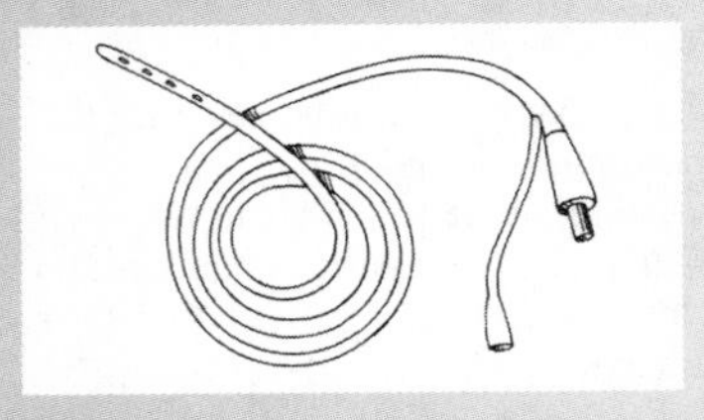

Moss tube, which has a triple lumen, is usually inserted during surgery. (See *Types of nasogastric tubes*.)

◆ The NG tube must be removed carefully to prevent injury or aspiration.

Equipment

Inserting an NG tube

NG tube (usually #12, #14, #16, or #18 French for a normal adult) ◆ towel or linen-saver pad ◆ facial tissues ◆ emesis basin ◆ penlight ◆ 1″ or 2″ hypoallergenic tape ◆ gloves ◆ water-soluble lubricant ◆ cup of water with straw (if appropriate) ◆ pH indicator paper ◆ tongue blade ◆ catheter-tip or bulb syringe or irrigation set ◆ safety pin ◆ ordered suction equipment ◆ optional: ice, alcohol pad, warm water, and rubber band

Removing an NG tube

Gloves ◆ catheter-tip syringe ◆ normal saline solution ◆ towel or linen-saver pad ◆ adhesive remover ◆ optional: clamp

Implementation

◆ Whether an NG tube is being inserted or removed, provide privacy, wash your hands, and put on gloves before the procedure.

Inserting an NG tube

◆ Check the physician's order to determine the type of tube that should be inserted.

◆ Inspect the NG tube for defects, such as rough edges or partially closed lumens. Check the patency of the tube by flushing it with water.

◆ To ease insertion, increase the flexibility of a stiff tube by coiling it around your gloved fingers for a few seconds or by dipping it into warm water.
◆ Stiffen a limp rubber tube by briefly chilling it in ice.
◆ Verify the patient's identity using two patient identifiers. Explain the procedure to the patient to ease her anxiety and promote cooperation. Explain that she may have some nasal discomfort, that she may gag, and that her eyes may water. Tell her that swallowing will ease advancement of the tube.
◆ Agree on a signal that the patient can use if she wants you to stop briefly during the procedure.
◆ Gather and prepare all needed equipment.
◆ Help the patient into high Fowler's position, unless contraindicated.
◆ Stand at the patient's right side if you're right-handed or at her left side if you're left-handed, to ease insertion.
◆ Drape the towel or linen-saver pad over the patient's chest to protect her gown and bed linens from spills.
◆ Have the patient blow her nose gently to clear her nostrils.
◆ Place the facial tissues and emesis basin within the patient's reach.
◆ Help the patient to face forward, with her neck in a neutral position.
◆ To determine how long the NG tube must be to reach the patient's stomach, hold the end of the tube at the tip of her nose, and then extend the tube to the her earlobe and then down to the xiphoid process.
◆ Use tape to mark this distance on the tubing.
– Average measurements for an adult range from 22″ to 26″ [56 to 66 cm].
– You may need to add 2″ (5 cm) to this measurement for tall patients, to ensure entry into the stomach.
◆ To determine which nostril will allow easier access, use a penlight to look for a deviated septum or other abnormalities. Ask the patient if she has had nasal surgery or a nasal injury. Determine airflow in both nostrils by occluding one nostril at a time while the patient breathes through her nose. Choose the nostril with better airflow.
◆ Lubricate the first 3″ (7.6 cm) of the tube with a water-soluble lubricant.
– Doing so minimizes injury to the nasal passages.
– Using a water-soluble lubricant prevents lipoid pneumonia, which may result from aspiration of an oil-based lubricant or from accidental slippage of the tube into the trachea.
◆ Instruct the patient to hold her head straight and upright.
◆ Grasp the tube with the end pointing downward, curve it, if needed, and carefully insert it into the more patent nostril (as shown below).

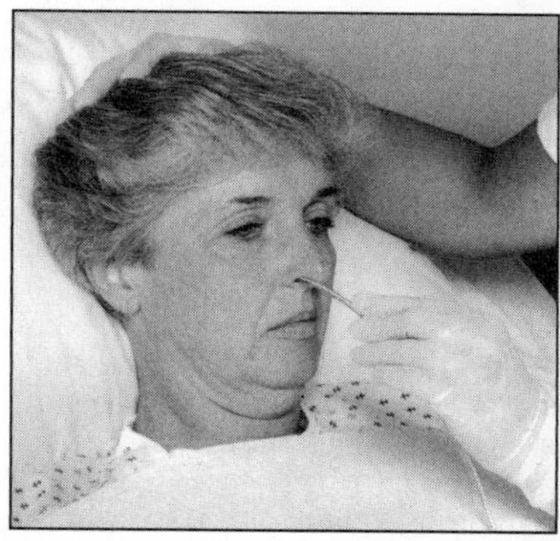

◆ Aim the tube downward and toward the ear closer to the chosen nostril. Advance it slowly to avoid pressure on the turbinates, pain, and bleeding.
◆ When the tube reaches the nasopharynx, you'll feel resistance. Tell the patient to lower her head slightly to close the trachea and open the esophagus. Rotate the tube 180 degrees toward the opposite nostril to redirect it so that it won't enter the patient's mouth.
◆ Unless contraindicated, offer the patient a cup of water with a straw. Direct her to sip and swallow as you

slowly advance the tube (as shown below). This helps the tube to pass to the esophagus. If you aren't using water, ask the patient to swallow.

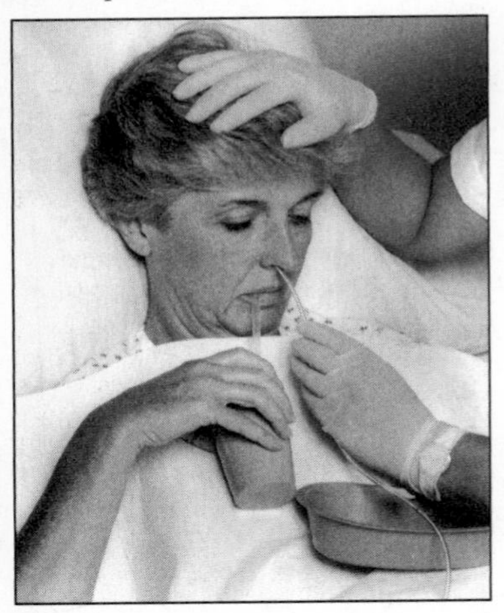

Ensuring proper tube placement

◆ Use a tongue blade and penlight to examine the patient's mouth and throat for signs of a coiled section of tubing (especially in an unconscious patient). Coiling indicates an obstruction.

◆ Keep an emesis basin and facial tissues readily available for the patient.

◆ As you carefully advance the tube and the patient swallows, watch for signs of respiratory distress, which may indicate that the tube is in the bronchus and must be removed immediately.

◆ Stop advancing the tube when the tape mark reaches the patient's nostril.

◆ Attach a catheter-tip or bulb syringe to the tube, and try to aspirate the stomach contents. If you don't obtain stomach contents, position the patient on her left side to move the contents into the greater curvature of the stomach, and aspirate again.

Alert When confirming tube placement, never place the end of the tube in a container of water. If the tube is mispositioned in the trachea, the patient may aspirate water. Furthermore, water without bubbles doesn't confirm proper placement. Instead, the tube may be coiled in the trachea or the esophagus.

◆ If you still can't aspirate the stomach contents, advance the tube 1″ to 2″ (2.5 to 5 cm), then aspirate again.

◆ Check the aspirate for pH using the pH indicator paper.

- A pH of 5 or less with a clear, slightly yellow, or grassy-green color aspirate generally confirms gastric placement.
- A pH of 6 or more with light to golden yellow or brownish-green color aspirate indicates small bowel placement.
- A pH greater than 6 with clear aspirate with white mucus shreds may indicate pulmonary placement.

◆ Patients on stomach acid-reducing medications, those with GI bleeding, and those on continuous feedings may require initial and periodic radiographic placement confirmation as the pH test may not be accurate. Check your facility guidelines.

◆ If these tests don't confirm proper tube placement, you'll need X-ray verification.

◆ Don't start feeding until placement is confirmed, per your facility's policy.

◆ Secure the NG tube to the patient's nose with hypoallergenic tape (or another designated tube holder).

- If the patient's skin is oily, wipe the bridge of her nose with an alcohol pad, and let it dry.
- You'll need about 4″ (10.2 cm) of 1″ tape.
- Split one end of the tape up the center about 1½″ (3.8 cm). Make tabs on the split ends by folding the sticky sides together.
- Stick the uncut end of the tape on the patient's nose so that the split in

the tape starts about ½″ (1.3 cm) to 1½″ from the tip of her nose.
- Crisscross the tabbed ends around the tube (as shown below).
- Apply another piece of tape over the bridge of the nose to secure the tube.

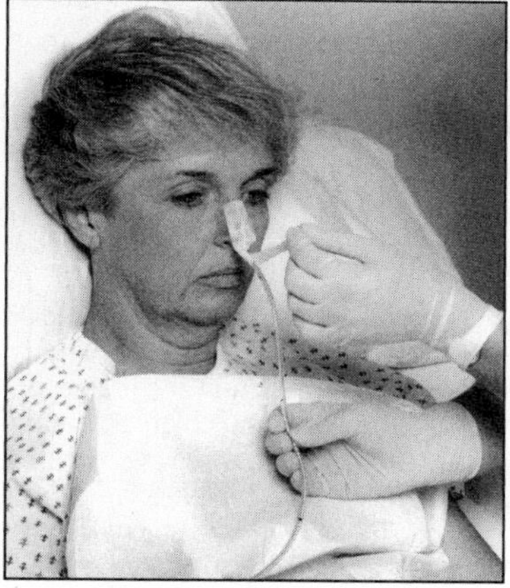

◆ Alternatively, stabilize the tube with a prepackaged product that secures and cushions it at the nose.
◆ To reduce discomfort from the weight of the tube, tie a slipknot around the tube with a rubber band. Secure the rubber band to the patient's gown with a safety pin, or wrap another piece of tape around the end of the tube and leave a tab. Fasten the tape tab to the patient's gown.
◆ Attach the tube to suction equipment, if ordered, and set the designated suction pressure.
◆ Provide frequent nose and mouth care while the tube is in place.
◆ Continue to check tube placement before each tube feeding, before giving drugs, and at least once daily if the patient is on continuous feeding.
◆ To maintain patency, flush the feeding tube with up to 60 ml of normal saline solution or water before and after giving drugs and feeding, or every 4 hours if on continuous tube feeding, per your facility's guidelines.

Removing an NG tube

◆ Explain the procedure to the patient, informing her that it may cause some nasal discomfort and sneezing or gagging.
◆ Check the patient's bowel function by auscultating for peristalsis or flatus.
◆ Help the patient into semi-Fowler's position.
◆ Drape a towel or linen-saver pad across her chest to protect her gown and bed linens from spills.
◆ Using a catheter-tip syringe, flush the tube with 10 ml of normal saline solution to make sure the tube doesn't contain stomach contents that could irritate tissues during removal.
◆ Untape the tube from the patient's nose, and unpin it from her gown.
◆ Clamp the tube by folding it in your hand.
◆ Ask the patient to hold her breath to close the epiglottis.
◆ Withdraw the tube gently and steadily. When the distal end of the tube reaches the nasopharynx, you can pull it quickly.
◆ As soon as possible, cover and remove the tube. Its sight and odor may nauseate the patient.
◆ Assist the patient with thorough mouth care, and clean the tape residue from her nose with adhesive remover.
◆ For the next 48 hours, monitor the patient for signs and symptoms of GI dysfunction, including nausea, vomiting, abdominal distention, and food intolerance. GI dysfunction may require reinsertion of the tube.

Special considerations

◆ Ross-Hanson tape is a helpful device for calculating the correct tube length. Place the narrow end of the tape at the tip of the patient's nose. Extend the tape to the patient's earlobe and down to the tip of the xiphoid process. Mark this distance on the edge of the tape labeled NOSE TO EAR TO XIPHOID. The corresponding measurement on the opposite edge of the tape is the proper insertion length.

◆ If the patient has a deviated septum or other nasal condition that prevents nasal insertion, pass the tube orally.
- Remove the patient's dentures, if needed.
- Slide the tube over the tongue, and proceed as you would for nasal insertion.
- Coil the end of the tube around your hand. This helps to curve and direct the tube downward at the pharynx.

◆ If the patient is unconscious, tilt her chin toward her chest to close the trachea. Advance the tube between respirations to make sure it doesn't enter the trachea.

◆ While advancing the tube in an unconscious patient or in a patient who can't swallow, stroke the patient's neck to encourage the swallowing reflex and facilitate passage down the esophagus.

◆ While advancing the tube, watch for signs that it has entered the trachea, such as choking or breathing difficulties in a conscious patient and cyanosis in an unconscious patient or a patient without a cough reflex. If these signs occur, remove the tube immediately. Allow the patient time to rest; then try to reinsert the tube.

◆ Vomiting after tube placement suggests tubal obstruction or incorrect position. Examine the patient immediately to determine the cause.

◆ An NG tube may be inserted or removed at home. Indications for insertion include gastric decompression and short-term feeding. A home care nurse or the patient may insert the tube, deliver the feeding, and remove the tube.

◆ Check the patient for complications of prolonged intubation, such as skin erosion at the nostril, sinusitis, esophagitis, esophagotracheal fistula, gastric ulceration, and pulmonary and oral infection. Additional complications that may result from suction include electrolyte imbalances and dehydration.

Documentation

◆ Record the type and size of the NG tube.

◆ Record the date, time, and route of insertion.

◆ Note the type and amount of suction, if used.

◆ Note a description of the drainage, including the amount, color, character, consistency, odor, and pH.

◆ Record whether tube placement was verified clinically or by radiograph.

◆ Note the patient's tolerance of the insertion procedure.

◆ Record the date and time of tube removal.

◆ Note color, consistency, and amount of gastric drainage at tube removal.

◆ Record the patient's tolerance of removal procedure.

Pulse oximetry

◆ Performed intermittently or continuously, oximetry is a relatively simple procedure that's used to monitor arterial oxygen saturation noninvasively.

◆ Two diodes send red and infrared light through a pulsating arterial vascular bed such as one in the fingertip or the earlobe.

◆ A photodetector measures the transmitted light as it passes through the vascular bed, detects the relative amount of color absorbed by the arterial blood, and calculates the exact mixed venous oxygen saturation without interference from surrounding venous blood, skin, connective tissue, or bone.

◆ The results of ear oximetry will be inaccurate if the patient's earlobe is poorly perfused, as from low cardiac output.

◆ Pulse oximeters usually denote arterial oxygen saturation values with the symbol Spo_2. Invasively measured arterial oxygen saturation values are denoted by the symbol Sao_2.

Equipment

Oximeter ◆ transducer (photodetector) for finger or ear probe ◆ alcohol pads ◆ nail polish remover, if needed

Implementation

◆ Explain the procedure to the patient.

Finger pulse oximetry

◆ Select a finger for the test. Although the index finger is commonly used, a smaller finger may be selected if the patient's fingers are too large for the equipment.

◆ Make sure that the patient isn't wearing false fingernails, and remove any nail polish from the test finger with nail polish remover.

◆ Place the transducer (photodetector) finger probe over the patient's finger so that light beams and sensors oppose each other and attach to the oximeter.

◆ If the patient has long fingernails, position the probe perpendicular to the finger, if possible, or clip the fingernail.

◆ the patient has a latex allergy, cover the finger with a clear bandage.

◆ Always position the patient's hand at heart level to eliminate venous pulsations and to promote accurate readings.

Age alert If you're testing a neonate or a small infant, wrap the probe around the foot so that the light beams and detectors oppose each other. For a large infant, use a probe that fits on the great toe, and secure it to the foot.

◆ Turn on the power switch. If the device is working properly, a beep will sound, a display will light momentarily, and the pulse searchlight will flash. The Spo_2 and pulse rate displays will show stationary zeros.

◆ After four to six heartbeats, the Spo_2 and pulse rate displays will supply information with each beat, and the pulse amplitude indicator will begin to track the pulse.

Ear pulse oximetry

◆ Using an alcohol pad, massage the patient's earlobe for 10 to 20 seconds. Mild erythema indicates adequate vascularization.

◆ Following the manufacturer's instructions, attach the ear probe to the patient's earlobe or pinna.

◆ Use the ear probe stabilizer for prolonged or exercise testing. Be sure to establish good contact on the ear; an unstable probe may set off the low-perfusion alarm.

◆ After the probe has been attached for a few seconds, a saturation reading and pulse waveform will appear on the screen.

◆ Leave the ear probe in place for 3 minutes or more, until readings stabilize at the highest point, or take three separate readings and average them, revascularizing the patient's earlobe each time.

◆ After the procedure, remove the probe, turn off and unplug the unit, and clean the probe by gently rubbing it with an alcohol pad.

Special considerations

◆ If oximetry has been performed properly, the readings are typically ac-

Diagnosing pulse oximeter problems

To maintain a continuous display of arterial oxygen saturation levels, you'll need to keep the monitoring site clean and dry. Make sure that the skin doesn't become irritated from adhesives used to keep disposable probes in place. You may need to change the site if this happens. Disposable probes that irritate the skin can be replaced by nondisposable models that don't need tape.

Another common problem with pulse oximeters is the failure of the devices to obtain a signal. If this happens, your first reaction should be to check the patient's vital signs. If they're sufficient to produce a signal, check for the following problems.

Poor connection

See if the sensors are properly aligned. Make sure that the wires are intact and securely fastened and that the pulse oximeter is plugged into a power source.

Inadequate or intermittent blood flow to the site

Check the patient's pulse rate and capillary refill time, and take corrective action if blood flow to the site is decreased. This may mean loosening restraints, removing tight-fitting clothes, taking off a blood pressure cuff, or checking arterial and I.V. lines. If these interventions don't work, you may need to find an alternate site. Finding a site with proper circulation may prove challenging when a patient is receiving a vasoconstrictor.

Equipment malfunction

Remove the pulse oximeter from the patient, set the alarm limits at 85% and 100%, and try the instrument on yourself or another healthy person. This will tell you if the equipment is working correctly.

curate. However, certain factors may interfere with accuracy.
- An elevated bilirubin level may falsely lower Spo_2 readings
- Elevated carboxyhemoglobin or methemoglobin levels, such as occur in heavy smokers and urban dwellers, can cause a falsely elevated Spo_2 reading. (See *Diagnosing pulse oximeter problems.*)
- Certain intravascular substances, such as lipid emulsions and dyes, can prevent accurate readings.
- Excessive light (as from phototherapy, surgical lamps, direct sunlight, and excessive ambient lighting), excessive patient movement, excessive ear pigment, hypothermia, hypotension, and vasoconstriction may interfere as well.

◆ If the patient has compromised circulation in his extremities, you can place a photodetector across the bridge of his nose.

◆ If Spo_2 is used to guide weaning of the patient from forced inspiratory oxygen, obtain arterial blood gas analysis occasionally to correlate Spo_2 readings with Sao_2 levels.

◆ If an automatic blood pressure cuff is used on the same extremity that's used to measure Spo_2, the cuff will interfere with Spo_2 readings during inflation.

◆ If light is a problem, cover the probes; if patient movement is a problem, move the probe or select a different probe; and if ear pigment is a problem, reposition the probe, revascularize the site, or use a finger probe.

◆ Normal Spo_2 levels for ear and pulse oximetry are 95% to 100% for adults and 94% to 100% by 1 hour after birth for healthy, full-term neonates.

◆ Lower levels may indicate hypoxemia that warrants intervention.
- For such patients, follow facility policy or the physician's orders, which may include increasing oxygen therapy.
- If SaO_2 levels decrease suddenly, you may need to resuscitate the patient immediately.
- Notify the physician of any significant change in the patient's condition.

Documentation

◆ Record the date, time, and type of procedure.

◆ Record the oximetric measurement and actions taken (in appropriate flowcharts, if indicated).

Seizure management

◆ Seizures are paroxysmal events caused by abnormal electrical discharges of neurons in the brain.

◆ Seizures may be partial or general.
- Partial seizures are usually unilateral, involving a localized, or focal, area of the brain.
- Generalized seizures involve the entire brain.

◆ When a patient has a generalized seizure, the goal of nursing care is to protect him from injury and prevent serious complications. Appropriate care also includes observation of the characteristics of the seizure to help determine the area of the brain involved.

◆ Patients who are considered at risk for seizures are those with a history of seizures and those with conditions that predispose them to seizures, such as:
- metabolic abnormalities, such as hypocalcemia, hypoglycemia, and pyridoxine deficiency
- brain tumors or other space-occupying lesions
- infections, such as meningitis, encephalitis, and brain abscess
- traumatic injury, especially if the dura mater was penetrated
- ingestion of toxins, such as mercury, lead, or carbon monoxide
- genetic abnormalities, such as tuberous sclerosis and phenylketonuria
- perinatal injuries
- stroke.

◆ Patients at risk for seizures need precautionary measures to help prevent injury if a seizure occurs. (See *Precautions for generalized seizures,* page 262.)

Equipment

Oral airway ◆ suction equipment ◆ side rail pads ◆ seizure activity record ◆ optional: I.V. line and normal saline solution, oxygen as ordered, endotracheal intubation, dextrose 50% in water, thiamine

Implementation

◆ If you're with a patient when he has an aura, take precautions to keep him safe during the impending seizure.
- Help him get into bed, raise the side rails, and adjust the bed flat.
- Use side rail pads and blankets to pad the rails securely.
- If he's away from his room, lower him to the floor and place a pillow, blanket, or other soft material under his head to keep it from hitting the floor.

◆ Stay with the patient during the seizure, and be ready to intervene if complications such as airway obstruction develop. If needed, have another staff member obtain the appropriate equipment and notify the physician of the obstruction.

◆ Provide privacy, if possible.

Alert During a seizure, don't try to hold the patient's mouth

Precautions for generalized seizures

By taking appropriate precautions, you can help to protect a patient from injury, aspiration, and airway obstruction in case he has a seizure. Plan your precautions using information obtained from the patient's history. What kind of seizure has the patient previously had? Is he aware of exacerbating factors? Sleep deprivation, missed doses of an anticonvulsant, and even upper respiratory tract infections can increase seizure frequency in some people who have had seizures. Was his previous seizure an acute episode, or did it result from a chronic condition?

Gather the equipment

Based on answers provided in the patient's history, you can tailor your precautions to his needs. Start by gathering the appropriate equipment, including a hospital bed with full-length side rails, commercial side rail pads or six bath blankets (four for a crib), adhesive tape, an oral airway, and oral or nasal suction equipment.

Bedside preparations

Carry out the precautions that you think are appropriate for the patient. Remember that a patient with preexisting seizures who's being admitted for a change in medication, treatment of an infection, or detoxification may have an increased risk of seizures.

◆ Explain the reasons for the precautions to the patient.

◆ To protect the patient's limbs, head, and feet from injury if he has a seizure while in bed, cover the side rails, headboard, and footboard with side rail pads or bath blankets. If you use blankets, keep them in place with adhesive tape. Be sure to keep the side rails raised while the patient is in bed to prevent falls. Keep the bed in a low position to minimize injuries that may occur if the patient climbs over the side rails.

◆ Place an airway at the patient's bedside, or tape it to the wall above the bed according to facility policy. Keep suction equipment nearby in case you need to establish a patent airway. Explain to the patient how the airway will be used.

◆ If the patient has frequent or prolonged seizures, prepare an I.V. saline lock to facilitate the administration of emergency medications.

open or place your hands inside his mouth. After the patient's jaw becomes rigid, don't force his airway into place because you could break his teeth or cause another injury. If needed, insert an oral airway after the seizure subsides.

◆ Move hard or sharp objects away from the patient, and loosen his clothing.

◆ Don't forcibly restrain the patient or restrict his movements during the seizure. The force of his movements against restraints could cause muscle strain or even joint dislocation.

◆ Time the seizure activity from beginning to end, and continually check the patient during the seizure.

◆ Observe the earliest sign, such as head or eye deviation, as well as how the seizure progresses, what form it takes, and how long it lasts.

◆ Document the seizure on the hospital seizure activity record. Your description may help determine the type and cause of the seizure.

◆ If this is the patient's first seizure, notify the physician immediately. If the patient has had seizures before, notify the physician only if the seizure activity is prolonged or if the patient doesn't regain consciousness. (See *Understanding status epilepticus*.)

◆ If ordered, establish an I.V. line and infuse normal saline solution at a keep-vein-open rate.

◆ If the seizure is prolonged and the patient becomes hypoxemic, give oxygen, as ordered. Some patients may require endotracheal intubation.

◆ If the patient has diabetes and hypoglycemia, obtain a blood glucose measurement via glucometer, then administer dextrose 50% in water by I.V. push, if ordered. If the patient has alcoholism, a bolus of thiamine may be ordered to stop the seizure.

◆ After the seizure, turn the patient on his side and apply suction, if needed, to facilitate drainage of secretions and maintain a patent airway. Insert an oral airway, if needed.

◆ Check the patient for injuries.

◆ Reorient and reassure the patient, as needed.

◆ When the patient is comfortable and safe, document what happened during the seizure.

◆ After the seizure, monitor the patient's vital signs and mental status every 15 to 20 minutes for 2 hours.

◆ Ask the patient about his aura and activities preceding the seizure. The type of aura (auditory, visual, olfactory, gustatory, or somatic) helps to pinpoint the site in the brain where the seizure originated.

Understanding status epilepticus

Status epilepticus is a continuous seizure state that has many causes including abrupt withdrawal of an anticonvulsant, hypoxic or metabolic encephalopathy, acute head trauma, or septicemia caused by encephalitis or meningitis. It's accompanied by respiratory distress and is always an emergency.

Status epilepticusis can occur with all types of seizures. The most dangerous is generalized tonic-clonic status epilepticus, which is a continuous generalized tonic-clonic seizure without intervening return of consciousness.

Emergency treatment of status epilepticus usually consists of phenobarbital, diazepam, or phenytoin; I.V. dextrose 50% (when seizures are caused by hypoglycemia); and I.V. thiamine (in patients with chronic alcoholism or withdrawal).

Special considerations

◆ Because a seizure may indicate an underlying disorder, such as meningitis or a metabolic or electrolyte imbalance, a complete diagnostic workup will be ordered if the cause of the seizure isn't evident.

◆ The patient who has a seizure may experience an injury, respiratory difficulty, and decreased mental capability.

- Common injuries include scrapes and bruises that occur when the patient hits objects during the seizure and traumatic injury to the tongue caused by biting.
- If you suspect a serious injury, such as a fracture or deep laceration, notify the physician and arrange for appropriate evaluation and treatment.

◆ Changes in respiratory function include aspiration, airway obstruction, and hypoxemia. After the seizure, complete a respiratory check and notify the physician if you suspect a problem.

◆ Expect most patients to experience a postictal period of decreased mental status lasting 30 minutes to 24 hours. Reassure the patient that this doesn't indicate incipient brain damage.

Documentation

- Record the reason for seizure precautions.
- Note all precautions taken.
- Record the date and the time that a seizure began, as well as its duration and any precipitating factors.
- Record the patient's description of anything that could have been an aura before the seizure.
- Note any involuntary behavior that occurred at the start of the seizure (such as lip smacking, chewing movements, or hand and eye movements), where the movement began, whether it showed any progression or pattern, and the parts of the body involved.
- Note whether the patient's eyes deviated to one side and whether the pupils changed in size, shape, equality, or reaction to light.
- Note whether the patient's teeth were clenched or open.
- Note any incontinence, vomiting, or salivation that occurred during the seizure.
- Record the patient's response to the seizure (Was the patient aware of what happened? Did he fall into a deep sleep after the seizure? Was he upset or ashamed?).
- Record all drugs given.
- Note complications experienced during the seizure, and all interventions performed.
- Record the patient's mental status after the seizure.

Sequential compression therapy

- Safe, effective, and noninvasive, sequential compression therapy helps prevent deep vein thrombosis (DVT) in surgical patients. This therapy massages the legs in a wavelike, milking motion that promotes blood flow and deters thrombosis.
- Typically, sequential compression therapy complements other preventive measures, such as antiembolism stockings and anticoagulant therapy. Although patients who are at low risk for DVT may require only antiembolism stockings, those who are at moderate to high risk may require both antiembolism stockings and sequential compression therapy. These preventive measures continue for as long as the patient remains at risk.
- Both antiembolism stockings and sequential compression sleeves are commonly used preoperatively and postoperatively because blood clots tend to form during surgery. About 20% of blood clots form in the femoral vein.
- Sequential compression therapy counteracts blood stasis and coagulation changes, two of the three major factors that promote DVT. It reduces stasis by increasing peak blood flow velocity, helping to empty the femoral vein's valve cusps of pooled or static blood. The compressions cause an anticlotting effect by increasing fibrinolytic activity, which stimulates the release of a plasminogen activator.

Equipment

Measuring tape and sizing chart for brand of sleeves being used ◆ pair of compression sleeves in correct size ◆ connecting tubing ◆ compression controller

Implementation

- Explain the procedure to the patient to increase his cooperation. Wash your hands and provide privacy.

Determining proper sleeve size

- Before applying the compression sleeve, determine the proper size of sleeve that you need.

◆ Measure the circumference of the patient's upper thigh while she rests in bed. Do this by placing the measuring tape under the thigh at the gluteal furrow (as shown below).

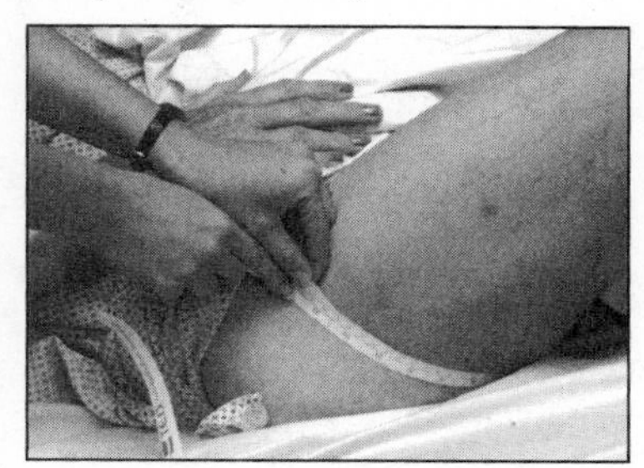

◆ Hold the tape snugly, but not tightly, around the patient's leg. Note the exact circumference.
◆ Find the patient's thigh measurement on the sizing chart, and locate the corresponding size of the compression sleeve.
◆ Remove the compression sleeves from the package and unfold them.
◆ Lay the unfolded sleeves on a flat surface with the cotton lining facing up (as shown below).

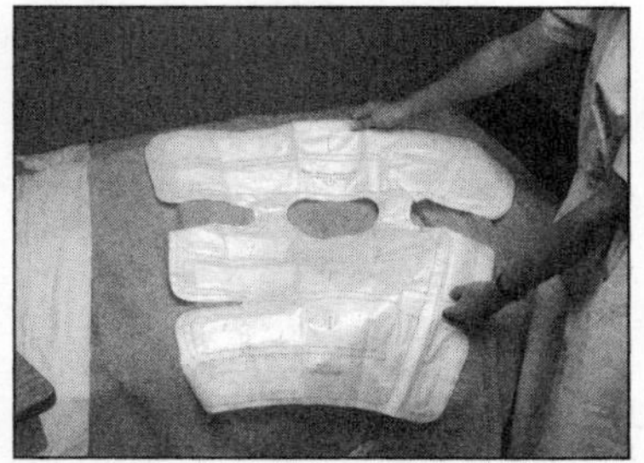

◆ Notice the markings on the lining denoting the ankle and the area behind the knee at the popliteal pulse point. Use these markings to position the sleeves at the appropriate landmarks.

Applying the sleeves
◆ Place the patient's leg on the lining of one of the sleeves. Position the back of the knee over the popliteal opening.
◆ Make sure that the back of the ankle is over the ankle marking.
◆ Starting at the side opposite the clear plastic tubing, wrap the sleeve snugly around the patient's leg.
◆ Fasten the sleeve securely with the Velcro fasteners. For the best fit, secure the ankle and calf sections, followed by the thigh section.
◆ The sleeve should fit snugly, but not tightly. Check the fit by inserting two fingers between the sleeve and the patient's leg at the knee opening. Loosen or tighten the sleeve by readjusting the Velcro fastener.
◆ Using the same procedure, apply the second sleeve (as shown below).

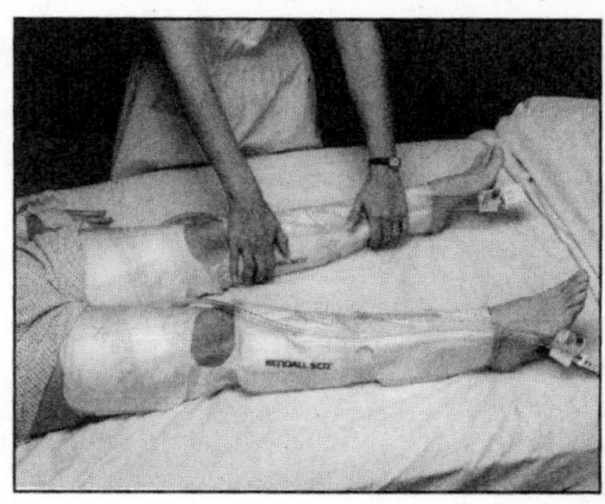

Operating the system
◆ Connect each sleeve to the tubing leading to the controller. Both sleeves must be connected to the compression controller for the system to operate.
◆ Line up the blue arrows on the sleeve connector with the arrows on the tubing connectors, and firmly push the ends together. Listen for a click, which signals a firm connection.
◆ Make sure that the tubing isn't kinked.
◆ Plug the compression controller into the proper wall outlet, and turn on the power.
◆ The controller automatically sets the compression sleeve pressure at 45 mm Hg, which is the midpoint of the normal range (35 to 55 mm Hg).

◆ Observe the patient to see how well he tolerates the therapy and the controller as the system completes its first cycle.
◆ Check the AUDIBLE ALARM key. The green light should be lit, indicating that the alarm is working.
◆ The compression sleeves should function continuously (24 hours per day) until the patient is fully ambulatory. Check the sleeves at least once each shift to ensure proper fit and inflation.

Removing the sleeves

◆ You may remove the sleeves when the patient is walking, bathing, or leaving the room for tests or other procedures, as long as you reapply them immediately after the tests and procedures are over.
◆ To disconnect the sleeves from the tubing, press the latches on each side of the connectors and pull the connectors apart.
◆ Store the tubing and the compression controller according to facility policy. This equipment isn't disposable.

Special considerations

◆ The compression controller also has a mechanism to help cool the patient.
◆ If you're applying only one sleeve — for example, if the patient has a cast — leave the unused sleeve folded in the plastic bag. Cut a small hole in the sealed bottom edge of the bag, and pull the sleeve connector (the part that holds the connecting tubing) through the hole. Then you can join both sleeves to the compression controller.
◆ If a malfunction triggers the instrument alarm, you'll hear beeping. The system shuts off whenever the alarm is activated.
◆ To respond to the alarm, remove the operator's card from the slot on the top of the compression controller. Follow the instructions printed on the card next to the matching code.
◆ Don't use this therapy in patients with any of these conditions:
- acute DVT or DVT diagnosed within the last 6 months
- severe arteriosclerosis or any other ischemic vascular disease
- massive edema of the legs because of pulmonary edema or heart failure
- any local condition that would likely be aggravated by the compression sleeves, such as dermatitis, vein ligation, gangrene, and recent skin grafting. A patient with a pronounced leg deformity would also be unlikely to benefit from compression sleeves.

Documentation

◆ Note the patient's understanding of the procedure.
◆ Record procedure activities.
◆ Record the patient's response to the procedure.
◆ Note the status of the alarm and cooling settings.

Surgical site verification

◆ Wrong-site surgery is a general term that refers to a surgical procedure performed on the wrong body part or side of the body, or even the wrong patient. This error may occur in the operating room or in other settings, such as during ambulatory care or interventional radiology.
◆ Several factors may contribute to an increased risk of wrong-site surgery:
- inadequate evaluation of the patient
- inadequate review of the medical records
- inaccurate communication among members of the health team
- involvement of multiple surgeons in the procedure

- failure to include the patient in the site-identification process
- relying solely on the physician for site identification.

◆ Because serious consequences may result from wrong-site surgery, the nurse must confirm that the correct site has been identified before surgery begins.

Equipment

Surgical consent ◆ medical record ◆ procedure schedule ◆ hypoallergenic, nonlatex permanent marker

Implementation

◆ Confirm the patient's identity using two patient identifiers.

◆ Before the procedure, check the patient's chart for documentation.

◆ Compare the information on the chart with the history and physical examination form, the nursing assessment, the preprocedure verification checklist, the signed informed consent form with the exact procedure site identified, the procedure schedule, and the patient's verbal confirmation of the correct site.

◆ After verbally confirming the site with the patient, the person performing the procedure — or another member of the surgical team who's fully informed about the patient and the intended procedure — marks the site with a permanent marker. The mark needs to be placed so that it's visible after the patient has been prepared and draped.

◆ The surgical team (surgeon, operating room or procedure staff, and anesthesia personnel) must identify the patient and verify the correct procedure and the correct site before they begin the surgery.

Special considerations

◆ If the patient's condition prevents him from verifying the correct site, the surgeon will identify and mark the site using history and physical examination forms, signed informed consent form, preprocedure verification checklist, procedure schedule, X-rays, and other imaging studies.

Documentation

◆ Record information on the preprocedure verification checklist used by your facility.

◆ Record confirmation that the correct site was verified and marked.

Transfusion of whole blood and packed cells

◆ An LPN assists an RN with this procedure.

◆ Whole blood transfusion replenishes the volume and the oxygen-carrying capacity of the circulatory system by increasing the mass of circulating red blood cells (RBCs).

◆ Transfusion of packed RBCs, from which 80% of the plasma has been removed, restores only the oxygen-carrying capacity.

◆ Whole blood without the plasma removed has a hematocrit of about 38%. After plasma is removed, the resulting component has a hematocrit of 65% to 80% and a usual volume of 300 to 350 ml.

◆ Each unit of whole blood or RBCs contains enough hemoglobin to raise the hemoglobin level in an average-sized adult 1 g/L, or by 3%.

◆ Both types of transfusion treat decreased hemoglobin levels and hematocrit.

◆ Whole blood is usually used only when decreased levels result from he-

morrhage; packed RBCs are used when depressed levels accompany normal blood volume, to avoid possible fluid and circulatory overload. (See *Transfusing blood and selected components,* pages 270 to 275.)
- Whole blood and packed RBCs contain cellular debris and require in-line filtration during administration.
- Washed packed RBCs, commonly used for patients who were previously sensitized to transfusions, are rinsed with a special solution that removes white blood cells and platelets, thus decreasing the chance of a transfusion reaction.

Alert To prevent errors and potentially fatal reactions, facility policy generally follows JCAHO policy, which requires that two nurses identify the patient and blood products before administering a transfusion.

Alert If the patient is a Jehovah's Witness, a transfusion requires special written permission.

Equipment and preparation

Blood administration set (including 170- to 260-micron filter and tubing with drip chamber for blood, or combined set) ◆ I.V. pole ◆ gloves ◆ gown ◆ face shield ◆ whole blood or packed RBCs ◆ 250 ml of normal saline solution ◆ venipuncture equipment, if needed (should include 20G or larger catheter) ◆ optional: ice bag and warm compresses

Implementation

- Prepare the equipment when you're ready to start the infusion.
- Verify the patient's identity using two patient identifiers. Explain the procedure to the patient. Make sure he has signed an informed consent form before any blood is transfused.
- Record the patient's baseline vital signs.
- If the patient doesn't have an I.V. line in place, perform a venipuncture, using a catheter with a diameter of 20G or larger. Avoid using an existing line if the needle or catheter lumen is smaller than 20G. Central venous access devices may also be used for transfusion therapy.
- Obtain whole blood or packed RBCs from the blood bank within 30 minutes of the transfusion start time.
  - Check the expiration date on the blood bag, and observe the bag for abnormal color, RBC clumping, gas bubbles, and extraneous material.
  - Return outdated or abnormal blood to the blood bank.
- Identification of blood and blood products is performed at the patient's bedside by two licensed professionals, according to facility policy.
  - Compare the name and number on the patient's wristband with the information on the label of the blood bag.
  - Check the blood bag identification number, the ABO blood group, and Rh compatibility.
  - Compare the patient's blood bank identification number, if present, with the number on the blood bag.
- Put on gloves, a gown, and a face shield.
- Use a Y-type set, and close all of the clamps on the set.
- Insert the spike of the line that you're using for the normal saline solution into the bag of saline solution.
- Open the port on the blood bag, and insert the spike of the line that you're using to administer the blood or cellular component into the port.
- Hang the bag of normal saline solution and blood or cellular component on the I.V. pole, open the clamp on the line of saline solution, and squeeze the drip chamber until it's half full.
- Remove the adapter cover at the tip of the blood administration set, open the main flow clamp, and prime the tubing with saline solution.

◆ If you're giving packed RBCs with a Y-type set, you can add saline solution to the bag to dilute the cells by closing the clamp between the patient and the drip chamber and opening the clamp from the blood. Lower the blood bag below the saline container and let 30 to 50 ml of saline solution flow into the packed cells. Close the clamp to the blood bag, rehang the bag, rotate it gently to mix the cells and saline solution, and close the clamp to the saline container.
◆ If you're giving whole blood, gently invert the bag several times to mix the cells.
◆ Attach the prepared blood administration set to the venipuncture device, and flush it with normal saline solution. Close the clamp to the saline solution, and open the clamp between the blood bag and the patient.
◆ Adjust the flow rate to no greater than 5 ml/minute for the first 15 minutes of the transfusion so that you can observe the patient for a possible transfusion reaction.
◆ If signs of a transfusion reaction develop, do the following:
- Stop the transfusion and record the patient's vital signs.
- Infuse saline solution at a moderately slow infusion rate, and notify the physician at once.
◆ If no signs of a reaction appear within 15 minutes, adjust the flow clamp to the ordered infusion rate.
◆ A unit of RBCs may be given over 1 to 4 hours, as ordered.
◆ After completing the transfusion, put on gloves and remove and discard the used infusion equipment.
◆ Reconnect the original I.V. fluid, if needed, or stop the I.V. infusion.
◆ Return the empty blood bag to the blood bank. Discard the tubing and filter.
◆ Record the patient's vital signs.

Special considerations

◆ Straight-line and Y-type blood administration sets are commonly used. The use of these filters can postpone sensitization to transfusion therapy.
◆ Administer packed RBCs with a Y type set. Using a straight-line set forces you to piggyback the tubing so that you can stop the transfusion, if necessary, but still keep the vein open. Piggybacking increases the chance that harmful microorganisms will enter the tubing as you're connecting the blood line to the established line.
◆ Multiple-lead tubing minimizes the risk of contamination, especially when multiple units of blood are transfused. (A straight-line set would require multiple piggybacking.) A Y-type set gives you the option of adding normal saline solution to packed cells — decreasing their viscosity — if the patient can tolerate the added fluid volume.
◆ Although some microaggregate filters can be used for up to 10 units of blood, replace the filter and tubing if more than 1 hour elapses between transfusions.
◆ When giving multiple units of blood under pressure, use a blood warmer to avoid hypothermia. Blood components may be warmed to no more than 107.6° F (42° C).
◆ For rapid blood replacement, you may need to use a pressure bag. Excessive pressure may develop, leading to broken blood vessels and extravasation, with hematoma and hemolysis of the infusing RBCs.
◆ If the transfusion stops, take the following steps, as needed:
- Check that the I.V. container is at least 3′ (0.9 m) above the level of the I.V. site.
- Make sure that the flow clamp is open and that the blood completely

(Text continues on page 274.)

Transfusing blood and selected components

BLOOD COMPONENT	INDICATIONS
Whole blood Complete (pure) blood *Volume: 500 ml*	◆ To restore blood volume lost as a result of hemorrhage, trauma, or burns
Packed red blood cells (RBCs) Same RBC mass as whole blood, but with 80% of the plasma removed *Volume: 250 ml*	◆ To restore or maintain oxygen-carrying capacity ◆ To correct anemia and blood loss that occurs during surgery ◆ To increase RBC mass
White blood cells (WBCs or leukocytes) Whole blood with all of the RBCs and about 80% of the supernatant plasma removed *Volume: usually 150 ml*	◆ To treat sepsis that's unresponsive to antibiotics (especially if patient has positive blood cultures or a persistent fever > 101° F [38.3° C]) and granulocytopenia (granulocyte count usually < 500/μl)
Leukocyte-poor RBCs Same as packed RBCs, with about 95% of the leukocytes removed *Volume: 200 ml*	◆ Same as for packed RBCs ◆ To prevent febrile reactions from leukocyte antibodies ◆ To treat immunocompromised patients

CROSSMATCHING	NURSING CONSIDERATIONS
◆ ABO identical: Type A receives A; type B receives B; type AB receives AB; type O receives O. ◆ Rh match is needed.	◆ Use a blood administration set to infuse blood over 2 to 4 hours. ◆ Avoid giving whole blood when the patient can't tolerate the circulatory volume. ◆ Reduce the risk of a transfusion reaction by adding a microfilter to the administration set to remove platelets. ◆ Warm blood if a large quantity is being given.
◆ Type A receives A or O. ◆ Type B receives B or O. ◆ Type AB receives AB, A, B, or O. ◆ Type O receives O. ◆ Rh match is needed.	◆ Use a blood administration set to infuse blood over 2 to 4 hours. ◆ Remember that packed RBCs provide the same oxygen-carrying capacity as whole blood, with less risk of volume overload. ◆ Give packed RBCs as ordered to prevent potassium and ammonia buildup, which may occur in stored plasma. ◆ Avoid giving packed RBCs for anemic conditions that are correctable with nutrition or drug therapy.
◆ Same as for packed RBCs ◆ Compatibility with human leukocyte antigen (HLA) is preferable, but not needed unless the patient is sensitized to HLA as a result of previous transfusions. ◆ Rh match is needed.	◆ Use a straight-line I.V. set with a standard in-line blood filter to provide 1 unit daily for 5 days or until the infection resolves. ◆ As prescribed, premedicate with diphenhydramine. ◆ Because a WBC infusion induces fever and chills, give an antipyretic if fever occurs. Don't stop the transfusion; instead, reduce the flow rate as ordered for patient comfort. ◆ Shake the container to prevent the WBCs from settling, thus preventing delivery of a bolus infusion of WBCs.
◆ Same as for packed RBCs ◆ Rh match is needed.	◆ Use a blood administration set to infuse blood over 1½ to 4 hours. ◆ Other considerations are the same as those for packed RBCs.

(continued)

Transfusing blood and selected components *(continued)*

BLOOD COMPONENT	INDICATIONS
Platelets Platelet sediment from RBCs or plasma *Volume: 35 to 50 ml/unit; 1 unit of platelets = 7 × 10^7 platelets*	◆ To treat thrombocytopenia caused by decreased platelet production, increased platelet destruction, or massive transfusion of stored blood ◆ To treat acute leukemia and marrow aplasia ◆ To improve platelet count preoperatively in a patient whose count is 100,000/µl or less
Fresh frozen plasma (FFP) Uncoagulated plasma separated from RBCs and rich in coagulation factors V, VIII, and IX *Volume: 200 to 250 ml*	◆ To expand plasma volume ◆ To treat postoperative hemorrhage or shock ◆ To correct an undetermined coagulation factor deficiency ◆ To replace a specific factor when that factor alone isn't available ◆ To correct factor deficiencies caused by hepatic disease
Albumin 5% (buffered saline); albumin 25% (salt poor) A small plasma protein prepared by fractionating pooled plasma *Volume: 5% = 12.5 g/250 ml; 25% = 12.5 g/50 ml*	◆ To replace volume lost because of shock from burns, trauma, surgery, or infections ◆ To replace volume and prevent marked hemoconcentration ◆ To treat hypoproteinemia (with or without edema)

CROSSMATCHING	NURSING CONSIDERATIONS
◆ ABO compatibility isn't needed, but is preferable with repeated platelet transfusions. ◆ Rh match is preferred.	◆ Use a filtered component drip administration set to infuse 100 ml over 15 minutes. ◆ As prescribed, premedicate with antipyretics and antihistamines if the patient's history includes a platelet transfusion reaction. ◆ Avoid giving platelets when the patient has a fever. ◆ Prepare to draw blood for a platelet count as ordered, 1 hour after the platelet transfusion, to determine the increments for platelet transfusion. ◆ Keep in mind that a physician seldom orders a platelet transfusion for conditions in which platelet destruction is accelerated, such as idiopathic thrombocytopenic purpura and drug-induced thrombocytopenia.
◆ ABO compatibility isn't needed, but is preferable with repeated platelet transfusions. ◆ Rh match is preferred.	◆ Use a blood administration set, and administer the infusion rapidly. ◆ Large-volume transfusions of FFP may require correction for hypocalcemia because citric acid in FFP binds calcium.
◆ Not needed	◆ Use the administration set supplied by the manufacturer, with the rate and volume dictated by the patient's condition and response. ◆ Reactions to albumin (fever, chills, nausea) are rare. ◆ Avoid mixing albumin with protein hydrolysates and alcohol solutions. ◆ Consider delivering albumin as a volume expander until the laboratory completes crossmatching for a whole blood transfusion. ◆ Albumin is contraindicated in severe anemia and given cautiously in cardiac and pulmonary disease because heart failure may result from circulatory overload.

(continued)

Transfusing blood and selected components *(continued)*

BLOOD COMPONENT	INDICATIONS
Factor VIII (cryoprecipitate) Insoluble portion of plasma recovered from FFP *Volume: about 30 ml (freeze-dried)*	◆ To treat a patient with hemophilia A ◆ To control bleeding associated with factor VIII deficiency ◆ To replace fibrinogen or a deficiency of factor VIII
Factors II, VII, IX, X complex (prothrombin complex) Lyophilized, commercially prepared solution drawn from pooled plasma	◆ To treat congenital factor V deficiency and other bleeding disorders resulting from acquired deficiency of factors II, VII, IX, and X

covers the filter. If it doesn't, squeeze the drip chamber until it does.
- Gently rock the bag back and forth, agitating blood cells that may have settled.
- Untape the dressing over the I.V. site to check cannula placement. Reposition the cannula, if necessary.
- Flush the line with saline solution, and restart the transfusion. Using a Y-type set, close the flow clamp to the patient and lower the blood bag. Open the saline clamp and allow some saline solution to flow into the blood bag. Rehang the blood bag, open the flow clamp to the patient, and reset the flow rate.
- If a hematoma develops at the I.V. site, stop the infusion immediately. Remove the I.V. cannula. Notify the physician, and expect to place ice on the site intermittently for 8 hours; then apply warm compresses. Follow facility policy.
- If the blood bag empties before the next one arrives, administer normal saline solution slowly. If you're using a Y-type set, close the blood line clamp, open the saline clamp, and let the saline run slowly until the new blood arrives. Decrease the flow rate or clamp the line before attaching the new unit of blood.

◆ Despite improvements in cross-matching precautions, transfusion reactions can still occur.

◆ Unlike a transfusion reaction, an infectious disease that's transmitted during a transfusion may go undetected until days, weeks, or even months later, when it produces signs and symptoms.
- Measures to prevent disease transmission include laboratory testing of

CROSSMATCHING	NURSING CONSIDERATIONS
◆ ABO compatibility isn't needed, but is preferable.	◆ Use the administration set supplied by the manufacturer. Administer factor VIII with a filter. The standard dose recommended for the treatment of acute bleeding episodes in hemophilia is 15 to 20 units/kg. ◆ The half-life of factor VIII (8 to 10 hours) requires repeated transfusions at specified intervals to maintain normal levels.
◆ ABO compatibility and Rh match aren't needed.	◆ Use the administration set supplied by the manufacturer. Base the dose on the desired factor level and the patient's body weight. ◆ Recognize that a high risk of hepatitis accompanies this type of transfusion. ◆ Arrange to draw blood for a coagulation assay to be performed before administration and at suitable intervals during treatment. ◆ This type of transfusion is contraindicated when the patient has hepatic disease resulting in fibrinolysis and when the patient has disseminated intravascular coagulation and isn't undergoing heparin therapy.

blood products and careful screening of potential donors, neither of which is guaranteed.

– Hepatitis C accounts for most cases of posttransfusion hepatitis. The tests that detect hepatitis B and hepatitis C can produce false-negative results and may allow some cases of hepatitis to go undetected.

– When testing for antibodies to human immunodeficiency virus (HIV), remember that antibodies don't appear until 6 to 12 weeks after exposure. The estimated risk of acquiring HIV from blood products varies from 1 in 40,000 to 1 in 153,000.

– Many blood banks screen blood for cytomegalovirus (CMV). Blood with CMV is especially dangerous for an immunosuppressed, seronegative patient.

– Blood banks also test blood for syphilis, but refrigerating blood virtually eliminates the risk of transfusion-related syphilis.

◆ Circulatory overload and hemolytic, allergic, febrile, and pyogenic reactions can result from any transfusion, particularly those given over 4 hours from the infusion start time. Coagulation disturbances, citrate intoxication, hyperkalemia, acid-base imbalance, loss of 2,3-diphosphoglycerate, ammonia intoxication, and hypothermia can result from massive transfusion.

Documentation

◆ Record the date and time of the transfusion.

◆ Record type and amount of transfusion product.

◆ Note patient's vital signs.

◆ Record that you and another nurse checked all identification data.

◆ Note the patient's response.
◆ Note any transfusion reaction and treatment.

Tube feedings

◆ Tube feedings involve delivery of a liquid feeding formula directly to the stomach (known as gastric gavage), duodenum, or jejunum.
◆ Gastric gavage is typically indicated for a patient who can't eat normally because of dysphagia or oral or esophageal obstruction or injury. Gastric feedings may also be given to an unconscious or intubated patient or to a patient who's recovering from GI tract surgery and can't ingest food orally.
◆ Duodenal or jejunal feedings decrease the risk of aspiration because the formula bypasses the pylorus. Jejunal feedings result in reduced pancreatic stimulation; thus, the patient may require an elemental diet.
◆ Patients usually receive gastric feedings on an intermittent schedule. For duodenal or jejunal feedings, most patients seem to better tolerate a continuous slow drip.
◆ Liquid nutrient solutions come in various formulas for administration through a nasogastric tube, a small-bore feeding tube, a gastrostomy or jejunostomy tube, a percutaneous endoscopic gastrostomy or jejunostomy tube, or a gastrostomy feeding button.
◆ Tube feeding is contraindicated in patients who have no bowel sounds or have a suspected intestinal obstruction.

Equipment

Gastric feedings

Feeding formula ◆ 120 ml of water ◆ gavage bag with tubing and flow regulator clamp ◆ towel or linen-saver pad ◆ 60-ml syringe or bulb syringe ◆ optional: infusion controller and gavage bag tubing set (for continuous administration) and adapter to connect gavage tubing to feeding tube

Duodenal or jejunal feedings

Feeding formula ◆ enteral administration set, containing gavage container, drip chamber, roller clamp or flow regulator, and tube connector ◆ I.V. pole ◆ 60-ml syringe with adapter tip ◆ water ◆ optional: volumetric pump administration set (for enteral infusion pump) and Y-connector

Implementation

◆ Provide privacy, and wash your hands.
◆ Verify the patient's identity using two patient identifiers. Tell the patient that he'll receive nourishment through the tube, and explain the procedure to him. If possible, give him a schedule of subsequent feedings.
◆ If the patient has a nasal or an oral tube, cover his chest with a towel or linen-saver pad to protect him and the bed linens from spills.
◆ Check the patient's abdomen for bowel sounds and distention.
◆ Let the formula to warm to room temperature before giving it. Cold formula increases the chance of diarrhea.
– Never warm formula over direct heat or in a microwave.
– Heat may curdle the formula or change its chemical composition, and hot formula may injure the patient.
◆ Pour 60 ml of water into the graduated container. After you close the flow clamp on the administration set, pour the appropriate amount of formula into the gavage bag.
◆ Hang no more than a 4- to 6-hour supply at one time to prevent bacterial growth.
◆ Open the flow clamp on the administration set to remove air from the lines. This keeps air from entering the

patient's stomach and causing distention and discomfort.

Gastric feeding

◆ Elevate the bed to semi-Fowler's or high Fowler's position to prevent aspiration by gastroesophageal reflux and to promote digestion.

◆ Check the placement of the feeding tube to ensure that it hasn't slipped out since the last feeding.

– Never give a tube feeding until you're certain that the tube is properly positioned in the patient's stomach.

– Giving a feeding through a misplaced tube can cause the feeding formula to enter the patient's lungs.

◆ To check the patency and position of the tube, gently try to aspirate gastric secretions.

– If no gastric secretions return, the tube may be not be lying near any pooled gastric secretions. Reposition the patient on his left side to move the tube into pooled gastric secretions, and aspirate again.

– Placement may need to be verified by radiograph.

◆ Check the aspirate for pH using the pH indicator paper.

– A pH of 5 or less with a clear, slightly yellow, or grassy-green color aspirate generally confirms gastric placement.

– A pH of 6 or more with light to golden yellow or brownish-green color aspirate indicates small bowel placement.

– A pH greater than 6 with clear aspirate with white mucus shreds may indicate pulmonary placement.

◆ Patients on stomach acid-reducing medications, those with GI bleeding, and those on continuous feedings may require initial and periodic radiographic placement confirmation as the pH test may not be accurate. Check your facility guidelines.

◆ Report any problems verifying placement to the clinical supervisor at once, and notify the physician as appropriate.

◆ To determine gastric emptying, aspirate and measure the residual gastric contents.

– Withhold feedings if the residual volume is greater than the predetermined amount specified in the physician's order (usually 50 to 100 ml).

– Reinstill any aspirate obtained.

◆ Connect the gavage bag tubing to the feeding tube. Depending on the type of tube used, you may need to use an adapter to connect the two.

◆ If you're using a bulb or catheter-tip syringe, remove the bulb or plunger. Attach the syringe to the pinched-off feeding tube to prevent excess air from entering the patient's stomach, causing distention.

◆ If you're using an infusion controller, thread the tube from the formula container through the controller, according to manufacturer directions. Blue food dye can be added to the feeding to allow you to identify aspiration quickly. Purge the tubing of air, and attach it to the feeding tube.

◆ Open the flow regulator clamp on the gavage bag tubing, and adjust the flow rate, as appropriate. When using a bulb syringe, fill the syringe with formula and release the feeding tube to allow formula to flow through it. The height at which you hold the syringe determines the flow rate. When the syringe is three-quarters empty, pour more formula into it.

◆ To prevent air from entering the tube and the patient's stomach, never allow the syringe to empty completely. If you're using an infusion controller, set the flow rate according to manufacturer directions.

◆ Always give a tube feeding slowly — typically, 200 to 350 ml over 15 to 30 minutes, depending on the patient's tolerance and the physician's order— to prevent sudden stomach distention, which can cause nausea, vomiting, cramps, or diarrhea.

◆ After giving the appropriate amount of formula, flush the tubing by adding about 60 ml of water to the gavage bag or bulb syringe, or manually flush it with a barrel syringe. This maintains the patency of the tube by removing excess formula, which could occlude the tube.

◆ If you're administering a continuous feeding, flush the feeding tube every 4 hours to help prevent occlusion of the tube. Monitor gastric emptying every 4 hours.

◆ To stop a gastric feeding (depending on the equipment you're using), close the regulator clamp on the gavage bag tubing, disconnect the syringe from the feeding tube, or turn off the infusion controller.

◆ Cover the end of the feeding tube with its plug or cap to prevent leakage and contamination.

◆ Leave the patient in semi-Fowler's or high Fowler's position for at least 30 minutes.

◆ Rinse all reusable equipment with warm water. Dry it and store it in a convenient place for the next feeding. Change the equipment every 24 hours or according to facility policy.

Duodenal or jejunal feeding

◆ Elevate the head of the bed, and place the patient in low Fowler's position.

◆ Open the enteral administration set, and hang the gavage container on the I.V. pole.

◆ If you're using a nasoduodenal tube, measure its length to check tube placement. You may not obtain any residual contents when you aspirate the tube. However, check any aspirate obtained for color and character and pH with the pH indicator paper.

– A pH of 5 or less with a clear, slightly yellow, or grassy-green color aspirate generally confirms gastric placement.

– A pH of 6 or more with light to golden yellow or brownish-green color aspirate indicates small bowel placement.

– A pH greater than 6 with clear aspirate with white mucus shreds may indicate pulmonary placement.

◆ Open the roller clamp, and regulate the flow to the desired rate. To regulate the rate with a volumetric infusion pump, follow manufacturer directions for setting up the equipment. Most patients receive small amounts initially, with volumes increasing gradually once tolerance is established.

◆ Flush the tube with water every 4 hours to maintain patency and provide hydration. A needle catheter jejunostomy tube may need to be flushed every 2 hours to prevent buildup of formula inside the tube. A Y-connector may be useful for frequent flushing. Attach the continuous feeding tube to the main port, and use the side port for flushes.

◆ Change the equipment every 24 hours or according to facility policy.

Special considerations

◆ Refrigerate formulas that are prepared in the dietary department or pharmacy. Refrigerate commercial formulas only after they have been opened. Check the date on all formula containers. Discard expired commercial formula. Use powdered formula within 24 hours of mixing. Shake the container vigorously to mix the solution thoroughly.

◆ A bulb syringe or large catheter-tip syringe may be substituted for a gavage bag after the patient shows tolerance for a gravity drip infusion. The physician may order an infusion pump to ensure accurate delivery of the prescribed formula.

◆ If the feeding solution doesn't initially flow through a bulb syringe, attach the bulb and squeeze it gently to start the flow. Then remove the bulb. Never use the bulb to force the formula through the tube.

◆ If the patient becomes nauseated or vomits, stop the feeding immediately. He may vomit if his stomach becomes distended because of overfeeding or delayed gastric emptying.

◆ To reduce oropharyngeal discomfort from the tube, allow the patient to brush his teeth or care for his dentures regularly, and encourage frequent gargling. If the patient is unconscious, administer oral care swabs every 2 hours. Use petroleum jelly on dry, cracked lips.

Alert Dry mucous membranes may indicate dehydration, which requires increased fluid intake. Clean the patient's nostrils with cotton-tipped applicators, apply lubricant along the mucosa, and check the skin for signs of breakdown.

◆ During continuous feedings, check the patient often for abdominal distention.

◆ Flush the tubing by adding about 50 ml of water to the gavage bag or bulb syringe. This maintains the patency of the tube by removing excess formula, which could occlude the tube.

◆ If the patient has diarrhea, give him small, frequent, less concentrated feedings, or give bolus feedings over a longer period.

◆ Make sure that the formula isn't cold and that proper storage and sanitation practices have been followed.

◆ The loose stools associated with tube feedings make extra perineal skin care necessary. Giving paregoric, tincture of opium, or diphenoxylate hydrochloride may improve the condition, if ordered. Changing to a formula with more fiber may eliminate liquid stools.

◆ If the patient becomes constipated, the physician may increase the fruit, vegetable, or sugar content of the formula. Check the patient's hydration status because dehydration may produce constipation. Increase fluid intake, as needed. If the condition persists, give an appropriate drug or enema, as ordered.

◆ Drugs can be given through the feeding tube.

– Except for enteric-coated, time-released, or sustained-release medications, crush tablets or open and dilute capsules in water before giving them.

– Make sure that you flush the tubing afterward to ensure full instillation of medication.

– Some drugs may change the osmolarity of the feeding formula and cause diarrhea.

◆ Small-bore feeding tubes may kink, making instillation impossible. If you suspect this problem, try changing the patient's position, or withdraw the tube a few inches and restart. Never use a guide wire to reposition the tube.

◆ Constantly monitor the flow rate of a blended or high-residue formula to determine if the formula is clogging the tubing as it settles. To prevent such clogging, squeeze the bag frequently to agitate the solution.

◆ Collect blood samples, as ordered.

– Monitor blood glucose levels to determine glucose tolerance. (A serum glucose level of less than 200 mg/dl is considered stable.)

– Hyperglycemia and diuresis may indicate an excessive carbohydrate level, which could lead to fatal hyperosmotic dehydration.

– Also monitor serum levels of electrolytes, blood urea nitrogen, and glucose as well as serum osmolality and other pertinent findings to determine the patient's response to therapy and check his hydration status.

◆ Special pulmonary formulas are available for patients who are prone to carbon dioxide retention.

◆ Check the flow rate hourly to ensure correct infusion. (With an improvised administration set, use a time tape to record the rate because it's difficult to obtain precise readings from an irrigation container or enema bag.)

◆ For duodenal or jejunal feeding, most patients tolerate a continuous drip better than bolus feedings. Bolus feedings can cause such complications as hyperglycemia and diarrhea.

◆ Until the patient acquires a tolerance for the formula, you may need to dilute it to one-half or three-quarters strength to start, and increase it gradually. Patients who are under stress or who are receiving a steroid may experience a pseudodiabetic state. Examine these patients frequently to determine the need for insulin.

◆ If the physician orders blue dye added to the enteral feeding, be aware of the possible complications. FD&C Blue No. 1 has been linked to bluish discoloration of body fluids and skin and more serious adverse events, including death. Patients at risk for increased intestinal permeability (those with sepsis, burns, trauma, shock, surgical interventions, renal failure, celiac sprue, or inflammatory bowel disease) appear to be at increased risk for absorbing Blue No. 1 from Blue No. 1–tinted enteral feedings.

– Blue No. 1–tinted enteral feedings may interfere with the results of Hemoccult tests.

◆ Erosion of the esophageal, tracheal, nasal, and oropharyngeal mucosa can result if tubes are left in place for a long time. If possible, use smaller-lumen tubes to prevent such irritation. Check facility policy regarding the frequency of changing feeding tubes to prevent complications.

◆ With the gastric route, frequent or large-volume feedings can cause bloating and retention. Dehydration, diarrhea, and vomiting can cause metabolic disturbances. Cramping and abdominal distention usually indicate intolerance.

◆ With the duodenal or jejunal route, clogging of the feeding tube is common.

◆ The patient may have metabolic, fluid, and electrolyte abnormalities, including hyperglycemia, hyperosmolar dehydration, coma, edema, hypernatremia, and essential fatty acid deficiency. Monitor signs and symptoms and laboratory resports regularly.

◆ The patient may also experience dumping syndrome, in which a large amount of hyperosmotic solution in the duodenum causes excessive diffusion of fluid through the semipermeable membrane and results in diarrhea. In a patient with low serum albumin levels, these signs and symptoms may result from low oncotic pressure in the duodenal mucosa. (See *Managing tube feeding problems*.)

Patient teaching tip For home tube feedings, teach the patient about the infusion control device; use of the syringe or bag and tubing; care of the tube and insertion site; and formula mixing. Explain that formula may be mixed in an electric blender according to package directions. Formula that isn't used within 24 hours must be discarded. If the formula must hang longer than 8 hours, advise the patient or caregiver to use a gavage or pump administration set with an ice pouch to decrease the incidence of bacterial growth. Tell him to use a new bag daily. Teach family members which signs and symptoms to report to the physician or home

Managing tube feeding problems

COMPLICATIONS	INTERVENTIONS
Aspiration of gastric secretions	◆ Stop feeding immediately. ◆ Perform tracheal suction of the aspirated contents, if possible. ◆ Notify the physician. Prophylactic antibiotics and chest physiotherapy may be ordered. ◆ Check tube placement before feeding to prevent complications.
Tube obstruction	◆ Flush the tube with warm water. If needed, replace the tube. ◆ Flush the tube with 50 ml of water after each feeding to remove excess sticky formula, which could occlude the tube.
Oral, nasal, or pharyngeal irritation or necrosis	◆ Provide frequent oral hygiene using mouthwash or lemon-glycerin swabs. Use petroleum jelly on cracked lips. ◆ Change the position of the tube. If necessary, replace the tube.
Vomiting, bloating, diarrhea, or cramps	◆ Reduce the flow rate. ◆ Give metoclopramide to increase GI motility. ◆ Warm the formula to prevent GI distress. ◆ For 30 minutes after feeding, position the patient on his right side with his head elevated to facilitate gastric emptying. ◆ Notify the physician, who may want to reduce the amount of formula being given during each feeding.
Constipation	◆ Provide additional fluids if the patient can tolerate them. ◆ Give a bulk-forming laxative. ◆ Increase the fruit, vegetable, or sugar content of the feeding.
Electrolyte imbalance	◆ Monitor serum electrolyte levels. ◆ Notify the physician, who may want to adjust the formula content to correct the deficiency.
Hyperglycemia	◆ Monitor blood glucose levels. ◆ Notify the physician of elevated levels. ◆ Give insulin, if ordered. ◆ The physician may adjust the glucose content of the formula.

care nurse as well as what measures to take in an emergency.

Documentation

- Record date, volume of formula, and volume of water (on the intake and output sheet).
- Note findings of abdominal examination, including the tube exit site, if appropriate.
- Note amount of residual gastric contents.
- Record verification of tube placement and patency.
- Note amount, type, and time of feeding.
- Note patient's tolerance of feeding, including nausea, vomiting, cramping, diarrhea, and distention.
- Record results of blood and urine tests.
- Note hydration status.
- Record any drugs given through the tube.
- Note date and time of administration set changes.
- Note oral and nasal hygiene performed.
- Record results of specimen collections.

Urinary catheter insertion, indwelling

- Also known as a *Foley* or *retention* catheter, an indwelling urinary catheter remains in the bladder to provide continuous urine drainage. A balloon inflated at the catheter's distal end prevents it from slipping out of the bladder after insertion.
- Indwelling catheters are used most commonly to relieve bladder distention caused by urine retention and to allow continuous urine drainage when the urinary meatus is swollen from childbirth, surgery, or local trauma.
- Other indications for an indwelling catheter include urinary tract obstruction (by a tumor or enlarged prostate), infection from neurogenic bladder paralysis caused by spinal cord injury or disease, and any illness in which the patient's urine output must be monitored closely.
- During bladder retraining for patients with neurologic disorders, such as stroke or spinal cord injury, bladder ultrasound scanning may be used to determine postvoid residual urine volume and determine the need for intermittent catheterization, with a smaller diameter, non-permanent catheter.
- An indwelling catheter is inserted using sterile technique and only when absolutely necessary. Insertion should be performed with extreme care to prevent injury and infection.

Equipment

Sterile indwelling catheter (latex or silicone #10 to #22 French [average adult sizes are #16 to #18 French]) ◆ syringe filled with 5 to 10 ml of sterile water ◆ washcloth ◆ towel ◆ soap and water ◆ two linen-saver pads ◆ sterile gloves ◆ sterile drape ◆ sterile fenestrated drape ◆ sterile cotton-tipped applicators (or cotton balls and plastic forceps) ◆ povidone-iodine or other antiseptic cleaning agent ◆ urine receptacle ◆ sterile water-soluble lubricant ◆ sterile drainage collection bag ◆ intake and output sheet ◆ adhesive tape ◆ optional: urine specimen container and laboratory request form, leg band with Velcro closure, gooseneck lamp or flashlight, pillows or rolled blankets or towels

Implementation

- Prepackaged sterile disposable kits that usually contain all the necessary equipment are available. The syringes

in these kits are prefilled with 10 ml of normal saline solution.
◆ Check the order on the patient's chart to determine if a catheter size or type has been specified. Select the appropriate equipment, and assemble it at the patient's bedside.
◆ Explain the procedure to the patient and provide privacy. Check his chart and ask when he voided last.
◆ Wash your hands and put on clean gloves. Make sure the patient doesn't have a latex allergy.
◆ Drape the patient with a sheet to provide privacy but enable the procedure.
◆ Have a coworker hold a flashlight or place a gooseneck lamp next to the patient's bed so that you can see the urinary meatus clearly.
◆ Place a female patient in the supine position, with her knees flexed and separated and her feet flat on the bed, about 2′ (61 cm) apart. If she finds this position uncomfortable, have her flex one knee and keep the other leg flat on the bed.

Alert If needed, use pillows or rolled towels or blankets to provide support with positioning.

◆ You may need help keeping the patient in position or directing the light.
◆ Place the male patient in the supine position with his legs extended and flat on the bed. Ask the patient to hold the position to give you a clear view of the urinary meatus and to prevent contamination of the sterile field.
◆ Use the washcloth to clean the patient's genital area and perineum thoroughly with soap and water. Dry the area with a towel, and then remove gloves and wash your hands.
◆ Place the linen-saver pads on the bed between the patient's legs and under the hips.
◆ To create the sterile field, open the prepackaged kit or equipment tray and place it between the female patient's legs or next to the male patient's hip. If the sterile gloves are the first item on the top of the tray, put them on. Then drape the patient's lower abdomen with the sterile fenestrated drape so that only the genital area remains exposed. Take care not to contaminate your gloves.
◆ Open the rest of the kit or tray while maintaining sterile technique. All items provided in the kit are sterile and may be handled using the sterile gloves.
◆ Make sure the patient isn't allergic to iodine solution; if he *is* allergic, another antiseptic cleaning agent must be used.
◆ Tear open the packet of povidone-iodine or other antiseptic cleaning agent, and use it to saturate the sterile cotton balls or applicators. Be careful not to spill the solution on the equipment.
◆ Open the packet of water-soluble lubricant and apply it to the catheter tip; attach the drainage bag to the other end of the catheter. (If you're using a commercial kit, the drainage bag may be attached.) Make sure all tubing ends remain sterile, and be sure the clamp at the emptying port of the drainage bag is closed to prevent urine leakage from the bag. Some drainage systems have an air-lock chamber to prevent bacteria from traveling to the bladder from urine in the drainage bag.

Note: Some urologists and nurses use a syringe prefilled with water-soluble lubricant and instill the lubricant directly into the male urethra, instead of on the catheter tip. This method helps prevent trauma to the urethral lining as well as possible urinary tract infection. Check your facility's policy.
◆ Before inserting the catheter, inflate the balloon with normal saline solution to inspect it for leaks. To do this, attach the saline-filled syringe to the luer-lock, then push the plunger and check for seepage as the balloon expands. Aspirate the saline to deflate

the balloon. Also inspect the catheter for resiliency. Rough, cracked catheters can injure the urethral mucosa during insertion, which can predispose the patient to infection.

◆ For a female patient, separate the labia majora and labia minora as widely as possible with the thumb, middle, and index fingers of your nondominant hand so you have a full view of the urinary meatus. Sterile technique is now broken with this hand. Keep the labia well separated throughout the procedure, so they don't obscure the urinary meatus or contaminate the area when it's cleaned.

◆ With your dominant hand, use a sterile, cotton-tipped applicator (or pick up a sterile cotton ball with the plastic forceps) and wipe one side of the urinary meatus with a single downward motion. Wipe the other side with another sterile applicator or cotton ball in the same way. Then wipe directly over the meatus with still another sterile applicator or cotton ball. Take care not to contaminate your sterile glove.

◆ For a male patient, hold the penis with your nondominant hand. Sterile technique is now broken with this hand. If he's uncircumcised, retract the foreskin. Then gently lift and stretch the penis to a 60- to 90-degree angle. Hold the penis this way throughout the procedure to straighten the urethra and maintain a sterile field.

◆ Use your dominant hand to clean the glans with a sterile cotton-tipped applicator or a sterile cotton ball held in the forceps. Clean in a circular motion, starting at the urinary meatus and working outward.

◆ Repeat the procedure, using another sterile applicator or cotton ball and taking care not to contaminate your sterile glove.

◆ Pick up the catheter with your dominant hand and prepare to insert the lubricated tip into the urinary meatus. To facilitate insertion by relaxing the sphincter, ask the patient to cough as you insert the catheter. Tell him to breathe deeply and slowly to further relax the sphincter and minimize spasms. Hold the catheter close to its tip to ease insertion and control its direction.

Alert Never force a catheter during insertion. Maneuver it gently as the patient bears down or coughs. If you still meet resistance, stop and notify the registered nurse. Sphincter spasms, strictures, misplacement in the vagina (in females), or an enlarged prostate (in males) may cause resistance.

◆ For a female patient, advance the catheter 2″ to 3″ (5 to 7.5 cm)—while continuing to hold the labia apart—until urine begins to flow. If the catheter is inadvertently inserted into the vagina, leave it there as a landmark. Then begin the procedure over again using new supplies.

◆ For a male patient, advance the catheter to the bifurcation and check for urine flow. If the foreskin was retracted, replace it to prevent compromised circulation and painful swelling.

◆ When urine stops flowing, attach the saline-filled syringe to the luer-lock.

◆ Push the plunger and inflate the balloon to keep the catheter in place in the bladder.

Alert Never inflate a balloon without first establishing urine flow, which assures you that the catheter is in the bladder.

◆ Hang the collection bag below bladder level to prevent urine reflux into the bladder, which can cause infection, and to facilitate gravity drainage of the bladder.

◆ Make sure the tubing doesn't get tangled in the bed's side rails.

◆ Tape the catheter to a female patient's thigh to prevent possible tension on the urogenital trigone.

◆ Tape the catheter to a male patient's abdomen or thigh to prevent pressure on the urethra at the penoscrotal junction, which can lead to formation of urethrocutaneous fistulas. Taping this way also prevents traction on the bladder.
◆ As an alternative, secure the catheter to the patient's thigh using a leg band with a Velcro closure. This decreases skin irritation, especially in patients with long-term indwelling catheters.
◆ Dispose of all used supplies properly.

Special considerations

◆ Several types of catheters are available with balloons of various sizes. Each type has its own method of inflation and closure. The balloon size determines the amount of solution needed for inflation, and the exact amount is usually printed on the distal extension of the catheter used for inflating the balloon.
◆ If needed, ask a female patient to lie on her side with her knees drawn up to her chest during the catheterization procedure. This position may be especially helpful for elderly or disabled patients, such as those with severe contractures.
◆ If the physician orders a urine specimen for laboratory analysis, obtain it from the urine receptacle with a specimen collection container at the time of catheterization, and send it to the laboratory with the appropriate laboratory request form. Connect the drainage bag when urine stops flowing.
◆ Explain the basic principles of gravity drainage so that the patient realizes the importance of keeping the drainage tubing and collection bag lower than his bladder at all times.
◆ Inspect the catheter and tubing periodically while they're in place to detect compression or kinking that could obstruct urine flow.
◆ For monitoring purposes, empty the collection bag at least every 8 hours.
– Excessive fluid volume may require more frequent emptying to prevent traction on the catheter, which would cause the patient discomfort, and to prevent injury to the urethra and bladder wall.
– Some facilities encourage changing catheters at regular intervals if the patient will have long-term continuous drainage. Check your facility's policy.

Alert **Observe the patient carefully for adverse reactions caused by removing excessive volumes of residual urine such as hypovolemic shock. Check your facility's policy to determine the maximum amount of urine that may be drained at one time (some facilities limit the amount to 700 to 1,000 ml). Whether to limit the amount of urine drained is currently controversial. Clamp the catheter at the first sign of an adverse reaction, and notify the physician.**

◆ Urinary tract infection can result from the introduction of bacteria into the bladder. Improper insertion can cause traumatic injury to the urethral and bladder mucosa. Bladder atony or spasms can result from rapid decompression of a severely distended bladder.

Documentation

◆ Record the date and time of catheterization.
◆ Note the size and type of indwelling catheter used.
◆ Note the characteristics of urine emptied from the bladder, including amount and color.
◆ Record the patient's tolerance for the procedure (if large volumes of urine have been emptied).
◆ Record fluid-balance data, if required, on the intake and output sheet.

◆ Note whether a urine specimen was sent for laboratory analysis.

Urinary catheter maintenance and removal

◆ Intended to prevent infection and other complications by keeping the catheter insertion site clean, routine catheter care typically is performed daily after the patient's morning bath and immediately after perineal care. (Bedtime catheter care may have to be performed before perineal care.)
◆ Because some studies suggest that catheter care increases the risk of infection and other complications rather than lowers it, many health care facilities don't recommend daily catheter care. Thus, individual facility policy dictates whether or not a patient receives such care.
◆ Regardless of the catheter care policy, the equipment and the patient's genitalia require inspection twice daily.
◆ An indwelling urinary catheter should be removed when bladder decompression is no longer needed, when the patient can resume voiding, or when the catheter is obstructed.
◆ Depending on the length of the catheterization, the physician may order bladder retraining before catheter removal.

Equipment

Catheter care

Povidone-iodine (or other antiseptic cleaning agent) ◆ sterile gloves ◆ eight sterile 4″ × 4″ gauze pads ◆ basin ◆ sterile absorbent cotton balls or cotton-tipped applicators ◆ leg bag ◆ collection bag ◆ adhesive tape ◆ waste receptacle ◆ optional: safety pin, rubber band, gooseneck lamp or flashlight, adhesive remover, antibiotic ointment, specimen container

Perineal cleaning

Washcloth ◆ additional basin ◆ soap and water

Commercially prepared catheter care kits containing all necessary supplies are available.

Catheter removal

Absorbent cotton ◆ gloves ◆ alcohol pad ◆ 10-ml syringe with a luer-lock ◆ bedpan ◆ optional: clamp for bladder retraining

Implementation

◆ Explain the procedure and its purpose to the patient.
◆ Provide privacy.

Catheter care

◆ Wash your hands and bring all equipment to the patient's bedside. Open the gauze pads, place several in the first basin, and pour some povidone-iodine or other cleaning agent over them.
◆ Some facilities specify that, after wiping the urinary meatus with cleaning solution, you should wipe it off with wet, sterile gauze pads to prevent possible irritation from the cleaning solution. If this is your facility's policy, pour water into the second basin, and moisten three more gauze pads.
◆ Make sure the lighting is adequate so that you can see the perineum and catheter tubing clearly. Place a gooseneck lamp at the bedside if needed.
◆ Inspect the catheter for any problems, and check the urine drainage for mucus, blood clots, sediment, and turbidity. Then pinch the catheter between two fingers to determine if the lumen contains any material.
◆ If you notice any of these conditions (or if your facility's policy requires it), obtain a urine specimen (about 6 oz [180 ml]) and notify the physician.

◆ Inspect the outside of the catheter where it enters the urinary meatus for encrusted material and suppurative drainage. Also inspect the tissue around the meatus for irritation or swelling.
◆ Remove any adhesive tape securing the catheter to the patient's thigh or abdomen. Inspect the area for signs of adhesive burns — redness, tenderness, or blisters. If necessary, clean residue from the previous tape site with adhesive remover.
◆ Put on the sterile gloves.
◆ Use a saturated, sterile gauze pad or cotton-tipped applicator to clean the outside of the catheter and the tissue around the meatus. To avoid contaminating the urinary tract, always clean by wiping away from — never toward — the urinary meatus.
◆ Use a dry gauze pad to remove encrusted material.

Alert Don't pull on the catheter while you're cleaning it. This can injure the urethra and the bladder wall. It can also expose a section of the catheter that was inside the urethra, so that when you release the catheter, the newly contaminated section will reenter the urethra, introducing potentially infectious organisms.

◆ Remove your gloves and tear a piece of adhesive tape from the roll.
◆ To prevent skin hypersensitivity or irritation, retape the catheter on the opposite side.

Alert Provide enough slack before securing the catheter to prevent tension on the tubing, which could injure the urethral lumen or bladder wall.

◆ Most drainage bags have a plastic clamp on the tubing to attach them to the sheet. If this isn't available, wrap a rubber band around the drainage tubing, insert the safety pin through a loop of the rubber band, and pin the tubing to the sheet below bladder level. Then attach the collection bag, below bladder level, to the bed frame.
◆ Dispose of all used supplies in a waste receptacle.

Catheter removal

◆ Wash your hands. Assemble the equipment at the patient's bedside. Explain the procedure and tell him that he may feel slight discomfort.
◆ Tell him that you'll check him periodically during the first 6 to 24 hours after catheter removal to make sure he resumes voiding.
◆ Put on gloves. Attach the syringe to the luer-lock mechanism on the catheter.
◆ Pull back on the plunger of the syringe. This deflates the balloon by aspirating the injected fluid. The amount of fluid injected is usually indicated on the tip of the catheter's balloon lumen and on the care plan or Kardex and the patient's chart.
◆ Grasp the catheter with the absorbent cotton and gently pull it from the urethra. Before doing so, offer the patient a bedpan.
◆ Measure and record the amount of urine in the collection bag before discarding it.

Special considerations

◆ Some facilities require the use of specific cleaning agents for catheter care, so check your facility's policy manual before beginning this procedure.
◆ A physician's order is needed if applying antibiotic ointments to the urinary meatus after cleaning.
◆ Avoid raising the drainage bag above bladder level. This prevents reflux of urine, which may contain bacteria.
◆ To avoid damaging the urethral lumen or bladder wall, always disconnect the drainage bag and tubing from

the bed linen and bed frame before helping the patient out of bed.

◆ When possible, attach a leg bag to allow the patient greater mobility. If the patient will be discharged with an indwelling catheter, teach him how to use a leg bag.

◆ Encourage patients with unrestricted fluid intake to increase intake to at least 3,000 ml per day. This helps flush the urinary system and reduces sediment formation.

◆ To prevent urinary sediment and calculi from obstructing the drainage tube, some patients are placed on an acid-ash diet to acidify the urine. Cranberry juice, for example, may help to promote urinary acidity.

◆ After catheter removal, check the patient for incontinence (or dribbling), urgency, persistent dysuria or bladder spasms, fever, chills, or palpable bladder distention. Report these to the physician.

◆ When changing catheters after long-term use, you may need a larger size catheter because the meatus enlarges, causing urine to leak around the catheter.

◆ Watch carefully for complications.

- Acute renal failure may result from a catheter obstructed by sediment. Be alert for sharply reduced urine flow from the catheter. Check the patient for bladder discomfort or distention.
- Urinary tract infection can result from catheter insertion or from intraluminal or extraluminal migration of bacteria up the catheter. Signs and symptoms may include cloudy urine, foul-smelling urine, hematuria, fever, malaise, tenderness over the bladder, and flank pain.
- Major complications in removing an indwelling catheter are failure of the balloon to deflate and rupture of the balloon. If the balloon ruptures, cystoscopy is usually performed to ensure removal of any balloon fragments.

Documentation

◆ Record care you performed, any modifications, and patient complaints.

◆ Note the condition of the perineum and urinary meatus.

◆ Note the character of the urine in the drainage bag, and any sediment buildup.

◆ Record whether a specimen was sent for laboratory analysis.

◆ Note fluid intake and output (hourly record is usually needed for critically ill patients and those with renal insufficiency who are hemodynamically unstable).

◆ Record bladder retraining activities, the date and time the catheter was clamped, time it was released, and volume and appearance of urine.

◆ Document catheter removal activities, the date and time, patient's tolerance of the procedure, when and how much the patient voided after catheter removal, and any associated problems.

7 Specimen collection

Blood, fecal occult

- Used to detect occult blood (hidden GI bleeding) and for distinguishing between true melena and melena-like stools, which may result from certain drugs, such as iron supplements and bismuth compounds
- Two common screening tests: Hematest (an orthotolidine reagent tablet) and the Hemoccult slide (filter paper impregnated with guaiac)
- Easily performed on collected specimens or smears from a digital rectal examination
- A blue reaction in a fecal smear if occult blood loss exceeds 5 ml in 24 hours
- No fecal smear needed for ColoCARE or EZ-Detect, two newer tests
- Important for early detection of colorectal cancer because 80% of affected patients test positive with Hemoccult slides, 24% with ColoCARE
- Three positive test results (with patient following prescribed diet) required to confirm GI bleeding
- Additional tests required to confirm cause, including colorectal cancer

Equipment

Test kit ◆ gloves ◆ glass or porcelain plate ◆ tongue blade or other wooden applicator

Implementation

- Explain the test to the patient including dietary guidelines. Tell him to maintain a high-fiber diet and to avoid red meat, poultry, fish, turnips, beets, and horseradish for 48 to 72 hours before the test as well as throughout the collection period because these substances may alter test results.
- As ordered, have the patient stop iron preparations, bromides, iodides, rauwolfia derivatives, indomethacin, colchicine, salicylates, potassium, phenylbutazone, oxyphenbutazone, bismuth compounds, steroids, and ascorbic acid for 48 to 72 hours before the test and during it to ensure accurate results and avoid possible bleeding, which some of these compounds may cause.

Hematest reagent tablet test

- Put on gloves and collect a stool specimen.
- Use a wooden applicator to smear a bit of the stool specimen on the filter paper supplied with the test kit. Or, after performing a digital rectal examination, wipe the finger you used for the examination on a square of the filter paper.
- Place the filter paper with the stool smear on a glass plate.
- Remove a reagent tablet from the bottle, and immediately replace the cap tightly.
- Place the tablet in the center of the stool smear on the filter paper.
- Add one drop of water to the tablet, and let it soak in for 5 to 10 seconds.
- Add a second drop, letting it run from the tablet onto the specimen and filter paper.
- If needed, tap the plate gently to dislodge any water from the top of the tablet.
- After 2 minutes, the filter paper will turn blue if the test is positive.

Alert Don't read the color that appears on the tablet itself or that develops on the filter paper after the 2-minute period.

- Note the results and discard the filter paper.
- Remove and discard your gloves, and wash your hands thoroughly.

Hemoccult slide test

- Put on gloves and collect a stool specimen.

◆ Open the flap on the slide packet, and use a wooden applicator to apply a thin smear of the stool specimen to the guaiac-impregnated filter paper exposed in box A. Or, after performing a digital rectal examination, wipe the finger you used for the examination on a square of the filter paper.
◆ Apply a second smear from another part of the specimen to the filter paper exposed in box B because some parts of the specimen may not contain blood.
◆ Let the specimens dry for 3 to 5 minutes.
◆ Open the flap on the reverse side of the slide package, and place 2 drops of Hemoccult developing solution on the paper over each smear.
◆ A blue reaction will appear in 30 to 60 seconds if the test is positive.
◆ Record the results and discard the slide package.
◆ Remove and discard your gloves, and wash your hands thoroughly.

ColoCARE and EZ-Detect tests

◆ Drop the test paper in the toilet with the stool.
◆ After the manufacturer's specified time period, check the test paper in the toilet for color change to blue or green. Record the results in the patient's chart.

Special considerations

◆ Make sure the stool specimen isn't contaminated with urine, soap solution, disinfectant, or toilet tissue, and test as soon as possible after collection.
◆ Test samples from several portions of the same specimen because occult blood from the upper GI tract isn't always evenly dispersed throughout the formed stool; likewise, blood from colorectal bleeding may occur mostly on the outer stool surface.
◆ Check the condition of the reagent tablets and note their expiration date. Use only fresh tablets and discard outdated ones.
◆ Protect Hematest tablets from moisture, heat, and light.
◆ If repeat testing is needed after a positive screening test, re-explain the test to the patient and remind him to carefully follow the dietary guidelines.
◆ Report positive results to the physician.

Documentation

◆ Record the time and date of each test.
◆ Record the type of screening test used and the result of the test.
◆ Note any unusual characteristics of the stool tested.

Blood, venous

◆ Involves venipuncture—piercing a vein with a needle and collecting blood in a syringe or evacuated tube
◆ Typically done in antecubital fossa
◆ May be done in a vein in the dorsal forearm, the dorsum of the hand or foot, or another accessible location
◆ Not done in inner wrist because doing so may damage underlying structures
◆ Usually performed by laboratory staff in a hospital, but is done by medical assistants and nurses in physician's offices and home care settings

Equipment

Tourniquet ◆ gloves ◆ syringe or evacuated tubes and needle holder ◆ antiseptic pads ◆ 20G or 21G needle for the forearm or 25G needle for the wrist, hand, ankle, or a child ◆ color-coded collection tubes containing appropriate additives ◆ labels ◆ laboratory request

Guide to color-top collection tubes

TUBE COLOR	DRAW VOLUME	ADDITIVE	PURPOSE
Red	2 to 20 ml	None	Serum studies
Lavender	2 to 10 ml	EDTA	Whole-blood studies
Green	2 to 15 ml	Heparin (sodium, lithium, or ammonium)	Plasma studies
Blue	2.7 or 4.5 ml	Sodium citrate and citric acid	Coagulation studies on plasma
Black	2.7 or 4.5 ml	Sodium oxalate	Coagulation studies on plasma
Gray	3 to 10 ml	Glycolytic inhibitor, such as sodium fluoride, powdered oxalate, or glycolytic-microbial inhibitor	Glucose determinations on serum or plasma
Yellow	12 ml	Acid-citrate-dextrose	Whole-blood studies

form and laboratory biohazard transportation bag ◆ 2″ × 2″ gauze pads ◆ adhesive bandage (see *Guide to color-top collection tubes*)

Preparation of equipment

◆ If you're using evacuated tubes, open the needle packet, attach the needle to its holder, and select the appropriate tubes.
◆ If you're using a syringe, attach the appropriate needle to it. Make sure the syringe can hold all the blood required for the test.
◆ Label all collection tubes clearly with the patient's name, date of birth, the physician's name, the date and time of collection, and initials of the person performing the venipuncture.

Implementation

◆ Wash your hands thoroughly, and put on gloves.
◆ Confirm the patient's identity using two patient identifiers and tell him that you're about to collect a blood sample.
◆ Explain the procedure to ease the patient's anxiety and ensure cooperation.
◆ Ask if the patient has ever felt faint, sweaty, or nauseated when having blood drawn.
◆ If the patient is on bed rest, ask him to lie in a supine position with his head slightly elevated and his arms at his sides.
◆ If the patient is ambulatory, ask him to sit in a chair and support his arm securely on an armrest or a table.
◆ Examine the patient's veins to determine the best puncture site. (See *Common venipuncture sites*.) Look for

the vein's blue color, or palpate the vein to find a firm rebound sensation.

◆ Tie a tourniquet 2″ (5 cm) proximal to the area chosen. By impeding venous return to the heart while still allowing arterial flow, a tourniquet produces venous dilation. If arterial perfusion remains adequate, you'll be able to feel the radial pulse.

◆ Clean the venipuncture site with an antiseptic pad.

◆ Apply it with friction for 30 seconds or until the final pad comes away clean.

◆ Let the skin dry before performing the venipuncture.

◆ If the vein hasn't dilated, have the patient open and close his fist a few times. Then ask him to close his fist as you insert the needle and to open it again when the needle is in place.

◆ Immobilize the vein by pressing just below the venipuncture site with your thumb and drawing the skin taut.

◆ Position the needle holder or syringe with the needle bevel up and the shaft parallel to the path of the vein, at a 30-degree angle to the arm.

◆ Insert the needle into the vein.

◆ If you're using a syringe, venous blood will appear in the hub. Withdraw the blood slowly, pulling the plunger of the syringe gently to create steady suction until you obtain the required sample.

Alert Pulling the plunger too forcibly may collapse the vein.

◆ If you're using a needle holder and an evacuated tube, grasp the holder securely to stabilize it in the vein, and push down on the collection tube until the needle punctures the rubber stopper. Blood will flow into the tube automatically.

◆ Remove the tourniquet as soon as blood flows adequately to prevent stasis and hemoconcentration, which can impair test results.

Common venipuncture sites

These illustrations show the anatomic locations of veins commonly used for venipuncture. The most commonly used sites are on the forearm, followed by those on the hand.

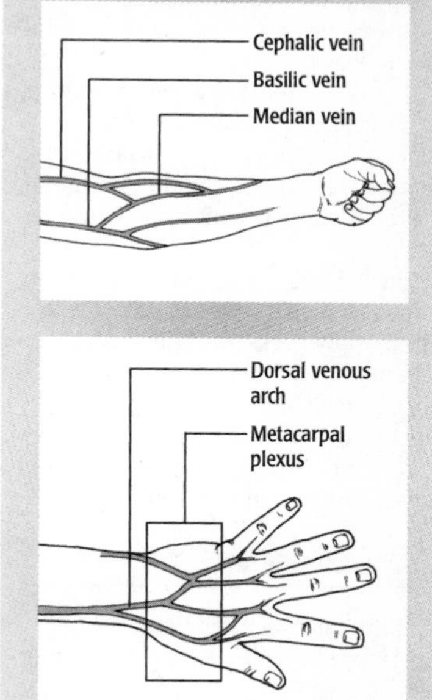

◆ If the flow is sluggish, leave the tourniquet in place longer, but always remove it before withdrawing the needle. Don't leave the tourniquet on for more than 3 minutes.

◆ Continue to fill the required tubes, removing one and inserting another.

◆ Gently rotate each tube as you remove it to help mix the additive with the sample.

◆ After you've drawn the sample, place a gauze pad over the puncture site and slowly and gently remove the needle from the vein.

Alert When using an evacuated tube, remove it from the needle holder to release the vacuum before withdrawing the needle from the vein.

◆ Apply gentle pressure to the puncture site for 2 to 3 minutes or until bleeding stops. This prevents extravasation into the surrounding tissue, which can cause a hematoma.

◆ After bleeding stops, apply an adhesive bandage.

◆ If you've used a syringe, transfer the sample to the collection tubes. Place the specimen tubes inside the biohazard transport bag, being careful to avoid foaming, which can cause hemolysis.

◆ Finally, check the venipuncture site to see if a hematoma has developed. If it has, apply pressure until you're sure bleeding has stopped (about 5 minutes), after which you may apply warm soaks to the site.

◆ Discard syringes, needles, and used gloves in the appropriate containers.

Special considerations

◆ Many manufacturers make safety-engineered blood collection sets; their use is recommended to prevent needle sticks.

◆ Never collect a venous sample from an arm or a leg that's already being used for I.V. therapy or blood administration because this may affect test results.

◆ Don't collect a venous sample from an infection site because this may introduce pathogens into the vascular system.

◆ Avoid collecting blood from edematous areas, arteriovenous shunts, an arm on the same side as a previous lymph node dissection, and sites of previous hematomas or vascular injury.

◆ If the patient has large, distended, highly visible veins, perform venipuncture without a tourniquet to minimize the risk of hematoma formation.

◆ If the patient has a clotting disorder or is receiving anticoagulant therapy, maintain firm pressure on the venipuncture site for at least 5 minutes after withdrawing the needle to prevent hematoma formation.

◆ Avoid using veins in the patient's legs for venipuncture, if possible, because this increases the risk of thrombophlebitis. Some facilities require a physician's order to collect blood from a leg or foot vein. Check your facility's policy and procedure.

Complications

◆ A hematoma at the needle insertion site is the most common complication of venipuncture.

◆ Infection may result from poor technique.

Documentation

◆ Record the date, time, and site of the venipuncture.

◆ Record the name of the test.

◆ Note the time the sample was sent to the laboratory.

◆ Note the amount of blood collected.

◆ Note any adverse reactions to the procedure.

Sputum

◆ May be cultured for identification of respiratory pathogens

◆ Secreted by mucous membranes lining the bronchioles, bronchi, and trachea

◆ Carries saliva, nasal and sinus secretions, dead cells, and normal oral bacteria from the respiratory tract

◆ Usual method of collection: expectoration

◆ May require ultrasonic nebulization, hydration, or chest percussion and postural drainage
◆ Less common methods: tracheal suctioning and, rarely, bronchoscopy
◆ Tracheal suctioning: Requires caution in patients with heart disease (may precipitate arrhythmias); contraindicated within 1 hour of eating and in patients with esophageal varices, nausea, facial or basilar skull fractures, laryngospasm, or bronchospasm

Equipment

Expectoration

Sterile specimen container with tight-fitting cap ◆ gloves ◆ label ◆ laboratory request form and laboratory biohazard transport bag ◆ aerosol (10% sodium chloride, propylene glycol, acetylcysteine, or sterile or distilled water), as ordered ◆ facial tissues ◆ emesis basin

Tracheal suctioning

#12 to #14 French sterile suction catheter ◆ water-soluble lubricant ◆ laboratory request form and laboratory biohazard transport bag ◆ sterile gloves ◆ mask ◆ goggles ◆ sterile in-line specimen trap (Lukens trap) ◆ normal saline solution ◆ portable suction machine, if wall unit is unavailable ◆ oxygen therapy equipment ◆ optional: nasal airway, to obtain a nasotracheal specimen with suctioning, if needed

Alert Commercial suction kits have all equipment except the suction machine and an in-line specimen container.

Preparation of equipment

◆ Equipment and preparation depend on the method of collection.
◆ Gather the appropriate equipment for the task.

Implementation

◆ If possible, collect the specimen early in the morning, before breakfast, to obtain an overnight accumulation of secretions.
◆ Confirm the patient's identity using two patient identifiers.
◆ Tell the patient that you need to collect a specimen of sputum.
◆ Explain the difference between sputum and saliva.
◆ Explain the procedure to promote cooperation.

Expectoration

◆ Instruct the patient to sit in a chair or at the edge of the bed. If he can't sit up, place him in high Fowler's position.
◆ Ask the patient to rinse his mouth with water to reduce specimen contamination.

Alert Avoid mouthwash or toothpaste because they may affect the mobility of organisms in the sputum sample.

◆ Tell him to cough deeply and expectorate directly into the specimen container. Ask him to produce at least 15 ml of sputum, if possible.
◆ Put on gloves.
◆ Cap the container and, if needed, clean its exterior.
◆ Remove and discard your gloves, and wash your hands thoroughly.
◆ Label the container with the patient's name and room number, physician's name, date and time of collection, and initial diagnosis.
◆ Include on the laboratory request form whether the patient was febrile or taking antibiotics and whether sputum was induced (because such specimens commonly appear watery and may resemble saliva).
◆ Send the specimen to the laboratory immediately in a laboratory biohazard transport bag.

Tracheal suctioning

◆ If the patient can't produce an adequate specimen by coughing, prepare to suction him to obtain the specimen.
◆ Explain the suctioning procedure to him and tell him that he may cough, gag, or feel short of breath during the procedure.
◆ Check the suction machine to make sure it's functioning properly.
◆ Place the patient in high Fowler's or semi-Fowler's position.
◆ Give oxygen to the patient before starting the procedure.
◆ Wash your hands thoroughly.
◆ Place a mask and goggles over your face.
◆ Put on sterile gloves. Consider one hand sterile and the other hand clean to prevent cross-contamination.
◆ Connect the suction tubing to the male adapter of the in-line specimen trap.
◆ Attach the sterile suction catheter to the rubber tubing of the trap.
◆ Tell the patient to tilt his head back slightly.
◆ Lubricate the catheter with normal saline solution, and gently pass it through the patient's nostril without suction.
◆ When the catheter reaches the larynx, the patient will cough. As he does, quickly advance the catheter into the trachea. Tell him to take several deep breaths through his mouth to ease insertion.
◆ To obtain the specimen, apply suction for 5 to 10 seconds but never longer than 15 seconds because prolonged suction can cause hypoxia.
◆ If the procedure must be repeated, let the patient rest for four to six breaths.
◆ When collection is completed, stop the suction, gently remove the catheter, and give oxygen.
◆ Detach the catheter from the in-line trap, gather it up in your dominant hand, and pull the glove cuff inside out and down around the used catheter to enclose it for disposal.
◆ Remove and discard the other glove and your mask and goggles.
◆ Detach the trap from the tubing connected to the suction machine. Seal the trap tightly by connecting the rubber tubing to the male adapter of the trap.
◆ Examine the specimen to make sure it's actually sputum, not saliva, because saliva will produce inaccurate test results.
◆ Label the trap's container as an expectorated specimen, place in a laboratory biohazard transport bag, and send it to the laboratory immediately with a completed laboratory request form.
◆ Offer the patient a glass of water or mouthwash.

Special considerations

◆ If you can't obtain a sputum specimen through tracheal suctioning, perform chest percussion to loosen and mobilize secretions, and position the patient for optimal drainage. After 20 to 30 minutes, repeat the tracheal suctioning procedure.
◆ Because expectorated sputum is contaminated by normal mouth flora, tracheal suctioning provides a more reliable specimen for diagnosis.
◆ If the patient becomes hypoxic or cyanotic during suctioning, remove the catheter immediately and give oxygen.
◆ If the patient has asthma or chronic bronchitis, watch for aggravated bronchospasms with the use of more than a 10% concentration of sodium chloride or acetylcysteine in an aerosol.
◆ If he may have tuberculosis, don't use more than 20% propylene glycol with water when inducing a sputum specimen because a higher concentration inhibits growth of the pathogen and causes erroneous test results. If propylene glycol isn't available, use

10% to 20% acetylcysteine with water or sodium chloride.

Complications

◆ Patients with cardiac disease may develop arrhythmias during the procedure as a result of coughing, especially when the specimen is obtained by suctioning.
◆ Other potential complications include tracheal trauma or bleeding, vomiting, aspiration, and hypoxemia.

Documentation

◆ Record the collection method used.
◆ Record the time and date of collection.
◆ Note how the patient tolerated the procedure.
◆ Note the color and consistency of the specimen.
◆ Record the disposition of the specimen to the laboratory for analysis.

Stool

◆ Collected to determine the presence of blood, ova, parasites, bile, fat, pathogens, or such substances as ingested drugs
◆ Collected randomly or for specific periods such as 72 hours
◆ Requires careful instruction to ensure proper collection and an uncontaminated specimen
◆ Conditions such as GI bleeding and steatorrhea revealed by gross examination of stool characteristics, such as color, consistency, and odor

Equipment

Specimen container with lid ◆ gloves ◆ two tongue blades ◆ paper towel or paper bag ◆ bedpan or portable commode ◆ three patient-care reminders (for timed specimens) ◆ laboratory request form and laboratory biohazard transport bag

Implementation

◆ Confirm the patient's identity using two patient identifiers.
◆ Explain the procedure to the patient and his family, if possible, to ensure their cooperation and prevent inadvertent disposal of timed stool specimens.

Random specimen

◆ Tell the patient to notify you when he has the urge to defecate.
◆ Have him defecate into a clean, dry bedpan or commode.
◆ Caution him not to contaminate the specimen with urine or toilet tissue because urine inhibits fecal bacterial growth and toilet tissue contains bismuth, which interferes with test results.
◆ Put on gloves.
◆ Using a tongue blade, transfer the most representative stool specimen from the bedpan to the container, and cap the container.
◆ If the stool contains visible blood, mucus, or pus, be sure to include it with the specimen.
◆ Wrap the tongue blade in a paper towel and discard it.
◆ Remove and discard your gloves, and wash your hands thoroughly to prevent cross-contamination.

Timed specimen

◆ Place a patient-care reminder stating "save all stool" over the patient's bed, in his bathroom, and in the utility room.
◆ Obtain the timed specimen as you would a random specimen, but remember to transfer *all stool* to the specimen container.
◆ After putting on gloves, collect the first specimen, and include it in the total specimen.

◆ If stool must be obtained with an enema, use only tap water or normal saline solution.
◆ As ordered, send each specimen to the laboratory immediately with a laboratory request form or, if permitted, refrigerate the specimens collected during the test period and send them when collection is complete.
◆ All specimens must be stored and transported in an approved laboratory biohazard container.
◆ Make sure the patient is comfortable after the procedure and that he has the opportunity to thoroughly clean his hands and perianal area. Some patients may need perineal care.
◆ When specimen collection is completed, remove and discard your gloves.

Special considerations

◆ To prevent contamination, never place a stool specimen in a refrigerator that contains food or drugs.
◆ Notify the physician if the stool specimen looks unusual.

Documentation

◆ Record the time of specimen collection and transport to the laboratory.
◆ Note the stool color, odor, and consistency.
◆ Note any unusual stool characteristics.
◆ Note whether the patient had trouble passing the stool.

Urine

Random specimen
◆ Usually collected as part of the physical examination or at various times during hospitalization
◆ Permits laboratory screening for urinary and systemic disorders as well as for drug screening

Clean-catch midstream specimen
◆ Replacing random collection because it provides a virtually uncontaminated specimen
◆ No need for catheterization

Indwelling catheter specimen
◆ Obtained either by clamping the drainage tube and emptying the accumulated urine into a container or by aspirating a specimen with a syringe
◆ Requires sterile collection technique to prevent catheter contamination and urinary tract infection
◆ Contraindicated after genitourinary surgery

Equipment

Random specimen
Bedpan or urinal with cover, if needed ◆ gloves ◆ graduated container ◆ specimen container with lid ◆ label ◆ laboratory request form and laboratory biohazard transport bag

Clean-catch midstream specimen
Basin ◆ soap and water ◆ towel ◆ gloves ◆ graduated container ◆ antiseptic wipes ◆ sterile specimen container with lid ◆ label ◆ bedpan or urinal, if needed ◆ laboratory request form and laboratory biohazard transport bag

Alert Commercial clean-catch kits containing antiseptic towelettes, sterile specimen container with lid and label, and instructions for use in several languages are widely used.

Indwelling catheter specimen
Gloves ◆ alcohol pad ◆ 10-ml syringe ◆ 21G or 22G 1¼″ needle or needleless cannula ◆ tube clamp ◆ sterile specimen container with lid ◆ label ◆ laboratory request form and laboratory biohazard transport bag

Implementation

◆ Confirm the patient's identity using two patient identifiers.
◆ Tell the patient that you need a urine specimen for laboratory analysis.
◆ Explain the procedure to him and his family, if needed, to promote cooperation and prevent accidental disposal of specimens.

Random specimen

◆ Provide privacy.
◆ If the patient is on bed rest, tell him to void into a clean bedpan or urinal.
◆ If the patient is ambulatory, tell him to void into either a urinal or bedpan in the bathroom.
◆ Put on gloves.
◆ Pour at least 120 ml of urine into the specimen container, and cap the container securely.
◆ If the patient's urine output must be measured and recorded, pour the remaining urine into the graduated container. Otherwise, discard the remaining urine.
◆ If you inadvertently spill urine on the outside of the container, clean and dry it to prevent cross-contamination.
◆ After you label the specimen container with the patient's name and room number and the date and time of collection, attach the laboratory request form, place it in the laboratory biohazard transport bag, and send it the laboratory immediately.

Alert Delayed transport of the specimen may alter test results.

◆ Clean the graduated container and urinal or bedpan, and return them to their proper storage area. Discard disposable items.
◆ Wash your hands thoroughly to prevent cross-contamination.
◆ Instruct an ambulatory patient to wash his hands. If the patient is on bed rest, offer a washcloth and soap and water so he can wash his hands.

Clean-catch midstream specimen

◆ Because the goal is a virtually uncontaminated specimen, explain the procedure to the patient carefully. Provide illustrations to emphasize the correct collection technique, if possible.

Female patient

◆ Tell the patient to remove all clothing from the waist down and to sit back on the toilet seat and spread her legs.
◆ Have the patient clean the labial folds, vulva, and urinary meatus with soap and water.
◆ Tell the patient to separate her labial folds with her thumb and forefinger.
◆ Instruct her to wipe the area three times, using three fresh wipes. Tell her to wipe down one side with the first pad and discard it, to wipe the other side with the second pad and discard it and, finally, to wipe down the center over the urinary meatus with the third pad and discard it.
◆ Stress the importance of cleaning from front to back to avoid contaminating the genital area with fecal matter.
◆ Tell the patient to straddle the bedpan or toilet and to keep her labia separated while voiding.
◆ Instruct the patient to begin voiding into the bedpan or toilet. Then, without stopping the urine stream, the patient should move the collection container into the stream, collecting 30 to 50 ml at the midstream portion of the voiding. The patient can then finish voiding into the bedpan or toilet.

Male patient

◆ Tell the patient to remove all clothing from the waist down and stand in front of the toilet as he normally would to urinate.
◆ Have the patient clean the tip of his penis with soap and water.
◆ Tell him to wipe the area three times, each time with a fresh wipe provided in a commercial kit.

◆ If the patient is uncircumcised, stress the need to retract his foreskin to effectively clean the meatus and to keep it retracted while voiding.
◆ Instruct the patient to begin voiding into the bedpan, urinal, or toilet. Then, without stopping the urine stream, the patient should move the collection container into the stream, collecting 30 to 50 ml at the midstream portion of the voiding. The patient can then finish voiding into the bedpan, urinal, or toilet.

Specimen preparation
◆ Put on gloves before discarding the first and last portions of the voiding, and measure the remaining urine in a graduated container for intake and output records, if needed. Be sure to include the amount in the specimen container when recording the total amount voided.
◆ Take the sterile container from the patient, and cap it securely. Avoid touching the inside of the container or the lid. If the outside of the container is soiled, clean it and wipe it dry.
◆ Remove your gloves and discard them properly.
◆ Wash your hands thoroughly. Instruct the patient to do the same.
◆ Label the container with the patient's name and room number, name of test, type of specimen, collection time, and suspected diagnosis, if known.
◆ If a urine culture has been ordered, note any current antibiotic therapy on the laboratory request form.
◆ Place the specimen in a laboratory biohazard transport bag and send the container to the laboratory immediately or place it on ice to prevent specimen deterioration and altered test results.

Indwelling catheter specimen
◆ About 30 minutes before collecting the specimen, clamp the drainage tube to allow urine to accumulate.
◆ Just before you obtain the specimen, put on gloves.
◆ If the drainage tube has a built-in sampling port, wipe the port with an alcohol pad.
◆ Uncap the needle or needleless cannula on the syringe; insert the needle or needleless cannula into the sampling port at a 90-degree angle to the tubing.
◆ Aspirate the specimen into the syringe.
◆ If the drainage tube doesn't have a sampling port and the catheter is made of rubber, obtain the specimen from the catheter.
Alert Other types of catheters will leak after you withdraw the needle.
◆ To withdraw the specimen from a rubber catheter, wipe it with an alcohol pad just above where it connects to the drainage tube. Insert the needle into the rubber catheter at a 45-degree angle and withdraw the specimen.
Alert Never insert the needle into the shaft of the catheter because this may puncture the lumen leading to the catheter balloon.
◆ Transfer the specimen to a sterile container, label it, and send it to the laboratory immediately in a laboratory biohazard transport bag or place it on ice.
◆ If a urine culture will be performed, be sure to list any current antibiotic therapy on the laboratory request form.
Alert Make sure you unclamp the drainage tube after collecting the specimen to prevent urine backflow, which may cause bladder distention and infection.

Documentation

◆ Record times of specimen collection and transport to the laboratory.
◆ Record the test to be performed.
◆ Note the appearance, odor, and color of the specimen.

◆ Note any unusual characteristics of the specimen.
◆ Record urine volume (in the intake and output record), if needed.

Urine, timed

◆ Typically used to measure hormones, proteins, and electrolytes, which are excreted in small, variable amounts over an extended period
◆ Most common: 24-hour specimen, because it gives an average excretion rate for substances eliminated during this period
◆ May be collected for a shorter period, such as 2 or 12 hours, depending on the specific information needed
◆ May be collected after a challenge dose of a chemical — insulin, for example — to detect various renal disorders

Equipment

Large collection bottle with a cap or stopper, or a commercial plastic container ◆ preservative, if needed ◆ gloves ◆ bedpan or urinal if patient doesn't have an indwelling catheter ◆ graduated container if patient is on intake and output measurement ◆ ice-filled container if a refrigerator isn't available ◆ label ◆ laboratory request form and laboratory biohazard transport container ◆ four patient-care reminders

Alert **Check with the laboratory to find out which preservatives may need to be added to the specimen or whether a dark collection bottle is required.**

Implementation

◆ Confirm the patient's identity using two patient identifiers.
◆ Explain the procedure to the patient and family, as needed, to enlist their cooperation and prevent accidental disposal of urine during the collection period.
◆ Explain that failure to collect even one specimen during the collection period invalidates the test and requires that it begin again.
◆ Place patient-care reminders over the patient's bed, in his bathroom, on the bedpan hopper in the utility room, and on the urinal or indwelling catheter collection bag. Include the patient's name and room number, the date, and the collection interval.
◆ Instruct the patient to save all urine during the collection period, to notify you after each voiding, and to avoid contaminating the urine with stool or toilet tissue.
◆ Explain any diet or drug restrictions, and make sure the patient understands and is willing to comply with them.

2-hour collection

◆ If possible, have the patient drink two to four 8-oz (480 to 960 ml) glasses of water about 30 minutes before collection begins.
◆ After 30 minutes, tell the patient to void.
◆ Put on gloves and discard this specimen so the patient starts the collection period with an empty bladder.
◆ If ordered, give a challenge dose of medication (such as glucose solution or corticotropin), and record the time.
◆ If possible, offer the patient a glass of water at least every hour during the collection period to stimulate urine production.
◆ After each voiding, put on gloves and add the specimen to the collection bottle.
◆ Instruct the patient to void about 15 minutes before the end of the collection period, if possible, and add this specimen to the collection bottle.
◆ At the end of the collection period, send the appropriately labeled collection bottle to the laboratory immediate-

ly in an approved laboratory biohazard transport container, along with a properly completed laboratory request form.

12- and 24-hour collection

◆ Put on gloves and ask the patient to void.
◆ Discard this urine so the patient starts the collection period with an empty bladder. Record the time.
◆ After putting on gloves and pouring the first urine specimen into the collection bottle, add the required preservative. Then refrigerate the bottle or keep it on ice until the next voiding, as appropriate.
◆ Collect all urine voided during the prescribed period.
◆ Just before the collection period ends, ask the patient to void again, if possible.
◆ Add this last specimen to the collection bottle, and pack it in ice to inhibit deterioration of the specimen.
◆ Label the collection bottle, place it in an approved laboratory biohazard transport container, and send it to the laboratory with a properly completed laboratory request form.

Special considerations

◆ Keep the patient well hydrated before and during the test to ensure adequate urine flow.
◆ Before collection of a timed specimen, make sure the laboratory will be open when the collection period ends to help ensure prompt, accurate results.
◆ To avoid contamination, never store a specimen in a refrigerator that contains food or drugs.
◆ If the patient has an indwelling catheter in place, put the collection bag in an ice-filled container at his bedside.
◆ Instruct the patient to avoid exercise and ingestion of coffee, tea, or any drugs (unless directed otherwise by the physician) before the test to avoid altering test results.
◆ If a specimen is discarded accidentally during the collection period, you'll need to restart the collection. This may result in an additional day of hospitalization, which may cause the patient personal and financial hardship. Therefore, emphasize the need to save all the patient's urine during the collection period to everyone involved in his care as well as to his family and other visitors.

Documentation

◆ Record the date and intervals of specimen collection.
◆ Note when the collection bottle was sent to the laboratory.

8 Common laboratory tests

Alanine aminotransferase

Purpose

◆ To detect acute hepatic disease, especially hepatitis and cirrhosis without jaundice, and evaluate its treatment
◆ To distinguish between myocardial and hepatic tissue damage (with aspartate aminotransferase)
◆ To assess the hepatotoxicity of some drugs

Reference values

Adults and children (> age 6 months)
Females: 7 to 35 units/L (SI, 0.12 to 0.6 µkat/L)
Males: 10 to 40 units/L (SI, 0.17 to 0.68 µkat/L)

Neonates
13 to 45 units/L (SI, 0.22 to 0.77 µkat/L)

Special considerations

◆ Alanine aminotransferase (ALT) is needed for energy production and is found mainly in the liver, with lesser amounts in the kidneys, heart, and skeletal muscles.
◆ ALT levels may be increased slightly in acute myocardial infarction. They may be increased slightly to moderately in active cirrhosis and drug-induced or alcoholic hepatitis. And they may be very high in viral hepatitis, severe drug-induced hepatitis, or other hepatic disease with extensive necrosis.

Aldosterone, serum

Purpose

◆ To aid in diagnosing primary and secondary aldosteronism, adrenal hyperplasia, hypoaldosteronism, and salt-losing syndrome

Reference values

Upright position
Adults: 7 to 30 nanogram/dl (SI, 0.19 to 0.83 nmol/L)
Adolescents: 4 to 48 nanogram/dl (SI, 0.11 to 1.33 nmol/L)

Special considerations

◆ Aldosterone regulates ion transport across cell membranes to promote reabsorption of sodium and chloride in exchange for potassium and hydrogen ions.
◆ It helps maintain blood pressure and volume and regulate fluid and electrolyte imbalance.
◆ Values vary with time of day and patient's posture.
◆ Excessive aldosterone secretion may indicate a primary (Conn's syndrome) or secondary (renovascular hypertension, heart failure, cirrhosis) disease. Low levels may indicate primary hypoaldosteronism, salt-losing syndrome, eclampsia, or Addison's disease.
◆ Urge the patient to eat a low-carbohydrate, normal-sodium diet, and to avoid licorice for at least 2 weeks before this test.
◆ Withhold all drugs that alter fluid, sodium, and potassium balance — especially diuretics, antihypertensives, steroids, hormonal contraceptives, and estrogens — for at least 2 weeks before the test, as ordered.
◆ Withhold all renin inhibitors for 1 week before the test, as ordered.

Alkaline phosphatase

Purpose

◆ To detect and identify skeletal diseases characterized mainly by osteoblastic activity
◆ To detect focal hepatic lesions that cause biliary obstruction, such as a tumor or abscess
◆ To assess the patient's response to vitamin D in the treatment of rickets
◆ To supplement information from other liver function studies and GI enzyme tests

Reference values

Females
Ages 1 to 12: < 350 units/L
Age > 15: 25 to 100 units/L

Males
Ages 1 to 12: < 350 units/L
Ages 12 to 14: < 500 units/L
Age > 20: 25 to 100 units/L

Special considerations

◆ Alkaline phosphatase (ALP) is an enzyme that affects bone calcification and lipid and metabolite transport.
◆ An elevated ALP level usually indicates skeletal disease or extrahepatic or intrahepatic biliary obstruction causing cholestasis.
◆ Tell the patient to fast for at least 8 hours before the test.

Amylase, serum

Purpose

◆ To diagnose acute pancreatitis
◆ To distinguish between acute pancreatitis and other causes of abdominal pain that warrant immediate surgery
◆ To evaluate possible pancreatic injury caused by abdominal trauma or surgery

Reference values

Adults
25 to 125 units/L (SI, 0.4 to 2.1 µkat/L)

Elderly (> age 60)
24 to 151 units/L (SI, 0.4 to 2.5 µkat/L)

Neonates
6 to 65 units/L (SI, 0.1 to 1.1 µkat/L)

Special considerations

◆ Amylase (AML) helps digest starch and glycogen in the mouth, stomach, and intestine.
◆ Measurement of serum or urinary AML is the most important laboratory test in cases of suspected acute pancreatic disease.
◆ After the onset of acute pancreatitis, AML levels rise within 2 hours, peak within 12 to 48 hours, and return to normal within 3 to 4 days.
◆ Levels may be increased moderately in obstruction of the common bile duct, pancreatic duct, or ampulla of Vater; pancreatic injury from a perforated peptic ulcer; pancreatic cancer; or acute salivary gland disease.

Arterial blood gas analysis

Purpose

◆ To evaluate the efficiency of pulmonary gas exchange
◆ To assess the integrity of the ventilatory control system

◆ To determine the acid-base level of the blood
◆ To monitor respiratory therapy

Reference values

Adults

Pao_2: > 80 mm Hg (SI, > 10.6 kPa)
$Paco_2$: 35 to 45 mm Hg (SI, 4.6 to 5.9 kPa)
pH: 7.35 to 7.45
O_2 content: 15 to 22 vol % (SI, 6.6 to 9.7 mmol/L)
Sao_2: > 94% (SI, > 0.94)
HCO_3^-: 22 to 26 mEq/L (SI, 22 to 26 mmol/L)

Special considerations

◆ Arterial blood gas (ABG) analysis measures the partial pressure of arterial oxygen (Pao_2), partial pressure of arterial carbon dioxide ($Paco_2$), pH of an arterial sample, oxygen content (O_2CT), arterial oxygen saturation (Sao_2), and bicarbonate (HCO_3^-) level.
◆ ABG analysis may be drawn by percutaneous arterial puncture or with an arterial line.
◆ Low Pao_2, O_2CT, and Sao_2 levels and a high $Paco_2$ may result from conditions that impair respiratory function and airway obstruction.
◆ Low readings may result from obstruction of the bronchioles, an abnormal ventilation to perfusion ratio, or alveoli that are damaged or filled with fluid.
◆ Low O_2CT — with normal Pao_2, Sao_2 and, possibly, $Paco_2$ values — may result from severe anemia, decreased blood volume, and reduced capacity to carry hemoglobin oxygen.
◆ ABG values also give information about acid-base disorders.

Aspartate aminotransferase

Purpose

◆ To aid detection and differential diagnosis of acute hepatic disease
◆ To monitor the progress and prognosis of patients with cardiac and hepatic diseases
◆ To aid diagnosis of myocardial infarction (MI) along with creatine kinase and lactate dehydrogenase levels

Reference values

Adults

Females: 10 to 36 units/L (SI, 0.17 to 0.6 µkat/L)
Males: 14 to 20 units/L (SI, 0.23 to 0.33 µkat/L)

Children

9 to 80 units/L (SI, 0.15 to 1.3 µkat/L)

Neonates

47 to 150 units/L (SI, 0.78 to 2.5 µkat/L)

Special considerations

◆ Aspartate aminotransferase (AST) is essential to energy production and is found in many cells, mainly in the liver, heart, skeletal muscles, kidneys, pancreas, and red blood cells.
◆ AST is released into serum in proportion to cellular damage. Levels increase early in a disease process, are most increased during the most acute phase, and decrease as the disease resolves.
◆ Moderate to high levels (5 to 10 times normal) may indicate dermatomyositis, Duchenne's muscular dystrophy, or chronic hepatitis.
◆ High levels (10 to 20 times normal) may indicate severe MI, severe infec-

tious mononucleosis, or alcoholic cirrhosis.
◆ Extreme elevations (more than 20 times normal) may indicate acute viral hepatitis, severe skeletal muscle trauma, extensive surgery, drug-induced hepatic injury, or severe passive liver congestion.
◆ Tell the patient that the test usually involves three venipunctures over 3 days.

Bilirubin

Purpose

◆ To evaluate liver function
◆ To aid in diagnosing jaundice and monitoring its progress
◆ To aid in diagnosing biliary obstruction and hemolytic anemia
◆ To determine whether a neonate needs an exchange transfusion or phototherapy because of dangerously high levels of unconjugated bilirubin

Reference values

Adults
Total: 0.3 to 1 mg/dl (SI, 5 to 17 μmol/L)
Conjugated (direct): 0 to 0.2 mg/dl (SI, 0 to 3.4 μmol/L)

Neonates
Total: 1 to 10 mg/dl (SI, 17 to 170 μmol/L)
Conjugated (direct): 0 to 0.8 mg/dl (SI, 0 to 136 μmol/L)
Unconjugated (indirect): 0 to 10 mg/dl (SI, 0 to 170 μmol/L)

Special considerations

◆ Bilirubin is the main bile pigment and major product of hemoglobin catabolism.
◆ Unconjugated bilirubin may accumulate in a neonate's brain, causing irreparable damage.
◆ Increased indirect serum bilirubin levels may indicate hepatic damage, severe hemolytic anemia, and congenital enzyme deficiencies.
◆ Increased direct serum bilirubin levels usually indicate biliary obstruction.
◆ In neonates, increased total bilirubin levels may indicate the need for an exchange transfusion.
◆ Adults should fast for at least 4 hours before the test.

Blood urea nitrogen

Purpose

◆ To evaluate kidney function and diagnose renal disease
◆ To aid in assessing hydration

Reference values

Adults
6 to 20 mg/dl (SI, 2.1 to 7.1 mmol/L)

Children
5 to 18 mg/dl (SI, 1.8 to 6.4 mmol/L)

Elderly (> age 60)
8 to 23 mg/dl (SI, 2.9 to 8.2 mmol/L)

Special considerations

◆ Blood urea nitrogen (BUN), the chief end-product of protein metabolism, is formed in the liver from ammonia and excreted by the kidneys.
◆ BUN level reflects protein intake and renal excretory capacity but is a less reliable indicator of uremia than the serum creatinine level.
◆ BUN levels are increased in renal disease, reduced renal blood flow, uri-

nary tract obstruction, and increased protein catabolism.
◆ BUN levels are decreased in severe hepatic damage, malnutrition, and overhydration.

Calcium, serum

Purpose

◆ To evaluate endocrine function, calcium metabolism, and acid-base balance
◆ To guide therapy in patients with renal failure, renal transplant, endocrine disorders, malignancies, cardiac disease, and skeletal disorders

Reference values

Adults
Total calcium: 8.8 to 10.4 mg/dl (SI, 2.2 to 2.6 mmol/L)
Ionized calcium: 4.65 to 5.28 mg/dl (SI, 1.16 to 1.32 mmol/L)

Children (varies with age)
Total calcium: 8.8 to 10.7 mg/dl (SI, 2.2 to 2.7 mmol/L)
Ionized calcium: 4.8 to 5.52 mg/dl (SI, 1.2 to 1.38 mmol/L)

Special considerations

◆ About 1% of the body's total calcium circulates in the blood; of this, about 50% is bound to plasma proteins and 40% is ionized, or free.
◆ The serum calcium level reflects the total amount of calcium in the blood; the ionized calcium level reflects the fraction of serum calcium in ionized form.
◆ Hypercalcemia may occur in hyperparathyroidism and parathyroid tumors, Paget's disease of the bone, multiple myeloma, metastatic carcinoma, multiple fractures, prolonged immobilization, inadequate calcium excretion, excessive calcium ingestion, and overuse of antacids.
◆ Hypocalcemia may result from hypoparathyroidism, total parathyroidectomy, malabsorption, Cushing's syndrome, renal failure, acute pancreatitis, peritonitis, malnutrition with hypoalbuminemia, renal failure, and blood transfusions.
◆ In the patient with hypocalcemia, be alert for circumoral and peripheral numbness and tingling, muscle twitching, Chvostek's sign (facial muscle spasm), tetany, muscle cramping, Trousseau's sign (carpopedal spasm), seizures, arrhythmias, laryngeal spasm, decreased cardiac output, prolonged bleeding time, fractures, and prolonged QT interval.

Carcinoembryonic antigen

Purpose

◆ To monitor the effectiveness of cancer therapy
◆ To assist in the staging of colorectal cancers, assess the adequacy of surgical resection, and test for recurrence of colorectal cancers

Reference values

Adults
< 5 nanogram/ml (SI, < 5 mg/L)

Special considerations

◆ Carcinoembryonic antigen (CEA) is a protein normally found in fetal tissue; however, production may begin again later if a neoplasm develops.
◆ High CEA levels are characteristic of various malignant and certain nonmalignant conditions.

- Persistent elevation of CEA levels suggests residual or recurrent tumor.
- If CEA levels exceed normal before surgical resection, chemotherapy, or radiation therapy, a return to normal within 6 weeks suggests successful treatment.

Cerebrospinal fluid analysis

Purpose

- To measure cerebrospinal fluid (CSF) pressure
- To aid diagnosis of viral or bacterial meningitis, subarachnoid or intracranial hemorrhage, tumors, and brain abscesses
- To aid diagnosis of neurosyphilis and chronic central nervous system infections
- To check for Alzheimer's disease

Reference values

See *Findings in cerebrospinal fluid analysis*.

Special considerations

- CSF is commonly obtained by lumbar puncture but also may be obtained during other neurologic tests such as myelography.
- Explain that a headache is the most common adverse effect of a lumbar puncture but that cooperation during the test helps minimize this effect.
- Make sure the patient or legal guardian has signed the appropriate consent form.

Chloride, serum

Purpose

- To detect an acid-base imbalance (acidosis or alkalosis)
- To aid evaluation of fluid status and extracellular cation-anion balance

Reference values

Adults and children
96 to 106 mEq/L (SI, 96 to 106 mmol/L)

Neonates
96 to 113 mEq/L (SI, 96 to 113 mmol/L)

Special considerations

- Chloride, the major extracellular fluid anion, helps regulate blood volume and arterial pressure, and it affects acid-base balance.
- Chloride is absorbed from the intestines and excreted mainly by the kidneys.
- Excessive loss of gastric juices or other chloride-containing secretions may cause hypochloremic metabolic alkalosis; excessive retention or ingestion of chloride may lead to hyperchloremic metabolic acidosis.
- Hyperchloremia occurs with severe dehydration, complete renal shutdown, head injury, and primary aldosteronism.
- Hypochloremia occurs with low sodium and potassium levels as a result of prolonged vomiting, gastric suctioning, intestinal fistula, chronic renal failure, and Addison's disease.

Findings in cerebrospinal fluid analysis

TEST	NORMAL	ABNORMAL	IMPLICATIONS
Pressure	90 to 180 mm H_2O	Increase	◆ Increased intracranial pressure
		Decrease	◆ Spinal subarachnoid obstruction above puncture site
Appearance	Clear, colorless	Cloudy	◆ Infection
		Xanthochromic or bloody	◆ Subarachnoid, intracerebral, or intraventricular hemorrhage; spinal cord obstruction; traumatic tap (usually noted only in initial specimen)
		Brown, orange, or yellow	◆ Elevated protein levels, red blood cell (RBC) breakdown (blood present for at least 3 days)
Protein	15 to 45 mg/dl (SI, 150 to 450 mg/L)	Marked increase	◆ Tumors, trauma, hemorrhage, diabetes mellitus, polyneuritis, blood in cerebrospinal fluid (CSF)
		Marked decrease	◆ Rapid production of CSF
Gamma globulin	3% to 12% of total protein	Increase	◆ Demyelinating disease, neurosyphilis, Guillain-Barré syndrome
Glucose	40 to 70 mg/dl (SI, 2.2 to 3.9 mmol/L)	Increase	◆ Systemic hyperglycemia
		Decrease	◆ Systemic hypoglycemia, bacterial or fungal infection, meningitis, mumps, postsubarachnoid hemorrhage
Cell count	0 to 5 white blood cells	Increase	◆ Active disease: meningitis, acute infection, onset of chronic illness, tumor, abscess, infarction, demyelinating disease

(continued)

Findings in cerebrospinal fluid analysis *(continued)*

TEST	NORMAL	ABNORMAL	IMPLICATIONS
Cell count *(continued)*	No RBCs	RBCs	◆ Hemorrhage or traumatic lumbar puncture
Venereal Disease Research Laboratories test for syphilis, and other serologic tests	Nonreactive	Positive	◆ Neurosyphilis
Chloride	115 to 130 mEq/L	Decrease	◆ Infected meninges
Gram stain	No organisms	Gram-positive or gram-negative organisms	◆ Bacterial meningitis

Cholesterol, total

Purpose

◆ To assess the risk of coronary artery disease (CAD)
◆ To evaluate fat metabolism
◆ To aid diagnosis of nephrotic syndrome, pancreatitis, hepatic disease, hypothyroidism, and hyperthyroidism
◆ To assess the efficacy of lipid-lowering drug therapy

Reference values

Adults

Desirable: 140 to 199 mg/dl (SI, 3.63 to 5.15 mmol/L)
Borderline high: 200 to 239 mg/dl (SI, 5.18 to 6.19 mmol/L)
High: > 240 mg/dl (SI, > 6.20 mmol/L)

Children and adolescents (ages 12 to 18 years)

Desirable: < 170 mg/dl (SI, < 4.39 mmol/L)
Borderline high: 170 to 199 mg/dl (SI, 4.4 to 5.16 mmol/L)
High: > 200 mg/dl (SI, > 5.18 mmol/L)

Special considerations

◆ Total cholesterol test measures the circulating levels of free cholesterol and cholesterol esters.
◆ Instruct the patient not to eat or drink for 12 hours before the test.
◆ Elevated serum cholesterol levels may indicate a risk of CAD as well as incipient hepatitis, lipid disorders, bile duct blockage, nephrotic syndrome, obstructive jaundice, pancreatitis, and hypothyroidism.
◆ Low serum cholesterol levels commonly reflect malnutrition, cellular

necrosis of the liver, or hyperthyroidism.

Creatine kinase

Purpose

◆ To detect and diagnose acute myocardial infarction (MI) and reinfarction (mainly using the CK-MB isoenzyme)
◆ To evaluate causes of chest pain and monitor the severity of myocardial ischemia after cardiac surgery, cardiac catheterization, and cardioversion (mainly using CK-MB)
◆ To detect early dermatomyositis and musculoskeletal disorders that aren't neurogenic in origin, such as Duchenne's muscular dystrophy (mainly using total CK)

Reference values

Adults

Females: 26 to 140 units/L (SI, 0.46 to 2.38 µkat/L)
Males: 38 to 174 units/L (SI, 0.63 to 2.9 µkat/L)

Infants

2 to 3 times adult values

Isoenzymes

CK-MM (CK_3)*:* 96 to 100%
CK-MB (CK_2)*:* 0 to 6%
CK-BB (CK_1)*:* 0%

Special considerations

◆ Creatine kinase (CK) reflects normal tissue catabolism; increased serum levels indicate trauma to cells.
◆ Measuring CK isoenzymes localizes the site of tissue destruction: CK-BB is mostly found in brain tissue, CK-MM and CK-MB in skeletal and heart muscle. CK-MB and CK-MM isoenzymes can be assayed to increase the sensitivity of the test.
◆ Tell a patient being evaluated for musculoskeletal disorders to avoid exercising for 24 hours before the test.
◆ Detectable CK-BB isoenzyme may indicate brain tissue injury, widespread malignant tumors, severe shock, or renal failure.
◆ CK-MM values increase after skeletal muscle trauma; with dermatomyositis, muscular dystrophy, and hypothyroidism; and following muscle activity caused by agitation, such as during acute psychosis.
◆ CK-MB levels $> 5\%$ of the total CK level indicate MI, especially if the lactate dehydrogenase isoenzyme ratio is > 1. In acute MI, CK-MB increases in 2 to 4 hours, peaks in 12 to 24 hours, and returns to normal in 24 to 48 hours; total CK level follows a similar pattern but increases slightly later.
◆ Total CK levels may increase in severe hypokalemia, carbon monoxide poisoning, malignant hyperthermia, and alcoholic cardiomyopathy; after a seizure; and, occasionally, with pulmonary or cerebral infarction.

Creatinine clearance

Purpose

◆ To assess renal function (mainly glomerular filtration)
◆ To monitor the progression of renal insufficiency

Reference values

Urine

Females: 11 to 20 mg/kg/24 hours (SI, 97 to 177 µmol/kg/day)
Males: 14 to 26 mg/kg/24 hours (SI, 124 to 230 µmol/kg/day)

Blood
0.8 to 1.2 mg/dl (SI, 71 to 106 µmol/L)

Special considerations

◆ Creatinine is the main end-product of creatine, and its production is proportional to total muscle mass.
◆ Creatinine clearance is an excellent diagnostic indicator of renal function and becomes abnormal when more than 50% of the nephrons have been damaged.
◆ Low creatinine clearance may result from reduced renal blood flow, acute tubular necrosis, acute or chronic glomerulonephritis, advanced bilateral chronic pyelonephritis, advanced bilateral renal lesions, nephrosclerosis, heart failure, or severe dehydration
◆ Before the test, tell the patient to avoid meat, poultry, fish, tea, and coffee for 6 hours; to avoid strenuous physical exercise during the test; and to expect a timed urine specimen and at least one blood sample.

Creatinine, serum

Purpose

◆ To assess glomerular filtration
◆ To screen for renal damage

Reference values

Adults
Females: 0.6 to 1.1 mg/dl (SI, 53 to 97 µmol/L)
Males: 0.9 to 1.3 mg/dl (SI, 80 to 115 µmol/L)

Children (ages 3 to 18 years)
0.5 to 1 mg/dl (SI, 44 to 88 µmol/L)

Special considerations

◆ Creatinine is an end-product of creatine metabolism that appears in serum in amounts proportional to muscle mass and provides a more sensitive measure of renal damage than BUN levels.
◆ Elevated serum creatinine levels usually indicate renal disease that has seriously damaged 50% or more of nephrons.

Erythrocyte sedimentation rate

Purpose

◆ To monitor inflammatory or malignant disease
◆ To aid in detecting and diagnosing such diseases as tuberculosis, tissue necrosis, and connective tissue disease

Reference values

Adults
Females: 0 to 20 mm/hour (> age 50: 0 to 30 mm/hour)
Males: 0 to 15 mm/hour (> age 50: 0 to 20 mm/hour)

Children
0 to 10 mm/hour

Special considerations

◆ Erythrocyte sedimentation rate (ESR) measures the degree of erythrocyte settling that occurs in a blood sample during a specified amount of time and is a sensitive but nonspecific early indicator of disease.
◆ ESR usually increases significantly in widespread inflammatory disorders.
◆ It also increases in pregnancy, anemia, acute or chronic inflammation, tuberculosis, paraproteinemias, rheumat-

ic fever, rheumatoid arthritis, and some cancers.
◆ ESR may be depressed in polycythemia, sickle cell anemia, hyperviscosity, and low plasma fibrinogen or globulin levels.

Estrogens

Purpose

◆ To determine sexual maturation and fertility
◆ To aid in diagnosing gonadal dysfunction, such as precocious or delayed puberty, menstrual disorders (especially amenorrhea), and infertility
◆ To determine fetal well-being
◆ To aid in diagnosing estrogen-secreting tumors

Reference values

Serum total estrogens
Females
60 to 400 pg/ml (SI, 60 to 400 nanogram/L)
Postmenopausal women: < 130 pg/ml (SI, < 130 nanogram/L)
Prepubertal women: < 25 pg/ml (SI, < 25 nanogram/L)
Pubertal women: 30 to 280 pg/ml (SI, 30 to 280 nanogram/L)

Males
20 to 80 pg/ml (SI, 20 to 80 nanogram/L)

Special considerations

◆ Estrogens promote development of secondary female sexual characteristics and normal menstruation.
◆ Estrogens are secreted by ovarian follicular cells during the first half of the menstrual cycle and by the corpus luteum during the luteal phase; in menopause, secretion drops to a constant, low level.
◆ Decreased estrogen levels may indicate primary hypogonadism, ovarian failure, secondary hypogonadism, or menopause.
◆ Abnormally high estrogen levels may occur with estrogen-producing tumors, precocious puberty, severe hepatic disease, and congenital adrenal hyperplasia
◆ Withhold all steroid and pituitary-based hormones before testing, as ordered.

Glucose, fasting plasma

Purpose

◆ To screen for diabetes mellitus
◆ To monitor drug or diet therapy in patients with diabetes mellitus

Reference values

Adults
≤ 110 mg/dl (SI, ≤ 6.1 mmol/L)

Children (ages 2 to 18 years)
60 to 100 mg/dl (SI, 3.3 to 5.6 mmol/L)

Special considerations

◆ Fasting plasma glucose test measures plasma glucose levels after a 12- to 14-hour fast.
◆ Fasting plasma glucose levels of 126 mg/dl (SI, 7 mmol/L) or more obtained on two or more occasions confirms diabetes mellitus.
◆ A 2-hour postprandial plasma glucose test or an oral glucose tolerance test may be performed to confirm the diagnosis in a patient with borderline or transiently elevated levels.

Glucose, 2-hour postprandial plasma

Purpose

◆ To aid in diagnosing diabetes mellitus
◆ To monitor drug or diet therapy in patients with diabetes mellitus

Reference values

Patients without diabetes
< 145 mg/dl (SI, < 8 mmol/L)

Patients > age 50
Levels slightly elevated

Special considerations

◆ The 2-hour postprandial blood glucose test is performed when the patient shows symptoms of diabetes (polydipsia and polyuria) or when the results of the fasting plasma glucose test suggest diabetes.
◆ Two 2-hour postprandial blood glucose values of 200 mg/dl (SI, 11.1 mmol/L) or above indicate diabetes mellitus.
◆ Tell the patient to eat a balanced meal or one containing 100 g of carbohydrates before the test and then to fast for 2 hours. Instruct him to avoid smoking and strenuous exercise after the meal.

Glucose tolerance test, oral

Purpose

◆ To confirm the diagnosis of diabetes mellitus in selected patients
◆ To aid in diagnosing hypoglycemia and malabsorption syndrome

Reference values

Adults
30-minute plasma glucose level: 110 to 170 mg/dl (SI, 6.1 to 9.4 mmol/L)
1-hour plasma glucose level after glucose load: < 184 mg/dl (SI, < 10.2 mmol/L)
2-hour plasma glucose level after glucose load: < 138 mg/dl (SI, < 7.7 mmol/L)
3-hour plasma glucose level after glucose load: 70 to 120 mg/dl (SI, 3.9 to 6.7 mmol/L)

Children
2-hour plasma glucose level after glucose load: < 140 mg/dl (SI, < 7.8 mmol/L)

Special considerations

◆ The oral glucose tolerance test is the most sensitive method of evaluating borderline cases of diabetes mellitus.
◆ Plasma and urine glucose levels are monitored for 3 hours after the patient ingests a challenge dose of glucose.
◆ Decreased glucose tolerance, in which glucose levels peak sharply before falling slowly to fasting levels, may confirm diabetes mellitus or result from Cushing's disease, hemochromatosis, pheochromocytoma, or central nervous system lesions.
◆ Increased glucose tolerance, in which levels may peak at less than normal, may indicate insulinoma, malabsorption syndrome, adrenocortical insufficiency, hypothyroidism, or hypopituitarism
◆ Instruct the patient to maintain a high-carbohydrate diet for 3 days and then fast for 10 to 16 hours before the test.
◆ Tell the patient not to smoke, drink coffee or alcohol, or exercise strenu-

ously for 8 hours before or during the test.

Hematocrit

Purpose

- To aid in diagnosing polycythemia, anemia, or abnormal states of hydration
- To aid in calculating red blood cell (RBC) indices

Reference values

Adults

Females: 36% to 48% (SI, 0.36 to 0.48)
Males: 42% to 52% (SI, 0.42 to 0.52)

Children

Ages 0 to *2 weeks:* 44% to 64% (SI, 0.44 to 0.64)
Ages 2 to *8 weeks:* 39% to 59% (SI, 0.39 to 0.59)
Ages 2 to *6 months:* 35% to 49% (SI, 0.35 to 0.49)
Ages 6 months to *1 year:* 29% to 43% (SI, 0.29 to 0.43)
Ages 1 to *6:* 30% to 40% (SI, 0.3 to 0.4)
Ages 6 to *16:* 32% to 42% (SI, 0.32 to 0.42)
Ages 16 to *18:* 34% to 44% (SI, 0.34 to 0.44)

Special considerations

- Hematocrit (HCT) measures the percentage of packed RBCs by volume in a sample of whole blood.
- Decreased HCT suggests anemia, hemodilution, or massive blood loss.
- Increased HCT indicates polycythemia or hemoconcentration from blood loss or dehydration.

Hemoglobin, glycosylated

Purpose

- To assess control of diabetes mellitus

Reference values

All populations

4% to 6.7% of total hemoglobin H

Special considerations

- Glycosylated hemoglobin (HbA_{1C}) levels provide information about the average blood glucose level during the preceding 2 to 3 months to evaluate the long-term effectiveness of diabetes therapy.
- HbA_{1C} values are reported as a percentage of the total hemoglobin in an RBC; a value greater than 10% indicates poor control, less than 8% indicates good control.

Hemoglobin, total

Purpose

- To measure the severity of anemia or polycythemia and monitor the response to therapy
- To obtain data to calculate mean corpuscular hemoglobin (MCH) and mean corpuscular hemoglobin concentration (MCHC)

Reference values

Adults

Females: 12 to 16 g/dl (SI, 120 to 160 g/L)
Males: 14 to 17.4 g/dl (SI, 140 to 174 g/L)

Children

Ages 0 to 2 weeks: 14.5 to 24.5 g/dl (SI, 145 to 245 g/L)
Ages 2 to 8 weeks: 12.5 to 20.5 g/dl (SI, 125 to 205 g/L)
Ages 2 to 6 months: 10.7 to 17.3 g/dl (SI, 107 to 173 g/L)
Ages 6 months to 1 year: 9.9 to 14.5 g/dl (SI, 99 to 145 g/L)
Ages 1 to 6: 9.5 to 14.1 g/dl (SI, 95 to 141 g/L)
Ages 6 to 16: 10.3 to 14.9 g/dl (SI, 103 to 149 g/L)
Ages 16 to 18: 11.1 to 15.7 g/dl (SI, 111 to 157 g/L)

Special considerations

◆ Total hemoglobin (Hb) level is used to measure the amount of Hb in a deciliter of whole blood and is usually part of a complete blood count.
◆ Hb level correlates closely with the red blood cell (RBC) count and affects the Hb-RBC ratio (MCH and MCHC).
◆ A decreased Hb level may indicate anemia, recent hemorrhage, or fluid retention, causing hemodilution.
◆ An increased Hb level suggests hemoconcentration from polycythemia or dehydration.

Hepatitis B surface antigen

Purpose

◆ To screen blood donors for hepatitis B infection
◆ To screen people at high risk for contracting hepatitis B
◆ To aid in the differential diagnosis of viral hepatitis

Reference values

All populations

Negative results for hepatitis B surface antigen (HBsAg)

Special considerations

◆ HBsAg appears in the sera of patients with hepatitis B virus.
◆ If HBsAg is found in donor blood, that blood must be discarded because it carries a risk of transmitting hepatitis.

Human chorionic gonadotropin, serum

Purpose

◆ To detect early pregnancy
◆ To determine the adequacy of hormone production in high-risk pregnancies
◆ To aid in diagnosing trophoblastic tumors, such as hydatidiform moles and choriocarcinoma, and tumors that secrete human chorionic gonadotropin (hCG) ectopically
◆ To monitor treatment for the induction of ovulation and conception

Reference values

Females

Nonpregnant: < 5 IU/L
Pregnant: Levels vary widely, depending in part on the number of days since the patient's last normal menstrual period

Special considerations

◆ hCG is a hormone produced in the placenta. Levels increase steadily during the first trimester and peak at about 10 weeks' gestation.

◆ hCG may be detected in the blood 9 days after ovulation. Along with progesterone, it maintains the corpus luteum during early pregnancy.
◆ Elevated hCG beta-subunit levels are present in pregnancy, hydatidiform mole, trophoblastic neoplasms of the placenta, and nontrophoblastic carcinomas that secrete hCG (including gastric, pancreatic, and ovarian adenocarcinomas).

Human chorionic gonadotropin, urine

Purpose

◆ To detect and confirm pregnancy
◆ To aid in diagnosing hydatidiform mole or human chorionic gonadotropin (hCG) to secreting tumors, threatened abortion, or dead fetus

Reference values

Females
Qualitative
Nonpregnant: Negative
Pregnant: Positive

Quantitative
Pregnant:
- First trimester: Up to 500,000 IU/24 hours
- Second trimester: 10,000 to 25,000 IU/24 hours
- Third trimester: 5,000 to 15,000 IU/24 hours

Special considerations

◆ Qualitative analysis of urine levels of hCG allows detection of pregnancy as early as 14 days after ovulation.
◆ During pregnancy, increased urine hCG levels may indicate multiple pregnancy or erythroblastosis fetalis; decreased urine hCG levels may indicate threatened abortion or ectopic pregnancy.
◆ Measurable levels of hCG in men and nonpregnant women may indicate choriocarcinoma, ovarian or testicular tumors, melanoma, multiple myeloma, or gastric, hepatic, pancreatic, or breast cancer.
◆ Inform the patient that the test requires a first-voided morning specimen (qualitative test) or urine collection over a 24-hour period (quantitative test).

Human immunodeficiency virus antibodies

Purpose

◆ To screen for human immunodeficiency virus (HIV) infection in high-risk patients
◆ To screen donated blood for HIV

Reference values

All populations
Negative results

Special considerations

◆ The HIV antibody test detects antibodies to HIV in the serum.
◆ Initial identification of HIV is usually achieved through the enzyme-linked immunosorbent assay. Positive findings are confirmed by Western blot test and immunofluorescence.
◆ Provide the patient with counseling about the reasons for performing the test.
◆ The test detects previous exposure to the virus; however, it doesn't identify patients who have been exposed to the virus but haven't yet made antibodies.

Human leukocyte antigen test

Purpose

◆ To specify the types of human leukocyte antigen (HLA) on a patient's white blood cells (WBCs)
◆ To provide histocompatibility typing of transplant recipients and donors
◆ To aid genetic counseling
◆ To aid paternity testing

Reference values

All populations
Presence of HLA types (which include HLA-A, HLA-B, HLA-C, and HLA-D), which must then be compared between donor and recipient

Special considerations

◆ HLA is essential to immunity and determines the degree of histocompatibility between transplant recipients and donors.
◆ Specific HLA types have been linked to specific diseases, such as rheumatoid arthritis and multiple sclerosis, but HLA findings have little diagnostic significance on their own.
◆ If the patient has had a recent blood transfusion, HLA testing may need to be postponed.

International normalized ratio

Purpose

◆ To evaluate the effectiveness of oral anticoagulant therapy

Reference values

Patients taking warfarin
2 to 3

Patients with mechanical prosthetic heart valves
2.5 to 3.5

Special considerations

◆ International normalized ratio (INR) is the best method for standardizing measurement of prothrombin time to monitor oral anticoagulant therapy.
◆ An increased INR may indicate disseminated intravascular coagulation, cirrhosis, hepatitis, vitamin K deficiency, salicylate intoxication, uncontrolled oral anticoagulation, or massive blood transfusion.

Lactate dehydrogenase

Purpose

◆ To aid in differential diagnosis of myocardial infarction (MI), pulmonary infarction, anemias, and hepatic disease
◆ To support the results of creatine kinase (CK) isoenzyme tests in diagnosing MI or to provide a diagnosis when CK-MB samples are obtained too late to show an increase
◆ To monitor patient response to some forms of chemotherapy

Reference values

Normal values vary with the testing method used. Check with your laboratory for applicable reference values.

Adults
140 to 280 units/L

Children
60 to 170 units/L

Neonates
160 to 450 units/L

Special considerations

◆ Because lactate dehydrogenase (LD) is present in most body tissues, cellular damage increases the total serum LD level, limiting its diagnostic usefulness.
◆ Five tissue-specific isoenzymes can be measured: LD_1 and LD_2 appear mainly in the heart, red blood cells, and kidneys; LD_3 is found mainly in the lungs; and LD_4 and LD_5 occur in the liver, skin, and skeletal muscles.
◆ In an acute MI, the concentration of LD_1 is greater than that of LD_2 within 12 to 48 hours after the onset of symptoms (flipped LD).
◆ LD_2, LD_3, LD_4 may be increased in granulocytic leukemia, lymphomas, and platelet disorders
◆ If the patient may have had an MI, tell him that he will have retests for 2 days to monitor progressive changes.

Lipoprotein-cholesterol fractionation

Purpose

◆ To assess the risk of coronary artery disease (CAD)
◆ To determine the efficacy of lipid-lowering drug therapy

Reference values

Adults

Low-density lipoprotein level
Desirable: < 130 mg/dl (SI, < 3.4 mmol/L)
Borderline high-risk: 140 to 159 mg/dl (SI, 3.4 to 4.1 mmol/L)
High-risk: > 160 mg/dl (SI, > 4.1 mmol/L)

High-density lipoprotein level
Females: 35 to 80 mg/dl (SI, 0.91 to 2.07 mmol/L)
Males: 35 to 65 mg/dl (SI, 0.91 to 1.68 mmol/L)

Special considerations

◆ Cholesterol fractionation tests measure low-density lipoprotein (LDL) and high-density lipoprotein (HDL) levels.
◆ The American College of Cardiology recommends an HDL level of 40 mg/dl or greater, with women maintaining an HDL level of at least 45 mg/dl. An HDL level greater than 60 mg/dl is considered heart healthy.
◆ LDL level should be less than 100 mg/dl, with levels of 160 mg/dl or greater considered high.
◆ HDL level is inversely related to the risk of CAD; the higher the HDL level, the lower the risk of CAD. In contrast, the higher the LDL level, the higher the risk of CAD.
◆ Instruct the patient to maintain a normal diet for 2 weeks before the test, to avoid alcohol for 24 hours before the test, and to fast and avoid exercise for 12 to 14 hours before the test.

Lyme disease serology

Purpose

◆ To confirm the diagnosis of Lyme disease

Reference values

All populations

Negative for IgG and IgM Lyme antibodies by enzyme-linked immunosorbent assay and Western blot test

Special considerations

◆ Serologic tests for Lyme disease measure antibody response to the spirochete *Borrelia burgdorferi* and indicate current infection or previous exposure.

◆ Serologic tests identify 50% of patients with early-stage Lyme disease and all patients with later complications of carditis, neuritis, and arthritis as well as patients in remission.

◆ A positive test result helps confirm the diagnosis, but isn't definitive.

Magnesium, serum

Purpose

◆ To evaluate electrolyte status

◆ To assess neuromuscular and renal function

Reference values

Adults

1.8 to 2.6 mg/dl (SI, 0.74 to 1.07 mmol/L)

Children

1.7 to 2.1 mg/dl (SI, 0.7 to 0.86 mmol/L)

Neonates

1.5 to 2.2 mg/dl (SI, 0.62 to 0.91 mmol/L)

Special considerations

◆ Magnesium, vital to neuromuscular function, is found mostly in bone and intracellular fluid; it's absorbed by the small intestine and excreted in urine and stool.

◆ Hypermagnesemia occurs in renal failure, with inadequate renal excretion of magnesium, with the administration or ingestion of magnesium and in adrenal insufficiency.

◆ Observe a patient with hypermagnesemia for lethargy; flushing; diaphoresis; decreased blood pressure; slow, weak pulse; muscle weakness; diminished deep tendon reflexes; slow, shallow respiration; and electrocardiogram (ECG) changes.

◆ Hypomagnesemia results from chronic alcoholism, malabsorption syndrome, diarrhea, faulty absorption after bowel resection, prolonged bowel or gastric aspiration, acute pancreatitis, primary aldosteronism, severe burns, hypercalcemic conditions, malnutrition, and certain diuretics.

◆ Watch the patient with hypomagnesia for leg and foot cramps, hyperactive deep tendon reflexes, arrhythmias, muscle weakness, seizures, twitching, tetany, tremors, and ECG changes.

◆ Instruct the patient not to use magnesium salts for at least 3 days before the test.

Myoglobin

Purpose

◆ As a nonspecific test, to estimate damage to skeletal or cardiac muscle tissue

◆ To predict flare-ups of polymyositis

◆ Specifically, to determine if a myocardial infarction (MI) has occurred

Reference values

All populations

5 to 70 nanogram/ml (SI, 5 to 70 μg/L)

Special considerations

◆ Myoglobin, usually found in skeletal and cardiac muscle, is released into the bloodstream in ischemia, trauma, and muscle inflammation.

◆ Increased myoglobin levels may occur in MI, acute alcohol intoxication, dermatomyositis, hypothermia (with prolonged shivering), muscular dystrophy, polymyositis, rhabdomyolysis, severe burn injuries, trauma, severe renal failure, and systemic lupus erythematosus.

Occult blood, fecal

Purpose

- To detect GI bleeding
- To aid in the early diagnosis of colorectal cancer

Reference values

All populations
Negative for blood

Special considerations

- This test is particularly important for the early diagnosis of colorectal cancer.
- A positive test result indicates GI bleeding.
- Instruct the patient to eat a high-fiber diet and refrain from eating red meat, turnips, and horseradish for 48 to 72 hours before the test and during the collection period.

Partial thromboplastin time

Purpose

- To screen for deficiencies of clotting factors in the intrinsic pathways
- To monitor response to heparin therapy

Reference values

All populations
21 to 35 seconds

Special considerations

- Partial thromboplastin time (PTT) evaluates the clotting factors of the intrinsic pathway — except platelets.
- If the patient is receiving anticoagulant therapy, ask the physician to specify the reference values for the therapy that's being delivered.
- Prolonged PTT may indicate a deficiency of certain plasma clotting factors, the presence of heparin, or the presence of fibrin split products, fibrinolysins, or circulating anticoagulants that are antibodies to specific clotting factors.

Phosphate, serum

Purpose

- To aid in diagnosing renal disorders and acid-base imbalance
- To detect endocrine, skeletal, and calcium disorders

Reference values

Adults
2.7 to 4.5 mg/dl (SI, 0.87 to 1.45 mmol/L)

Children
4.5 to 5.5 mg/dl (SI, 1.45 to 1.78 mmol/L)

Neonates
4.5 to 9 mg/dl (SI, 1.45 to 2.91 mmol/L)

Special considerations

- Phosphates are essential in energy storage and use, calcium regulation, red blood cell function, acid-base balance, bone formation, and carbohydrate, protein, and fat metabolism.

◆ The intestines absorb most phosphates from dietary sources; the kidneys excrete phosphates and serve as a regulatory mechanism.
◆ Calcium and phosphate levels have an inverse relationship; if one is increased, the other is decreased.
◆ Hypophosphatemia may result from renal tubular acidosis, malnutrition, malabsorption syndromes, hyperparathyroidism, treatment of diabetic ketoacidosis, and in children, suppressed growth.
◆ Hyperphosphatemia may result from skeletal disease, healing fractures, hypoparathyroidism, acromegaly, diabetic ketoacidosis, high intestinal obstruction, lactic acidosis, and renal failure.
◆ Symptoms of hypophosphatemia include anemia, prolonged bleeding, bone demineralization, decreased white blood cell count, and anorexia.
◆ Symptoms of hyperphosphatemia include tachycardia, muscle weakness, diarrhea, cramping, and hyperreflexia.

Platelet count

Purpose

◆ To evaluate platelet production
◆ To assess the effects of chemotherapy or radiation therapy on platelet production
◆ To diagnose and monitor severe thrombocytosis or thrombocytopenia
◆ To confirm a visual estimate of the number and morphologic features of platelets from a stained blood film

Reference values

Adults
140 to 400 × 10^3/µl (SI, 140 to 400 × 10^9/L)

Children
150 to 450 × 10^3/µl (SI, 150 to 450 × 10^9/L)

Special considerations

◆ Platelets promote coagulation and the formation of a hemostatic plug in vascular injury.
◆ A decreased platelet count (thrombocytopenia) can result from aplastic or hypoplastic bone marrow, infiltrative bone marrow disease, megakaryocytic hypoplasia, folic acid or vitamin B_{12} deficiency, pooling of platelets in an enlarged spleen, increased platelet destruction, disseminated intravascular coagulation, or mechanical injury to platelets.
◆ An increased platelet count (thrombocytosis) can result from hemorrhage, infectious disorders, iron deficiency anemia, recent surgery, pregnancy, splenectomy, inflammatory disorders, primary thrombocythemia, myelofibrosis with myeloid metaplasia, polycythemia vera, and chronic myelogenous leukemia.

Potassium, serum

Purpose

◆ To evaluate the clinical signs of potassium excess (hyperkalemia) or potassium depletion (hypokalemia)
◆ To monitor renal function, acid-base balance, and glucose metabolism
◆ To evaluate neuromuscular and endocrine disorders
◆ To detect the origin of arrhythmias

Reference values

Adults
3.5 to 5.2 mEq/L (SI, 3.5 to 5.2 mmol/L)

Children

Ages 1 to 18 years: 3.4 to 4.7 mEq/L (SI, 3.4 to 4.7 mmol/L)
Ages 7 days to 1 year: 4.1 to 5.3 mEq/L (SI, 4.1 to 5.3 mmol/L)

Neonates

*Ages 0 to 7 days:*3.7 to 5.9 mEq/L (SI, 3.7 to 5.9 mmol/L)

Special considerations

◆ Potassium helps maintain osmotic equilibrium in the cells and regulate muscle activity, enzyme activity, and acid-base balance. It also affects renal function.
◆ Hyperkalemia may occur in burn injuries, crush injuries, diabetic ketoacidosis, transfusions of large amounts of blood, myocardial infarction, renal failure, or Addison's disease.
◆ Findings in hyperkalemia include electrocardiogram (ECG) changes, weakness, malaise, nausea, diarrhea, colicky pain, and muscle irritability that progresses to flaccid paralysis, oliguria, and bradycardia.
◆ Hypokalemia may result from aldosteronism or Cushing's syndrome, loss of body fluids (as from long-term diuretic therapy, vomiting, or diarrhea), and excessive ingestion of licorice.
◆ Findings in hypokalemia include decreased reflexes; ECG changes; a rapid, weak, irregular pulse; mental confusion; hypotension; anorexia; muscle weakness; and paresthesia.

Prostate-specific antigen

Purpose

◆ To screen for prostate cancer in men older than age 50
◆ To monitor the course of prostate cancer and aid in evaluating treatment

Reference values

Males

0 to 4 nanograms/ml (SI, 0 to 4 μg/L)

Special considerations

◆ Measurement of serum prostate-specific antigen (PSA) levels, along with a digital rectal examination, is recommended as a screening test for prostate cancer in men older than age 50.
◆ About 80% of patients with prostate cancer have pretreatment PSA values greater than 4 nanograms/ml; about 20% of patients with benign prostatic hyperplasia also have levels greater than 4 nanograms/ml.
◆ Further assessment and testing, including tissue biopsy, are needed to confirm the diagnosis of prostate cancer.

Protein, urine

Purpose

◆ To aid in the diagnosis of pathologic states characterized by proteinuria, primarily renal disease

Reference values

24-hour urine collection

Females: 30 to 100 mg/L (SI, 3 to 10 mg/dl)
Males: 10 to 140 mg/L (SI, 1 to 14 mg/dl)
Children < age 10: 10 to 100 mg/L (SI, 1 to 10 mg/dl)

Special considerations

◆ Proteinuria is a chief characteristic of renal disease; when present in a single specimen, a 24-hour urine collec-

tion is required to identify specific renal abnormalities.
- ◆ Moderate proteinuria occurs in several types of renal disease and in diseases in which renal failure develops as a late complication (such as diabetes or heart failure.
- ◆ Heavy proteinuria is commonly linked to nephrotic syndrome.
- ◆ Tell the patient that the test usually requires a 24-hour urine collection; random collection can be done.

Protein electrophoresis, serum

Purpose

- ◆ To aid diagnosis of hepatic disease, protein deficiency, renal disorders, and GI and neoplastic diseases

Reference values

Adults
Total serum protein: 6 to 8 g/dl (SI, 60 to 80 g/L)
Albumin: 3.8 to 5 g/dl (SI, 38 to 50 g/L)
Alpha$_1$-globulin: 0.1 to 0.3 g/dl
Alpha$_2$-globulin: 0.6 to 1 g/dl
Beta-globulin: 0.7 to 1.4 g/dl
Gamma-globulin: 0.7 to 1.6 g/dl

Special considerations

- ◆ Protein electrophoresis measures the levels of serum albumin and globulins, which are the major blood proteins. This test identifies five protein fractions: albumin and alpha$_1$, alpha$_2$, beta, and gamma proteins.

Prothrombin time

Purpose

- ◆ To evaluate the extrinsic coagulation system (factors V, VII, and X and prothrombin and fibrinogen)
- ◆ To monitor the response to oral anticoagulant therapy

Reference values

All populations
11 to 13 seconds (may vary by laboratory)

Special considerations

- ◆ In a patient taking oral anticoagulants, prothrombin time is usually maintained at 1 to 2½ times the normal control value.

Red blood cell count

Purpose

- ◆ To provide data for calculating mean corpuscular volume and mean corpuscular hemoglobin, which show red blood cell (RBC) size and hemoglobin content
- ◆ To support other hematologic tests that are used to diagnose anemia or polycythemia

Reference values

Adults
Females: 3.6 to 5 $\times$ 10^6/µl (SI, 3.6 to 5 $\times$ 10^{12}/L)
Males: 4.2 to 5.4 $\times$ 10^6/µl (SI, 4.2 to 5.4 $\times$ 10^{12}/L)

Children (ages 6 to 16 years)
4 to 5.2 × 10^6/µl (SI, 4 to 5.2 × 10^{12}/L)

Special considerations

◆ Normal RBC values may be higher in patients who live at high altitudes or are very active.
◆ An elevated RBC count may indicate absolute or relative polycythemia.
◆ A depressed count may indicate anemia, fluid overload, or hemorrhage more than 24 hours ago.

Red blood cell indices

Purpose

◆ To aid in diagnosing and classifying anemias

Reference values

Mean corpuscular volume (MCV)
82 to 98 µl (SI, 82 to 98 fL)

Mean corpuscular hemoglobin (MCH)
26 to 34 pg/cell (SI, 0.4 to 0.53 fmol/cell)

Mean corpuscular hemoglobin concentration (MCHC)
32 to 36 g/dl (SI, 320 to 360 g/L)

Special considerations

◆ MCV indicates the average red blood cell (RBC) size (microcytic, macrocytic, or normocytic).
◆ MCH gives the weight of hemoglobin (Hb) in an average RBC.
◆ MCHC is the concentration of Hb in 100 ml of packed RBCs and helps distinguish normally colored (normochromic) RBCs from paler (hypochromic) RBCs.
◆ Low MCV and MCHC indicate microcytic, hypochromic anemias caused by iron deficiency anemia, pyridoxine-responsive anemia, or thalassemia.
◆ High MCV suggests macrocytic anemia caused by megaloblastic anemia, folic acid or vitamin B_{12} deficiency, inherited disorders of DNA synthesis, or reticulocytosis.

Sodium, serum

Purpose

◆ To evaluate the fluid-electrolyte balance and the acid-base balance and related neuromuscular, renal, and adrenal functions

Reference values

Adults and children ages 1 to 16 years
136 to 145 mEq/L (SI, 136 to 145 mmol/L)

Full-term neonates
133 to 142 mEq/L (SI, 133 to 142 mmol/L)

Special considerations

◆ Sodium (Na^+) affects the distribution of water in the body, maintains the osmotic pressure of extracellular fluid, helps promote neuromuscular function, helps maintain the acid-base balance, and influences chloride and potassium levels.
◆ Hypernatremia may be caused by inadequate water intake, water loss in excess of sodium loss (such as diabetes insipidus, impaired renal function, prolonged hyperventilation and, occasionally, severe vomiting or diarrhea), sodi-

um retention (such as aldosteronism), and excessive sodium intake.
◆ Check the patient with hypernatremia for signs of thirst, restlessness, dry mucous membranes, flushed skin, oliguria, and diminished reflexes. If increased total body sodium causes water retention, observe for hypertension, dyspnea, edema, and heart failure.
◆ Hyponatremia may result from inadequate sodium intake or from excessive sodium loss as a result of profuse sweating, GI suctioning, diuretic therapy, diarrhea, vomiting, adrenal insufficiency, burns, and chronic renal insufficiency with acidosis.
◆ Check the patient with hyponatremia for apprehension, lassitude, headache, decreased skin turgor, abdominal cramps, and tremors that may progress to seizures.

Thyroid-stimulating immunoglobulin

Purpose

◆ To aid in evaluating suspected thyroid disease
◆ To aid in diagnosing suspected thyrotoxicosis, especially in patients with exophthalmos
◆ To monitor thyrotoxicosis treatment

Reference values

All populations
Thyroid-stimulating immunoglobulin (TSI) doesn't normally appear in serum. However, it's considered normal at levels equal to or greater than the 1.3 index.

Special considerations

◆ TSI appears in the blood of most patients with Graves' disease.
◆ TSI stimulates the thyroid gland to produce and excrete excessive amounts of thyroid hormone.
◆ Increased TSI levels are associated with exophthalmos, Graves' disease (thyrotoxicosis), and recurrence of hyperthyroidism.

Thyroxine

Purpose

◆ To evaluate thyroid function
◆ To aid in diagnosing hyperthyroidism and hypothyroidism
◆ To monitor the response to antithyroid drugs in hyperthyroidism or to thyroid replacement therapy in hypothyroidism (Thyroid-stimulating hormone estimates are needed to confirm hypothyroidism.)

Reference values

Adults
5.4 to 11.5 µg/dl (SI, 57 to 148 nmol/L)

Children
6.4 to 13.3 µg/dl (SI, 83 to 172 nmol/L)

Neonates
11.8 to 22.6 µg/dl (SI, 152 to 292 nmol/L)

Special considerations

◆ Thyroxine (T_4) is secreted by the thyroid gland in response to thyroid-stimulating hormone (TSH) and, indirectly, thyrotropin-releasing hormone.
◆ Only a fraction of T_4 circulates freely in the blood; the rest binds strongly to plasma proteins, primarily T_4-binding globulin (TBG). This

minute fraction is responsible for the clinical effects of thyroid hormone.

- Elevated T_4 levels occur with primary and secondary hyperthyroidism, including excessive T_4 (levothyroxine) replacement therapy.
- Low levels suggest primary or secondary hypothyroidism or possibly T_4 suppression by normal, elevated, or replacement levels of triiodothyronine (T_3).
- If the diagnosis of hypothyroidism is in doubt, TSH levels may be obtained.

Thyroxine, free, and triiodothyronine, free

Purpose

- To measure the metabolically active form of the thyroid hormones
- To aid in diagnosing hyperthyroidism and hypothyroidism when T_4-binding globulin (TBG) levels are abnormal

Reference values

Free thyroxine (FT_4)
0.7 to 2 nanogram/dl (SI, 10 to 26 pmol/L)

Free triiodothyronine (FT_3)
260 to 480 pg/dl (SI, 4 to 7.4 pmol/L)

Special considerations

- FT_4 and FT_3 tests measure the minute portions of T_4 and T_3 that aren't bound to TBG and other serum proteins; these unbound hormones are responsible for the thyroid's effects on cellular metabolism.
- Measurement of these free hormone levels is the best indicator of thyroid function.
- Elevated FT_4 and FT_3 levels indicate hyperthyroidism, unless peripheral resistance to thyroid hormone is present.
- T_3 toxicosis, a form of hyperthyroidism, yields high FT_3 levels with normal or low FT_4 values.
- Low FT_4 levels indicate hypothyroidism, except in patients receiving T_3 replacement therapy.
- Patients receiving thyroid therapy may have varying levels of FT_4 and FT_3, depending on the preparation used and the time of sample collection.

Triglycerides

Purpose

- To screen for hyperlipidemia or pancreatitis
- To help identify nephrotic syndrome and patients with poorly controlled diabetes mellitus
- To determine the risk of coronary artery disease
- To calculate the low-density lipoprotein cholesterol level using the Friedewald equation

Reference values

Adults (≥ age 25)
Desirable: < 150 mg/dl (SI, < 1.70 mmol/L)
Borderline high: 150 to 199 mg/dl (SI, 1.70 to 2.25 mmol/L)
High: 200 to 499 mg/dl (SI, 2.26 to 5.64 mmol/L)
Very high: ≥ 500 mg/dl (SI, ≥ 5.65 mmol/L)

Females (< age 25)
Ages 20 to 24 years: 32 to 100 mg/dl (SI, 0.36 to 1.13 mmol/L)
Ages 15 to 20 years: 39 to 124 mg/dl (SI, 0.44 to 1.4 mmol/L)

Ages 10 to 14 years: 37 to 131 mg/dl (SI, 0.42 to 1.48 mmol/L)
< 9 years: 35 to 110 mg/dl (SI, 0.4 to 1.24 mmol/L)

Males (< age 25)
Ages 20 to 24 years: 34 to 137 mg/dl (SI, 0.38 to 1.55 mmol/L)
Ages 15 to 20 years: 37 to 148 mg/dl (SI, 0.42 to 1.67 mmol/L)
Ages 10 to 14 years: 32 to 125 mg/dl (SI, 0.36 to 1.41 mmol/L)
< 9 years: 30 to 100 mg/dl (SI, 0.34 to 1.13 mmol/L)

Special considerations

- A mild to moderate increase in serum triglyceride levels indicates biliary obstruction, diabetes mellitus, nephrotic syndrome, endocrinopathies, or overconsumption of alcohol.
- A marked increase in levels without an identifiable cause reflects congenital hyperlipoproteinemia and warrants lipoprotein phenotyping to confirm the diagnosis.
- Instruct the patient to fast for at least 12 hours before the test and to avoid alcohol for 24 hours.

Triiodothyronine

Purpose

- To aid in the diagnosis of triiodothyronine (T_3) toxicosis
- To aid in the diagnosis of hypothyroidism and hyperthyroidism
- To monitor the clinical response to thyroid replacement therapy in hypothyroidism

Reference values

Adults
80 to 200 nanograms/dl (SI, 1.2 to 3.1 nmol/L)

Children (ages 1 to 14 years)
105 to 245 nanograms/dl (SI, 1.6 to 3.8 nmol/L)

Pregnant patients
116 to 247 nanograms/dl (SI, 1.8 to 3.8 nmol/L)

Special considerations

- The T_3 test is highly specific and measures the total (bound and free) serum content of T_3. It is a more accurate diagnostic indicator of hyperthyroidism than T_4.
- In T_3 toxicosis, T_3 levels rise, while total and free T_4 levels remain normal.
- T_3 levels surpass T_4 levels in patients receiving thyroid replacement therapy containing more T_3 than T_4.
- Withhold drugs, such as steroids, propranolol, and cholestyramine, which may affect thyroid function, as ordered.

Triiodothyronine uptake

Purpose

- To aid in diagnosing hypothyroidism and hyperthyroidism when the T_4-binding globulin level is normal
- To aid in the diagnosis of primary disorders of thyroid-binding globulin levels

Reference values

All populations
Ratio between patient specimen and standard control: 0.9 to 1.1
Uptake: 25% to 35% (arbitrary units)

Special considerations

- High triiodothyronine (T_3) uptake percentage with elevated T_4 levels indicates hyperthyroidism.

◆ Low T_3 uptake percentage with low T_4 levels, indicates hypothyroidism.

◆ High T_3 uptake percentage and a low or normal free triiodothyronine (FT_4) level may result from protein loss (as in nephrotic syndrome), decreased production (as a result of excess androgen or genetic or idiopathic causes), or competition for T_4 binding sites by certain drugs (salicylates, phenylbutazone, and phenytoin).

◆ Low T_3 uptake percentage and a high or normal FT_4 level may be caused by exogenous or endogenous estrogen (pregnancy) or from idiopathic causes.

◆ Withhold drugs, such as estrogens, androgens, phenytoin, salicylates, and thyroid preparations, that may interfere with test results, as ordered.

Troponin

Purpose

◆ To detect and diagnose acute myocardial infarction (MI) and reinfarction

◆ To evaluate possible causes of chest pain

Reference values

Qualitative

Negative

Troponin I

< 0.35 nanogram/ml (SI, < 0.35 µg/L)

Troponin T

< 0.2 nanogram/ml (SI, < 0.2 µg/L)

Special considerations

◆ Cardiac troponin I (cTnI) and cardiac troponin T (cTnT) are proteins in the striated cells that are specific markers of cardiac damage.

◆ Elevations in troponin levels can be seen within 1 hour of MI and persist for a week or longer. As long as tissue injury continues, the troponin levels will remain high.

◆ Levels of cTnI aren't detectable in people who don't have cardiac injury.

Uric acid, serum

Purpose

◆ To confirm the diagnosis of gout

◆ To help detect renal dysfunction

Reference values

Adults

Females: 2.4 to 6 mg/dl (SI, 143 to 357 µmol/L)

Males: 3.4 to 7 mg/dl (SI, 202 to 416 µmol/L)

Children

2 to 5.5 mg/dl (SI, 119 to 327 µmol/L)

Special considerations

◆ Increased uric acid levels may occur with gout, impaired kidney function, heart failure, glycogen storage disease, infections, hemolytic and sickle cell anemia, polycythemia, neoplasms, and psoriasis.

◆ Low uric acid levels may indicate defective tubular absorption (such as Fanconi's syndrome) or acute hepatic atrophy.

◆ Instruct the patient to fast for 8 hours before the test.

Normal findings in routine urinalysis

ELEMENT	FINDINGS
Macroscopic	
Color	◆ Pale yellow to amber
Odor	◆ Slightly aromatic
Appearance	◆ Clear to slightly hazy
Specific gravity	◆ 1.005 to 1.025
pH	◆ 4.5 to 8
Protein	◆ Negative
Glucose	◆ Negative
Ketone bodies	◆ Negative
Bilirubin	◆ Negative
Urobilinogen	◆ 0.5 to 4 mg/day
Hemoglobin	◆ Negative
Erythrocytes (RBCs)	◆ Negative
Nitrites (bacteria)	◆ Negative
Leukocytes (WBCs)	◆ Negative
Microscopic	
RBCs	◆ Negative or rare
WBCs	◆ Negative or rare
Epithelial cells	◆ Few: hyaline casts 0 to 1/lpf (low-power field)
Casts	◆ Negative: occasional hyaline casts
Crystals	◆ Negative (none)
Bacteria	◆ None
Yeast cells	◆ None
Parasites	◆ None

Urinalysis, routine

Purpose

◆ To screen for renal or urinary tract disease

◆ To detect metabolic or systemic disease unrelated to renal disorders

◆ To detect substance (drug) use

Reference values

See *Normal findings in routine urinalysis*.

Special considerations

Urinalysis allows evaluation of several important urine characteristics.

◆ *Color:* Color change can result from diet, drugs, and many diseases.

◆ *Odor:* In diabetes mellitus, starvation, and dehydration, a fruity odor accompanies the formation of ketone bodies. In urinary tract infection (UTI), a fetid odor commonly is caused by *Escherichia coli*. Maple syrup urine disease and phenylketonuria also cause distinctive odors. Other abnormal odors include those similar to a brewery, sweaty feet, cabbage, fish, and sulfur.

◆ *Turbidity:* Turbid urine may contain red or white blood cells, bacteria, fat, or chyle and may reflect renal infection.

◆ *Specific gravity:* Low specific gravity (< 1.005) is characteristic of diabetes insipidus, nephrogenic diabetes insipidus, acute tubular necrosis, and pyelonephritis. Fixed specific gravity, in which the value remains 1.010 regardless of fluid intake, occurs in chronic glomerulonephritis with severe renal damage. High specific gravity (> 1.035) occurs in nephrotic syndrome, dehydration, acute glomerulonephritis, heart failure, liver failure, and shock.

◆ *pH:* Alkaline urine pH may result from Fanconi's syndrome, UTI, and metabolic or respiratory alkalosis. Acid urine pH may reflect renal tuberculosis, pyrexia, phenylketonuria, alkaptonuria, or acidosis.

◆ *Protein:* Proteinuria suggests renal failure or disease (including nephrosis, glomerulosclerosis, glomerulonephritis, nephrolithiasis, nephrotic syndrome, and polycystic kidney disease) or multiple myeloma.

◆ *Glucose:* Glycosuria usually indicates diabetes mellitus but may result from pheochromocytoma, Cushing's syndrome, impaired tubular reabsorption, advanced renal disease, increased intracranial pressure, and I.V. solutions containing glucose and total parenteral nutrition containing 10% to 50% glucose.

◆ *Ketones:* Ketonuria occurs in diabetes mellitus when cellular energy needs exceed available cellular glucose and may also occur in starvation states, low- or no-carbohydrate diets, and after diarrhea or vomiting.

◆ *Bilirubin:* Bilirubin in urine may occur in liver disease resulting from obstructive jaundice or hepatotoxic drugs or toxins or from fibrosis of the biliary canaliculi (which may occur in cirrhosis).

◆ *Urobilinogen*: Increased urobilinogen in the urine may indicate liver damage, hemolytic disease, or severe infection. Decreased levels may occur with biliary obstruction, inflammatory disease, antimicrobial therapy, severe diarrhea, or renal insufficiency.

◆ *Cells:* Hematuria indicates bleeding in the genitourinary tract and may result from infection, obstruction, inflammation, trauma, tumors, glomerulonephritis, renal hypertension, lupus nephritis, renal tuberculosis, renal vein thrombosis, renal calculi, hydronephrosis, pyelonephritis, scurvy, malaria, parasitic infection of the bladder, subacute bacterial endocarditis, polyarteritis nodosa, hemorrhagic disorders, strenuous exercise, or exposure to toxic chemicals. Excess white blood cells (WBCs) in the urine implies urinary tract inflammation, especially cystitis or pyelonephritis. The finding of WBC and WBC casts in the urine suggests renal infection or noninfective inflammatory disease. Numerous epithelial cells suggest renal tubular degeneration, such as heavy metal poisoning, eclampsia, and kidney transplant rejection.

◆ *Casts:* Excessive numbers of casts indicate renal disease.

- Hyaline casts may reflect renal parenchymal disease, inflammation, trauma to the glomerular capillary membrane, and some physiologic states (such as after exercise).
- Epithelial casts may reflect renal tubular damage, nephrosis, eclampsia, amyloidosis, and heavy metal poisoning.
- Coarse and fine granular casts may reflect acute or chronic renal failure, pyelonephritis, and chronic lead intoxication.
- Fatty and waxy casts may reflect nephrotic syndrome, chronic renal disease, and diabetes mellitus.
- RBC casts may reflect renal parenchymal disease (especially glomerulonephritis), renal infarction, subacute bacterial endocarditis, vascular disorders, sickle cell anemia, scurvy, blood dyscrasias, malignant hypertension, collagen disease, and acute inflammation.
- WBC casts may reflect acute pyelonephritis and glomerulonephritis, nephrotic syndrome, pyogenic infection, and lupus nephritis.

◆ *Crystals:* Numerous calcium oxalate crystals suggest hypercalcemia or ingestion of ethylene glycol. Cystine crystals (cystinuria) reflect an inborn error of metabolism.

◆ *Other components*: Bacteria, yeast cells, and parasites in urine sediment reflect genitourinary tract infection or contamination of external genitalia. The most common parasite in sediment is *Trichomonas vaginalis,* which causes vaginitis, urethritis, and prostatovesiculitis.

White blood cell count

Purpose

- To identify infection or inflammation
- To determine the need for further tests, such as white blood cell (WBC) differential or bone marrow biopsy
- To monitor the response to chemotherapy or radiation therapy

Reference values

Adults
4,500 to 10,500 cells/µl (SI, 4,500 to 10,500 cells/µl)

Children (ages 6 to 18 years)
4,800 to 10,800 cells/µl (SI, 4,800 to 10,800 cells/µl)

Special considerations

- An increased WBC count (leukocytosis) may occur with infection as well as leukemia, tissue necrosis from burns, myocardial infarction, or gangrene.
- A decreased WBC count (leukopenia) indicates bone marrow depression that may result from viral infection or a toxic reaction, such as after antineoplastic treatment, ingestion of mercury or other heavy metals, or exposure to benzene or arsenicals.
- Leukopenia typically accompanies influenza, typhoid fever, measles, infectious hepatitis, mononucleosis, and rubella.
- Tell the patient to avoid strenuous exercise for 24 hours and to avoid eating a heavy meal before the test.

White blood cell differential

Purpose

- To evaluate the body's capacity to resist and overcome infection
- To detect and identify various types of leukemia
- To determine the stage and severity of an infection
- To detect allergic reactions and parasitic infections and assess their severity (eosinophil count)
- To distinguish viral infections from bacterial infections

Reference values

Adults (> age 18)
Neutrophils (segmented): 50% to 62%
Eosinophils: 0 to 3%
Basophils: 0 to 1%
Lymphocytes: 25% to 40%
Monocytes: 3% to 7%

Children (ages 6 to 16 years)
Neutrophils (segmented): 32% to 54%
Eosinophils: 0 to 3%
Basophils: 0 to 1%
Lymphocytes: 27% to 57%
Monocytes: 0 to 5%

Special considerations

- White blood cells (WBCs) are classified as one of five major types — neutrophils, eosinophils, basophils, lymphocytes, and monocytes — and the percentage of each type is determined.
- Abnormal differential patterns provide evidence of a wide range of disease states and other conditions.
- For accurate diagnosis, differential test results must be interpreted in relation to the total WBC count.
- Tell the patient to refrain from strenuous exercise for 24 hours before the test.

9 Care of pressure ulcers and traumatic wounds

Care of pressure ulcers

◆ Pressure ulcers are ischemic lesions that result when pressure against the tissues impairs circulation and delivery of oxygen and other life-sustaining nutrients, damaging the skin and underlying structures.

◆ The pressure may be applied with great force for a short period or with less force over a longer period.

◆ Most pressure ulcers develop over bony prominences, where pressure, friction, and shearing force combine to break down skin and underlying tissues.

◆ Common sites include the sacrum, coccyx, ischial tuberosities, and greater trochanters. (See *Pressure points: Common sites for ulcers.*)

◆ Particularly in bedridden and relatively immobile patients, other common sites include the skin over the vertebrae, scapulae, ears, elbows, knees, and heels.

Alert Untreated, pressure ulcers can lead to serious infection.

◆ Successful treatment involves relieving pressure, restoring circulation and, if possible, resolving or managing related disorders.

◆ Typically, the duration and effectiveness of treatment depend on the characteristics of the pressure ulcer. (See *Staging pressure ulcers,* pages 338 and 339.)

Pressure points: Common sites for ulcers

Ulcers may develop at pressure points, which are shown in these illustrations. To help prevent ulcers, stress the importance of repositioning the patient often and checking the skin carefully for changes.

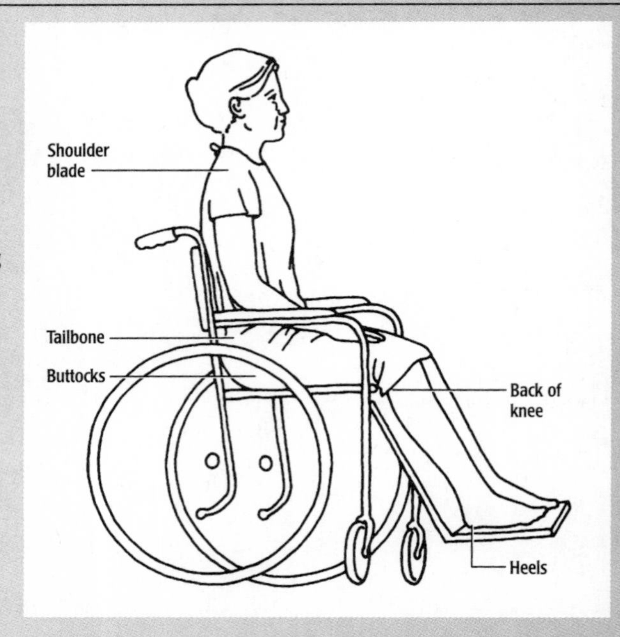

◆ Ideally, prevention is the key to avoiding extensive therapy.
◆ Preventive measures include:
– ensuring adequate nourishment
– maintaining mobility to relieve pressure and promote circulation.
◆ When a pressure ulcer develops despite preventive efforts, treatment includes:
– frequent repositioning to relieve pressure
– pressure-reduction devices, such as beds, mattresses, mattress overlays, and chair cushions. (See *Pressure-reduction devices,* page 340.)
◆ Treatment also includes:
– topical drugs
– wound cleaning
– debridement
– moist dressings to support wound healing.
◆ The nurse usually performs or coordinates treatments according to facility policy. The procedures described here address cleaning and dressing pressure ulcers. Always follow standard precautions.

Equipment

Hypoallergenic tape or elastic netting ◆ piston-type irrigating system ◆ two pairs of gloves ◆ normal saline solution, as ordered ◆ sterile 4″ × 4″ gauze pads ◆ selected topical dressing (moist saline gauze, hydrocolloid, transparent,

(Text continues on page 340.)

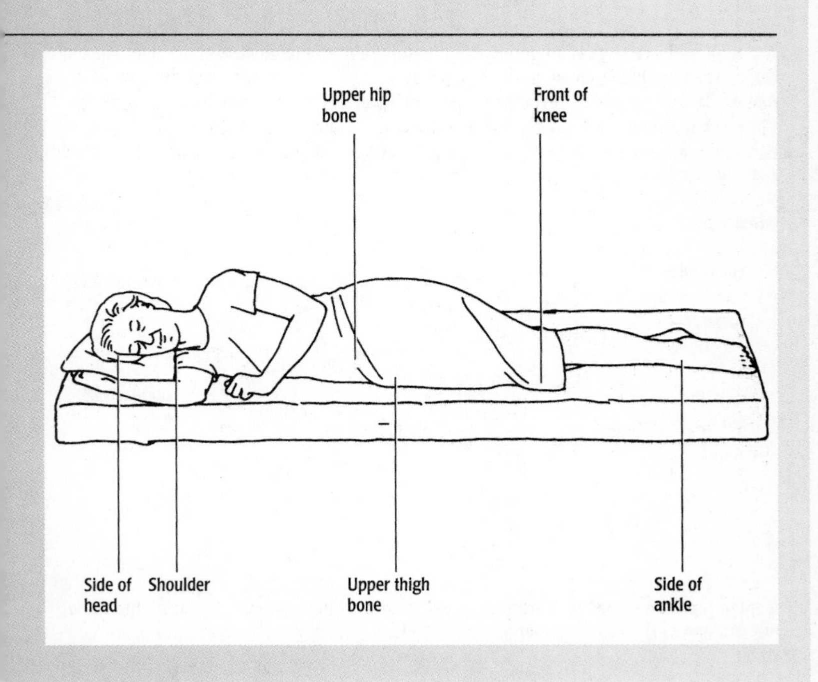

Staging pressure ulcers

The staging system described here is based on the recommendations of the National Pressure Ulcer Advisory Panel (NPUAP) (Consensus Conference, 1991) and the Agency for Health Care Policy and Research (Clinical Practice Guidelines for Treatment of Pressure Ulcers, 1992, 1994). The definition of a stage I pressure ulcer was updated by the NPUAP in 1998.

Stage I

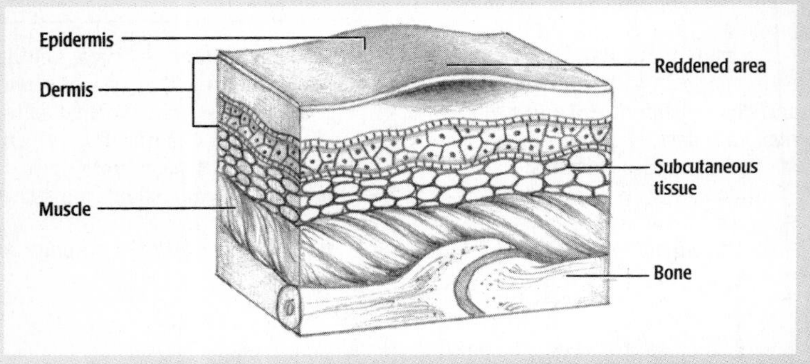

A stage I pressure ulcer is an observable pressure-related alteration of intact skin. The indicators, compared with the adjacent or opposite area of the body, may include changes in one or more of these features: Skin temperature (warmth or coolness), tissue consistency (firm or boggy feel), or sensation (pain or itching). The ulcer appears as a defined area of persistent redness in lightly pigmented skin; in darker skin, the ulcer may have a persistent red, blue, or purple hue.

Stage II

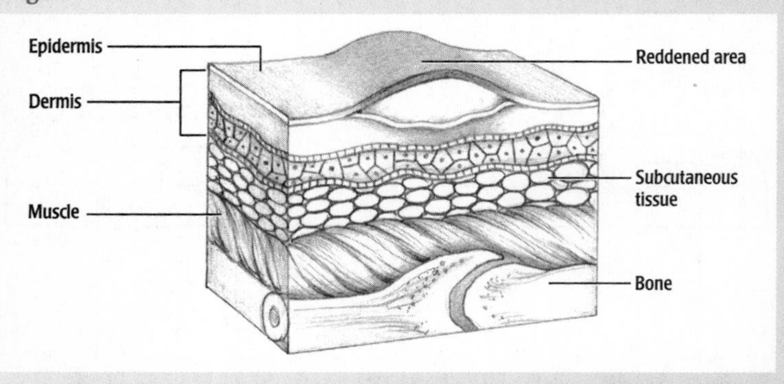

A stage II pressure ulcer is characterized by partial-thickness skin loss involving the epidermis or dermis. The ulcer is superficial and appears as an abrasion, a blister, or a shallow crater.

Stage III

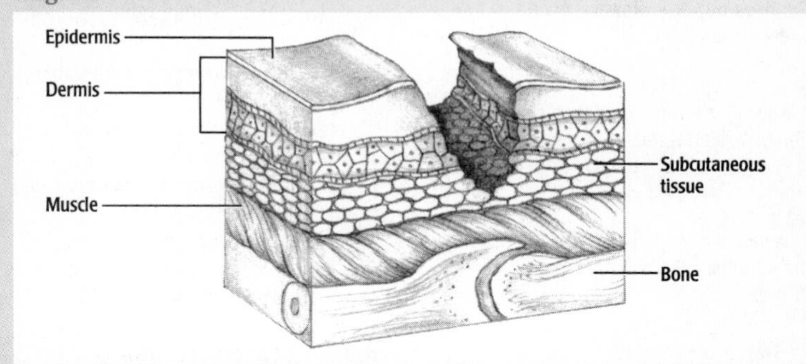

A stage III pressure ulcer is characterized by full-thickness skin loss that involves damage or necrosis of the subcutaneous tissue that may extend down to, but not through, the underlying fascia. The ulcer appears as a deep crater that may undermine the adjacent tissue.

Stage IV

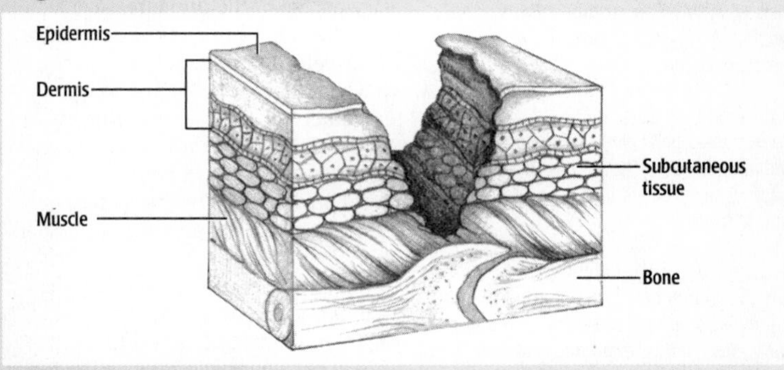

A stage IV pressure ulcer is characterized by full-thickness skin loss and extensive destruction, tissue necrosis, or damage to the muscle, bone, or support structures (for example, tendon or joint capsule). Stage IV pressure ulcers may also be associated with tunneling or sinus tracts (channeling that extends from the wound).

alginate, foam, or hydrogel) ◆ linen-saver pads ◆ impervious plastic trash bag ◆ disposable wound-measuring device ◆ sterile cotton swabs ◆ optional: 21G needle and syringe, alcohol pad, pressure-reducing device, turning sheet

Implementation

◆ Assemble the equipment at the patient's bedside.
◆ Cut the tape into strips for securing dressings.
◆ Loosen the lids on cleaning solutions and drugs for easy removal.
◆ Make sure that the impervious plastic trash bag is within reach.
◆ Before performing any dressing change, wash your hands and implement standard precautions.

Cleaning the pressure ulcer

◆ Provide privacy and explain the procedure to the patient to reduce fear and promote cooperation.
◆ Position the patient in a way that maximizes his comfort while giving easy access to the pressure ulcer.
◆ Cover the bed linens with a linen-saver pad to prevent soiling.
◆ Open the normal saline solution container and the piston syringe.
◆ Carefully pour normal saline solution into an irrigation container to avoid splashing. (The container may be clean or sterile, depending on facility policy.)
◆ Insert the piston syringe into the opening in the irrigation container.
◆ Open the packages of supplies.
◆ Put on gloves and remove the old dressing from the pressure ulcer.
◆ Discard the soiled dressing in the impervious plastic trash bag to avoid contaminating the sterile field and spreading infection.
◆ Inspect the wound. Note the color, amount, and odor of drainage and necrotic debris. (See *Tailoring wound care to wound color.*)

Pressure-reduction devices

The use of special pads, mattresses, and beds can help relieve pressure when a patient is unable to move himself.

Gel pads
Gel pads disperse pressure over a wider surface area.

Water mattress or pads
A wave effect provides even distribution of body weight.

Alternating-pressure air mattress
Alternating deflation and inflation of the mattress tubes changes the areas of pressure.

Foam mattress or pads
Foam areas, which must be at least 3" (7.5 cm) thick, cushion skin and minimize pressure.

Low–air-loss beds
The surface of low–air-loss beds consists of inflated air cushions. Each section is adjusted to provide optimal pressure relief.

Air-fluidized beds
Air-fluidized beds contain beads that move under an airflow to support the patient, thus reducing shearing force and friction.

Mechanical lifting devices
Lift sheets and other mechanical lifting devices prevent shearing by lifting the patient rather than dragging him across the bed.

Padding
Pillows, towels, and soft blankets can reduce pressure in body hollows.

Foot cradle
A foot cradle lifts the bed linens to relieve pressure over the feet.

Tailoring wound care to wound color

You can promote healing by keeping a wound moist, clean, and free from debris. For open wounds, you can use wound color to guide the specific management approach that will aid healing

WOUND COLOR	MANAGEMENT TECHNIQUE
Red	◆ Cover the wound, keep it moist and clean, and protect it from trauma. ◆ Use a transparent dressing (such as Tegaderm or OpSite) over a gauze dressing moistened with normal saline solution. Or use a hydrogel, foam, or hydrocolloid dressing to insulate and protect the wound.
Yellow	◆ Clean the wound and remove the yellow layer. ◆ Cover the wound with a moisture-retaining dressing, such as a hydrogel or foam dressing, or a moist gauze dressing with or without a debriding enzyme. ◆ Consider hydrotherapy with whirlpool or pulsatile lavage.
Black	◆ Debride the wound as ordered. Use an enzyme product (such as Accuzyme or Panafil) or hydrotherapy with whirlpool or pulsatile lavage. ◆ Don't debride noninfected heel ulcers or wounds with an inadequate blood supply. Keep them clean and dry.

◆ Measure the perimeter of the wound with the disposable wound-measuring device (a square, transparent card with concentric circles arranged in a bull's-eye fashion and bordered with a straightedge ruler).
◆ Using the piston syringe, apply full force to irrigate the pressure ulcer to remove necrotic debris and help to decrease bacteria in the wound.
◆ Remove and discard the soiled gloves and put on a fresh pair.
◆ Insert a sterile cotton swab into the wound to gauge the depth of wound tunneling or undermining. Tunneling usually signals extension of the wound along fascial planes.
◆ Look at the condition of the skin and the ulcer. Note the character of the clean wound bed and the surrounding skin.

Alert If you observe adherent necrotic material, notify a wound care specialist or a physician to ensure that appropriate debridement is performed.

◆ Prepare to apply the selected topical dressing. Directions for application of topical moist saline gauze, hydrocolloid, transparent, alginate, foam, and hydrogel dressings follow. For other dressings or topical agents, follow facility protocol or manufacturer instructions. (See *Wound care dressings,* page 342.)

Applying a moist saline gauze dressing

◆ Irrigate the pressure ulcer with normal saline solution. Blot the surrounding skin dry with a sterile 4″ × 4″ gauze pad.

Wound care dressings

Some dressings absorb moisture from a wound bed, whereas others add moisture. Use the scale below to quickly determine the category of dressing that's appropriate for the patient.

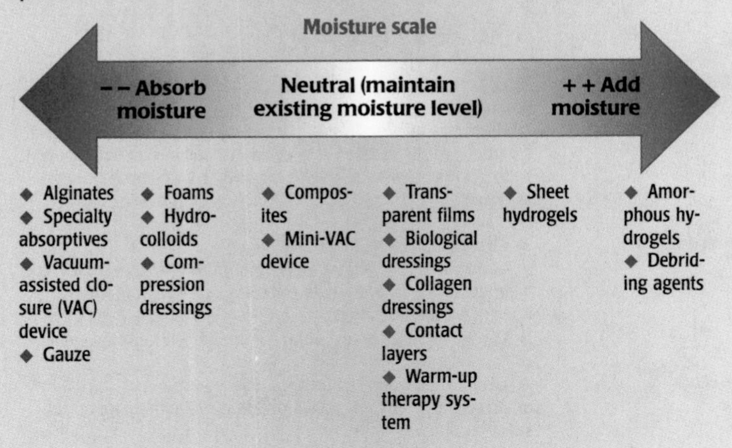

◆ Moisten the gauze dressing with normal saline solution.
◆ Gently place the dressing over the surface of the ulcer. To separate surfaces within the wound, gently place a dressing between opposing wound surfaces.
◆ To avoid damage to tissues, don't pack the gauze tightly.
◆ Change the dressing often enough to keep the wound moist. (See *Choosing a wound dressing*.)

Applying a hydrocolloid dressing

◆ Irrigate the pressure ulcer with normal saline solution. Blot the surrounding skin dry with a sterile 4″ × 4″ gauze pad.
◆ Choose a clean, dry, pre-sized dressing, or cut one to overlap the pressure ulcer by about 1″ (2.5 cm).
◆ Pull the release paper from the adherent side of the dressing and apply the dressing to the wound. To minimize irritation, carefully smooth out wrinkles as you apply the dressing.
◆ If the edges of the dressing must be secured with hypoallergenic tape, apply a skin sealant to the intact skin around the ulcer. The sealant protects the skin and promotes adherence of the tape.
◆ After the area dries, tape the dressing to the skin. Avoid using tension or pressure when applying the tape.
◆ Remove your gloves and discard them in the impervious plastic trash bag. Dispose of refuse according to facility policy and wash your hands.
◆ Change a hydrocolloid dressing every 2 to 7 days as needed — for example, if the patient complains of pain, if the dressing no longer adheres, or if leakage occurs.

Applying a transparent dressing

◆ Irrigate the pressure ulcer with normal saline solution. Blot the surround-

Choosing a wound dressing

Use the information below to determine the type of dressing that's appropriate for the patient.

Alginate dressings

Made from seaweed, alginate dressings are nonwoven, absorptive dressings that are available as soft, white sterile pads or ropes. They absorb excessive exudate and may be used on infected wounds. As these dressings absorb exudate, they turn into a gel that keeps the wound bed moist and promotes healing. When exudate is no longer excessive, switch to another type of dressing.

Antimicrobials

These dressings are infused with silver, iodine, or polyhexethylene biguanide. They come in many forms and types and are designed to reduce or prevent wound infection. Antimicrobials are used in draining, exudating, and nonhealing wounds as a primary or secondary dressing.

Collagens

These are absorbent, nonadherent dressings made of collagen – which encourages new collagen fiber growth and tissue development as well as wound debridement. They're available as sheets, pads, particles, and gels. They conform well to a wound surface and can be used with topical agents. They can be used for wounds with minimal to heavy exudate. A secondary dressing is required.

Foam dressings

Foam dressings are spongelike polymer dressings that may be impregnated or coated with other materials. They're somewhat absorptive and may be have an adhesive border. These dressings promote moist wound healing and are useful when a nonadherent surface is desired.

Gauze dressings

Made of absorptive cotton or synthetic fabric, gauze dressings are permeable to water, water vapor, and oxygen and may be impregnated with hydrogel or another agent. If you're uncertain about which type of dressing to use, you may apply a gauze dressing moistened with saline solution until a wound specialist recommends definitive treatment.

Hydrocolloid dressings

Hydrocolloid dressings are adhesive, moldable wafers made of a carbohydrate-based material. They usually have waterproof backings. These dressings are impermeable to oxygen, water, and water vapor, and most have some absorptive properties.

Hydrogel dressings

Water-based and nonadherent, hydrogel dressings are polymer-based dressings that have some absorptive properties. They're available as a gel in a tube, as flexible sheets, and as saturated gauze packing strips. They may have a cooling effect that eases pain, and they're used when the wound needs moisture.

Transparent film dressings

Transparent film dressings are clear, adherent, and nonabsorptive. These polymer-based dressings are permeable to oxygen and water vapor but not to water. Their transparency allows inspection of the wound. Because they can't absorb drainage, they're used on partial-thickness wounds with minimal exudate.

ing skin dry with a sterile 4″ × 4″ gauze pad.

- Select a dressing to overlap the ulcer by 2″ (5 cm).
- Gently lay the dressing over the ulcer. To prevent shearing force, don't stretch the dressing.
- Press firmly on the edges of the dressing to promote adherence. Although this type of dressing is self-adhesive, you may need to tape the edges to prevent them from curling.
- Change the dressing every 3 to 7 days, depending on the amount of drainage.

Applying an alginate dressing

- Irrigate the pressure ulcer with normal saline solution. Blot the surrounding skin dry with a sterile 4″ × 4″ gauze pad.
- Apply the alginate dressing to the surface of the ulcer.
- Cover the area with a secondary dressing (such as gauze pads) as ordered.
- Secure the dressing with hypoallergenic tape or elastic netting.
- If the wound is draining heavily, change the dressing once or twice daily for the first 3 to 5 days. As the drainage decreases, change the dressing less often — every 2 to 4 days, or as ordered.
- When the drainage stops or the wound bed looks dry, stop using an alginate dressing.

Applying a foam dressing

- Irrigate the pressure ulcer with normal saline solution. Blot the surrounding skin dry with a sterile 4″ × 4″ gauze pad.
- Gently lay the foam dressing over the ulcer.
- Use hypoallergenic tape, elastic netting, or gauze to hold the dressing in place.
- Change the dressing when the foam no longer absorbs the exudate.

Applying a hydrogel dressing

- Irrigate the pressure ulcer with normal saline solution. Blot the surrounding skin dry with a sterile 4″ × 4″ gauze pad.
- Apply gel to the wound bed.
- Cover the area with a secondary dressing.
- If the dressing that you select comes in sheet form, cut the dressing to match the wound base. Otherwise, the surrounding intact skin can become macerated.
- Change the dressing daily or as needed to keep the wound bed moist.
- Hydrogel dressings also come in a prepackaged, saturated gauze for wounds that need to have "dead space" filled. Follow the manufacturer's directions.

Preventing pressure ulcers

- Turn and reposition the patient every 1 to 2 hours, unless contraindicated.
- When turning the patient, lift rather than slide him because sliding increases friction and shear. Use a turning sheet and get help from coworkers, if needed. (See *Preventing skin tears.*)
- Adapt position changes to the patient's needs.
- Emphasize the importance of regular position changes to the patient and family.
- Encourage family participation in treating and preventing pressure ulcers by having family members perform a position change correctly after you've shown them how.
- Post a turning schedule at the patient's bedside.
- Use pillows to position the patient in proper body alignment to increase comfort.
- Remove wrinkles from the sheets because they can increase pressure and cause discomfort.

◆ Avoid placing the patient directly on the trochanter. Instead, place him on his side at about a 30-degree angle.
◆ For a patient who can't turn himself or who's turned on a schedule, use a pressure-reducing device, such as air, gel, or a 4" (10 cm) foam-mattress overlay.
◆ Low- or high-air-loss therapy may be needed to reduce excessive pressure and promote evaporation of excess moisture.
◆ As appropriate, implement active or passive range-of-motion exercises to relieve pressure and promote circulation. To save time, combine these exercises with bathing, if applicable.
◆ Except for brief periods, avoid raising the head of the bed more than 30 degrees to prevent shearing pressure.
◆ If the patient is confined to a chair or wheelchair, tell him to shift his weight every 15 minutes to promote blood flow to compressed tissues.
- Show a paraplegic patient how to shift his weight by doing push-ups in the wheelchair.
- If he needs help, sit next to him and help him shift his weight to one buttock for 60 seconds. Repeat the procedure on the other side.
- Provide him with pressure-relieving cushions, as appropriate.
- Avoid seating the patient on a rubber or plastic doughnut because it may increase localized pressure at vulnerable points.
◆ Adjust or pad appliances, casts, or splints, as needed, to ensure proper fit and avoid increased pressure and impaired circulation.
◆ Tell the patient to avoid heat lamps and harsh soaps because they dry the skin. Applying lotion after bathing will help to keep his skin moist.
◆ Also tell him to avoid vigorous massage because it can damage capillaries.
◆ If the patient's condition permits, recommend a diet that includes adequate calories, protein, and vitamins.

Preventing skin tears

With aging, the risk of skin tearing increases. By taking these precautions, you can substantially reduce a patient's risk.

Prevent skin tears by:
◆ using proper techniques for lifting, positioning, transferring, and turning the patient to reduce or eliminate friction or shear
◆ padding support surfaces where risk is greatest, such as bed rails and limb supports on a wheelchair
◆ using pillows or cushions to support the patient's arms and legs
◆ telling the patient to add protection by wearing long-sleeved shirts and long pants, as weather permits
◆ using nonadhering dressings or those with minimal adherent, such as paper tape, and using a skin barrier wipe before applying dressings
◆ removing tape cautiously using the push-pull technique
◆ using wraps, such as a stockinette or soft gauze, to protect areas of skin where the risk of tearing is high
◆ telling the patient to avoid sudden or sharp movements that can pull the skin and possibly cause a skin tear
◆ applying moisturizing lotion twice daily to areas at risk.

Dietary therapy may involve nutritional consultation and the use of food supplements, enteral feeding, or total parenteral nutrition.
◆ If diarrhea develops or if the patient is incontinent, clean and dry the soiled skin. Then apply a protective moisture barrier to prevent skin maceration.
◆ Make sure the patient, his family, and caregivers learn strategies for preventing and treating pressure ulcers so that they understand the importance of care, the choices available, the rationales for treatment, and their own role in selecting pressure ulcer prevention

goals and shaping the patient's care plan.

◆ Recheck pressure ulcers at least weekly.

Special considerations

◆ Avoid using elbow or heel protectors that fasten with a single narrow strap or that contain elastic too tight for the diameter of the patient's arm or foot. The strap or tight elastic may impair neurovascular function in the involved hand, arm, or foot.

◆ Avoid using artificial sheepskin. It doesn't reduce pressure and it may create a false sense of security.

◆ Repair of stage III and stage IV ulcers may require surgical intervention (such as direct closure, skin grafting, and flaps), depending on the patient's needs.

◆ Infection may cause foul-smelling drainage, persistent pain, severe erythema, induration, and elevated skin and body temperatures. Advancing infection or cellulitis can lead to septicemia.

◆ Severe erythema may signal worsening cellulitis, which indicates that the offending organisms have invaded the tissue and are no longer localized.

Documentation

◆ Record date and time of all treatments.

◆ Record specific treatments given.

◆ Note preventive strategies performed.

◆ Note the location and size (length, width, and depth) of the pressure ulcer.

◆ Note the color and appearance of the wound bed.

◆ Record the amount, odor, color, and consistency of drainage.

◆ Note the condition of the surrounding skin.

◆ Make any updates to the care plan.

◆ Note any change in the condition or size of the pressure ulcer (on the clinical record).

◆ Record any elevation of skin temperature (on the clinical record).

◆ Note when the physician was notified of pertinent abnormal observations.

◆ Record the patient's daily temperature (on the graphic sheet) to allow easy review of body temperature patterns.

Care of traumatic wounds

◆ Traumatic wounds include abrasions, lacerations, bites, and penetrating wounds.

- In an abrasion, the skin is scraped and the skin surface partially lost.
- In a laceration, tearing of the skin causes jagged, irregular edges. The severity of a laceration depends on its size, depth, and location.
- Traumatic bite wounds may be caused by animals or humans.
- A penetrating wound can occur when a pointed object, such as a knife or glass fragment, penetrates the skin.

Equipment

Sterile basin ◆ normal saline solution ◆ sterile 4″ × 4″ gauze pads ◆ sterile gloves ◆ clean gloves ◆ surgical brush ◆ nonadherent pads ◆ petroleum gauze ◆ antibacterial ointment ◆ 50-ml catheter-tip syringe ◆ porous tape ◆ linen-saver pad

Implementation

◆ Place a linen-saver pad under the area to be cleaned.

◆ Remove any clothing covering the wound.

◆ Assemble the needed equipment at the patient's bedside.

◆ Fill a sterile basin with normal saline solution.

Caring for a traumatic wound

When caring for a patient with a traumatic wound, begin by checking the ABCs: airway, breathing, and circulation. Move on to the wound itself only after the ABCs are stable. Here are the basic steps to follow in caring for each type of traumatic wound.

Abrasion

- Flush the area of the abrasion with normal saline solution or a wound-cleaning solution.
- Use a sterile 4″ × 4″ gauze pad moistened with normal saline solution to remove dirt or gravel. Gently rub toward the entry point to work contaminants back out the way they entered.
- If the wound is extremely dirty, you may need to assist in scrubbing it with a surgical brush. This process is painful for the patient.
- Allow a small wound to dry and form a scab. Cover a larger wound with a nonadherent pad or petroleum gauze and a light dressing. Apply antibacterial ointment, if ordered.

Laceration

- Moisten a sterile 4″ × 4″ gauze pad with normal saline solution or a wound-cleaning solution. Gently clean the wound, beginning at the center and working out to about 2″ (5 cm) beyond the edge of the wound.
- When the pad becomes soiled, discard it and use a new one. Continue until the wound looks clean.
- If needed, irrigate the wound with a 50-ml catheter-tip syringe and normal saline solution.
- Assist the physician in suturing the wound, if needed; apply sterile strips of porous tape if suturing isn't needed.
- Apply antibacterial ointment, as ordered, to prevent infection.
- Apply a dry sterile dressing over the wound to absorb drainage and help prevent bacterial contamination.

Bite

- Immediately irrigate the wound with copious amounts of normal saline solution. Don't immerse and soak the wound because this may let bacteria float back into the tissue.
- Clean the wound with sterile 4″ × 4″ gauze pads and an antiseptic solution such as povidone-iodine.
- Assist with debridement, if ordered.
- Apply a loose dressing. If the bite is located on an extremity, elevate the area to reduce swelling.
- Ask the patient what bit him to determine whether he's at risk for rabies. Give rabies and tetanus shots, as needed.

Penetrating wound

- If the wound is minor, allow it to bleed for a few minutes before cleaning it. A larger puncture wound may require irrigation.
- Cover the wound with a dry dressing.
- If the wound contains an embedded foreign object, such as a shard of glass or metal, stabilize the object until the physician can remove it.
- When the object is removed and bleeding is under control, clean the wound as you would a laceration.

- Depending on the nature and location of the wound, wear sterile or clean gloves to avoid spreading infection.
- Give pain medication, if ordered.
- Wash your hands and apply appropriate protective equipment.
- For a description of the specific care of a traumatic wound, see *Caring for a traumatic wound.*

Special considerations

- When irrigating a traumatic wound, avoid using more than 8 pounds per square inch of pressure. High-pressure irrigation with a 3 cc or 10 cc syringe and small gauge needle can deter healing and let bacteria infiltrate the tissue.
- Avoid cleaning a traumatic wound with alcohol because doing so causes pain and tissue dehydration. Also avoid antiseptics for wound cleaning because they can impede healing.
- Observe the patient for signs and symptoms of infection, such as warm, red skin at the site or purulent discharge.
- Observe all dressings. If edema is present, adjust the dressing to avoid impairing circulation to the area.

Documentation

- Record the date and time of the procedure.
- Note the size and condition of the wound.
- Record drug administration.
- Note specific wound care measures taken.
- Note patient teaching provided.

10 Pain and its management

Understanding pain

◆ Pain is a subjective experience unique to the person experiencing it. Any report of pain must be investigated and addressed.
◆ The Joint Commission on Accreditation of Healthcare Organizations (JCAHO) has designated pain level as "the fifth vital sign." Nurses are required to determine each patient's pain on admission and frequently thereafter, and to address pain in the care plan.
◆ Pain has a sensory component and a reaction component.
- The sensory component involves an electrical impulse that travels to the central nervous system, where it's perceived as pain.
- The response to this perception is the reaction component.
◆ Pain may be acute, chronic, or both. (See *Differentiating acute and chronic pain.*)
- Acute pain is caused by tissue damage from injury, disease, or surgical or diagnostic procedures. It varies in intensity from mild to severe and lasts briefly. It's considered a protective mechanism because it warns of current or potential damage or organ disease.
- Chronic pain is pain that has lasted 6 months or longer and is ongoing. Although it may be as intense as acute pain, it isn't a warning of tissue damage.
◆ It's important for you to understand how pain is determined.
◆ The most valid identification of pain comes from the patient's own reports. (See *PQRST: The alphabet of pain identification.*)
◆ Many pain identification tools are available. The chosen tool should be used consistently so that everyone on the health care team is speaking the same language when addressing the patient's pain.
◆ The three most common pain identification tools used by clinicians are the visual analog scale (see *Visual analog scale*), the numeric rating scale (see *Numeric rating scale,* page 352), and the FACES scale (see *Wong-Baker FACES scale,* page 352).
◆ Pain may cause many physiological and psychological responses; watch

Differentiating acute and chronic pain

Acute pain may cause certain physiologic and behavioral changes that you won't observe in a patient with chronic pain.

TYPE OF PAIN	PHYSIOLOGIC EVIDENCE	BEHAVIORAL EVIDENCE
Acute	◆ Increased respirations ◆ Increased pulse ◆ Increased blood pressure ◆ Dilated pupils ◆ Diaphoresis	◆ Restlessness ◆ Distraction ◆ Worry ◆ Distress
Chronic	◆ Normal respirations, pulse, blood pressure, and pupil size ◆ No diaphoresis	◆ Reduced or absent physical activity ◆ Despair or depression ◆ Hopelessness

PQRST: The alphabet of pain identification

The PQRST mnemonic device is commonly used to obtain more information about the patient's pain. It includes the following questions to help elicit important details.

Provocative or palliative

- What provokes or worsens your pain?
- What relieves your pain or causes it to subside?

Quality or quantity

- What does the pain feel like? For example, is it aching, intense, knifelike, burning, or cramping?
- Are you having pain right now? If so, is it more or less severe than usual?
- To what degree does the pain affect your normal activities?
- Do you have other symptoms along with the pain, such as nausea or vomiting?

Region and radiation

- Where is your pain?
- Does the pain radiate to other parts of your body?

Severity

- How severe is your pain? How would you rate it on a scale of 0 to 10, with 0 being no pain and 10 being the worst pain imaginable?
- How would you describe the intensity of your pain at its best? At its worst? Right now?

Timing

- When did your pain begin?
- At what time of day is your pain least? At what time of day is it greatest?
- Is the onset sudden or gradual?
- Is the pain constant or intermittent?

Visual analog scale

With the visual analog scale, have the patient place a mark on the scale to indicate his current level of pain, as shown here.

NO PAIN ——————————————X———— **PAIN AS BAD AS IT CAN BE**

Numeric rating scale

A numeric rating scale can help the patient quantify his pain. To use this scale, the patient chooses a number from 0 (indicating no pain) to 10 (indicating the worst pain imaginable) to reflect his current level of pain. He can either circle the number on the scale or state the number that best describes his pain.

NO PAIN	0	1	2	3	4	5	6	7	8	9	10	PAIN AS BAD AS IT CAN BE

Wong-Baker FACES scale

A child or an adult with language difficulties may not be able to express the pain he's feeling. In such instances, a pain intensity scale such as the one shown below may be helpful. To use this scale, the patient chooses the face that best represents the severity of his pain.

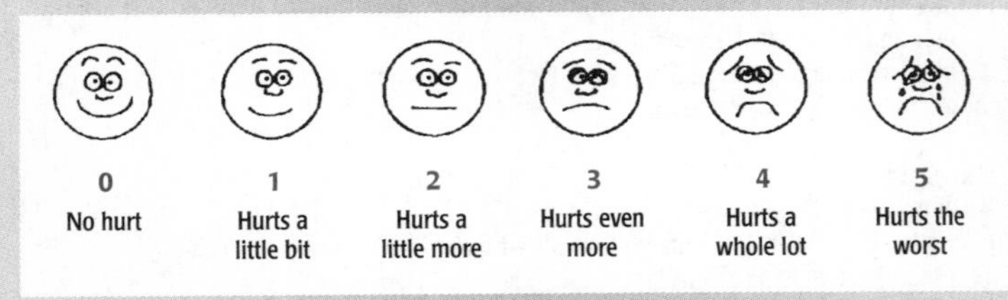

From Hockenberry MJ, Wilson D, Winkelstein ML: *Wong's Essentials of Pediatric Nursing,*, ed. 7, St. Louis, 2005, p. 1259. Used with permission. Copyright, Mosby.

carefully for them whenever you care for the patient. (See *Pain behavior checklist.*)

Understanding pain management

◆ Adequate pain control depends on effective identification and interventions, including drug therapy. To provide the best care possible, work with physicians and other members of the health care team to carry out an individualized pain management program for each patient.

◆ Two drug classes are commonly used for pain management:
- nonopioids
- opioids

◆ Nonopioids are the first choice for managing mild pain. They decrease pain by inhibiting inflammation at the injury site or by blocking the entrance of pain signals to the brain. Examples of nonopioids are:
- acetaminophen
- nonsteroidal anti-inflammatory drugs

Pain behavior checklist

A patient often communicates pain, distress, or suffering through pain behaviors. Place a check in the box next to each behavior that you observe or infer while talking with the patient.

- ☐ Grimacing
- ☐ Moaning
- ☐ Sighing
- ☐ Clenching the teeth
- ☐ Holding or supporting the painful body area
- ☐ Sitting rigidly
- ☐ Shifting posture or position often
- ☐ Moving in a guarded or protective manner
- ☐ Moving very slowly
- ☐ Taking medication
- ☐ Using a cane, a cervical collar, or another prosthetic device
- ☐ Requesting help with walking
- ☐ Stopping often while walking
- ☐ Lying down during the day
- ☐ Avoiding physical activity
- ☐ Being irritable
- ☐ Asking such questions as, "Why did this happen to me?"
- ☐ Asking to be relieved from tasks or activities

Controlled substance schedules

Drugs regulated by the Controlled Susbtances Act of 1970 are divided into the following groups or schedules:

◆ Schedule I (C-I): High abuse potential and no accepted medical use. Examples include heroin, cocaine, and LSD.
◆ Schedule II (C-II): High abuse potential with severe dependence potential. Examples include opioids, amphetamines, and some barbiturates.
◆ Schedule III (C-III): Less abuse potential than schedule II drugs and moderate dependence potential. Examples include nonbarbiturate sedatives, nonamphetamine stimulants, anabolic steroids, dronabinol, and limited amounts of certain opioids.
◆ Schedule IV (C-IV): Less abuse potential than schedule III drugs and limited dependence potential. Examples include some sedatives, anxiolytics, and nonopioid analgesics
◆ Schedule V (C-V): Limited abuse potential. This category includes mainly small amounts of opioids, such as codeine, used as antitussives or antidiarrheals. Under federal law, limited quantities of certain C-V drugs may be purchased without a prescription directly from a pharmacist if allowed under specific state laws. The purchaser must be at least age 18 and must furnish suitable identification. All such transactions must be recorded by the dispensing pharmacist.

– salicylates such as aspirin.
◆ Opioids contain either a derivative of the opium plant or a synthetic drug that imitates such a derivative. Opioids work by blocking the release of neurotransmitters that help transmit pain signals to the brain. The Food and Drug Administration (FDA) regulates the prescription of these drugs by categorizing them into controlled substance schedules. (See *Controlled substance schedules*.)

◆ Some of the most common pain management drugs include acetaminophen, aspirin, codeine, fentanyl, hydromorphone, ibuprofen, ketorolac, and morphine. (See *Common pain management drugs.*)

Common pain management drugs

DRUG	INDICATIONS	ADVERSE EFFECTS
acetaminophen Acephen, Anacin Aspirin Free, Tylenol	◆ Mild pain ◆ Fever	◆ Leukopenia, neutropenia, pancytopenia, thrombocytopenia ◆ Severe liver damage ◆ Hypoglycemia
aspirin ASA, Ascriptin, Bufferin	◆ Mild pain ◆ Fever ◆ Transient ischemic attacks and thromboembolic disorders ◆ Treatment or reduction of the risk of myocardial infarction (MI) in a patient with previous MI or unstable angina ◆ Pericarditis after an acute MI ◆ Prevention of reocclusion in coronary revascularization procedures ◆ Stent implantation	◆ Hearing loss, tinnitus ◆ Dyspepsia, GI bleeding, GI distress, nausea, occult bleeding ◆ Acute renal insufficiency ◆ Leukopenia, prolonged bleeding time, thrombocytopenia ◆ Hepatitis, liver dysfunction ◆ Rash ◆ Angioedema, hypersensitivity reactions (anaphylaxis, asthma), Reye's syndrome
codeine phosphate, codeine sulfate	◆ Mild to moderate pain ◆ Nonproductive cough	◆ Clouded sensorium, dizziness, euphoria, light-headedness, sedation ◆ Bradycardia, hypotension ◆ Constipation, dry mouth, ileus, nausea, vomiting ◆ Urine retention ◆ Respiratory depression ◆ Diaphoresis

◆ Sometimes, combining analgesics can provide added pain relief. (See *Common nonopioid analgesic combinations,* pages 358 to 360, and *Common opioid analgesic combinations,* pages 360 to 362.)

SPECIAL CONSIDERATIONS

◆ Use cautiously in patients with a history of chronic alcohol abuse because hepatotoxicity may occur with therapeutic doses. Also use cautiously in patients with hepatic or cardiovascular disease, impaired renal function, or viral infection.
◆ Know the patient's total daily acetaminophen intake from all sources, including combination drugs, such as Percocet (acetaminophen and oxycodone). Toxicity can occur.
◆ Monitor prothrombin time (PT) and International Normalized Ratio in patients who take oral anticoagulants or long-term acetaminophen.

◆ Contraindicated in patients with glucose-6–phosphate dehydrogenase deficiency or bleeding disorders, such as hemophilia, von Willebrand's disease, or telangiectasia. Also contraindicated in patients with sensitivity reactions to nonsteroidal anti-inflammatory drugs (NSAIDs).
◆ Use cautiously in patients with GI lesions, impaired renal function, hypoprothrombinemia, vitamin K deficiency, thrombotic thrombocytopenic purpura, or hepatic impairment.
◆ Use cautiously in patients with a history of GI disease (especially peptic ulcer disease), increased risk of GI bleeding, or decreased renal function.
◆ Give 8 oz (237 ml) of water or milk with salicylates to ensure passage into the stomach. Have the patient sit up for 15 to 30 minutes after taking salicylates to prevent lodging in the esophagus.
◆ Monitor the patient's vital signs often, especially temperature.
◆ Salicylates may mask evidence of acute infection (fever, myalgia, erythema); carefully observe patients who are at risk for infection, such as those with diabetes.
◆ Monitor the complete blood count, platelet count, PT, blood urea nitrogen level, serum creatinine level, and the results of liver function studies periodically during salicylate therapy to detect abnormalities.
◆ Check the patient for evidence of hemorrhage, such as petechiae, bruising, coffee-ground vomitus, and black, tarry stools.

◆ Use cautiously in elderly or debilitated patients and in those with impaired renal or hepatic function, head injuries, increased intracranial pressure (ICP), increased cerebrospinal fluid (CSF) pressure, hypothyroidism, Addison's disease, acute alcoholism, central nervous system depression, bronchial asthma, chronic obstructive pulmonary disease (COPD), respiratory depression, or shock.
◆ Don't mix with other solutions because codeine phosphate is incompatible with many drugs.
◆ Patients who become physically dependent on the drug may have acute withdrawal symptoms if given an opioid antagonist.
◆ The drug may delay gastric emptying, increase biliary tract pressure resulting from contraction of the sphincter of Oddi, and interfere with hepatobiliary imaging studies.

(continued)

Common pain management drugs *(continued)*

DRUG	INDICATIONS	ADVERSE EFFECTS
fentanyl citrate Sublimaze; Fentanyl Transdermal System (Duragesic-25, Duragesic-50, Duragesic-75, Duragesic-100)	◆ Preoperative analgesic ◆ Adjunct to general anesthetic; low-dose regimen for minor procedures; moderate-dose regimen for major procedures; high-dose regimen for complicated procedures ◆ Postoperative analgesic ◆ Management of chronic pain in a patient who can't be managed by lesser means ◆ Management of breakthrough cancer pain	◆ Asthenia, clouded sensorium, confusion, sedation, somnolence ◆ Arrhythmias ◆ Constipation, dry mouth, nausea, vomiting ◆ Urine retention ◆ Apnea, respiratory depression
hydromorphone hydrochloride Dilaudid	◆ Moderate to severe pain ◆ Cough	◆ Clouded sensorium, dizziness, euphoria, sedation, somnolence ◆ Bradycardia, hypotension ◆ Constipation, nausea, vomiting ◆ Urine retention ◆ Bronchospasm, respiratory depression
ibuprofen Advil, Motrin, Motrin IB, Nuprin	◆ Arthritis, gout ◆ Mild to moderate pain, headache, backache, minor aches from the common cold ◆ Fever reduction	◆ Acute renal failure ◆ Agranulocytosis, aplastic anemia, leukopenia, neutropenia, pancytopenia, thrombocytopenia ◆ Bronchospasm ◆ Stevens-Johnson syndrome

SPECIAL CONSIDERATIONS

- Use cautiously in elderly or debilitated patients and in those with head injuries, increased CSF pressure, COPD, decreased respiratory reserve, compromised respirations, arrhythmias, or hepatic, renal, or cardiac disease.
- Give an anticholinergic, such as atropine or glycopyrrolate, to minimize the possible bradycardic effect of fentanyl.
- Gradually adjust the dosage in patients using the transdermal system. Reaching steady-state levels of a new dose may take up to 6 days; delay dose adjustment until after at least two applications.
- When reducing opioid therapy or switching to a different analgesic, expect to withdraw the transdermal system gradually. Because the serum fentanyl level decreases very gradually after removal, give half of the equianalgesic dose of the new analgesic 12 to 18 hours after removal.

- Contraindicated in patients with intracranial lesions caused by increased ICP, and whenever ventilator function is depressed, such as in status asthmaticus, COPD, cor pulmonale, emphysema, and kyphoscoliosis.
- Use cautiously in elderly or debilitated patients and in those with hepatic or renal disease, Addison's disease, hypothyroidism, prostatic hyperplasia, or urethral strictures.
- For a better analgesic effect, give the drug before the patient has intense pain.
- Give by direct injection over at least 2 minutes, and monitor the patient constantly. Keep resuscitation equipment available. Respiratory depression and hypotension can occur with I.V. use.
- Drug may worsen or mask gallbladder pain. Increased biliary tract pressure resulting from contraction of the sphincter of Oddi may interfere with hepatobiliary imaging studies.

- Contraindicated in patients who have the syndrome of nasal polyps, angioedema, and bronchospastic reaction to aspirin or other NSAIDs. Contraindicated during the last trimester of pregnancy because it may cause problems with the fetus or complications during delivery.
- Use cautiously in patients with impaired renal or hepatic function, GI disorders, peptic ulcer disease, cardiac decompensation, hypertension, or coagulation defects. Because chewable tablets contain aspartame, use cautiously in patients with phenylketonuria.
- Monitor auditory and ophthalmic functions periodically during ibuprofen therapy.
- Observe the patient for possible fluid retention.
- Patients older than age 60 may be more susceptible to the toxic effects of ibuprofen, especially adverse GI reactions. Use the lowest possible effective dose. The effect of the drug on renal prostaglandins may cause fluid retention and edema, a significant drawback for elderly patients, especially those with heart failure.

(continued)

Common pain management drugs *(continued)*

DRUG	INDICATIONS	ADVERSE EFFECTS
ketorolac tromethamine Toradol	◆ Short-term management of severe, acute pain ◆ Short-term management of moderately severe, acute pain when switching from parenteral to oral route	◆ Dizziness, drowsiness, headache, sedation ◆ Arrhythmias ◆ Dyspepsia, GI pain, nausea ◆ Renal failure ◆ Thrombocytopenia
morphine Astramorph PF, Avinza, Duramorph, Infumorph, Kadian, MS Contin, MSIR, MS/L, MS/S, OMS Concentrate, Oramorph SR, RMS Uniserts, Roxanol	◆ Severe pain ◆ Severe, chronic pain related to cancer ◆ Preoperative sedation and adjunct to anesthesia ◆ Postoperative analgesia ◆ Control of pain caused by an acute MI ◆ Control of angina pain ◆ Adjunctive treatment of acute pulmonary edema	◆ Dizziness, light-headedness, nightmares (with long-acting oral forms), seizures (with large doses) ◆ Bradycardia, cardiac arrest, hypotension, shock ◆ Anorexia, biliary tract spasms, constipation, dry mouth, ileus, nausea, vomiting ◆ Urine retention ◆ Thrombocytopenia ◆ Apnea, respiratory arrest, respiratory depression ◆ Diaphoresis, edema ◆ Decreased libido, physical dependence

Common nonopioid analgesic combinations

TRADE NAME	GENERIC DRUGS
Anacin, P-A-C Analgesic Tablets	◆ aspirin 400 mg ◆ caffeine 32 mg
Ascriptin, Magnaprin	◆ aspirin 325 mg ◆ magnesium hydroxide 50 mg ◆ aluminum hydroxide 50 mg ◆ calcium carbonate 50 mg
Ascriptin A/D, Magnaprin Arthritis Strength Caplets	◆ aspirin 325 mg ◆ magnesium hydroxide 75 mg ◆ aluminum hydroxide 75 mg ◆ calcium carbonate 75 mg

SPECIAL CONSIDERATIONS

- Contraindicated in patients with active peptic ulcer disease, recent GI bleeding or perforation, advanced renal impairment, risk of renal impairment as a result of volume depletion, suspected or confirmed cerebrovascular bleeding, hemorrhagic diathesis, incomplete hemostasis, or an increased risk of bleeding.
- Use cautiously in patients with impaired renal or hepatic function.
- The combined duration of ketorolac therapy (I.M., I.V., oral) shouldn't exceed 5 days. Oral use is only for continuation of I.V. or I.M. therapy.

- Contraindicated in patients with conditions that would preclude delivery of opioids by the I.V. route, such as acute bronchial asthma and upper airway obstruction.
- Use cautiously in elderly or debilitated patients and in those with head injury, increased ICP, seizures, pulmonary disease, prostatic hyperplasia, hepatic or renal disease, acute abdominal conditions, hypothyroidism, Addison's disease, or urethral strictures.
- Long-term therapy in patients with advanced renal disease may lead to toxicity from accumulation of the active metabolite.

Common nonopioid analgesic combinations *(continued)*

TRADE NAME	GENERIC DRUGS
Aspirin Free Anacin PM, Extra Strength Tylenol PM, Sominex Pain Relief	◆ acetaminophen 500 mg ◆ diphenhydramine 25 mg
Cama Arthritis Pain Reliever	◆ aspirin 500 mg ◆ magnesium oxide 150 mg ◆ aluminum hydroxide 125 mg
Esgic-Plus	◆ acetaminophen 500 mg ◆ caffeine 40 mg ◆ butalbital 50 mg

(continued)

Common nonopioid analgesic combinations *(continued)*

TRADE NAME	GENERIC DRUGS
Excedrin Extra Strength, Excedrin Migraine	◆ aspirin 250 mg ◆ acetaminophen 250 mg ◆ caffeine 65 mg
Excedrin P.M. Caplets	◆ acetaminophen 500 mg ◆ diphenhydramine citrate 38 mg
Sinutab Regular*	◆ acetaminophen 325 mg ◆ chlorpheniramine 2 mg ◆ pseudoephedrine hydrochloride 30 mg
Tecnal*	◆ aspirin 330 mg ◆ caffeine 40 mg ◆ butalbital 50 mg
Vanquish	◆ aspirin 227 mg ◆ acetaminophen 194 mg ◆ caffeine 33 mg ◆ aluminum hydroxide 25 mg ◆ magnesium hydroxide 50 mg

*Available in Canada only

Common opioid analgesic combinations

TRADE NAME AND CONTROLLED SUBSTANCE SCHEDULE	GENERIC DRUGS
Aceta with Codeine *CSS III*	◆ acetaminophen 300 mg ◆ codeine phosphate 30 mg
Anexsia 7.5/650, Lorcet Plus *CSS III*	◆ acetaminophen 650 mg ◆ hydrocodone bitartrate 7.5 mg
Capital with Codeine, Tylenol with Codeine Elixir *CSS V*	◆ acetaminophen 120 mg ◆ codeine phosphate 12 mg/5 ml
Darvocet-N 50 *CSS IV*	◆ acetaminophen 325 mg ◆ propoxyphene napsylate 50 mg
Darvocet-N 100, Propacet 100 *CSS IV*	◆ acetaminophen 650 mg ◆ propoxyphene napsylate 100 mg

Common opioid analgesic combinations *(continued)*

TRADE NAME AND CONTROLLED SUBSTANCE SCHEDULE	GENERIC DRUGS
Empirin With Codeine No. 3 *CSS III*	◆ aspirin 325 mg ◆ codeine phosphate 30 mg
Empirin With Codeine No. 4 *CSS III*	◆ aspirin 325 mg ◆ codeine phosphate 60 mg
Fioricet With Codeine *CSS III*	◆ acetaminophen 325 mg ◆ butalbital 50 mg ◆ caffeine 40 mg ◆ codeine phosphate 30 mg
Fiorinal With Codeine *CSS III*	◆ aspirin 325 mg ◆ butalbital 50 mg ◆ caffeine 40 mg ◆ codeine phosphate 30 mg
Lorcet 10/650 *CSS III*	◆ acetaminophen 650 mg ◆ hydrocodone bitartrate 10 mg
Lortab 2.5/500 *CSS III*	◆ acetaminophen 500 mg ◆ hydrocodone bitartrate 2.5 mg
Lortab 5/500 *CSS III*	◆ acetaminophen 500 mg ◆ hydrocodone bitartrate 5 mg
Lortab 7.5/500 *CSS III*	◆ acetaminophen 500 mg ◆ hydrocodone bitartrate 7.5 mg
Percocet 5/325 *CSS II*	◆ acetaminophen 325 mg ◆ oxycodone hydrochloride 5 mg
Percodan-Demi *CSS II*	◆ aspirin 325 mg ◆ oxycodone hydrochloride 2.25 mg ◆ oxycodone terephthalate 0.19 mg
Percodan, Roxiprin *CSS II*	◆ aspirin 325 mg ◆ oxycodone hydrochloride 4.5 mg ◆ oxycodone terephthalate 0.38 mg
Roxicet *CSS II*	◆ acetaminophen 325 mg ◆ oxycodone hydrochloride 5 mg
Roxicet 5/500, Roxilox *CSS II*	◆ acetaminophen 500 mg ◆ oxycodone hydrochloride 5 mg

(continued)

Common opioid analgesic combinations *(continued)*

TRADE NAME AND CONTROLLED SUBSTANCE SCHEDULE	GENERIC DRUGS
Roxicet Oral Solution *CSS II*	◆ acetaminophen 325 mg ◆ oxycodone hydrochloride 5 mg/5 ml
Talacen *CSS IV*	◆ acetaminophen 650 mg ◆ pentazocine hydrochloride 25 mg
Talwin Compound *CSS IV*	◆ aspirin 325 mg ◆ pentazocine hydrochloride 12.5 mg
Tylenol with Codeine No. 2 *CSS III*	◆ acetaminophen 300 mg ◆ codeine phosphate 15 mg
Tylenol with Codeine No. 3 *CSS III*	◆ acetaminophen 300 mg ◆ codeine phosphate 30 mg
Tylenol with Codeine No. 4 *CSS III*	◆ acetaminophen 300 mg ◆ codeine phosphate 60 mg
Tylox *CSS II*	◆ acetaminophen 500 mg ◆ oxycodone hydrochloride 5 mg
Vicodin, Zydone *CSS III*	◆ acetaminophen 500 mg ◆ hydrocodone bitartrate 5 mg
Vicodin ES *CSS III*	◆ acetaminophen 750 mg ◆ hydrocodone bitartrate 7.5 mg

11 Infection control

The Hospital Infection Control Practices Advisory Committee of the Centers for Disease Control and Prevention (CDC) has developed guidelines for isolation precautions in hospitals. These guidelines have two levels of precautions:
- ◆ Standard precautions
- ◆ Transmission-based precautions, which include airborne precautions, droplet precautions, and contact precautions.

Standard precautions

- ◆ Standard precautions decrease the risk of transmitting microorganisms from recognized and unrecognized sources of infection.
- ◆ Recognized sources of infection include the following:
  - blood
  - body fluids, secretions, and excretions (except sweat)
  - nonintact skin
  - mucous membranes.
- ◆ Because not all sources of infection can be recognized, standard precautions must be followed at all times and with every patient.

Implementation

- ◆ Wash your hands immediately if they become contaminated with blood or body fluids, secretions, or excretions; also wash your hands before and after providing patient care and after removing gloves.
- ◆ Use nonantimicrobial soap, if available, for routine hand washing.
- ◆ Wear gloves if you will or may come in contact with blood, specimens, tissue, body fluids, secretions, excretions, or contaminated surfaces or objects.
- ◆ Change your gloves between tasks and procedures performed on the same patient if you touch anything that might have a high concentration of microorganisms.
- ◆ Change your gloves and wash your hands between patient contacts to avoid cross-contamination.

Alert Wear vinyl or nitrile gloves if you're allergic to latex.

- ◆ Wear a gown, eye protection (goggles or glasses), and a mask during procedures that are likely to generate droplets of blood or body fluids, secretions, or excretions, such as extubation, surgery, endoscopic procedures, and dialysis.
- ◆ Carefully handle used patient care equipment that's soiled with blood, body fluids, secretions, or excretions to prevent exposure to skin and mucous membranes, contamination of clothing, and transfer of microorganisms to other patients and environments.
- ◆ Clean patient-care equipment with a facility-approved disinfectant between patients.
- ◆ Discard disposable equipment appropriately.
- ◆ Make sure that procedures for routine care, cleaning, and disinfection of environmental surfaces and equipment are followed.
- ◆ Keep contaminated linens away from your body to prevent contamination and transfer of microorganisms.
- ◆ Place linens in properly labeled containers and make sure that the linens are transported according to facility policy.
- ◆ Handle used needles and other sharps carefully. Don't bend them, break them, reinsert them into their original sheaths, or handle them unnecessarily.
- ◆ Use sharps with safety features whenever available.
- ◆ Immediately after use, discard sharps intact in an impervious disposal box.
- ◆ Use mouthpieces, resuscitation bags, or other ventilation devices in

place of mouth-to-mouth resuscitation whenever possible.

◆ Place a patient who can't maintain appropriate hygiene or who contaminates the environment in a private room. Notify infection control personnel.

◆ If you have an exudative lesion, avoid direct patient contact until the condition has resolved and your employee health provider clears you.

◆ Because precautions can't be specified for every clinical situation, use your judgment in individual cases. Refer to your facility's infection control manual or check with infection control personnel when you need more information.

◆ If occupational exposure to blood is likely, get vaccinated with the HBV vaccine series.

Transmission-based precautions

◆ Whenever a patient is known or suspected to be infected with highly contagious or epidemiologically important pathogens that are transmitted by air, droplet, or contact with dry skin or other contaminated surfaces, add transmission-based precautions to standard precautions.

◆ Examples of such pathogens include those that cause measles (air); influenza (droplet); and GI tract, respiratory tract, skin, and wound infections (contact).

◆ One or more types of transmission-based precautions may be combined and followed when a patient has a disease with multiple routes of transmission.

Airborne precautions

◆ Add these steps to standard precautions.

◆ Place the patient in a private room with these features:
- monitored negative air pressure in relation to surrounding areas
- 6 to 12 air exchanges per hour
- appropriate outdoor air discharge or high-efficiency filtration of room air.

◆ Keep the patient's room door closed.

◆ If a private room isn't available, consult with infection control personnel. As an alternative, the patient may share a room with a patient who has an active infection with the same microorganism. (See *Diseases requiring airborne precautions,* page 366.)

◆ Wear respiratory protection, such as a surgical mask or N-95 respirator (for tuberculosis [TB]), when entering the room of a patient with a known or suspected respiratory tract infection. If you're immune to measles and varicella, you don't need to wear respiratory protection in the room of a patient with these illnesses.

◆ Limit patient transport and movement out of the room. If the patient must leave the room, have him wear a surgical mask.

Droplet precautions

◆ Add these steps to standard precautions.

◆ Place the patient in a private room. Special ventilation isn't needed.

◆ If a private room isn't available, consult with infection control personnel. As an alternative, the patient may share a room with a patient who has an active infection with the same microorganism. (See *Diseases requiring droplet precautions,* page 367.)

◆ Wear a mask when working within 38″ (0.9 m) of the infected patient. If the patient has TB, wear an N-95 respirator.
- The N-95 respirator has been approved by the National Institute for Oc-

Diseases requiring airborne precautions

DISEASE	PRECAUTIONARY PERIOD
Chickenpox (varicella)	Until lesions are crusted and no new lesions appear
Herpes zoster (disseminated)	Duration of illness; susceptible persons should avoid entering room
Herpes zoster (localized in immunocompromised patient)	Duration of illness
Measles (rubeola)	Duration of illness
Tuberculosis (TB) (pulmonary or laryngeal, confirmed or suspected)	Depends on clinical response; patient must be receiving effective therapy, be improving clinically (decreased cough and fever and improved findings on chest radiograph), and have three consecutive negative sputum smears collected on different days; or TB must be ruled out

cupational Safety and Health and the Occupational Safety and Health Administration (OSHA) for caring for a patient with known or suspected infectious pulmonary TB.

- If the respirator fits correctly and has minimal leakage at the face seal, this respirator protects the wearer from at least 95% of particles the size of TB droplet nuclei.
- Fit testing, which detects leakage at the face seal, is mandatory when you start wearing the respirator. (See *Respirator seal check,* page 368.)

◆ Instruct visitors to stay at least 38″ away from the infected patient.

◆ Limit movement of the patient from the room. If the patient must leave the room, have him wear a surgical mask.

Contact precautions

◆ Add these steps to standard precautions.

◆ Place the patient in a private room.

◆ If a private room isn't available, consult with infection control personnel. As an alternative, the patient may share a room with a patient who has an active infection with the same microorganism. (See *Diseases requiring contact precautions,* pages 369 and 370.)

◆ Wear gloves whenever you enter the patient's room.

◆ Wear a gown when entering the patient's room if you think your clothing will have extensive contact with the patient or anything in the room or if the patient has diarrhea or is incontinent.

◆ Always change gloves after contact with infected material. Remove them before leaving the room.

◆ Remove your gown before leaving the room.

◆ Wash your hands immediately with an antimicrobial soap, or rub them with a waterless antiseptic. Then, avoid touching contaminated surfaces.

◆ Limit the patient's movement from the room and check with infection control personnel whenever he must leave it.

Diseases requiring droplet precautions

DISEASE	PRECAUTIONARY PERIOD
Invasive *Haemophilus influenzae* type b disease, including epiglottitis, meningitis, pneumonia, and sepsis	Until 24 hours after start of effective therapy
Invasive *Neisseria meningitidis* disease, including epiglottiditis, meningitis, pneumonia, and sepsis	Until 24 hours after start of effective therapy
Diphtheria (pharyngeal)	Until off antibiotics and two cultures taken at least 24 hours apart are negative
***Mycoplasma pneumoniae* infection**	Duration of illness
Pertussis	Until 5 days after start of effective therapy
Pneumonic plague	Until 72 hours after start of effective therapy
Streptococcal pharyngitis, pneumonia, or scarlet fever in infants and young children	Until 24 hours after start of effective therapy
Adenovirus infection in infants and young children	Duration of illness
Influenza	Duration of illness
Mumps	For 9 days after onset of swelling
Parvovirus B19	Duration of hospitalization when chronic disease occurs in an immunocompromised patient; for patients with transient aplastic crisis or red-cell crisis, maintain precautions for 7 days
Rubella (German measles)	Until 7 days after onset of rash

Reportable diseases

- The CDC, OSHA, the Joint Commission on Accreditation of Healthcare Organizations, and the American Hospital Association all require health care facilities to document and report certain diseases acquired in the community or in hospitals and other health care facilities. (See *Reportable diseases and infections*, page 371.)
- Typically, the health care facility reports diseases to the appropriate local authorities.
- These authorities notify the state health department, which reports the diseases to the appropriate federal agency or national organization.

Respirator seal check

Always check the respirator seal before using a respirator. To do this, place both of your hands over the respirator and exhale. If air leaks around your nose, adjust the nosepiece. If air leaks at the respirator's edges, adjust the straps along the side of your head. Recheck the respirator's fit after making any adjustments.

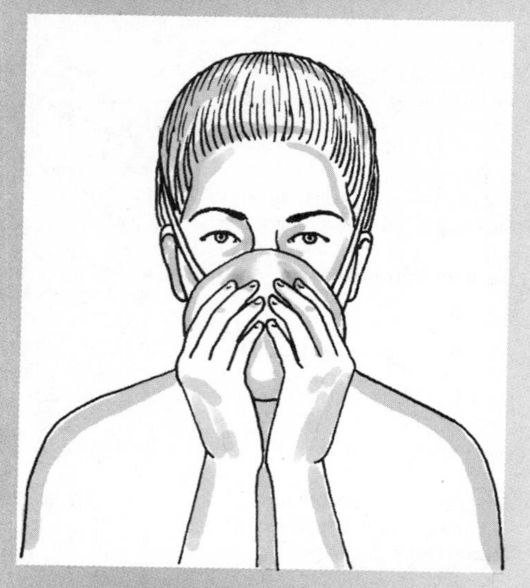

Basic procedures

Washing your hands

- Hand hygiene is a general term that refers to hand washing, antiseptic hand washing, surgical hand antisepsis, and antiseptic hand rubs.
- As defined by the CDC, hand washing refers to washing the hands with plain (not antimicrobial) soap and water. (See *Proper hand washing technique*, page 372.)
- Wash your hands between patients and whenever they're soiled or contaminated with infectious material.
- When you use an antiseptic agent (such as chlorhexidine, triclosan, or iodophor) you're performing an antiseptic hand wash.
- Surgical personnel perform surgical hand antisepsis preoperatively to eliminate transient bacteria and reduce resident hand flora.
- Whether it involves plain soap or an antiseptic agent, hand washing is the single most effective method for preventing the spread of infection.

Using a hand rub or sanitizer

- Hand rubs and sanitizers are appropriate after minimal contamination, when your hands aren't visibly soiled, and when running water isn't available.
- An antiseptic hand rub involves use of an antiseptic, alcohol-containing product that's designed to reduce the number of viable microorganisms on the skin.

Diseases requiring contact precautions

DISEASE	PRECAUTIONARY PERIOD
Infection or colonization with multidrug-resistant bacteria	Until antibiotics completed and culture negative
***Clostridium difficile* enteric infection**	Duration of illness
***Escherichia coli* disease in diapered or incontinent patient**	Duration of illness
Shigellosis in diapered or incontinent patient	Duration of illness
Hepatitis A in diapered or incontinent patient	Duration of illness
Rotavirus infection in diapered or incontinent patient	Duration of illness
Respiratory syncytial virus infection in infants and young children	Duration of illness
Parainfluenza virus infection in infants and young children	Duration of illness
Enteroviral infection in infants and young children	Duration of illness
Adenovirus infection in infants and young children	Duration of illness
Scabies	Until 24 hours after start of effective therapy
Diphtheria (cutaneous)	Until antibiotics completed and culture negative
Herpes simplex virus infection (neonatal or mucocutaneous)	Duration of illness
Impetigo	Until 24 hours after start of effective therapy
Major abscesses, cellulitis, or pressure ulcer	Until antibiotics completed and culture negative
Pediculosis (lice)	Until 24 hours after start of effective therapy

(continued)

Diseases requiring contact precautions *(continued)*

DISEASE	PRECAUTIONARY PERIOD
Rubella, congenital syndrome	During any admission until age 1, unless nasopharyngeal and urine cultures are negative for virus after age 3 months
Staphylococcal furunculosis in infants and young children	Duration of illness
Acute viral (acute hemorrhagic) conjunctivitis	Duration of illness
Viral hemorrhagic infection (Ebola, Lassa, Marburg)	Duration of illness
Zoster (chickenpox, disseminated zoster, or localized zoster in immunocompromised patient)	Until all lesions are crusted; requires airborne precautions as well
Smallpox	Duration of illness; requires airborne precautions as well

- Apply the solution to all surfaces of your hands and rub them until the product has dried (usually within 30 seconds).
- These products are also called waterless antiseptic agents because no water is needed.
- Alcohol-containing hand rubs usually contain emollients to prevent skin drying and chapping.

Putting on and removing a gown

- Handling isolation clothing properly is an important part of protecting yourself and avoiding contamination.
- Put on the gown and wrap it around the back of your clothing.
- Tie the strings or fasten the snaps or pressure-sensitive tabs at the neck.
- Make sure your clothing is completely covered and secure the gown at the waist.
- Because the outside surfaces of barrier clothing are contaminated, keep your gloves on when taking the clothing off.
- First, untie the waist strings of the gown and then untie the neck straps. Grasp the outside of the gown at the back of the shoulders and pull it down over your arms, turning it inside out to contain pathogens as you remove it.
- Holding the gown well away from you, fold it inside out.
- Discard the gown in the laundry if it's cloth and in a trash container if it's paper.

Reportable diseases and infections

This list contains the Centers for Disease Control and Prevention's list of nationally notifiable infectious diseases for 2005. Each state also keeps a list of reportable diseases appropriate to its region.

- Acquired immunodeficiency syndrome
- Anthrax
- Botulism (food-borne, infant, other [wound and unspecified])
- Brucellosis
- Chancroid
- *Chlamydia trachomatis,* genital infections
- Cholera
- Coccidioidomycosis
- Cryptosporidiosis
- Cyclosporiasis
- Diphtheria
- Ehrlichiosis (human granulocytic, human monocytic, human [other or unspecified agent])
- Encephalitis/meningitis (arboviral neuroinvasive and non-neuroinvasive diseases): California serogroup viral, eastern equine, Powassan, St. Louis, West Nile, western equine)
- Enterohemorrhagic *Escherichia coli* (O157:H7, Shiga toxin positive [serogroup non-O157], Shiga toxin positive [not serogrouped])
- Giardiasis
- Gonorrhea
- *Haemophilus influenzae,* invasive disease
- Hansen disease (leprosy)
- Hantavirus pulmonary syndrome
- Hemolytic uremic syndrome, postdiarrheal
- Hepatitis, viral, acute (hepatitis A acute, hepatitis B acute, hepatitis B virus perinatal infection, hepatitis C acute)
- Hepatitis, viral, chronic (chronic hepatitis B, hepatitis C virus infection [past or current])
- Human immunodeficiency virus (adult [≥13 years], pediatric [< 13 years])
- *Legionella* infections (legionnaires' disease)
- Influenza-associated pediatric mortality
- Listeriosis
- Lyme disease
- Malaria
- Measles
- Meningococcal disease
- Mumps
- Pertussis
- Plague
- Poliomyelitis (paralytic)
- Psittacosis (ornithosis)
- Q fever
- Rabies (animal, human)
- Rocky Mountain spotted fever
- Rubella (German measles) and congenital syndrome
- Salmonellosis
- Severe Acute Respiratory Syndrome-associated Corona Virus (SARS-CoV) disease
- Shigellosis
- Smallpox
- Streptococcal disease, invasive, group A
- Streptococcal toxic-shock syndrome
- *Streptococcus* pneumoniae, drug-resistant, invasive disease
- S. pneumoniae, invasive, in children ages younger than age 5
- Syphilis (primary, secondary, latent, early latent, late latent, latent unknown duration, neurosyphilis, late nonneurologic)
- Syphilis, congenital (syphilitic stillbirth)
- Tetanus
- Toxic-shock syndrome
- Trichinellosis (Trichinosis)
- Tuberculosis
- Tularemia
- Typhoid fever
- Vancomycin (intermediate *Staphylococcus aureus* [VISA], resistant *Staphylococcus aureus* [VRSA])
- Varicella (morbidity)
- Varicella (deaths only)
- Yellow fever

Proper hand washing technique

Hand rubs and sanitizers are appropriate for decontaminating your hands when they aren't visibly soiled or running water isn't available.

To minimize the spread of infection when hands are visibly soiled, follow these basic hand-washing instructions.

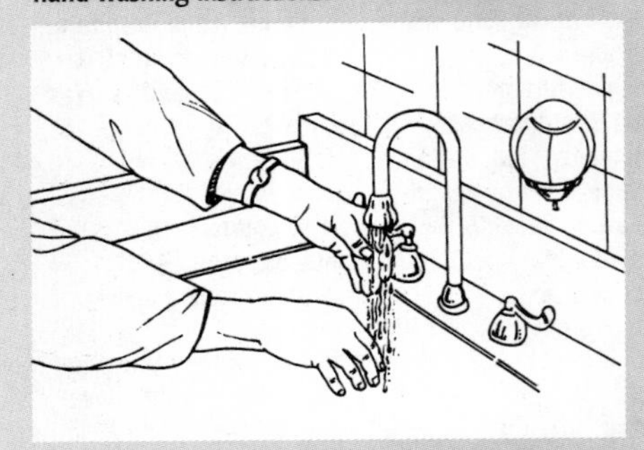

With your hands angled downward under the faucet, adjust the water temperature until it's comfortably warm.

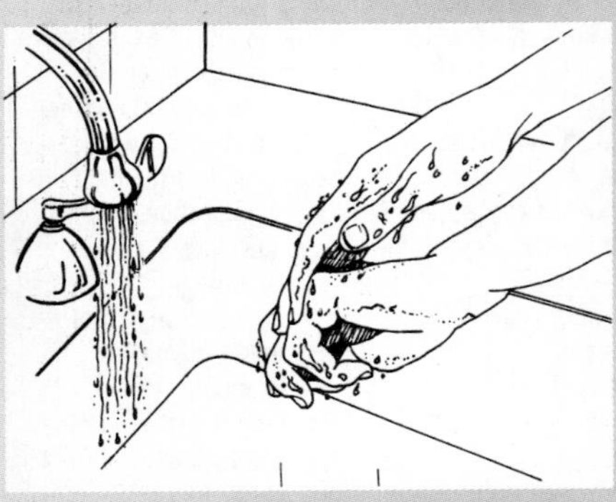

Add soap and work up a generous lather by scrubbing vigorously for at least 15 seconds. Make sure to clean beneath fingernails, around knuckles, and along the sides of fingers and hands.

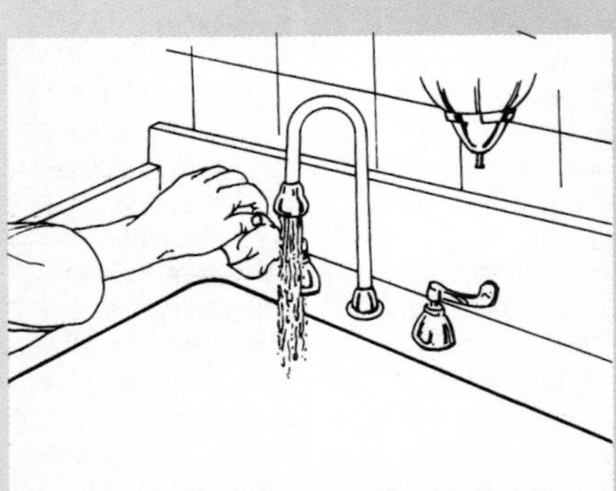

Rinse your hands completely to wash away suds and microorganisms. Pat dry with a paper towel. To prevent recontaminating your hands on the faucet handles, cover each one with a dry paper towel when turning off the water.

Putting on and removing a mask

◆ Wear a facemask to avoid inhaling airborne particles.
◆ Place the mask snugly over your nose and mouth. Secure the ear loops or tie the strings behind your head high enough so the mask won't slip off.
◆ If the mask has a metal strip, squeeze it to fit the bridge of your nose firmly but comfortably. If you wear eyeglasses, tuck the mask under their lower edge.
◆ To remove your mask, untie it, holding it by the strings. Discard it in the trash container.
◆ If the patient's disease is spread by airborne pathogens, consider removing the mask last.

Putting on sterile gloves

◆ To maintain sterility, it is important to use proper technique when putting on sterile gloves. (See *How to put on sterile gloves,* page 374.)

Removing contaminated gloves

◆ Using your nondominant hand, pinch the glove of the dominant hand near the top, as shown below. Don't let the outer surface of the glove buckle inward against your skin.

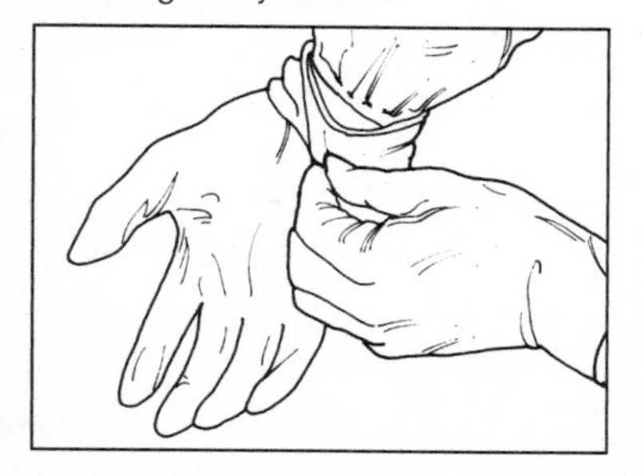

◆ Pull downward so that the glove turns inside out as it comes off, as shown below.

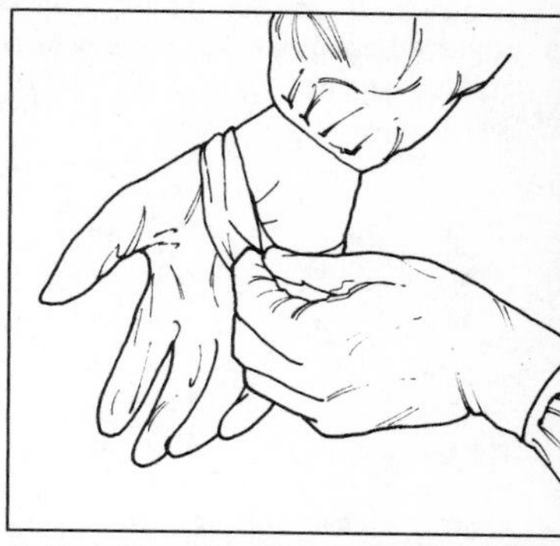

◆ Keep the glove from your dominant hand in your nondominant hand after removing it.
◆ Insert the first two fingers of your ungloved dominant hand under the edge of the nondominant glove, as shown below. Avoid touching the outer surface of the glove or folding it against the wrist of your nondominant hand.

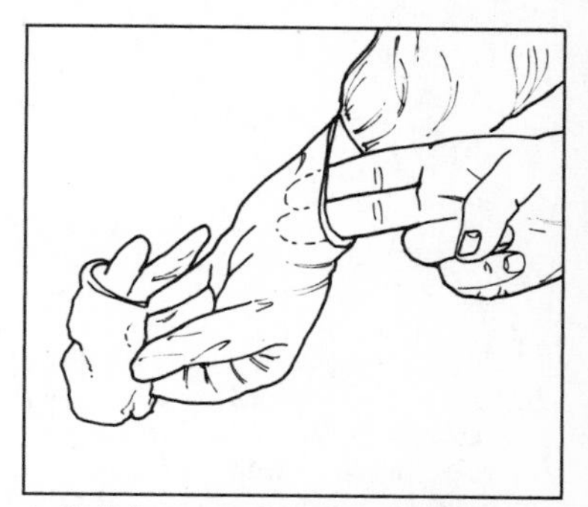

◆ Pull downward so that the glove turns inside out as it comes off, as shown. Continue pulling until the glove completely encloses the glove from your dominant hand and has its uncontaminated inner surface facing out, as shown at top of left column on page 375.

How to put on sterile gloves

Using your nondominant hand, pick up the opposite glove by grasping the exposed inside of the cuff.

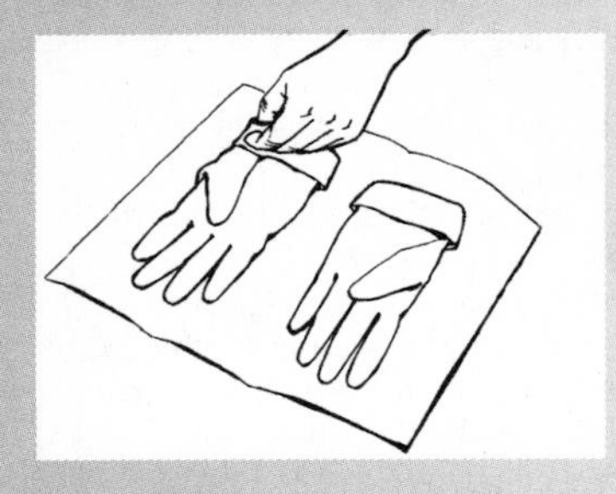

Pull the glove onto your dominant hand. Be sure to keep your thumb folded inward to avoid touching the sterile part of the glove. Allow the glove to come uncuffed as you finish inserting your hand, but don't touch the outside of the glove.

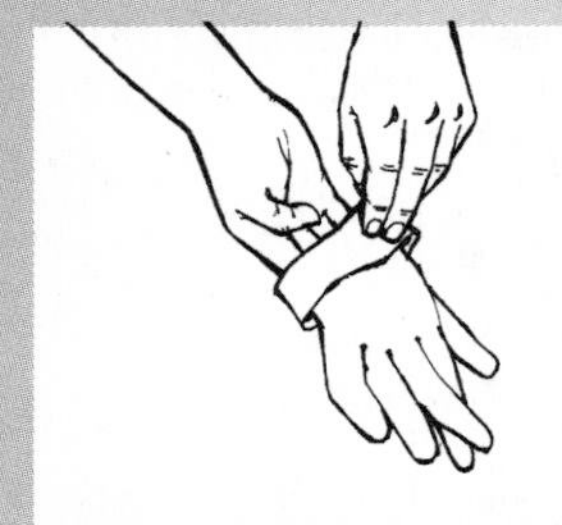

Slip the gloved fingers of your dominant hand under the cuff of the loose glove to pick it up.

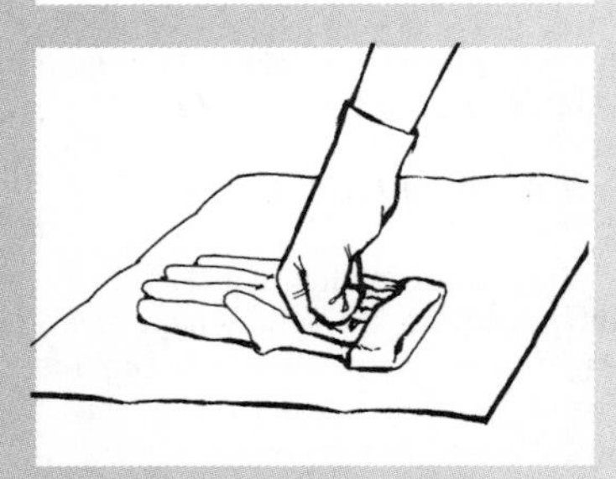

Slide your nondominant hand into the glove, holding your dominant thumb as far away as possible to avoid brushing against your arm. Allow the glove to come uncuffed as you finish putting it on, but don't touch the skin side of the cuff with your other gloved hand.

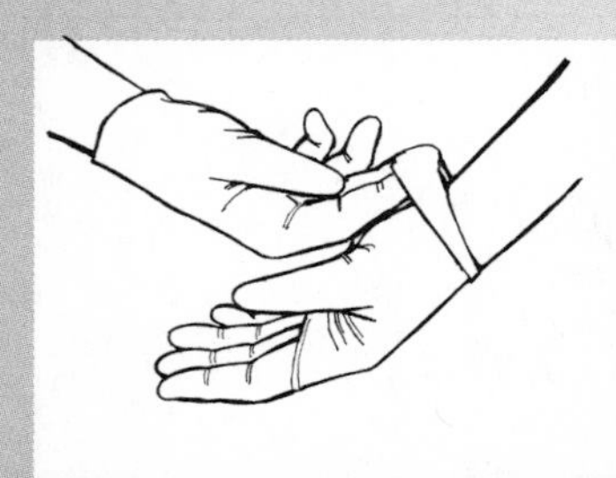

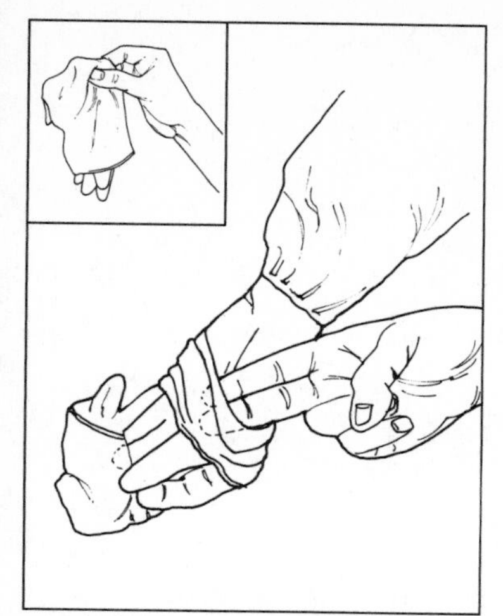

◆ Discard the gloves in the appropriate trash container and wash your hands.

Removing soiled linens

◆ All linens used in patient care settings are considered soiled. If you're handling visibly soiled linens, wear gloves.
◆ Handle linens as little as possible and with minimal agitation to avoid contaminating yourself.
◆ If the bed linens are saturated with blood, feces, urine, or other body fluids, wear a gown.
◆ If certain areas of the linens are heavily soiled, fold the fabric so that the soiled areas are on the inside of the folds. Then roll or fold the linens together in one bundle.
◆ When carrying linens, hold them away from your body to avoid contaminating your clothes.
◆ Bag the linens in the patient's room as soon as possible. Avoid placing them on chairs, tables, or the floor.
◆ Don't sort or rinse linens in patient care areas.
◆ Place soiled linens in a leakproof bag.
◆ After you put the linens in the bag, close the bag securely.
◆ Then remove your gloves and wash your hands before carrying the bag to its appropriate destination.

Disposing of soiled dressings

◆ Dispose of all wound dressings in a way that confines and contains blood or body fluids.
◆ Don't touch soiled areas of the dressing.
◆ Usually, you must wear nonsterile gloves to handle and remove soiled dressings.
◆ If the wound is large and draining, you'll also need to wear a gown.

Large dressings

◆ Immediately after removing a large dressing, fold the dressing inward to enclose the soiled areas.
◆ Wrap the large dressing in the disposable linen-saver pad used during the dressing change.
◆ Dispose of the dressing in a red-bagged biohazard container if the dressing is saturated with blood. Otherwise, it can be disposed of in the regular trash container.
◆ Remove your gloves and wash your hands.

Small dressings

◆ When removing a small dressing, enclose it in the disposable glove that you used to remove it. Holding the dressing in your gloved hand, pull the glove off with the inside surface facing out to contain the dressing.
◆ Don't touch the dressing with your bare hand.
◆ After you've sealed the dressing inside the disposable glove, discard both gloves and the dressing in the trash container in the patient's room.

Discarding contaminated equipment

- To protect yourself and the patient from infection, observe precautions when discarding soiled disposable or reusable equipment.
- Have a biohazard container available, as needed, to dispose of contaminated waste.
- Regulations for the disposal of contaminated waste vary from state to state and may change periodically.
- When disposing of a sharp object that's contaminated with potentially infectious materials, place it in an approved sharps container.
- Other contaminated disposable items should be placed in a red-bagged biohazard container if they contain large amounts of blood.
- Items with small amounts of dried blood can be discarded in the regular trash container.
- When transporting a waste bag, hold it away from your body to prevent inadvertent injury from sharp objects that may protrude through the bag.

Disposing of body fluids

- Check facility policy before handling infectious waste.
- Large amounts of secretions, excretions, or bulk blood may be carefully poured into a sanitary sewer.
- If you pour fluids into a hopper, you're required to wear a splash guard as well as personal protective equipment.

12 Drug administration

Administration guidelines

Precautions for drug administration

◆ Whenever you give a drug, observe these precautions to make sure you're giving the right drug in the right dose to the right patient.

Check the order

◆ Check the order on the patient's medication record against the physician's order.

Check the label

◆ Check the label on the drug three times before giving it to a patient to make sure you're giving the prescribed drug in the prescribed dose.

- Check it when you take the container from the shelf or drawer.
- Check it right before pouring the drug into a medication cup or drawing it into a syringe.
- Check it before returning the container to the shelf or drawer.

◆ If you're giving a unit-dose drug, check the label for the third time immediately after pouring it and again before discarding the wrapper.

◆ Don't open a unit-dose drug until you're at the patient's bedside.

Confirm the patient's identity

◆ Before giving the drug, confirm the patient's identity by checking his name and a second identifier on his wristband. Remember to check a second identifying characteristic (such as address, identification number, date of birth) other than the patient's room number. Then make sure that you have the correct drug.

◆ Explain the procedure to the patient and provide privacy.

Have a written order

◆ Make sure you have a written order for every drug to be given.

◆ If the order is verbal, make sure that the physician signs for it within the specified time.

Give labeled drugs

◆ Don't give drugs from poorly labeled or unlabeled containers.

◆ Also, don't attempt to label drugs or reinforce drug labels yourself; a pharmacist must do that.

Monitor drugs

◆ Never give a drug that someone else has poured or prepared.

◆ Never let the drug cart or tray out of your sight.

◆ Never return unwrapped or prepared drugs to stock containers. Instead, dispose of them and notify the pharmacy.

Answer patient questions

◆ If the patient questions you about a drug or dosage, check his medication record again. If the drug is correct, reassure him that it's correct.

◆ Make sure to tell him about changes in his drugs or dosages.

◆ Instruct him, as appropriate, about possible adverse reactions and encourage him to report any that he experiences.

Topical administration

Topical drugs

◆ Topical drugs, such as lotions and ointments, are applied directly to the patient's skin.

◆ They're commonly used for local, rather than systemic, effects.

◆ Typically, they must be applied two or three times daily to achieve a full therapeutic effect.

Equipment

Patient's medication record and chart ◆ prescribed medication ◆ sterile tongue blades ◆ gloves ◆ sterile 4″ × 4″ gauze pads ◆ transparent semipermeable dressing ◆ adhesive tape ◆ solvent (such as cottonseed oil) ◆ optional: cotton-tipped applicators, cotton gloves, or terry cloth scuffs

Implementation

◆ Explain the procedure to the patient because, after discharge, he may have to apply the drug by himself.

◆ Wash your hands to prevent cross-contamination and glove your dominant hand.

◆ Help the patient into a comfortable position and expose the area to be treated.

◆ Make sure that the skin or mucous membrane is intact (unless the drug has been ordered to treat a skin lesion). Applying a drug to broken or abraded skin may cause unwanted systemic absorption and further irritation.

◆ If needed, clean debris from the skin. You may need to change your glove if it becomes soiled.

To apply a paste, a cream, or an ointment

◆ Open the container. Place the cap upside down to avoid contaminating its inner surface.

◆ Remove a tongue blade from its sterile wrapper and cover one end of it with drug from the tube or jar.

◆ Transfer the drug from the tongue blade to your gloved hand.

◆ Apply the drug to the affected area with long strokes that follow the direction of hair growth, as shown above right. This technique avoids forcing drug into the hair follicles, which can cause irritation and lead to folliculitis.

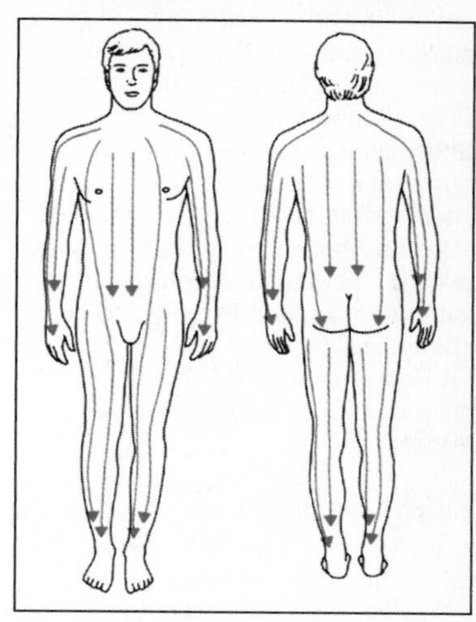

◆ Avoid using excessive pressure when applying the drug because it could abrade the skin or cause patient discomfort.

◆ When applying drug to a patient's face, use a cotton-tipped applicator for small areas such as under the eyes. For larger areas, use a sterile gauze pad and follow the directions shown below.

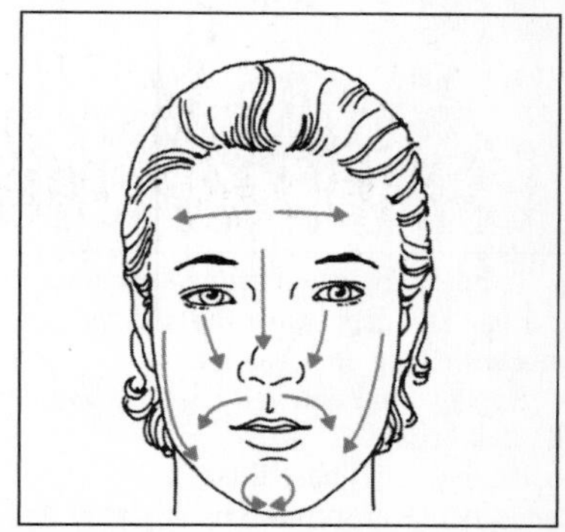

◆ To prevent contamination of the drug, use a new sterile tongue blade each time you remove drug from the container.

To remove an ointment

◆ Gently swab ointment from the patient's skin with a sterile 4″ × 4″ gauze pad. If the ointment has hardened or crusted, and cleansing with normal saline solution or other cleansing solution is ineffective, dab a cotton ball with a small amount of mineral oil to soften the ointment.

◆ Remove remaining oil by wiping the area with a clean sterile gauze pad. Don't wipe too hard because you could irritate the skin.

◆ Cleanse the area with normal saline solution or a prescribed wound care cleanser.

To apply other topical drugs

◆ To apply a medicated shampoo, follow package directions.

– Apply it with your fingertips, or instruct the patient to do so, as shown below.

– Massage it into the scalp, if appropriate.

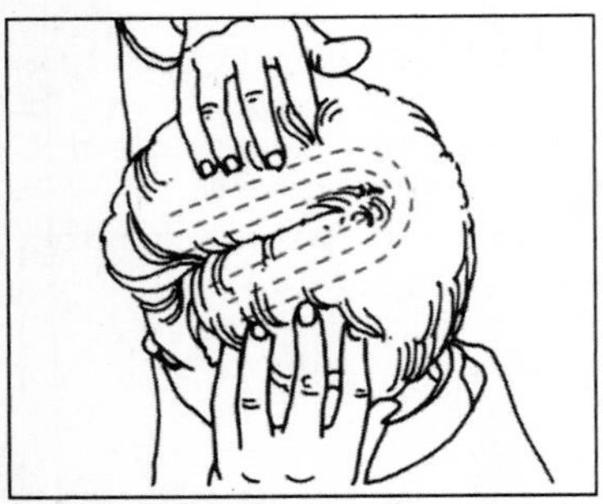

◆ To apply topical antifungal creams and nail lacquers, wash the affected area with soap and water.

– Apply cream and rub it gently into the nail beds.

– If the patient has athlete's foot, you can enhance absorption by applying the drug at night and covering the affected area with clean socks.

– Apply nail lacquers to the entire nail, starting at the nail bed.

– Let the lacquer dry thoroughly, about 5 to 10 minutes.

◆ To apply an aerosol spray, shake the container, if indicated, to mix the drug.

– Hold the container 6″ to 12″ (15 to 30.5 cm) from the skin or follow the manufacturer's recommendation.

– Spray the drug evenly over the treatment area to apply a thin film.

◆ To apply a powder, dry the skin surface and apply a thin layer of powder over the treatment area.

◆ To protect applied drugs and keep them from soiling the patient's clothes, tape a sterile gauze pad or a transparent semipermeable dressing over the treated area, if ordered. Avoid using an occlusive dressing, which may increase systemic absorption of the drug.

◆ If you're applying topical drug to the patient's hands, cover them with cotton gloves.

◆ If you're applying a topical drug to his feet, cover them with terrycloth scuffs or clean socks.

◆ Assess the patient's skin for signs of irritation, allergic reaction, or breakdown.

Special considerations

◆ To prevent skin irritation from accumulated drug, remove residue from previous applications before each new application.

◆ Always wear gloves to prevent your skin from absorbing the drug.

◆ Never apply ointment to the eyelids or ear canal unless ordered. The ointment may congeal and occlude the tear duct or ear canal.

◆ Inspect the treated area often for adverse or allergic reactions.

Transdermal drugs

◆ Given through an adhesive patch or a measured dose of ointment applied to the skin, transdermal drugs deliver constant, controlled drug directly into the bloodstream for a prolonged systemic effect.

◆ Drugs available in transdermal form include:
- nitroglycerin, which is used to control angina
- scopolamine, which is used to treat motion sickness
- estradiol, which is used for postmenopausal hormone replacement
- clonidine, which is used to treat hypertension
- fentanyl, which is used to control chronic pain.

◆ Nitroglycerin ointment is used to dilate the arteries and veins, thus improving cardiac perfusion in a patient with cardiac ischemia or angina pectoris.

◆ Nitroglycerin ointment dilates the coronary vessels for 2 to 12 hours; a patch can produce the same effect for as long as 24 hours.

◆ The scopolamine patch can relieve motion sickness for as long as 72 hours.

◆ Transdermal estradiol lasts 72 hours to 1 week.

◆ Transdermal clonidine lasts 7 days.

◆ Transdermal fentanyl lasts up to 72 hours.

Equipment

For a transdermal patch

Patient's medication record and chart ◆ prescribed drug ◆ optional: gloves

For transdermal ointment

Patient's medication record and chart ◆ ointment ◆ ruled application strip or measuring paper ◆ plastic wrap or transparent semipermeable dressing ◆ adhesive tape ◆ sphygmomanometer ◆ optional: gloves

Implementation

◆ Wash your hands and put on gloves.

◆ Make sure that previously applied drug has been removed from the skin.

◆ Locate a new site for application, different from the previous site.

To apply a transdermal patch

◆ Open the package and remove the patch.

◆ Without touching the adhesive surface, remove the clear plastic backing.

◆ Apply the patch to a dry, hairless area — behind the ear, for example, as with scopolamine.

◆ Avoid areas that may cause uneven absorption, such as skin folds or scars, or irritated or damaged skin.

◆ Don't apply the patch below the elbow or knee.

To apply transdermal ointment

◆ Nitroglycerin ointment is prescribed by the inch and comes with a rectangular piece of ruled paper to use in applying the drug.

◆ Put on gloves (optional) to avoid contact with the drug.

◆ Start by taking the patient's baseline blood pressure for comparison with later readings.

◆ Squeeze the prescribed amount of ointment onto the application strip or ruled paper, as shown below, taking care not to get any on your skin.

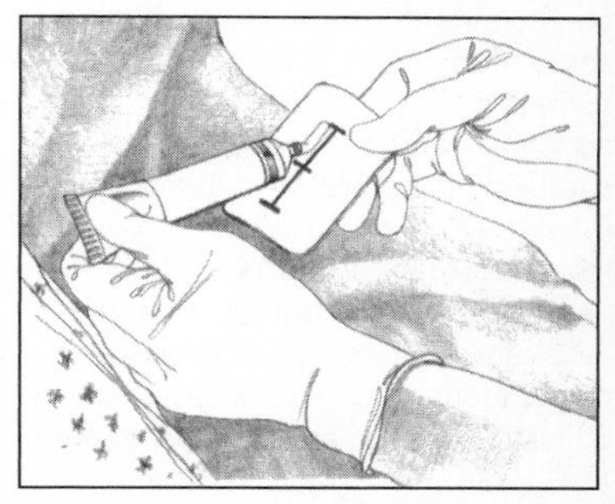

◆ After measuring the correct amount of ointment, tape the paper, drug side down, directly to the patient's skin on a dry, hairless area of the body.
◆ Don't rub the ointment into the skin.
◆ Tape the application strip and ointment to the skin.
◆ For increased absorption, the physician may request that you cover the site with plastic wrap or transparent semipermeable dressing and tape it in place, as shown below.

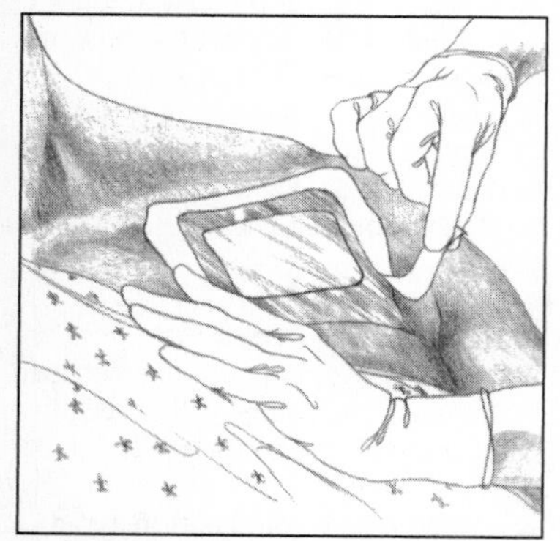

◆ Some health care facilities require you to use the paper to spread a thin layer of ointment over a 3″ (7.6-cm) area, usually on the patient's chest or arm.

After applying transdermal drugs
◆ Store the drug, as ordered.
◆ Instruct the patient to keep the area around the patch or ointment as dry as possible.
◆ Wash your hands immediately after applying the patch or ointment.

Special considerations
◆ Apply daily transdermal drugs at the same time every day to ensure a continuous effect, but alternate the application sites to avoid skin irritation.
◆ Five minutes after applying nitroglycerin ointment, obtain the patient's blood pressure reading.
– If his blood pressure has dropped significantly and he has a headache, notify the physician immediately.
– If his blood pressure has dropped but he has no symptoms, instruct him to lie still until his blood pressure returns to normal.
◆ Before reapplying nitroglycerin ointment, remove the plastic wrap, the application strip, and any ointment remaining on the skin at the previous site.
◆ When applying a scopolamine patch, instruct the patient not to drive or operate machinery until he knows how the drug affects him.
◆ If the patient is using a clonidine patch, encourage him to check with his physician before using over-the-counter cough preparations. They may counteract the effects of clonidine.

Eye drugs

◆ Eye drugs — drops or ointment — serve diagnostic and therapeutic purposes.
◆ During an eye examination, these drugs can be used to anesthetize the eye, dilate the pupil, and stain the cornea to identify anomalies.
◆ Therapeutic uses include lubrication of the eye and treatment of such conditions as glaucoma and infections.

Equipment
Patient's medication record and chart ◆ prescribed eye drug ◆ sterile cotton balls ◆ gloves ◆ warm water or normal saline solution ◆ sterile gauze pads ◆ facial tissue ◆ optional: ocular dressing

Implementation

◆ Make sure the drug is labeled for ophthalmic use. Then check the expiration date. Remember to date the container after the first use.

◆ Inspect ocular solutions for cloudiness, discoloration, and precipitation, but remember that some eye drugs are suspensions and normally appear cloudy. Don't use a solution that appears abnormal.

◆ Make sure that you know which eye to treat because different drugs or doses may be ordered for each eye.

◆ Keep in mind that "OD" means right eye, "OS" means left eye, and "OU" means both eyes.

◆ Put on gloves.

◆ If the patient has an ocular dressing, remove it by pulling it down and away from his forehead. Avoid contaminating your hands.

◆ To remove exudate or Meibomian gland secretions, clean around the eye with sterile cotton balls or sterile gauze pads moistened with warm water or normal saline solution.

– Have the patient close his eye and then gently wipe the eyelids from the inner to the outer canthus.

– Use a fresh cotton ball or gauze pad for each stroke.

◆ Have the patient sit or lie in the supine position.

◆ Instruct him to tilt his head back and toward his affected eye so that excess drug can flow away from the tear duct, minimizing systemic absorption through the nasal mucosa.

◆ Remove the dropper cap from the drug container and draw the drug into it.

◆ Before instilling eyedrops, instruct the patient to look up and away. This moves the cornea away from the lower lid and minimizes the risk of touching it with the dropper.

To instill eyedrops

◆ Steady the hand that's holding the dropper by resting it against the patient's forehead.

◆ With your other hand, pull down the lower lid of the affected eye and instill the drops in the conjunctival sac.

◆ Never instill eyedrops directly onto the eyeball.

Patient teaching tip When teaching an elderly patient how to instill eyedrops, keep in mind that he may have trouble feeling the drops enter the eye. Suggest chilling the drug slightly to enhance the sensation.

To apply eye ointment

◆ Pull down the lower lid of the affected eye.

◆ Squeeze a small ribbon of drug along the edge of the conjunctival sac, from the inner to the outer canthus, as shown below. Cut the ribbon by turning the tube.

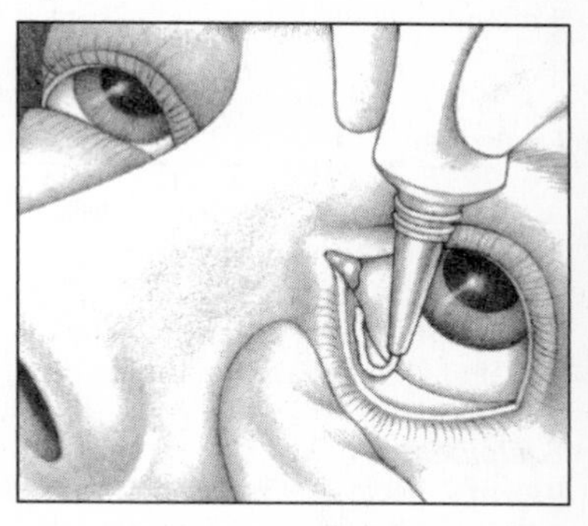

After instilling eyedrops or applying ointment

◆ Instruct the patient to close his eyes gently, without squeezing the lids shut.

◆ If you instilled drops, tell the patient to place a finger at the inner canthus for 2 to 3 minutes to block the tear duct.

◆ If you applied ointment, tell him to roll his eyes behind closed lids to help to distribute the drug over the eyeball.
◆ Use a clean facial tissue to remove excess drug leaking from the eye. Use a fresh tissue for each eye to prevent cross-contamination.
◆ Apply a new ocular dressing, if needed.
◆ Remove and discard your gloves and wash your hands.

Special considerations

◆ To maintain the sterility of the drug container, never touch the tip of the dropper or bottle to the eye area.

Alert If the dropper or bottle tip becomes contaminated, discard it and use another sterile dropper.

◆ If any solution remains in the dropper, discard it before returning the dropper to the bottle.
◆ If another drug is ordered for the same eye at the same time, wait 3 to 5 minutes before delivering the second drug.

Eardrops

◆ Eardrops may be instilled to treat infection or inflammation, to soften cerumen for later removal, to produce local anesthesia, or to facilitate the removal of an insect trapped in the ear.

Equipment

Patient's medication record and chart ◆ prescribed eardrops ◆ light source ◆ facial tissue or cotton-tipped applicator ◆ optional: cotton ball, bowl of warm water

Implementation

◆ Warm the drug to body temperature in the bowl of warm water or carry it in your pocket for 30 minutes before giving it.
◆ If needed, test the temperature by placing a drop on your wrist. (If the drug is too hot, it may burn the patient's eardrum.)
◆ To avoid injuring the ear canal, check the dropper before use to make sure that it isn't chipped or cracked.
◆ Wash your hands.
◆ Confirm the patient's identity.
◆ Confirm the correct drug.
– Compare the label on the eardrops with the order on the patient's medication record.
– Check the label again while drawing the drug into the dropper.
– Check the label for the final time before returning the eardrops to the shelf or drawer.
◆ Have the patient lie on the side opposite the affected ear.
◆ Straighten the patient's ear canal. For an adult, pull the auricle up and back.

Age alert For an infant or a child younger than age 3, gently pull the auricle down and back — the ear canal is straighter at this age.

◆ Using a light source, examine the ear canal for drainage.
– If you find any, clean the canal with a facial tissue or cotton-tipped applicator.
– Drainage can reduce the drug's effectiveness.
◆ To avoid damaging the ear canal with the dropper, gently rest the hand that's holding the dropper against the patient's head.
◆ Straighten the patient's ear canal again and instill the ordered number of drops.
◆ To avoid patient discomfort, aim the dropper so that the drops fall against the sides of the ear canal, not on the eardrum.
◆ Hold the ear canal in position until you see the drug disappear down the canal.

◆ After instilling the drops, lightly massage the tragus of the ear or apply gentle pressure.
◆ Instruct the patient to remain on his side for 5 to 10 minutes to let the drug finish running down the ear canal.
◆ Tuck the cotton ball (if ordered) loosely into the opening of the ear canal to prevent the drug from leaking out.
◆ Be careful not to insert the cotton ball too deep into the canal because doing so would prevent drainage of secretions and increase pressure on the eardrum.
◆ Clean and dry the outer ear.
◆ If ordered, repeat the procedure in the other ear after 5 to 10 minutes.
◆ Help the patient into a comfortable position.
◆ Wash your hands.

Special considerations

◆ Some conditions make the normally tender ear canal even more sensitive, so be especially gentle when performing this procedure.
◆ To prevent injury to the eardrum when inserting a cotton-tipped applicator, always keep the cotton tip in view.
◆ After instilling eardrops to soften cerumen, irrigate the ear, as ordered, to facilitate its removal.
◆ If the patient has vertigo, keep the side rails of his bed up, and help him as needed during the procedure. Move slowly and unhurriedly to avoid worsening his vertigo.
◆ If needed, teach the patient to instill eardrops correctly so he can continue treatment at home. Review the procedure and let the patient try it himself while you observe.

Nasal drugs

◆ Nasal drugs may be instilled through drops, a spray (using an atomizer), or an aerosol (using a nebulizer).
◆ Drops can be directed at a specific area; sprays and aerosols diffuse drug throughout the nasal passages.
◆ Nasal drugs include vasoconstrictors, antiseptics, anesthetics, hormones, vaccines, and corticosteroids.
◆ Most nasal drugs produce local rather than systemic effects.

Equipment

Patient's medication record and chart ◆ prescribed drug ◆ emesis basin (for nose drops) ◆ facial tissues ◆ optional: pillow, piece of soft rubber or plastic tubing, gloves

Implementation

◆ Wash your hands. Put on gloves, if needed.
◆ Have the patient blow his nose to clear secretions and enhance drug absorption.

To instill nose drops

◆ Draw some drug into the dropper.
◆ To reach the ethmoidal and sphenoidal sinuses, have the patient lie on his back with his neck hyperextended and his head tilted back over the edge of the bed. Support his head with one hand to prevent neck strain.
◆ To reach the maxillary and frontal sinuses, have the patient lie on his back, with his head toward the affected side and hanging slightly over the edge of the bed. Ask him to rotate his head laterally after hyperextension. Support his head with one hand to prevent neck strain.
◆ To relieve ordinary nasal congestion, help the patient into a reclining or supine position, with his head tilted slightly toward the affected side. Aim

the dropper upward, toward the patient's eye, rather than downward, toward his ear.

◆ Insert the dropper about ⅓″ (8 mm) into the nostril. Make sure it doesn't touch the sides of the nostril to avoid contaminating the dropper or making the patient sneeze.

Age alert For a child or an uncooperative patient, place a short piece of soft tubing on the end of the dropper to avoid damaging the mucous membranes.

◆ Instill the prescribed number of drops, observing the patient for signs of discomfort.

◆ Keep the patient's head tilted back for at least 5 minutes. Have him breathe through his mouth to keep the drops from leaking out and to allow time for the drug to work.

◆ Keep an emesis basin handy so the patient can expectorate drug that flows into the oropharynx and mouth.

◆ Use facial tissues to wipe excess drug from the patient's face.

◆ Instruct the patient not to blow his nose for several minutes after instillation.

◆ Return the dropper to the bottle and close it tightly.

To use a nasal spray

◆ Have the patient sit upright with his head erect.

◆ Remove the protective cap from the atomizer.

◆ Occlude one of the patient's nostrils and insert the atomizer tip about ½″ (1.3 cm) into the open nostril.

◆ Position the tip straight up, toward the inner canthus of the eye.

◆ Depending on the drug, have the patient hold his breath or inhale.

◆ Squeeze the atomizer once quickly and firmly—just enough to coat the inside of the nose.

Alert Excessive force may propel drug into the patient's sinuses and cause a headache.

◆ Repeat the procedure in the other nostril, as ordered.

◆ Tell the patient to keep his head tilted back for several minutes, to breathe slowly through his nose, and not to blow his nose for several minutes to make sure the drug has time to work.

To use a nasal aerosol

◆ Insert the drug cartridge according to the manufacturer's directions.

◆ Shake it well before each use and remove the protective cap.

◆ Hold the aerosol between your thumb and index finger, with the index finger on top of the cartridge.

◆ Tilt the patient's head back slightly and carefully insert the adapter tip into one nostril.

◆ Depending on the drug, tell the patient to hold his breath or to inhale.

◆ Press your fingers together firmly to release one measured dose.

◆ Shake the aerosol and repeat the procedure to instill medication into the other nostril.

◆ Remove the cartridge and wash the nasal adapter daily in lukewarm water.

◆ Let the adapter dry before reinserting the cartridge.

◆ Tell patient not to blow his nose for at least 2 minutes after receiving the drug.

Special consideration

◆ Calcitonin (Miacalcin), a hormone used for osteoporosis, should be given in only one nostril daily, the nostrils alternated each day. Make sure to document which nostril is used.

Vaginal drugs

◆ Vaginal drugs include suppositories, creams, gels, and ointments.

◆ Suppositories melt when they come in contact with the warm vaginal mucosa, and the drug diffuses topically—as effectively as creams, gels, and ointments.
◆ Vaginal drugs can be inserted as topical treatment for infection (particularly *Trichomonas vaginalis* and candidal vaginitis) or inflammation or as a contraceptive.
◆ Vaginal drugs usually come with a disposable applicator that allows placement of drug in the anterior and posterior fornices.
◆ Vaginal administration is most effective when the patient can remain lying down afterward, to retain the drug.

Equipment

Patient's medication record and chart ◆ prescribed medication and applicator, if needed ◆ gloves ◆ water-soluble lubricant ◆ cotton balls ◆ soap and warm water ◆ small sanitary pad

Implementation

◆ To minimize drug leakage, give vaginal drugs at bedtime when the patient is lying down whenever possible.
◆ Wash your hands, explain the procedure to the patient, and provide privacy.
◆ Ask the patient to void.
◆ Ask the patient if she would rather insert the drug herself. If so, provide appropriate instructions. If not, proceed with the following steps.
◆ Help her into the lithotomy position.
◆ Expose only the perineum.

To insert a suppository

◆ Remove the suppository from the wrapper and lubricate it with a water-soluble lubricant.
◆ Put on gloves and expose the vagina by spreading the labia.
◆ If you see discharge, wash the area with several cotton balls soaked in warm, soapy water. Clean each side of the perineum and then the center, using a fresh cotton ball for each stroke. While the labia are still separated, insert the suppository 3″ to 4″ (7.5 to 10 cm) into the vagina.

To insert an ointment, a cream, or a gel

◆ Fit the applicator to the tube of drug and gently squeeze the tube to fill the applicator with the prescribed amount of drug.
◆ Lubricate the applicator tip.
◆ Put on gloves and expose the vagina.
◆ Insert the applicator about 2″ (5 cm) into the patient's vagina and expel the drug by depressing the plunger on the applicator.
◆ Instruct the patient to remain in a supine position, with her knees flexed, for 5 to 10 minutes to let the drug flow into the posterior fornix.

After vaginal insertion

◆ Wash the applicator with soap and warm water and store or discard it, as appropriate. If it is to be reused, label it so it will be used for only one patient.
◆ Remove and discard your gloves.
◆ To keep drug from soiling the patient's clothing and bedding, provide a sanitary pad.
◆ Help the patient to return to a comfortable position and advise her to remain in bed as much as possible for the next several hours.
◆ Wash your hands thoroughly.

Special considerations

◆ Refrigerate vaginal suppositories that melt at room temperature.
◆ If possible, teach the patient how to insert the vaginal drug because she

may need to do so herself after discharge.

◆ Give her a patient-teaching sheet if one is available.

◆ Instruct the patient not to insert a tampon after inserting a vaginal drug because it will absorb the drug and decrease its effectiveness.

◆ Tell the patient that these drugs can weaken latex condoms and diaphragms if they're used within 72 hours of drug application.

Respiratory administration

Handheld oropharyngeal inhalers

◆ Handheld inhalers include the metered-dose inhaler or nebulizer, the turbo-inhaler, and the dry-powder, multidose inhaler.

◆ These devices deliver topical drugs to the respiratory tract, producing local and systemic effects.

◆ The mucosal lining of the respiratory tract absorbs the inhalant almost immediately.

◆ Examples of inhalants are bronchodilators, which are used to improve airway patency and facilitate drainage of mucus, and mucolytics, which liquefy tenacious bronchial secretions.

Equipment

Patient's medication record and chart ◆ metered-dose inhaler, turbo-inhaler, or dry-powder, multidose inhaler ◆ prescribed medications ◆ normal saline solution ◆ optional: spacer or extender

Implementation

To use a metered-dose inhaler

◆ Shake the inhaler bottle. Remove the cap and insert the stem into the small hole on the flattened portion of the mouthpiece, as shown below.

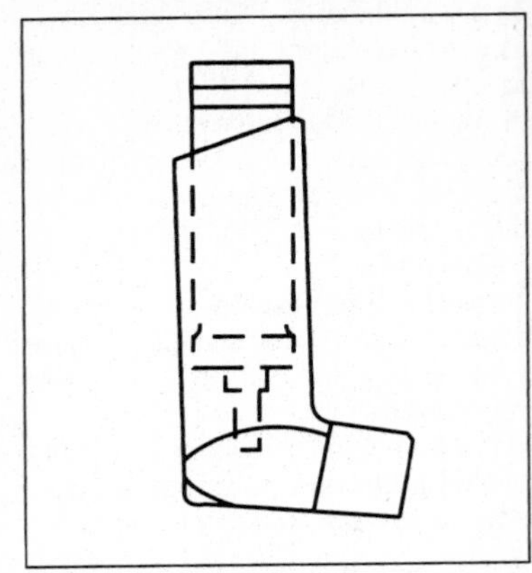

◆ Have the patient exhale.

◆ Place the inhaler about 1" (2.5 cm) in front of his open mouth.

◆ As you push the bottle down against the mouthpiece, instruct the patient to inhale slowly through his mouth and to keep inhaling until his lungs feel full.

◆ Compress the bottle against the mouthpiece only once.

◆ Remove the inhaler and tell the patient to hold his breath for several seconds.

◆ Then instruct him to exhale slowly through pursed lips to keep the distal bronchioles open, allowing increased absorption and diffusion of the drug.

◆ Have the patient gargle with tap water, if desired, to remove drug from his mouth and the back of his throat.

◆ Have the patient wait 1 to 3 minutes before another inhalation.

To use a turbo-inhaler

◆ Hold the mouthpiece in one hand. With the other hand, slide the sleeve away from the mouthpiece as far as possible, as shown at top of left column on next page.

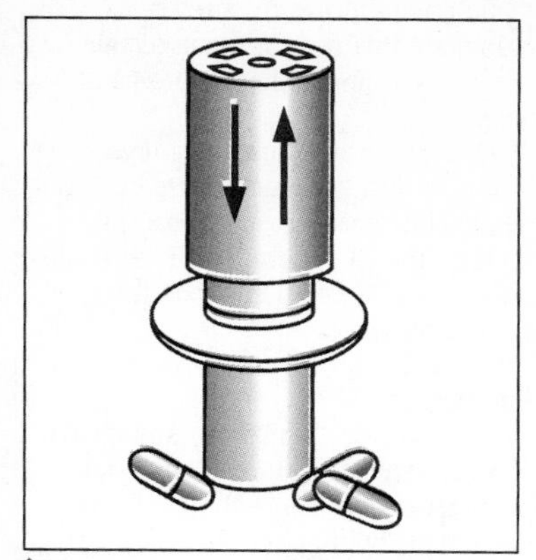

- Unscrew the tip of the mouthpiece by turning it counterclockwise.
- Press the colored portion of the drug capsule into the propeller stem of the mouthpiece. Screw the inhaler together again.
- Holding the inhaler with the mouthpiece at the bottom, slide the sleeve all the way down and then up again to puncture the capsule and release the drug. Do this only once.
- Have the patient exhale completely and tilt his head back.
- Instruct him to place the mouthpiece in his mouth, close his lips around it, and inhale once.
- Tell him to hold his breath for several seconds.
- Remove the inhaler from the patient's mouth and tell him to exhale as much air as possible.
- Repeat the procedure until all of the drug in the device has been inhaled.
- Have the patient gargle with normal saline solution, if desired.

To use a dry-powder, multidose inhaler

- The dry-powder, multidose inhaler is a nonaerosol device that delivers powdered drugs for inhalation.
- Holding the inhaler in one hand and putting the thumb of your other hand on the thumbgrip, push your thumb on the thumbgrip away from you until the mouthpiece appears and snaps into position.
- Holding the inhaler horizontal, slide the lever away from you until it clicks, activating a dose of the drug.
- Have the patient breathe out fully, then put the inhaler mouthpiece to his lips and have him breathe in quickly and deeply through the inhaler.
- Tell the patient to hold his breath about 10 seconds, and then have him breathe out slowly.
- Close the inhaler by sliding the thumbgrip back until it clicks shut.
- Never tilt the activated inhaler or allow the patient to exhale into it, and don't wash the inhaler; wipe it with a dry cloth.
- Remaining doses are shown on an indicator on the top of the inhaler, but the unit should be disposed of after 6 weeks even if all doses weren't used.

To use a holding chamber (InspirEase)

- Insert the inhaler into the mouthpiece of the holding chamber and shake the inhaler.
- Then place the mouthpiece into the opening of the holding device and twist the mouthpiece to lock it in place.
- Extend the holding device, have the patient exhale, and place the mouthpiece into his mouth.
- Press down on the inhaler once. Then have the patient inhale slowly and deeply, collapsing the bag completely. If he breathes incorrectly, the bag will make a whistling sound.
- Tell the patient to hold his breath for 5 to 10 seconds and then to exhale slowly into the bag.
- Then repeat the inhaling and exhaling steps.

◆ Have the patient wait 1 to 2 minutes and then repeat the procedure, if ordered.
◆ Disconnect the holding chamber from the mouthpiece, rinse both in lukewarm water, and let them air-dry.

Special considerations
◆ Teach the patient how to use the inhaler so he can continue treatments after discharge, if needed.
◆ Explain that an overdose can cause the drug to lose effectiveness.
◆ Tell the patient to record the date and time of each inhalation as well as his response.
◆ Some oral respiratory drugs can cause restlessness, palpitations, nervousness, other systemic effects, and hypersensitivity reactions, such as a rash, urticaria, and bronchospasm.
◆ If the patient has heart disease, use caution when giving an oral respiratory drug because it can potentiate coronary insufficiency, cardiac arrhythmias, or hypertension.
◆ If paradoxical bronchospasm occurs, stop the drug and call the physician.
◆ If the patient is using a bronchodilator and a corticosteroid, have him use the bronchodilator first, wait 5 minutes, and then use the corticosteroid.

Enteral administration

Oral drugs

◆ Most drugs are given orally because this route is usually the safest, most convenient, and least expensive.
◆ Drugs for oral use are available in many forms, including tablets, enteric-coated tablets, capsules, syrups, elixirs, oils, liquids, suspensions, powders, and granules.
◆ Some oral drugs require special preparation before use, such as mixing with juice to make them more palatable.
◆ Oral drugs are sometimes prescribed in higher dosages than their parenteral equivalents because, after absorption through the GI system, the liver breaks them down before they reach the systemic circulation.

Equipment
Patient's medication record and chart ◆ prescribed medication ◆ optional: medication cup; appropriate vehicle (such as jelly or applesauce) for crushed pills commonly used with children or elderly patients, or juice, water, or milk for liquid medications; and crushing or cutting device

Implementation
◆ Wash your hands.
◆ Assess the patient's condition, including his level of consciousness, ability to swallow, and vital signs, as needed. Changes in condition may warrant withholding a drug.
◆ Give the patient his drug and, as needed, liquid to aid swallowing, minimize adverse effects, or promote absorption.
◆ If appropriate, crush the drug to facilitate swallowing.
◆ Stay with the patient until he has swallowed the drug. If he seems confused or disoriented, check his mouth to make sure he has swallowed it.
◆ Return and check the patient's response within 1 hour after giving a drug.

Special considerations
◆ To avoid damaging or staining the patient's teeth, give acid or iron preparations through a straw.
◆ An unpleasant-tasting liquid can usually be made more palatable if tak-

en through a straw because the liquid contacts fewer taste buds.

◆ If the patient can't swallow a whole tablet or capsule, ask the pharmacist if the drug comes in liquid form or can be given by another route. If not, ask if you can crush the tablet or open the capsule and mix it with food.

Drugs given by nasogastric tube or gastrostomy button

◆ Besides providing an alternate means of nourishment, a nasogastric (NG) tube allows direct instillation of drugs into the GI system for a patient who can't take them orally.

◆ A gastrostomy button, inserted into an established stoma, lies flush with the skin and receives a feeding tube.

Equipment

Patient's medication record and chart ◆ prescribed drug ◆ towel or linen-saver pad ◆ 50- or 60-ml piston-type catheter-tip syringe ◆ feeding tubing ◆ two 4″ × 4″ gauze pads ◆ stethoscope ◆ gloves ◆ diluent (juice, water, or a nutritional supplement) ◆ cup for mixing medication and fluid ◆ spoon ◆ 50-ml cup of water ◆ gastrostomy tube and funnel, if needed ◆ optional: pill-crushing equipment, clamp (if not already attached to the tube)

Implementation

◆ Gather needed equipment at the patient's bedside.

◆ Liquids should be at room temperature to avoid abdominal cramping.

◆ Make sure that the cup, syringe, spoon, and gauze are clean.

Giving a drug by NG tube

◆ Wash your hands and put on gloves.

◆ Unpin the tube from the patient's gown.

◆ To avoid soiling the sheets during the procedure, fold back the bed linens and drape the patient's chest with a towel or linen-saver pad.

◆ Help the patient into Fowler's position, if her condition allows.

◆ Gently draw back on the piston of the syringe. The appearance of gastric contents implies that the tube is patent and in the stomach.

◆ Test the pH of the secretions using pH indicator paper. If the pH is 5 or less the NG tube placement is in the stomach. If the pH is 6 or more, the tube may be in the duodenum. Notify the supervisory nurse if you have difficulty verifying placement. If needed, the physician can order X-ray verification of placement.

◆ If no gastric contents appear or if you meet resistance, the tube may be lying against the gastric mucosa. Withdraw the tube slightly or turn the patient onto her left side to redirect the tube into pooled secretions.

◆ Clamp the tube, detach the syringe, and lay the end of the tube on a 4″ × 4″ gauze pad.

◆ If the drug is in tablet form, crush it before mixing it with the diluent.

Alert Make sure the particles are small enough to pass through the eyes at the distal end of the tube.

◆ If the drug is in capsule form, open it and pour the contents into the diluent.

◆ If the drug is liquid, pour it into the diluent and stir well.

◆ Reattach the syringe, without the piston, to the end of the tube.

◆ Holding the tube upright at a level slightly above the patient's nose, open the clamp and pour in the drug slowly and steadily, as shown at top of left column on next page.

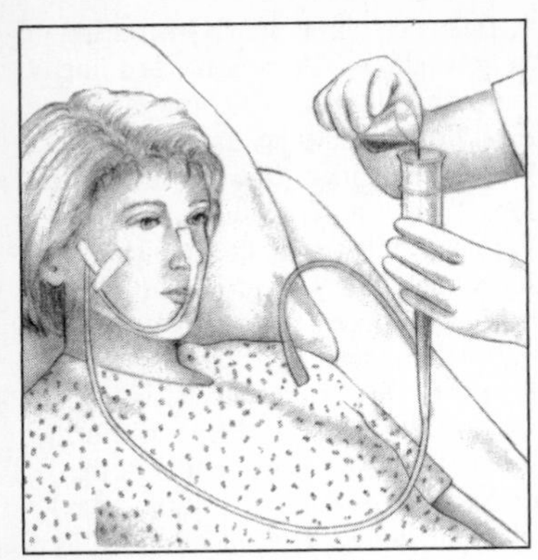

- To keep air from entering the patient's stomach, hold the tube at a slight angle, and add more drug before the syringe empties.
- If the drug flows smoothly, slowly give the entire dose. If it doesn't flow, it may be too thick. In this case, dilute it with water.
- If you think that the placement of the tube is inhibiting the flow, stop the procedure and recheck tube placement.
- If the patient shows signs of discomfort, stop giving the drug immediately.
- As the last of the drug flows out of the syringe, start to irrigate the tube by adding 30 to 50 ml of water (15 to 30 ml for a child).
- Irrigation clears drug from the tube and reduces the risk of clogging.
- When the water stops flowing, clamp the tube.
- Detach the syringe and discard it properly.
- Fasten the tube to the patient's gown and make sure that the patient is comfortable.
- Leave the patient in Fowler's position or on her right side, with her head partially elevated, for at least 30 minutes to facilitate flow and prevent esophageal reflux.

Giving a drug by gastrostomy button

- Help the patient into an upright position.
- Put on gloves and open the safety plug on top of the device.
- Attach the feeding tube set to the button.
- Remove the piston from the catheter-tipped syringe and insert the tip into the distal end of the feeding tube.
- Pour the prescribed drug into the syringe; let it flow into the stomach.
- After instilling all of the drug, pour 30 to 50 ml of water into the syringe and let it flow through the tube.
- When all of the water has been delivered, remove the feeding tube and replace the safety plug.
- Keep the patient in semi-Fowler's position for 30 minutes after giving the drug.

Special considerations

- If you must give a tube feeding and instill a drug, give the drug first to make sure the patient receives it all.
- If residual stomach contents exceed 100 ml, withhold the drug and feeding and notify the physician. Excessive stomach contents may indicate intestinal obstruction or paralytic ileus.
- If the NG tube is on suction, turn it off for 20 to 30 minutes after giving a drug.
- Document the amount of water and drug given.

Buccal and sublingual drugs

- Certain drugs are given buccally (between the patient's cheek and teeth) or sublingually (under the patient's tongue) to bypass the digestive tract and facilitate absorption into the bloodstream.
- Drugs given buccally include nicotine polacrilex gum.

◆ Drugs given sublingually include ergotamine tartrate, isosorbide dinitrate, and nitroglycerin.
◆ When using either method, observe the patient carefully to make sure he doesn't swallow the drug or develop mucosal irritation.

Equipment

Patient's medication record and chart ◆ prescribed drug ◆ drug cup

Implementation

◆ Wash your hands.
◆ For buccal delivery, place the tablet in the patient's buccal pouch, between the cheek and teeth.
◆ For sublingual delivery, place the tablet under the patient's tongue.
◆ To ensure absorption, instruct the patient to keep the drug in place until it dissolves completely.
◆ To prevent accidental swallowing, caution the patient against chewing the tablet or touching it with his tongue.
◆ Tell the patient not to smoke before the drug has dissolved because the vasoconstrictive effects of nicotine slow absorption.

Special considerations

◆ Don't give liquids; some buccal tablets take 1 hour to be absorbed.
◆ If the patient has angina, tell him to wet the nitroglycerin tablet with saliva and to keep it under his tongue until it's fully absorbed.

Rectal suppositories or ointment

◆ A rectal suppository is a small, solid, often cone-shaped, medicated mass, with a cocoa butter or glycerin base.
◆ The suppository inserted into the rectum to stimulate peristalsis and defecation or to relieve pain, vomiting, and local irritation.
◆ A rectal ointment is a semisolid drug that's used to produce local effects. It may be applied externally to the anus or internally to the rectum.

Equipment

Patient's medication record and chart ◆ rectal suppository or tube of ointment and ointment applicator ◆ gloves ◆ 4″ × 4″ gauze pads ◆ water-soluble lubricant ◆ optional: bedpan

Implementation

◆ Wash your hands.

To insert a rectal suppository

◆ Place the patient on his left side in Sims' position and drape him with the bedcovers, exposing only the buttocks.
◆ Put on gloves.
◆ Unwrap the suppository and lubricate it with water-soluble lubricant.
◆ Lift the patient's buttock with your nondominant hand to expose the anus.
◆ Tell the patient to take several deep breaths through his mouth to relax the anal sphincter during insertion.
◆ Insert the suppository with your index finger — tapered end first — about 3″ (7.6 cm), until it passes the internal anal sphincter, as shown below.

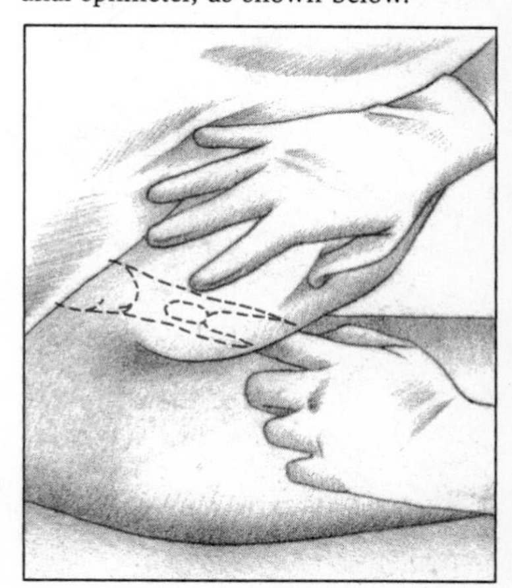

◆ Direct the tapered end of the suppository toward the side of the rectum so it contacts the membranes.
◆ Urge the patient to lie quietly and, if applicable, to retain the suppository for the correct length of time.
◆ Press on the anus with a gauze pad until the urge to defecate passes.
◆ Discard the used equipment and wash your hands thoroughly.

To apply an ointment
◆ For external use, wear gloves or use a gauze pad to spread drug over the anal area.
◆ For internal use, attach the applicator to the ointment tube and coat the applicator with water-soluble lubricant.
◆ Expect to use about 1″ (2.5 cm) of ointment. To gauge how much pressure to use during application, try squeezing a small amount from the tube before you attach the applicator.
◆ Lift the patient's buttock with your nondominant hand to expose the anus.
◆ Tell the patient to take several deep breaths through his mouth to relax the anal sphincter and reduce discomfort during insertion.
◆ Insert the applicator, directing it toward the umbilicus, as shown below.

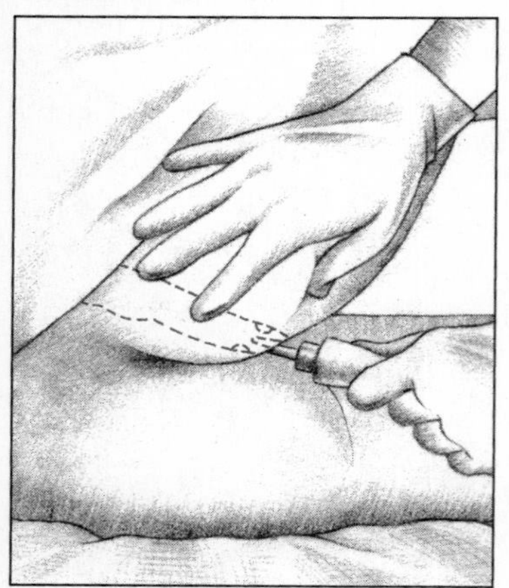

◆ Squeeze the tube to expel the drug.
◆ Remove the applicator and place a folded 4″ × 4″ gauze pad between the patient's buttocks to absorb excess ointment.
◆ Disassemble the tube and applicator and recap the tube.
◆ Clean the applicator with soap and warm water.
◆ Remove and discard your gloves and wash your hands thoroughly.

Special considerations
◆ To prevent softening and possible decreased effectiveness of the drug, store rectal suppositories in the refrigerator until they are needed.
◆ A softened suppository is difficult to handle and insert. To harden it again, hold the suppository (in its wrapper) under cold running water.
◆ Because the intake of food and fluid stimulates peristalsis, a suppository for relieving constipation should be inserted about 30 minutes before mealtime to help soften the stool and facilitate defecation.
◆ A medicated retention suppository should be inserted between meals.
◆ Tell the patient not to expel the suppository until the appropriate time. If he has trouble retaining it, put him on a bedpan.
◆ Make sure the patient's call bell is handy and watch for his signal because he may be unable to suppress the urge to defecate.
◆ Inform the patient that the suppository may discolor his next bowel movement.

Parenteral administration

Subcutaneous injection

◆ A subcutaneous injection allows slower, more sustained drug administration than an intramuscular injection.
◆ Drugs and solutions for subcutaneous injections are injected through a relatively short needle using meticulous sterile technique.

Equipment

Patient's medication record and chart ◆ prescribed drug ◆ needle of appropriate gauge and length ◆ gloves ◆ 1- to 3-ml syringe ◆ alcohol pads ◆ optional: antiseptic cleaner, filter needle, insulin syringe, insulin pump

Implementation

◆ Inspect the drug to make sure it isn't cloudy and doesn't contain precipitates.
◆ Wash your hands.
◆ Select a needle of the proper gauge and length.

Alert An average adult patient needs a 25G 5/8″ needle; an infant, a child, or an elderly or thin patient usually needs a 25G to 27G 1/2″ needle.

For single-dose ampules

◆ Wrap the neck of the ampule in an alcohol pad and snap off the top, away from you.
◆ If desired, attach a filter needle and withdraw the drug.
◆ Tap the syringe to clear air from it.
◆ Engage the needle safety device.
◆ Before discarding the ampule, check the label against the patient's medication record.
◆ Discard the filter needle and the ampule.
◆ Attach a needle of appropriate size and gauge to the syringe.

For single-dose or multidose vials

◆ Reconstitute powdered drugs according to the instructions on the label.
◆ Clean the rubber stopper of the vial with an alcohol pad.
◆ Pull the plunger of the syringe back until the volume of air in the syringe equals the volume of drug to be withdrawn from the vial.
◆ Insert the needle into the vial.
◆ Inject the air, invert the vial, and keep the bevel tip of the needle below the level of the solution as you withdraw the prescribed amount of drug.
◆ From a horizontal surface, scoop the safety cap back over the needle with one hand, then position the syringe vertically to click the cap tight.
◆ Tap the syringe to clear air from it.
◆ Check the drug label against the patient's medication record before returning a multidose vial to the shelf or drawer or before discarding a single-dose vial.

Giving the injection

◆ Select the injection site from those shown below and tell the patient where you'll be giving the injection.

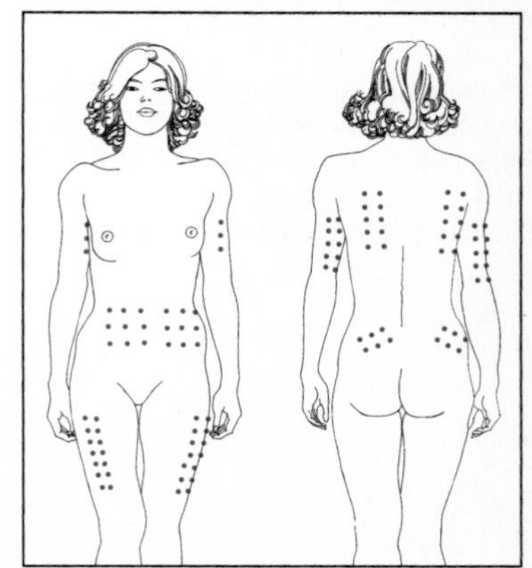

◆ Put on gloves.
◆ Position and drape the patient, as needed.
◆ Clean the injection site with an alcohol pad.
◆ Loosen the protective needle cover.
◆ With your nondominant hand, pinch the skin around the injection site firmly to elevate the subcutaneous tissue, forming a 1″ (2.5-cm) fat fold, as shown below.

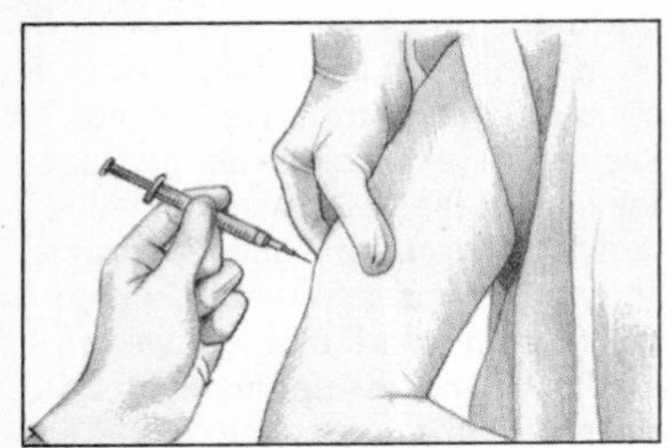

◆ Holding the syringe in your dominant hand (while pinching the skin around the injection site with the thumb and index finger of your nondominant hand), grip the needle sheath between the fourth and fifth fingers of your nondominant hand, and pull back to uncover the needle. Don't touch the needle.
◆ Position the needle with its bevel up.
◆ Tell the patient that she'll feel a prick as the needle is inserted.
◆ Insert the needle quickly in one motion at a 45- or 90-degree angle, as shown at the top of the next column, depending on the length of the needle, the drug, and the amount of subcutaneous tissue at the site.

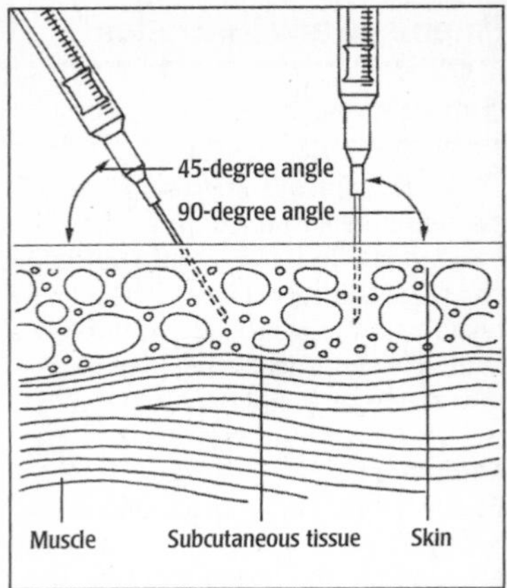

◆ Some drugs, such as heparin, must be injected at a 90-degree angle.
◆ Release the skin to avoid injecting the drug into compressed tissue and irritating the nerves.
◆ Pull the plunger back slightly to check for blood return. If none appears, slowly inject the drug.
◆ If blood appears on aspiration, withdraw the needle, prepare another syringe, and repeat the procedure.
◆ After injection, remove the needle at the same angle used for insertion.
◆ Cover the site with an alcohol pad and, if appropriate, massage the site gently.
◆ Remove the alcohol pad and check the injection site for bleeding or bruising.
◆ Dispose of injection equipment according to facility policy.
◆ Don't recap the needle; engage the needle safety device.

Special considerations

◆ Don't aspirate for blood return when giving insulin or heparin. It isn't needed with insulin and may cause a hematoma with heparin.
◆ Repeated injections in the same site can cause lipodystrophy. A natural im-

mune response, this complication can be minimized by rotating injection sites.

Intradermal injection

◆ Used mainly for diagnostic purposes, as in allergy or tuberculin testing, an intradermal substance is given in small amounts, usually 0.5 ml or less, into the outer layers of the skin.
◆ Because little systemic absorption takes place, this type of injection is used mainly to produce a local effect.
◆ The ventral forearm is the most commonly used site because of its easy access and lack of hair.
◆ In extensive allergy testing, the outer aspect of the upper arms may be used as well as the area of the back between the scapulae.

Equipment
Patient's medication record and chart ◆ prescribed drug ◆ tuberculin syringe with a 26G or 27G ½″ to ⅝″ needle ◆ gloves ◆ alcohol pads ◆ marking pen

Implementation
◆ Locate an injection site from those shown below and tell the patient where you'll be giving the injection.

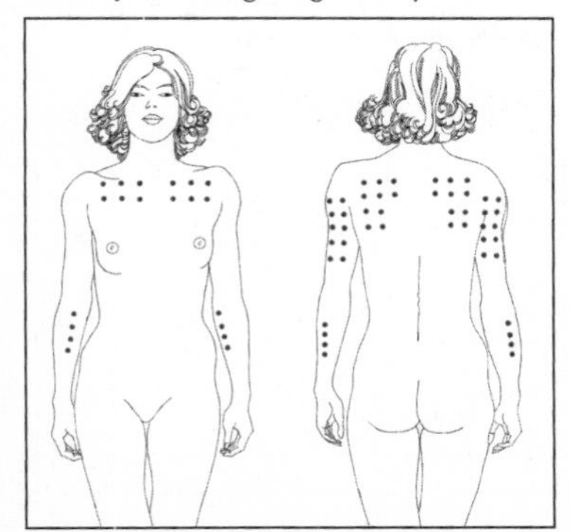

◆ Instruct the patient to sit up and to extend and support her arm on a flat surface, with the ventral forearm exposed.
◆ Put on gloves.
◆ With an alcohol pad, clean the surface of the ventral forearm about two or three fingerbreadths distal to the antecubital space.
◆ Make sure the test site is free from hair and blemishes.
◆ Let the skin dry completely before giving the injection.
◆ While holding the patient's forearm in your hand, stretch the skin taut with your thumb.
◆ With your free hand, hold the needle at a 15-degree angle to the patient's arm, bevel up.
◆ Insert the needle about ⅛″ (3 mm) below the epidermis.
◆ Stop when the bevel tip of the needle is under the skin and inject the antigen slowly.
◆ You should feel resistance as you do this and a wheal should form as you inject the antigen, as shown below.

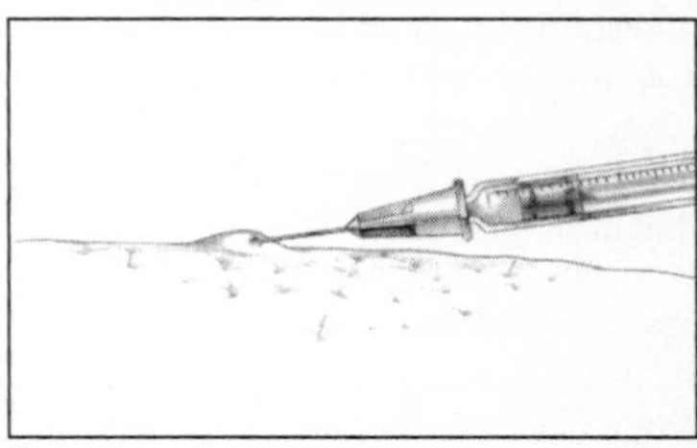

◆ If no wheal forms, you have injected the antigen too deeply. Withdraw the needle and give another test dose at least 2″ (5 cm) from the first site.
◆ Withdraw the needle at the same angle at which you inserted it.
◆ Don't rub the site. This could irritate the underlying tissue, which may affect the test results.
◆ Circle each test site with a marking pen and label each site according to the recall antigen given.
◆ Tell the patient not to wash the circles off until the test is completed.

◆ Dispose of needles and syringes according to facility policy.
◆ Remove and discard your gloves.
◆ In 24 to 48 hours, check the patient's response to skin testing.

Special considerations

◆ If the patient is hypersensitive to the test antigens, she could have a severe anaphylactic response.
◆ Be prepared to give an immediate epinephrine injection and other emergency resuscitation procedures.
◆ Be especially alert after giving a test dose of penicillin or tetanus antitoxin.

Intramuscular injection

◆ An intramuscular injection deposits drug deep into well-vascularized muscle for rapid systemic action and absorption of up to 5 ml.

Equipment

Patient's medication record and chart ◆ prescribed drug, which must be sterile ◆ diluent or filter needle, if needed ◆ 3- to 5-ml syringe ◆ 20G to 25G 1" to 3" needle ◆ gloves ◆ alcohol pads ◆ marking pen

Implementation

◆ Needles used for intramuscular injections are longer than subcutaneous needles because they need to reach deep into the muscle.
◆ Needle length also depends on the injection site, the patient's size, and the amount of subcutaneous fat covering the muscle.
◆ Larger needle gauges accommodate viscous solutions and suspensions.
◆ Needles may be packaged separately or already attached to the syringe.
◆ Check the drug for abnormal color and clarity. If in doubt, ask the pharmacist.
◆ Wipe the stopper of the vial with alcohol and draw the prescribed amount of drug into the syringe.
◆ Provide privacy, explain the procedure, and position and drape the patient; make sure the site is well lit and exposed.
◆ Wash your hands and select an appropriate injection site.
– Avoid a site that's inflamed, edematous, or irritated, or has moles, birthmarks, scar tissue, or other lesions.
– The dorsogluteal and ventrogluteal muscles are the most common sites (shown below).
– If the dorsogluteal site isn't properly identified, damage may be done to the sciatic nerve.

Dorsogluteal muscle

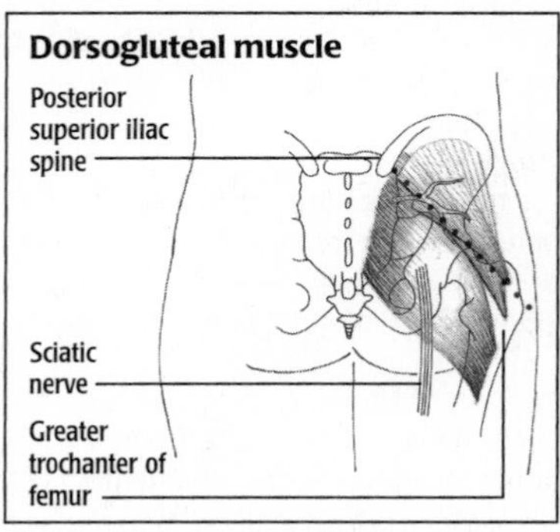

Ventrogluteal muscle

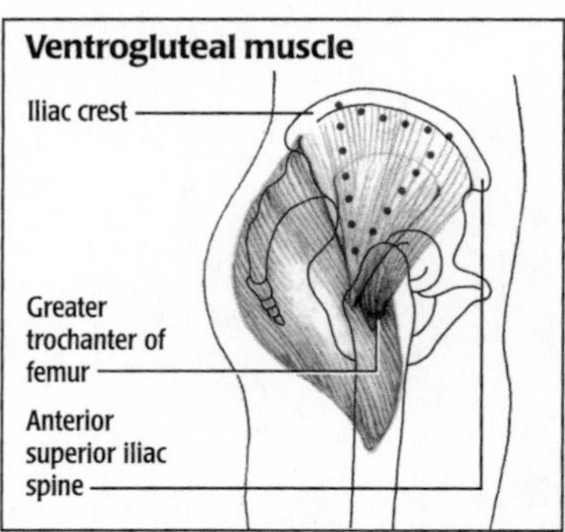

◆ The deltoid muscle (as shown at top of left column on next page) may be used for injections of 2 ml or less.

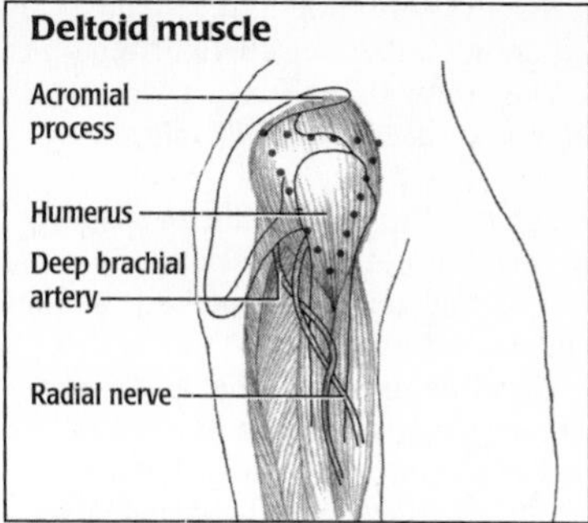

◆ The vastus lateralis muscle (shown below) is used most often in children; the rectus femoris muscle, also shown, may be used in infants.

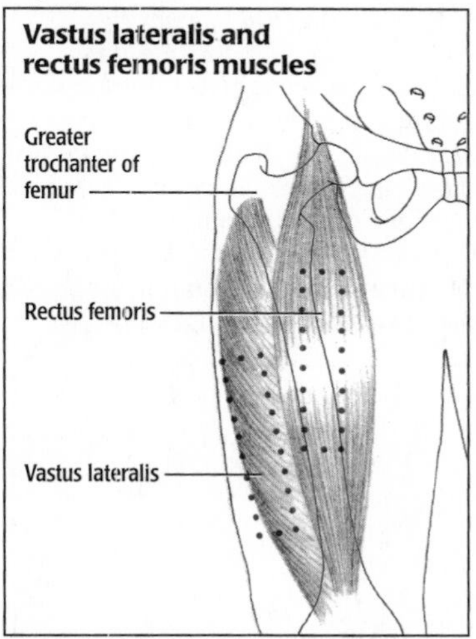

◆ If the patient needs repeated injections, remember to rotate injection sites.
◆ Position and drape the patient appropriately.
◆ Loosen, but don't remove, the needle sheath.
◆ Clean the site by moving an alcohol pad in circles of increasing diameter to about 2″ (5 cm).
◆ Let the skin dry; alcohol causes an unpleasant stinging sensation during injection.
◆ Put on gloves.
◆ With the thumb and index finger of your nondominant hand, gently stretch the skin, pulling it taut.
◆ With the syringe in your dominant hand, remove the needle sheath with the free fingers of your other hand.
◆ Position the syringe perpendicular to the skin surface and a couple of inches from the skin.
◆ Tell the patient that he'll feel a prick. Then quickly and firmly thrust the needle into the muscle.
◆ Pull back slightly on the plunger to aspirate for blood.
– If none appears, inject the drug slowly and steadily to let the muscle distend gradually. You should feel little or no resistance.
– If blood appears, the needle is in a blood vessel. Withdraw it, prepare a fresh syringe, and inject the drug at another site.
◆ Gently but quickly remove the needle at a 90-degree angle.
◆ Using a gloved hand, apply gentle pressure to the site with the used alcohol pad.
◆ Massage the relaxed muscle, unless contraindicated, to distribute the drug and promote absorption.
◆ Inspect the site for bleeding or bruising. Apply pressure or ice, as needed.
◆ Discard all equipment properly.
◆ Don't recap needles; put them in an appropriate biohazard container, after engaging the needle safety device, to avoid needle-stick injuries.

Special considerations

◆ Some drugs are dissolved in oil to slow absorption. Mix them well before use.

Age alert Never inject into the gluteal muscles of a child who has been walking for less than 1 year.

- If the patient needs repeated injections, consider numbing the area with ice before cleaning it.
- If you must inject more than 5 ml, divide the solution and inject it at two sites.
- Urge the patient to relax the muscles to reduce pain and bleeding.
- Intramuscular injections can damage local muscle cells and elevate the serum creatine kinase level, which can be confused with elevated levels caused by a myocardial infarction. Diagnostic tests can differentiate the two.

Z-track injection

- The Z-track intramuscular injection method prevents leakage, or tracking, into the subcutaneous tissue.
- Lateral displacement of the skin during the injection helps to seal the drug in the muscle.
- Typically, the Z-track method is used to give drugs that irritate and discolor subcutaneous tissue — mainly iron preparations such as iron dextran. It may also be used in elderly patients who have decreased muscle mass.
- This procedure requires careful attention to technique because leakage into subcutaneous tissue can cause the patient discomfort and may permanently stain some tissues.

Equipment

Patient's medication record and chart ◆ two 20G 1″ to 3″ needles ◆ prescribed medication ◆ gloves ◆ 3- to 5-ml syringe ◆ alcohol pad

Implementation

- Wash your hands.
- Make sure the needle you're using is long enough to reach the muscle. As a rule of thumb, a 200-lb (91-kg) patient requires a 2″ needle; a 100-lb (45-kg) patient, a $1\frac{1}{4}$″ to $1\frac{1}{2}$″ needle.
- Attach one needle to the syringe and draw up the prescribed drug.
- Then draw 0.2 to 0.5 cc of air (depending on facility policy) into the syringe.
- Remove the first needle and attach the second to prevent tracking the drug through the subcutaneous tissue as the needle is inserted.
- Place the patient in the lateral position, exposing the gluteal muscle to be used as the injection site. The patient may also be placed in the prone position. Put on gloves.
- Clean an area on the upper outer quadrant of the patient's buttock with an alcohol pad.
- Displace the skin laterally by pulling it away from the injection site. To do so, place your finger on the skin surface and pull the skin and subcutaneous layers out of alignment with the underlying muscle. In doing so, the skin should move about 1″ (2.5 cm).
- Insert the needle at a 90-degree angle in the site where you initially placed your finger, as shown below.

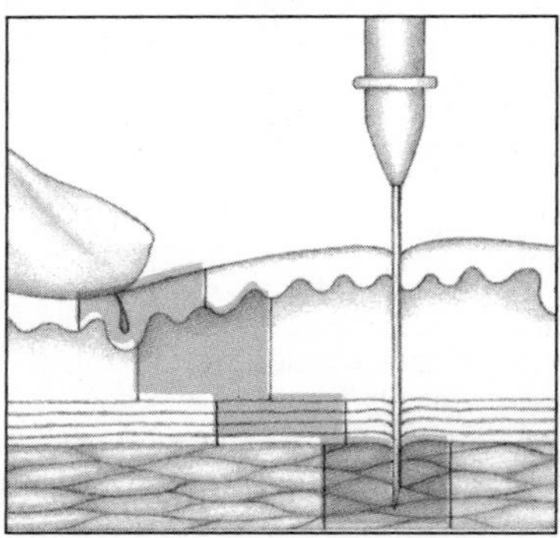

- Aspirate for blood return. If none appears, inject the drug slowly, followed by the air.
- Injecting air after the drug helps clear the needle and prevents tracking the drug through subcutaneous tissues as the needle is withdrawn.

◆ To ensure dispersion of the drug, wait 10 seconds before withdrawing the needle.
◆ Withdraw the needle slowly.
◆ Release the displaced skin and subcutaneous tissues to seal the needle track, as shown below.

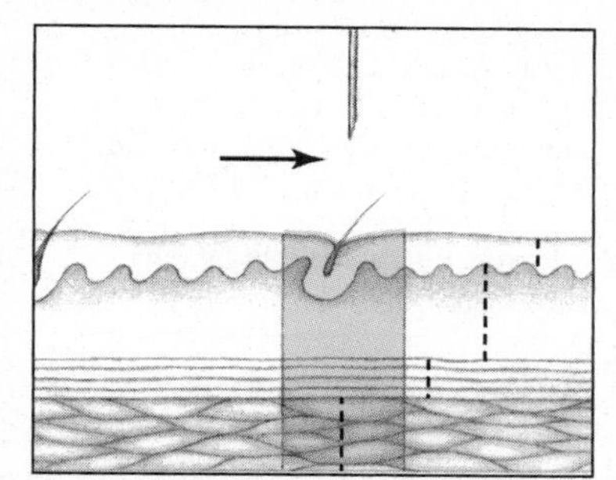

◆ Don't massage the injection site or let the patient wear a tight-fitting garment over the site; doing either could force drug into subcutaneous tissue.
◆ Encourage the patient to walk or move about in bed to facilitate absorption of the drug from the injection site.
◆ To avoid needle-stick injuries, don't recap needles; engage the needle safety device.
◆ Discard the needles and syringe in an appropriate biohazard container.
◆ Remove and discard your gloves.

Special considerations
◆ Never inject more than 5 ml of solution into a single site using the Z-track method. Alternate gluteal sites for repeat injections.
◆ If the patient is on bed rest, encourage active range-of-motion (ROM) exercises, or perform passive ROM exercises to facilitate absorption of the drug from the injection site.

Drug precautions

Drug-tobacco interactions

◆ Smoking — or living and working in a smoke-filled environment — can affect a patient's drug therapy, especially if he's taking one of the drugs listed here.
◆ For a patient using any of these drugs, monitor plasma drug levels closely and watch for possible adverse reactions.

ascorbic acid (vitamin C)
Possible effects
◆ Low serum levels of vitamin C
◆ Decreased oral absorption of vitamin C

Nursing consideration
◆ Tell the patient to increase his vitamin C intake.

chlordiazepoxide hydrochloride, chlorpromazine hydrochloride, diazepam
Possible effects
◆ Increased drug metabolism, which results in reduced plasma levels
◆ Decreased sedative effects

Nursing considerations
◆ Watch for a decrease in drug effectiveness.
◆ Adjust the patient's drug dosage, if ordered.

hormonal contraceptives that contain estrogen and progestogen
Possible effects
◆ Increased risk of adverse reactions, such as headache, dizziness, depression, altered libido, migraine, hypertension, edema, worsening of astigmatism or myopia, nausea, vomiting, and gallbladder disease

Nursing considerations
◆ Inform the patient of increased risk of myocardial infarction and stroke.
◆ Urge the patient to stop smoking or use a different birth control method.

propoxyphene hydrochloride
Possible effects
◆ Increased drug metabolism and decreased analgesic effects

Nursing consideration
◆ Watch for decreased drug effectiveness.

propranolol hydrochloride
Possible effects
◆ Increased metabolism, which decreases drug effectiveness
◆ Decreased drug effectiveness (Smoking increases heart rate, stimulates release of catecholamines from the adrenal medulla, raises arterial blood pressure, and increases myocardial oxygen consumption.)

Nursing considerations
◆ Monitor the patient's blood pressure and heart rate.
◆ To reduce the interaction between the drug and tobacco, the physician may order a selective beta-adrenergic blocker, such as atenolol.

theophylline
Possible effects
◆ Increased theophylline metabolism via induction of liver microsomal enzymes
◆ Lower plasma theophylline levels

Nursing considerations
◆ Monitor plasma theophylline levels and watch for a decreased therapeutic effect.
◆ Increase the drug dosage, if ordered.

Drug-alcohol interactions

◆ Drug-alcohol interactions are more than just potentiated central nervous system depression.
◆ Combined with nonsteroidal anti-inflammatory drugs, alcohol is highly irritating to the stomach.
◆ Combined with some diuretics and cardiac drugs, alcohol may cause a steep drop in blood pressure. (See *Effects of mixing drugs and alcohol.*)

Compatibility of drugs with tube feedings

◆ Some feeding formulas, such as Ensure, may break down chemically when combined with a drug such as Dimetapp Elixir.
◆ Increased formula viscosity and a clogged tube can occur as a result of giving Klorvess, Neo-Calglucon Syrup, or Phenergan Syrup with a feeding formula.
◆ Some drugs, such as ferrous sulfate and potassium chloride liquids, are incompatible with some formulas, causing clumping and other problems when mixed in a tube.
◆ Still other combinations may alter the bioavailability of some drugs, such as phenytoin.
◆ To avoid problems with incompatibility, follow these guidelines:
- Never add a drug to a feeding formula container.
- Always check the compatibility of an ordered drug and the feeding formula before giving it.
- Infuse 30 ml of water before and after giving a drug dose through the tube.
- Flush the feeding tube with 5 ml of water between drug doses if you're giving more than one drug.
- Dilute highly concentrated liquids with 60 ml of water before giving them.

Effects of mixing drugs and alcohol

DRUG	EFFECTS
Analgesics **Anxiolytics** **Antidepressants** **Antihistamines** **Antipsychotics** **Hypnotics**	Deepened central nervous system (CNS) depression
Monoamine oxidase inhibitors	Deepened CNS depression; possible hypertensive crisis with certain types of beer and wine that contain tyramine (Chianti, Alicante)
Oral antidiabetics	Disulfiram-like effects (facial flushing, headache), especially with chlorpropamide; inadequate food intake may trigger increased antidiabetic activity
Cephalosporins **metronidazole** **disulfiram**	Facial flushing, headache

- Instill drugs in liquid form when possible.
- If you must crush a tablet, crush it into fine dust and dissolve it in warm water.
- Never crush and liquefy enteric-coated tablets or timed-release capsules.
- Time the intervals for drug and formula administration appropriately.

Other precautions

Whenever you give a drug, keep the following precautions in mind.

◆ Many drugs have names that look and sound confusingly similar. (See *Look-alike and sound-alike drug names*, pages 404 to 407.)

◆ Some drugs shouldn't be combined in a syringe. (See *Compatibility of drugs combined in a syringe*, pages 408 and 409.)

◆ Some drugs shouldn't be crushed. (See *Drugs that shouldn't be crushed*, pages 410 to 412.)

◆ Certain drug combinations are known to have serious interactions. (See *Serious drug interactions*, pages 412 to 416.)

◆ Patients who take certain herbal supplements may receive drug-like effects from them and may need special follow-up care. (See *Monitoring patients using herbs*, pages 417 to 420.)

Teaching patients about drugs

◆ As the patient becomes more responsible for his own care, it's important that you supply him with all of the information that he needs to comply with his treatment plan. Accurate written information is crucial for any patient, but it's especially important for young patients, elderly patients, and those with cognitive impairments.

(Text continues on page 407.)

Look-alike and sound-alike drug names

Watch out for the following drug names that resemble other drug names either in the way they're spelled or in the way they sound. Don't confuse antivirals that use abbreviations for identification. Also, don't mix up different iron salts because their elemental content may vary.

abciximab and infliximab
acetazolamide and acetohexamide
acetylcholine and acetylcysteine
Aciphex and Aricept
Aggrastat and argatroban
albuterol and Albutein or atenolol
Aldactone and Aldactazide
Aldomet and Aldoril or Anzemet
alitretinoin and tretinoin
alprazolam and alprostadil
amantadine and rimantadine
Ambien and Amen
Amicar and Amikin
Amikin and Amicar
amiloride and amiodarone
aminophylline and amitriptyline or ampicillin
Aminosyn and Amikacin
amiodarone and amiloride
amitriptyline and aminophylline or nortriptyline
amlodipine and amiloride
Anafranil and alfentanil, enalapril, or nafarelin
anakinra and amikacin
Antabuse and Anturane
Anturane and Accutane or Artane
Anzemet and Aldomet
Apresoline and Apresazide
Aquasol A and AquaMEPHYTON
Aricept and Ascriptin
Artane and Anturane or Altace
Asacol and Os-Cal
atenolol and timolol or albuterol
Atrovent and Alupent
Avinza and Invanz
azathioprine and azidothymidine, Azulfidine, or azatadine
bacitracin and Bactroban
baclofen and Bactroban
BCG intravesical and BCG vaccine
Benadryl and Bentyl or Benylin
Benemid and Beminal
Bentyl and Aventyl or Benadryl
benztropine and bromocriptine or brimonidine
Betagan and Betagen or Betapen
Bumex and Buprenex
bupropion and buspirone
calcifediol and calcitriol
Carbatrol and carvedilol
carboplatin and cisplatin
Cardene and Cardura or codeine
Cardizem SR and Cardene SR
Cardura and Coumadin, K-Dur, Cardene, or Cordarone
Catapres and Cetapred or Combipres
Celebrex and Cerebyx or Celexa
Celexa and Celebrex or Cerebyx
Cerebyx and Cerezyme, Celexa, or Celebrex
Chloromycetin and chlorambucil
chlorpromazine and chlorpropamide
Ciloxan and Cytoxan or cinoxacin
cimetidine and simethicone
Citrucel and Citracal
clomiphene and clomipramine or clonidine
clonidine and quinidine or clomiphene
clorazepate and clofibrate
clotrimazole and co-trimoxazole
clozapine and Cloxapen, clofazimine, or Klonopin
codeine and Cardene, Lodine, or Cordran
corticotropin and cosyntropin
Cozaar and Zocor
cyclosporine and cycloserine
cyproheptadine and cyclobenzaprine
dacarbazine and Dicarbosil or procarbazine
Dantrium and Daraprim
Demerol and Demulen, Dymelor, or Temaril
desipramine and disopyramide or imipramine

Look-alike and sound-alike drug names *(continued)*

desmopressin and vasopressin
desonide and Desogen or Desoxyn
Desoxyn and digoxin or digitoxin
dexamethasone and desoximetasone
Dexedrine and dextran or Excedrin
Diamox and Diabinese
diazepam and diazoxide
diazoxide and Dyazide
diclofenac and Diflucan or Duphalac
dicyclomine and dyclonine or doxycycline
digoxin and doxepin, Desoxyn, or digitoxin
Dilantin and Dilaudid
dimenhydrinate and diphenhydramine
Diprivan and Ditropan
dipyridamole and disopyramide
disopyramide and desipramine or dipyridamole
Ditropan and diazepam
dobutamine and dopamine
doxapram and doxorubicin, doxepin, or doxazosin
doxepin and doxazosin, digoxin, doxapram, or Doxidan
doxycycline and doxylamine or dicyclomine
d-penicillamine and penicillin
dronabinol and droperidol
droperidol and dronabinol
DynaCirc and Dynacin
Elavil and Equanil or Mellaril
Eldepryl and enalapril
enalapril and Anafranil or Eldepryl
Endep and Depen
ephedrine and epinephrine
epinephrine and ephedrine or norepinephrine
Epogen and Neupogen
Estratab and Estratest
Ethmozine and Erythrocin
ethosuximide and methsuximide
etidronate and etretinate, etidocaine, or etomidate
Eurax and Serax or Urex
Femara and FemHRT
fentanyl and alfentanil
Flexeril and Floxin or Flaxedil
Flomax and Fosamax or Volmax
floxuridine and fludarabine or flucytosine
flunisolide and fluocinonide
fluorouracil and fludarabine, flucytosine, or floxuridine
fluoxetine and fluvoxamine or fluvastatin
fluticasone and fluconazole
fluvastatin and fluoxetine
folic acid and folinic acid
fosinopril and lisinopril
furosemide and torsemide
glimepiride and glyburide or glipizide
guanabenz and guanadrel or guanfacine
guaifenesin and guanfacine
Haldol and Halcion or Halog
hydralazine and hydroxyzine
hydrocortisone and hydroxychloroquine
hydromorphone and morphine
hydroxyzine and hydroxyurea or hydralazine
HyperHep and Hyperstat or Hyper-Tet
Hyperstat and Nitrostat
idarubicin and daunorubicin or doxorubicin
ifosfamide and cyclophosphamide
imipramine and desipramine
Imodium and Ionamin
Imuran and Inderal
Inderal and Inderide, Isordil, Adderall, or Imuran
Isoptin and Intropin
Isordil and Isuprel or Inderal
K-Phos-Neutral and Neutra-Phos-K
Lamictal and Lamisil
lamotrigine and lamivudine
Lanoxin and Levoxyl or levothyroxine
Lantus and Lente
Leukeran and leucovorin
Levatol or Lipitor
levothyroxine and liothyronine or liotrix
Lithobid and Levbid
Lithonate and Lithostat
Lithotabs and Lithobid or Lithostat
Lodine and codeine, iodine, or Iopidine
Lorabid and Lortab
lorazepam and alprazolam

(continued)

Look-alike and sound-alike drug names *(continued)*

Lotensin and Loniten or lovastatin
Luvox and Lasix
magnesium sulfate and manganese sulfate
Maxidex and Maxzide
Mellaril and Elavil
melphalan and Mephyton
Mestinon and Mesantoin or Metatensin
metaproterenol and metoprolol or metipranolol
methicillin and mezlocillin
methimazole and mebendazole or methazolamide
methocarbamol and mephobarbital
methylprednisolone and medroxyprogesterone
methyltestosterone and medroxyprogesterone
metoprolol and metaproterenol or metolazone
Mevacor and Mivacron
Micronor and Micro-K or Micronase
Minocin and niacin or Mithracin
mitomycin and mithramycin
Monopril and Monurol
Nalfon and Naldecon
naloxone and naltrexone
Navane and Nubain or Norvasc
nelfinavir and nevirapine
Nicoderm and Nitro-Dur
Nicorette and Nordette
nifedipine and nimodipine or nicardipine
Nitro-Bid and Nicobid
nitroglycerin and nitroprusside
norepinephrine and epinephrine
Noroxin and Neurontin
nortriptyline and amitriptyline
Nubain and Navane
nystatin and Nitrostat
Ocuflox and Ocufen
olsalazine and olanzapine
opium tincture and camphorated opium tincture
oxaprozin and oxazepam
oxymorphone and oxymetholone
pancuronium and pipecuronium
Parlodel and pindolol
paroxetine and paclitaxel
Paxil and Doxil, paclitaxel, or Taxol
pemoline and Pelamine
penicillin G benzathine and Polycillin, penicillamine, or other types of penicillin
penicillin G potassium and Polycillin, penicillamine, or other types of penicillin
penicillin G procaine and Polycillin, penicillamine, or other types of penicillin
penicillin G sodium and Polycillin, penicillamine, or other types of penicillin
penicillin V potassium and Polycillin, penicillamine, or other types of penicillin
pentobarbital and phenobarbital
pentostatin and pentosan
Persantine and Periactin
phentermine and phentolamine
phenytoin and mephenytoin
pindolol and Parlodel, Panadol, or Plendil
Pitocin and Pitressin
Plendil and pindolol
pralidoxime and pramoxine or pyridoxine
Pravachol and Prevacid or propranolol
prednisolone and prednisone
Premarin and Primaxin
Prilosec and Prozac, Prinivil, or Plendil
primidone and prednisone
Prinivil and Proventil or Prilosec
ProAmatine and protamine
probenecid and Procanbid
procainamide and probenecid
promethazine and promazine
propranolol and Pravachol
ProSom and Proscar or Prozac
protamine and Protopam or Protropin
Prozac and Proscar, Prilosec, or ProSom
pyridoxine and pralidoxime or Pyridium
Questran and Quarzan
quinidine and quinine or clonidine
ranitidine and ritodrine or rimantadine
Reminyl and Robinul
Restoril and Vistaril
riboflavin and ribavirin
rifabutin and rifampin or rifapentine
Rifater and Rifadin or Rifamate

Look-alike and sound-alike drug names *(continued)*

risperidone and reserpine or Risperdal
Ritalin and Rifadin
ritodrine and ranitidine
ritonavir and Retrovir
Sandimmune and Sandoglobulin or Sandostatin
saquinavir and saquinavir mesylate (the dosages are different)
Sarafem and Serophene
selegiline and Stelazine or Sertraline
Serentil and Serevent or Aventyl
simethicone and cimetidine
Sinequan and saquinavir
Solu-Cortef and Solu-Medrol
somatropin and somatrem or sumatriptan
sotalol and Stadol
streptozocin and streptomycin
sufentanil and alfentanil or fentanyl
sulfadiazine and sulfasalazine
sulfamethoxazole and sulfamethizole
sulfamethoxazole alone and combination products
sulfasalazine and sulfisoxazole, salsalate, or sulfadiazine
sulfisoxazole and sulfasalazine
sulfisoxazole alone and combination products
sulfonamide drugs
sumatriptan and somatropin
Survanta and Sufenta
Tegretol and Toradol
Tenex and Xanax, Entex, or Ten-K
terbinafine and terbutaline
terbutaline and tolbutamide or terbinafine
terconazole and tioconazole
Testoderm and Estraderm
testosterone and testolactone
thiamine and Thorazine
thioridazine and Thorazine
Tigan and Ticar
timolol and atenolol
Timoptic and Viroptic
tobramycin and Trobicin
Tobrex and TobraDex
tolnaftate and Tornalate
Toradol and Tegretol
Trandate and Trental
Trental and Trendar or Trandate
triamcinolone and Triaminicin or Triaminicol
triamterene and trimipramine
trifluoperazine and triflupromazine
trimipramine and triamterene or trimeprazine
Ultracet and Ultracef
Urispas and Urised
valacyclovir and valganciclovir
Vancenase and Vanceril
Vanceril and Vansil
Verelan and Vivarin, Feralyn, or Virilon
Versed and VePesid
vidarabine and cytarabine
vinblastine and vincristine, vindesine, or vinorelbine
Visine and Visken
Volmax and Flomax
Voltaren and Ventolin or Verelan
Wellbutrin and Wellcovorin or Wellferon
Xanax and Zantac, Tenex, or Zyrtec
Xenical and Xeloda
Zarontin and Zaroxolyn
Zaroxolyn and Zarontin
Zebeta and DiaBeta
Zestril and Zostrix
Zocor and Zoloft
Zofran and Zosyn, Zantac, or Zoloft
Zyrtec and Zyprexa

◆ When preparing your written medication teaching plan, it's important to include these points:
- name, dosage, and action of the drug
- frequency and times given
- special instructions for storage and preparation
- drugs (including over-the-counter products) and foods (including additives) to avoid

(Text continues on page 421.)

Compatibility of drugs combined in a syringe

KEY

- Y = compatible for at least 30 minutes
- P = provisionally compatible; administer within 15 minutes
- $P_{(5)}$ = provisionally compatible; administer within 5 minutes
- N = not compatible
- * = conflicting data

(A blank space indicates no available data.)

	atropine sulfate	butorphanol tartrate	chlorpromazine HCl	cimetidine HCl	codeine phosphate	dexamethasone sodium phosphate	dimenhydrinate	diphenhydramine HCl	droperidol	fentanyl citrate	glycopyrrolate	heparin Na	hydromorphone HCl	hydroxyzine HCl	meperidine HCl	metoclopramide HCl
atropine sulfate		Y	P	Y			P	P	P	P	Y	$P_{(5)}$	Y	P*	P	P
butorphanol tartrate	Y		Y	Y			N	Y	Y	Y				Y	Y	Y
chlorpromazine HCl	P	Y		N			N	P	P	P	Y	N	Y	P	P	P
cimetidine HCl	Y	Y	N					Y	Y	Y	Y	$P_{(5)}^*$	Y	Y	Y	
codeine phosphate											Y			Y		
dexamethasone sodium phosphate								N*			N		N*			Y
dimenhydrinate	P	N	N					P	P	P	N	$P_{(5)}$	Y	N	P	P
diphenhydramine HCl	P	Y	P	Y		N*	P		P	P	Y		Y	P	P	Y
droperidol	P	Y	P	Y			P	P		P	Y	N		P	P	P
fentanyl citrate	P	Y	P	Y			P	P	P			$P_{(5)}$	Y	P	P	P
glycopyrrolate	Y		Y	Y	Y	N	N	Y	Y				Y	Y	Y	
heparin Na	$P_{(5)}$		N	$P_{(5)}^*$			$P_{(5)}$		N	$P_{(5)}$					N	$P_{(5)}^*$
hydromorphone HCl	Y		Y	Y		N*	Y	Y		Y	Y			Y		
hydroxyzine HCl	P*	Y	P	Y	Y		N	P	P	P	Y		Y		P	P
meperidine HCl	P	Y	P	Y			P	P	P	P	Y	N		P		P
metoclopramide HCl	P	Y	P			Y	P	Y	P	P		$P_{(5)}^*$		P	P	
midazolam HCl	Y	Y	Y	Y			N	Y	Y	Y	Y		Y	Y	Y	Y
morphine sulfate	P	Y	P	Y			P	P	P	P	Y	N*		P	N	P
nalbuphine HCl	Y			Y				Y	Y		Y			Y		
pentazocine lactate	P	Y	P	Y			P	P	P	P	N	N	Y	P	P	P
pentobarbital Na	P	N	N	N			N	N	N	N	N		Y	N	N	
perphenazine	Y	Y	Y	Y			Y	Y	Y	Y				Y	Y	P*
phenobarbital Na												$P_{(5)}$	N			
prochlorperazine edisylate	P	Y	P	Y			N	P	P	P	Y		N*	P	P	P
promazine HCl	P		P	Y			N	P	P	P	Y			P	P	P
promethazine HCl	P	Y	P	Y			N	P	P	P	Y	N	Y	P	P	P*
ranitidine HCl	Y		N*			Y	Y	Y		Y	Y		Y	N	Y	Y
scopolamine HBr	P	Y	P	Y			P	P	P	P	Y		Y	P	P	P
secobarbital Na				N							N					
sodium bicarbonate											N					N
thiethylperazine maleate		Y											Y			
thiopental Na			N				N	N			N				N	

midazolam HCl	morphine sulfate	nalbuphine HCl	pentazocine lactate	pentobarbital Na	perphenazine	phenobarbital Na	prochlorperazine edisylate	promazine HCl	promethazine HCl	ranitidine HCl	scopolamine HBr	secobarbital Na	sodium bicarbonate	thiethylperazine maleate	thiopental Na	
Y	P	Y	P	P	Y		P	P	P	Y	P					atropine sulfate
Y	Y		Y	N	Y		Y		Y		Y			Y		butorphanol tartrate
Y	P		P	N	Y		P	P	P	N*	P				N	chlorpromazine HCl
Y	Y	Y	Y	N	Y		Y	Y	Y		Y	N				cimetidine HCl
																codeine phosphate
										Y						dexamethasone sodium phosphate
N	P		P	N	Y		N	N	N	Y	P				N	dimenhydrinate
Y	P	Y	P	N	Y		P	P	P	Y	P				N	diphenhydramine HCl
Y	P	Y	P	N	Y		P	P	P		P					droperidol
Y	P		P	N	Y		P	P	P	Y	P					fentanyl citrate
Y	Y	Y	N	N			Y	Y	Y	Y	Y	N	N		N	glycopyrrolate
	N*		N			$P_{(5)}$			N							heparin Na
Y			Y	Y		N	N*		Y	Y	Y			Y		hydromorphone HCl
Y	P	Y	P	N	Y		P	P	P	N	P					hydroxyzine HCl
Y	N		P	N	Y		P	P	P	Y	P				N	meperidine HCl
Y	P		P		P*		P	P	P*	Y	P		N			metoclopramide HCl
	Y	Y		N	N		N	Y	Y	N	Y			Y		midazolam HCl
Y			P	N*	Y		P*	P	P*	Y	P				N	morphine sulfate
Y				N			Y		N*	Y	Y			Y		nalbuphine HCl
	P			N	Y		P	P*	P*	Y	P					pentazocine lactate
N	N*	N	N		N		N	N	N	N	P		Y		Y	pentobarbital Na
N	Y		Y	N			Y		Y	Y	Y			N		perphenazine
										N						phenobarbital Na
N	P*	Y	P	N	Y			P	P	Y	P				N	prochlorperazine edisylate
Y	P		P*	N			P		P		P					promazine HCl
Y	P*	N*	P*	N	Y		P	P		Y	P				N	promethazine HCl
N	Y	Y	Y	N	Y	N	Y		Y		Y			Y		ranitidine HCl
Y	P	Y	P	P	Y		P	P	P	Y					Y	scopolamine HBr
																secobarbital Na
				Y											N	sodium bicarbonate
Y		Y			N					Y						thiethylperazine maleate
	N			Y			N		N		Y		N			thiopental Na

Drugs that shouldn't be crushed

Many drug forms, such as slow-release, enteric-coated, encapsulated beads, wax-matrix, sublingual, and buccal forms, are designed to release their active ingredients over a certain period or at preset intervals. The disruptions caused by crushing these drug forms can dramatically affect the absorption rate and increase the risk of adverse reactions.

Other reasons not to crush these drug forms include such considerations as taste, tissue irritation, and unusual formulation – for example, a capsule within a capsule, a liquid within a capsule, or a multiple-compressed tablet. Avoid crushing the following drugs, listed by brand name, for the reasons noted beside them.

Accutane (irritant)
Aciphex (delayed release)
Adalat CC (sustained release)
Advicor (extended release)
Aggrenox (extended release)
Allegra D (extended release)
Altocor (extended release)
Amnesteem (irritant)
Arthrotec (delayed release)
Asacol (delayed release)
Augmentin XR (extended release)
Avinza (extended release)
Azulfidine EN-tabs (enteric coated)
Bellergal-S (slow release)
Biaxin XL (extended release)
Bisacodyl (enteric coated)
Bontril Slow-Release (slow release)
Breonesin (liquid filled)
Brexin L.A. (slow release)
Bromfed (slow release)
Bromfed-PD (slow release)
Calan SR (sustained release)
Carbatrol (extended release)
Cardizem CD, LA, SR (slow release)
Cartia XT (extended release)
Ceclor CD (slow release)
Ceftin (strong, persistent taste)
Charcoal Plus DS (enteric coated)
Chloral Hydrate (liquid within a capsule, taste)
Chlor-Trimeton Allergy 8-hour and 12-hour (slow release)
Choledyl SA (slow release)
Cipro XR (extended release)
Claritin-D 12-hour (slow release)
Claritin-D 24-hour (slow release)
Colace (liquid within a capsule)
Colazal (granules within capsules must reach the colon intact)
Colestid (protective coating)
Compazine Spansules (slow release)
Concerta (extended release)
Congess SR (sustained release)
Contac 12 Hour, Maximum Strength 12 Hour (slow release)
Cotazym-S (enteric coated)
Covera-HS (extended release)
Creon (enteric coated)
Cytovene (irritant)
Dallergy, Dallergy-Jr (slow release)
Deconamine SR (slow release)
Depakene (slow release, mucous membrane irritant)
Depakote (enteric coated)
Depakote ER (extended release)
Desyrel (taste)
Dexedrine Spansule (slow release)
Diamox Sequels (slow release)
Dilacor XR (extended release)
Dilatrate-SR (slow release)
Dolobid (irritant)
Drisdol (liquid filled)
Dristan (protective coating)
Drixoral (slow release)
Dulcolax (enteric coated)
DynaCirc CR (slow release)
Easprin (enteric coated)
Ecotrin (enteric coated)
Ecotrin Maximum Strength (enteric coated)
E.E.S. 400 Filmtab (enteric coated)
Effexor XR (extended release)
Emend (hard gelatin capsule)
E-Mycin (enteric coated)
Entex LA (slow release)
Entex PSE (slow release)

Drugs that shouldn't be crushed *(continued)*

Eryc (enteric coated)
Ery-Tab (enteric coated)
Erythrocin Stearate (enteric coated)
Erythromycin Base (enteric coated)
Eskalith CR (slow release)
Extendryl JR, SR (slow release)
Feldene (mucous membrane irritant)
Feosol (enteric coated)
Feratab (enteric coated)
Fergon (slow release)
Fero-Folic 500 (slow release)
Fero-Grad-500 (slow release)
Ferro-Sequel (slow release)
Feverall Children's Capsules, Sprinkle (taste)
Flomax (slow release)
Fumatinic (slow release)
Geocillin (taste)
Glucophage XR (extended release)
Glucotrol XL (slow release)
Guaifed (slow release)
Guaifed-PD (slow release)
Guaifenex LA (slow release)
Guaifenex PSE (slow release)
Humibid DM, LA, Pediatric (slow release)
Hydergine LC (liquid within a capsule)
Hytakerol (liquid filled)
Iberet (slow release)
ICAPS Plus (slow release)
ICAPS Time Release (slow release)
Imdur (slow release)
Inderal LA (slow release)
Indocin SR (slow release)
InnoPran XL (extended release)
Ionamin (slow release)
Isoptin SR (sustained release)
Isordil Sublingual (sublingual)
Isordil Tembid (slow release)
Isosorbide Dinitrate Sublingual (sublingual)
Kaon-Cl (slow release)
K-Dur (slow release)
Klor-Con (slow release)
Klotrix (slow release)
K-Tab (slow release)
Levbid (slow release)
Levsinex Timecaps (slow release)
Lithobid (slow release)
Macrobid (slow release)
Mestinon Timespans (slow release)
Metadate CD, ER (extended release)
Methylin ER (extended release)
Micro-K Extencaps (slow release)
Motrin (taste)
MS Contin (slow release)
Mucinex (extended release)
Naprelan (slow release)
Nexium (sustained release)
Niaspan (extended release)
OxyContin (slow release)
Pancrease (enteric coated)
Pancrease MT (enteric coated)
Paxil CR (controlled release)
PCE (slow release)
Pentasa (controlled release)
Phazyme (slow release)
Phazyme 95 (slow release)
Phenytex (extended release)
Plendil (slow release)
Prelu-2 (slow release)
Prevacid, Prevacid SoluTab (delayed release)
Prilosec (slow release)
Prilosec OTC (delayed release)
Pro-Banthine (taste)
Procanbid (slow release)
Procardia (delayed absorption)
Procardia XL (slow release)
Protonix (delayed release)
Proventil Repetabs (slow release)
Prozac Weekly (slow release)
Quibron-T/SR (slow release)
Quinidex Extentabs (slow release)
Respaire SR (slow release)
Respbid (slow release)
Risperdal M-Tab (delayed release)
Ritalin-LA, -SR (slow release)
Rondec-TR (slow release)
Sinemet CR (slow release)
Slo-bid Gyrocaps (slow release)
Slo-Niacin (slow release)
Slo-Phyllin GG, Gyrocaps (slow release)
Slow FE (slow release)
Slow-K (slow release)
Slow-Mag (slow release)
Sorbitrate (sublingual)
Sotret (irritant)
Sudafed 12 Hour (slow release)
Sustaire (slow release)
Tegretol-XR (extended release)

(continued)

Drugs that shouldn't be crushed *(continued)*

Ten-K (slow release)
Tenuate Dospan (slow release)
Tessalon Perles (slow release)
Theobid Duracaps (slow release)
Theochron (slow release)
Theoclear LA (slow release)
Theolair-SR (slow release)
Theo-Sav (slow release)
Theospan-SR (slow release)
Theo-24 (slow release)
Theovent (slow release)
Theo-X (slow release)
Thorazine Spansules (slow release)
Tiazac (sustained release)
Topamax (taste)
Toprol XL (extended release)
T-Phyl (slow release)
Trental (slow release)
Trinalin Repetabs (slow release)
Tylenol Extended Relief (slow release)
Uniphyl (slow release)
Vantin (taste)
Verelan, Verelan PM (slow release)
Volmax (slow release)
Voltaren (enteric coated)
Voltaren-XR (extended release)
Wellbutrin SR (sustained release)
Xanax XR (extended release)
Zerit XR (extended release)
Zomig-ZMT (delayed release)
ZORprin (slow release)
Zyban (slow release)
Zyrtec-D 12 hour (extended release)

Serious drug interactions

When giving these drugs in combination, monitor the patient to prevent serious drug interactions.

DRUG	INTERACTING DRUG	POSSIBLE EFFECT
Aminoglycosides amikacin gentamicin kanamycin neomycin netilmicin streptomycin tobramycin	Parenteral cephalosporins ◆ ceftizoxime	May enhance nephrotoxicity
	Loop diuretics ◆ bumetanide ◆ ethacrynic acid ◆ furosemide	May enhance ototoxicity
Amphetamines amphetamine benzphetamine dextroamphetamine methamphetamine	Urine alkalinizers ◆ potassium citrate ◆ sodium acetate ◆ sodium bicarbonate ◆ sodium citrate ◆ sodium lactate ◆ tromethamine	Decreases urinary excretion of amphetamine

Serious drug interactions *(continued)*

DRUG	INTERACTING DRUG	POSSIBLE EFFECT
Angiotensin-converting enzyme (ACE) inhibitors captopril enalapril lisinopril benazepril fosinopril ramipril quinapril	indomethacin nonsteroidal anti-inflammatory drugs (NSAIDs)	Decreases or abolishes the effectiveness of the antihypertensive action of ACE inhibitors
Barbiturate anesthetics methohexital thiopental	Opiate analgesics	Enhances central nervous system and respiratory depression
Barbiturates amobarbital aprobarbital butabarbital mephobarbital pentobarbital phenobarbital primidone secobarbital	valproic acid	Increases serum barbiturate levels
Beta-adrenergic blockers acebutolol atenolol betaxolol carteolol esmolol levobunolol metoprolol nadolol penbutolol pindolol propranolol timolol	verapamil	Enhances the pharmacologic effects of both beta-adrenergic blockers and verapamil
carbamazepine	erythromycin	Increases the risk of carbamazepine toxicity
carmustine	cimetidine	Enhances the risk of bone marrow toxicity

(continued)

Serious drug interactions *(continued)*

DRUG	INTERACTING DRUG	POSSIBLE EFFECT
ciprofloxacin	Antacids that contain magnesium or aluminum hydroxide, iron supplements, sucralfate, multivitamins that contain iron or zinc	Decreases plasma levels as well as the effectiveness of ciprofloxacin
clonidine	Beta-adrenergic blockers	Enhances rebound hypertension after rapid withdrawal of clonidine
cyclosporine	carbamazepine, isoniazid, phenobarbital, phenytoin, rifabutin, rifampin	Reduces plasma levels of cyclosporine
Cardiac glycosides	Loop and thiazide diuretics	Increases the risk of cardiac arrhythmias as a result of hypokalemia
	Thiazide-like diuretics	Increases the therapeutic or toxic effects
digoxin	amiodarone	Decreases the renal clearance of digoxin
	quinidine	Enhances the clearance of digoxin
	verapamil	Elevates serum levels of digoxin
dopamine	phenytoin	Hypertension and bradycardia
epinephrine	Beta-adrenergic blockers	Increases systolic and diastolic pressures; causes a marked decrease in heart rate
erythromycin	astemizole	Increases the risk of arrhythmia
	carbamazepine	Decreases carbamazepine clearance
	theophylline	Decreases hepatic clearance of theophylline

Serious drug interactions *(continued)*

DRUG	INTERACTING DRUG	POSSIBLE EFFECT
ethanol	disulfiram furazolidone metronidazole	Causes an acute alcohol intolerance reaction
furazolidone	Amine-containing foods Anorexiants	Inhibits MAO, possibly leading to a hypertensive crisis
heparin	Salicylates NSAIDs	Enhances the risk of bleeding
levodopa	furazolidone	Enhances the toxic effects of levodopa
lithium	Thiazide diuretics NSAIDs	Decreases the excretion of lithium
meperidine	MAO inhibitors	Causes cardiovascular instability and increases toxic effects
methotrexate	probenecid	Decreases the elimination of methotrexate
	Salicylates	Increases the risk of methotrexate toxicity
Monoamine oxidase (MAO) inhibitors	Amine-containing foods Anorexiants meperidine	Risk of hypertensive crisis
Nondepolarizing muscle relaxants	Aminoglycosides Inhaled anesthetics	Enhances neuromuscular blockade
Potassium supplements	Potassium-sparing diuretics	Increases the risk of hyperkalemia
quinidine	amiodarone	Increases the risk of quinidine toxicity
Sympathomimetics	MAO inhibitors	Increased the risk of hypertensive crisis
Tetracyclines	Antacids containing magnesium, aluminum, or bismuth salts Iron supplements	Decreases plasma levels as well as the effectiveness of tetracyclines

(continued)

Serious drug interactions *(continued)*

DRUG	INTERACTING DRUG	POSSIBLE EFFECT
Theophylline	carbamazepine	Reduces theophylline levels
	cimetidine	Increases theophylline levels
	ciprofloxacin	Increases theophylline levels
	erythromycin	Increases theophylline levels
	phenobarbital	Reduces theophylline levels
	rifampin	Reduces theophylline levels
warfarin	testosterone	May enhance bleeding caused by increased hypoprothrombinemia
	Barbiturates carbamazepine	Reduces the effectiveness of warfarin
	amiodarone Certain cephalosporins chloral hydrate cholestyramine cimetidine clofibrate co-trimoxazole dextrothyroxine disulfiram	Increases the risk of bleeding
	erythromycin glucagon metronidazole phenylbutazone quinidine quinine Salicylates sulfinpyrazone Thyroid drugs Tricyclic antidepressants	Increases the risk of bleeding
	ethchlorvynol glutethimide griseofulvin	Decreases the pharmacologic effect
	rifampin trazodone	Decreases the risk of bleeding
	methimazole propylthiouracil	Increases or decreases the risk of bleeding

Monitoring patients using herbs

Altered laboratory values and changes in a patient's condition can help target your assessments and better meet the needs of a patient who takes herbal supplements.

HERB	WHAT TO MONITOR	EXPLANATION
aloe	◆ Serum electrolyte level ◆ Weight pattern ◆ Blood urea nitrogen (BUN) and creatinine levels ◆ Heart rate ◆ Blood pressure ◆ Urinalysis	Aloe has cathartic properties that inhibit water and electrolyte reabsorption, which may lead to potassium depletion, weight loss, and diarrhea. Long-term use may lead to nephritis, albuminuria, hematuria, and cardiac disturbances.
capsicum	◆ Liver function ◆ BUN and creatinine levels	Oral administration of capsicum may lead to gastroenteritis and hepatic or renal damage.
cat's claw	◆ Blood pressure ◆ Lipid panel ◆ Serum electrolyte level	Cat's claw may cause hypotension through inhibition of the sympathetic nervous system and its diuretic properties. It may also lower the cholesterol level.
chamomile (German, Roman)	◆ Menstrual changes ◆ Pregnancy	Chamomile may cause changes in the menstrual cycle and is a known teratogen in animals.
echinacea	◆ Temperature	When echinacea is used parenterally, dose-dependent, short-term fever, nausea, and vomiting can occur.
evening primrose	◆ Pregnancy ◆ Complete blood count (CBC) ◆ Lipid profile	Evening primrose elevates plasma lipid levels and reduces platelet aggregation. It may increase the risk of pregnancy complications, including premature rupture of the membranes, the need for oxytocin augmentation, arrest of descent, and the need for vacuum extraction.
fennel	◆ Liver function ◆ Blood pressure ◆ Serum calcium level ◆ Blood glucose level	Fennel contains trans-anethole and estragole. Trans-anethole has estrogenic activity, and estragole is a procarcinogen that can cause liver damage. Adverse effects include photodermatitis and allergic reactions, particularly in patients who are sensitive to carrots, celery, and mugwort.

(continued)

Monitoring patients using herbs *(continued)*

HERB	WHAT TO MONITOR	EXPLANATION
feverfew	◆ CBC ◆ Pregnancy ◆ Sleep pattern	Feverfew may inhibit blood platelet aggregation and decrease neutrophil and platelet secretory activity. It can cause uterine contractions in full-term, pregnant women. Adverse effects include mouth ulceration, tongue irritation and inflammation, abdominal pain, indigestion, diarrhea, flatulence, nausea, and vomiting. Post Feverfew syndrome includes nervousness, headache, insomnia, joint pain, stiffness, and fatigue.
flaxseed	◆ Lipid panel ◆ Blood pressure ◆ Serum calcium level ◆ Blood glucose level ◆ Liver function	Flaxseed has weak estrogenic and antiestrogenic activity. It may reduce platelet aggregation and the serum cholesterol level. Oral administration with inadequate fluid intake can cause intestinal blockage.
garlic	◆ Blood pressure ◆ Lipid panel ◆ Blood glucose level ◆ CBC ◆ Prothrombin time (PT) and partial thromboplastin time (PTT)	Garlic is associated with hypotension, leukocytosis, inhibition of platelet aggregation, and decreased blood glucose and cholesterol levels. Postoperative bleeding and prolonged bleeding time can occur.
ginger	◆ Blood glucose level ◆ Blood pressure ◆ Heart rate ◆ Respiratory rate ◆ Lipid panel ◆ Electrocardiogram	Ginger contains gingerols, which have positive inotropic properties. Adverse effects include platelet inhibition, hypoglycemia, hypotension, hypertension, and stimulation of respiratory centers. Overdoses cause central nervous system (CNS) depression and arrhythmias.
ginkgo	◆ Respiratory rate ◆ Heart rate ◆ PT and PTT	Consumption of ginkgo seed may cause difficulty breathing, weak pulse, seizures, loss of consciousness, and shock. Ginkgo leaf is associated with infertility as well as GI upset, headache, dizziness, palpitations, restlessness, lack of muscle tone, weakness, bleeding, subdural hematoma, subarachnoid hemorrhage, and a bleeding iris.

Monitoring patients using herbs *(continued)*

HERB	WHAT TO MONITOR	EXPLANATION
ginseng (American, Panax, Siberian)	◆ BUN and creatinine levels ◆ Blood pressure ◆ Serum electrolyte levels ◆ Liver function ◆ Serum calcium level ◆ Blood glucose level ◆ Heart rate ◆ Sleep pattern ◆ Menstrual changes ◆ Weight pattern ◆ PT, PTT, and International Normalized Ratio (INR)	Ginseng contains ginsenosides and eleutherosides that can affect blood pressure, CNS activity, platelet aggregation, and coagulation. Reduced glucose and glycosylated hemoglobin levels have also been reported. Adverse effects include drowsiness, mastalgia, vaginal bleeding, tachycardia, mania, cerebral arteritis, Stevens-Johnson syndrome, cholestatic hepatitis, amenorrhea, decreased appetite, diarrhea, edema, hyperpyrexia, pruritus, hypotension, palpitations, headache, vertigo, euphoria, and neonatal death.
goldenseal	◆ Respiratory rate ◆ Heart rate ◆ Blood pressure ◆ Liver function ◆ Mood pattern	Goldenseal contains berberine and hydrastine. Berberine improves bile secretion, increases coronary blood flow, and stimulates or inhibits cardiac activity. Hydrastine causes hypotension, hypertension, increased cardiac output, exaggerated reflexes, seizures, paralysis, and death as a result of respiratory failure. Other adverse effects include GI upset and constipation, excitatory states, hallucinations, delirium, nervousness, depression, dyspnea, and bradycardia.
kava	◆ Weight pattern ◆ Lipid panel ◆ CBC ◆ Blood pressure ◆ Liver function ◆ Urinalysis ◆ Mood changes	Kava contains arylethylene pyrone constituents that have CNS activity. It also has antianxiety effects. Long-term use may lead to weight loss, increased high-density lipoprotein cholesterol levels, hematuria, increased red blood cell count, decreased platelet count, decreased lymphocyte levels, reduced protein levels, and pulmonary hypertension.
milk thistle	◆ Liver function	Milk thistle contains flavonolignans, which have liver-protective and antioxidant effects.

(continued)

Monitoring patients using herbs *(continued)*

HERB	WHAT TO MONITOR	EXPLANATION
nettle	◆ Blood glucose level ◆ Blood pressure ◆ Weight pattern ◆ BUN and creatinine levels ◆ Serum electrolyte level ◆ Heart rate ◆ PT and INR	Nettle contains significant amounts of vitamin C, vitamin K, potassium, and calcium. Nettle may cause hyperglycemia, decreased blood pressure, decreased heart rate, weight loss, and diuretic effects.
passionflower	◆ Liver function ◆ Amylase level ◆ Lipase level	Passionflower may contain cyanogenic glycosides, which can cause liver and pancreas toxicity.
St. John's wort	◆ Vision ◆ Menstrual changes ◆ Excessive response to other medications administered concomitantly	St. John's wort may cause changes in menstrual bleeding and reduced fertility. Other adverse effects include GI upset, fatigue, dry mouth, dizziness, headache, delayed hypersensitivity, phototoxicity, and neuropathy. St. John's wort may also increase the risk of cataracts. St John's wort interferes with the metabolism of many drugs.
SAM-e	◆ Blood pressure ◆ Heart rate ◆ BUN and creatinine levels	SAM-e contains homocysteine, which requires folate, cyanocobalamin, and pyridoxine for metabolism. Increased levels of homocysteine are associated with cardiovascular and renal disease.
saw palmetto	◆ Liver function	Saw palmetto inhibits the conversion of testosterone to dihydrotestosterone and may inhibit growth factors. Adverse effects include cholestatic hepatitis, erectile or ejaculatory dysfunction, and altered libido.
valerian	◆ Blood pressure ◆ Heart rate ◆ Sleep pattern ◆ Liver function	Valerian contains valeric acid, which increases the level of gamma-butyric acid and decreases CNS activity. Adverse effects include cardiac disturbances, insomnia, chest tightness, and hepatotoxicity.

- special comfort measures or safety precautions
- adverse effects and possible signs and symptoms of a toxic reaction
- warnings about discontinuing the medication.

Reporting adverse drug reactions

◆ To meet the standards set by the Joint Commission on Accreditation of Healthcare Organizations (JCAHO), a facility must have a program for reporting adverse drug reactions, and a pharmacy and therapeutics committee at the facility must review all "significant" adverse reactions to ensure quality care.

◆ According to JCAHO, a "significant" reaction is one in which:
- the drug suspected of causing the reaction must be stopped
- the patient needs treatment with another drug, such as an antihistamine, a steroid, or epinephrine
- the patient's hospital stay is prolonged — for example, because surgery had to be delayed or more diagnostic tests had to be done.

◆ This type of reporting program offers three main benefits for the facility:
- When you know which patients are at increased risk for an adverse drug reaction and which drugs are most likely to cause them, you'll be more alert for early signs and symptoms and be prepared to intervene promptly.
- Lengthy stays and extra treatments caused by adverse drug reactions will be decreased.
- Fewer drug-induced injuries means fewer lawsuits brought against the facility and staff.

13 I.V. therapy

Fundamentals of I.V. therapy

Benefits of I.V. therapy

◆ I.V. therapy can be used to give fluids, drugs, nutrients, and other solutions when a patient can't take oral substances.
◆ I.V. drug delivery also allows more accurate dosing.
◆ Because the entire amount of a drug given I.V. reaches the bloodstream immediately, the drug begins to act almost instantaneously.

Risks of I.V. therapy

◆ Like other invasive procedures, I.V. therapy has risks, including:
- bleeding
- blood vessel damage
- infiltration (infusion of the I.V. solution into surrounding tissues rather than the blood vessel)
- infection
- overdose (because response to I.V. drugs is more rapid)
- incompatibility when drugs and I.V. solutions are mixed
- adverse or allergic responses to infused substances. (See *Risks and complications of peripheral I.V. therapy,* pages 424 to 431.)

◆ I.V. therapy also may have complications resulting from the needle or catheter (infection and phlebitis) or from the solution (circulatory overload, infiltration, sepsis, and allergic reaction).
◆ Patient activity can also be problematic. Simple tasks, such as transferring to a chair, ambulating, and washing oneself, can become complicated when the patient must cope with I.V. poles, I.V. lines, and dressings.
◆ I.V. therapy is more costly than oral, subcutaneous, or intramuscular routes of drug delivery.

Fluids, electrolytes, and I.V. therapy

◆ One of the primary objectives of I.V. therapy is to restore and maintain fluid and electrolyte balance.
◆ The human body is composed largely of liquid.
◆ These fluids account for about 60% of total body weight in an adult who weighs 155 lb (70.3 kg) and about 80% of total body weight in an infant.
◆ Body fluids are composed of water (a solvent) and dissolved substances (solutes).
◆ The solutes in body fluids include electrolytes (such as sodium) and nonelectrolytes (such as proteins).

Electrolytes

◆ Electrolytes are a major component of body fluids.
◆ There are six major electrolytes.
- Sodium
- Potassium
- Calcium
- Chloride
- Phosphorus
- Magnesium

◆ These vital substances are chemical compounds that dissociate in solution into electrically charged particles called ions.
◆ The electrical charges of ions conduct current needed for normal cell function. (See *Understanding electrolytes,* pages 432 and 433.)

Fluid and electrolyte balance

◆ Fluids and electrolytes are usually discussed in tandem, especially where I.V. therapy is concerned, because fluid balance and electrolyte balance are interdependent. Any change in one alters

(Text continues on page 433.)

Risks and complications of peripheral I.V. therapy

COMPLICATIONS	SIGNS AND SYMPTOMS
Local complications	
Cannula dislodgment	◆ Cannula partially backed out of vein ◆ Solution infiltrating
Hematoma	◆ Tenderness at the venipuncture site ◆ Bruised area around the site ◆ Inability to advance or flush the I.V. line
Infiltration	◆ Swelling at and above the I.V. site (may extend along the entire limb) ◆ Discomfort, burning, or pain at the site (may be painless) ◆ Tight feeling at the site ◆ Skin cool to the touch around the I.V. site ◆ Blanching at the site ◆ Continuing fluid infusion, even when the vein is occluded, although the rate may decrease
Nerve, tendon, or ligament damage	◆ Extreme pain (similar to electrical shock when the nerve is punctured) ◆ Numbness and muscle contraction ◆ Delayed effects, including paralysis, numbness, and deformity

POSSIBLE CAUSES	NURSING INTERVENTIONS
◆ Loosened tape, or tubing snagged in the bed linens, resulting in partial retraction of the cannula; cannula pulled out by a confused patient	◆ If no infiltration occurs, retape without pushing the cannula back into the vein. If it has pulled out, apply pressure to the I.V. site with a sterile dressing. ***Prevention*** ◆ Tape the venipuncture device securely on insertion.
◆ Puncture of the vein through the opposite wall at the time of insertion ◆ Leakage of blood as a result of needle displacement ◆ Application of inadequate pressure when the cannula is discontinued	◆ Remove the venous access device. ◆ Apply pressure and warm soaks to the affected area. ◆ Recheck for bleeding. ◆ Document the patient's condition and your interventions. ***Prevention*** ◆ Choose a vein that can accommodate the size of the venous access device. ◆ Release the tourniquet as soon as insertion is successful.
◆ Venous access device dislodged from the vein, or perforation of the vein	◆ Stop the infusion. ◆ Check the patient's pulse and capillary refill periodically to assess circulation. ◆ Restart the infusion above the infiltration site or in another limb. ◆ Document the patient's condition and your interventions. ***Prevention*** ◆ Check the I.V. site frequently. ◆ Don't obscure the area above the site with tape. ◆ Teach the patient to observe the I.V. site and to report pain or swelling.
◆ Improper venipuncture technique that causes injury to the surrounding nerves, tendons, or ligaments ◆ Tight taping or improper splinting with an arm board	◆ Stop the procedure. ***Prevention*** ◆ Don't penetrate the tissues repeatedly with the venous access device. ◆ Don't apply excessive pressure when taping; don't encircle the limb with tape. ◆ Pad the arm boards and secure them with tape, if possible.

(continued)

Risks and complications of peripheral I.V. therapy *(continued)*

COMPLICATIONS	SIGNS AND SYMPTOMS
Local complications *(continued)*	
Occlusion	◆ Infusion that doesn't flow ◆ Pump alarms indicating occlusion
Phlebitis	◆ Tenderness proximal to the venous access device ◆ Redness at the tip of the cannula and along the vein ◆ Vein that's hard on palpation ◆ Pain during infusion ◆ Possible blanching if vasospasm occurs ◆ Red skin over the vein during infusion ◆ Rapidly developing signs of phlebitis
Severed cannula	◆ Leakage from the shaft of the cannula

POSSIBLE CAUSES	NURSING INTERVENTIONS
◆ Interruption of the I.V. flow ◆ Failure to flush the heparin lock ◆ Backflow of blood in the line when the patient walks ◆ Line clamped for too long	◆ Use a mild flush injection. Don't force it. If unsuccessful, remove I.V. line and insert a new one. ***Prevention*** ◆ Maintain the I.V. flow rate. ◆ Flush promptly after intermittent piggyback administration. ◆ Have the patient walk with his arm bent at the elbow to reduce the risk of blood backflow.
◆ Poor blood flow around the venous access device ◆ Friction from movement of the cannula along the vein wall ◆ Venous access device left in the vein for too long ◆ Drug or solution with high or low pH or high osmolarity, such as phenytoin and some antibiotics (erythromycin, nafcillin, and vancomycin)	◆ Remove the venous access device. ◆ Apply warm soaks. ◆ Notify the physician if the patient has a fever. ◆ Document the patient's condition and your interventions. ◆ Decrease the flow rate. ◆ Try using an electronic flow device to achieve a steady flow. ***Prevention*** ◆ Restart the infusion using a larger vein for an irritating solution, or restart it with a smaller-gauge device to ensure adequate blood flow. ◆ Tape the device securely to prevent motion. ◆ If long-term therapy with an irritating drug is planned, ask the physician to use a central I.V. line. ◆ Dilute solutions before administration. For example, give antibiotics in a 250-ml solution rather than a 100-ml solution. If the drug has low pH, ask the pharmacist if the drug can be buffered with sodium bicarbonate. (Check facility policy.)
◆ Inadvertent cutting of the cannula by scissors ◆ Reinsertion of the needle into the cannula	◆ If the broken part is visible, attempt to retrieve it. If you're unsuccessful, notify the physician. ◆ If a portion of the cannula enters the bloodstream, place a tourniquet above the I.V. site to prevent progression of the broken part. ◆ Notify the physician and the radiology department. ◆ Document the patient's condition and your interventions. ***Prevention*** ◆ Don't use scissors near the I.V. site. ◆ Never reinsert the needle into the cannula. ◆ Remove the unsuccessfully inserted cannula and the needle together.

(continued)

Risks and complications of peripheral I.V. therapy *(continued)*

COMPLICATIONS	SIGNS AND SYMPTOMS
Local complications *(continued)*	
Thrombophlebitis	◆ Severe discomfort ◆ Reddened, swollen, and hardened vein
Thrombosis	◆ Painful, reddened, and swollen vein ◆ Sluggish or stopped I.V. flow
Vasovagal reaction	◆ Sudden pallor, sweating, faintness, dizziness, and nausea ◆ Decreased blood pressure
Venous spasm	◆ Pain along the vein ◆ Sluggish flow rate when the clamp is completely open ◆ Blanched skin over the vein
Systemic complications	
Air embolism	◆ Respiratory distress ◆ Unequal breath sounds ◆ Weak pulse ◆ Increased central venous pressure ◆ Decreased blood pressure ◆ Loss of consciousness

POSSIBLE CAUSES	NURSING INTERVENTIONS
◆ Thrombosis and inflammation	◆ Follow the procedure for thrombosis. ***Prevention*** ◆ Check the site frequently. Remove the venous access device at the first sign of redness and tenderness.
◆ Injury to the endothelial cells of the vein wall, allowing platelets to adhere and thrombi to form	◆ Remove the venous access device, and restart infusion in the opposite limb, if possible. ◆ Apply warm soaks. ◆ Watch for I.V. therapy–related infection; thrombi provide an excellent environment for bacterial growth. ***Prevention*** ◆ Use proper venipuncture techniques to reduce injury to the vein.
◆ Vasospasm as a result of anxiety or pain	◆ Lower the head of the bed. ◆ Instruct the patient to take deep breaths. ◆ Check the patient's vital signs. ***Prevention*** ◆ Prepare the patient for therapy to relieve his anxiety. ◆ Use a local anesthetic to prevent pain.
◆ Severe irritation of the vein from irritating drugs or fluids ◆ Administration of cold fluids or blood	◆ Apply warm soaks over the vein and the surrounding area. ◆ Decrease the flow rate. ***Prevention*** ◆ Use a blood warmer for blood or packed red blood cells.
◆ Solution container that's empty ◆ Solution container that's emptying, and an added container that's pushing air down the line (if the line isn't purged first) ◆ Tubing that's disconnected	◆ Discontinue the infusion. ◆ Place the patient on his left side in Trendelenburg's position to allow air to enter the right atrium and disperse by way of the pulmonary artery. ◆ Give oxygen. ◆ Notify the physician. ◆ Document the patient's condition and your interventions. ***Prevention*** ◆ Purge the tubing of air completely before starting the infusion. ◆ Use an air-detection device on the pump or an air-eliminating filter proximal to the I.V. site. ◆ Secure the connections.

(continued)

Risks and complications of peripheral I.V. therapy *(continued)*

COMPLICATIONS	SIGNS AND SYMPTOMS
Systemic complications *(continued)*	
Allergic reaction	◆ Itching ◆ Watery eyes and nose ◆ Bronchospasm ◆ Wheezing ◆ Urticarial rash ◆ Anaphylactic reaction (flushing, chills, anxiety, itching, palpitations, paresthesia, wheezing, seizures, cardiac arrest) up to 1 hour after exposure
Circulatory overload	◆ Discomfort ◆ Engorgement of the jugular veins ◆ Respiratory distress ◆ Increased blood pressure ◆ Crackles ◆ Increased difference between fluid intake and output
Systemic infection (septicemia or bacteremia)	◆ Fever, chills, and malaise for no apparent reason ◆ Contaminated I.V. site, usually with no visible signs of infection at the site

POSSIBLE CAUSES	NURSING INTERVENTIONS
◆ Allergens such as drugs	◆ If a reaction occurs, stop the infusion immediately. ◆ Maintain a patent airway. ◆ Notify the physician. ◆ Give an antihistaminic steroid, an anti-inflammatory, and an antipyretic as prescribed. ◆ Give 1:1,000 aqueous epinephrine subcutaneously as prescribed. Repeat at 3-minute intervals and as needed and prescribed. ***Prevention*** ◆ Obtain the patient's allergy history. Be aware of cross-allergies. ◆ Assist with test dosing, and document any new allergies. ◆ Monitor the patient carefully during the first 15 minutes of giving a new drug.
◆ Loosening of the roller clamp to allow run-on infusion ◆ Flow rate that's too rapid ◆ Miscalculation of fluid requirements	◆ Raise the head of the bed. ◆ Give oxygen as needed. ◆ Notify the physician. ◆ Give drugs (probably furosemide) as prescribed. ***Prevention*** ◆ Use a pump, controller, or rate minder for elderly or compromised patients. ◆ Recheck calculations of the fluid requirements. ◆ Monitor the infusion frequently.
◆ Failure to maintain sterile technique during insertion of the device or site care ◆ Severe phlebitis, which can set up ideal conditions for the growth of organisms ◆ Poor taping that permits the venous access device to move, which can introduce organisms into the bloodstream ◆ Prolonged indwelling time of the device ◆ Weak immune system	◆ Notify the physician. ◆ Give drugs as prescribed. ◆ Culture the site and the device. ◆ Monitor the patient's vital signs. ***Prevention*** ◆ Use sterile technique when handling solutions and tubing, inserting the venous access device, and discontinuing infusion. ◆ Secure all connections. ◆ Change the I.V. solutions, tubing, and venous access device at the recommended times.

Understanding electrolytes

Six major electrolytes play important roles in maintaining chemical balance: sodium, potassium, calcium, chloride, phosphorus, and magnesium. Electrolyte concentrations are expressed in milliequivalents per liter (mEq/L) and milligrams per deciliter (mg/dl).

ELECTROLYTE	PRINCIPAL FUNCTIONS	SIGNS AND SYMPTOMS OF IMBALANCE
Sodium (Na^+) ◆ Major cation in extracellular fluid (ECF) ◆ Normal serum level: 135 to 145 mEq/L	◆ Maintains appropriate ECF osmolarity ◆ Influences water distribution (with chloride) ◆ Affects concentration, excretion, and absorption of potassium and chloride ◆ Helps regulate acid-base balance ◆ Aids nerve- and muscle-fiber impulse transmission	*Hyponatremia:* muscle weakness, muscle twitching, decreased skin turgor, headache, tremor, seizures, coma *Hypernatremia:* thirst, fever, flushed skin, oliguria, disorientation, dry, sticky membranes
Potassium (K^+) ◆ Major cation in intracellular fluid (ICF) ◆ Normal serum level: 3.5 to 5 mEq/L	◆ Maintains cell electroneutrality ◆ Maintains cell osmolarity ◆ Assists in conduction of nerve impulses ◆ Directly affects cardiac muscle contraction ◆ Plays a major role in acid-base balance	*Hypokalemia:* decreased GI, skeletal muscle, and cardiac muscle function; decreased reflexes; rapid, weak, irregular pulse; muscle weakness or irritability; fatigue; decreased blood pressure; decreased bowel motility; paralytic ileus *Hyperkalemia:* muscle weakness, nausea, diarrhea, oliguria, paresthesia (altered sensation) of the face, tongue, hands, and feet
Calcium (Ca^{++}) ◆ Major cation found in ECF of teeth and bones ◆ Normal serum level: 8.9 to 10.1 mg/dl	◆ Enhances bone strength and durability (along with phosphorus) ◆ Helps maintain cell-membrane structure, function, and permeability ◆ Affects activation, excitation, and contraction of cardiac and skeletal muscles ◆ Participates in neurotransmitter release at synapses ◆ Helps activate specific steps in blood coagulation ◆ Activates serum complement in immune system function	*Hypocalcemia:* muscle tremor, muscle cramps, tetany, tonic-clonic seizures, paresthesia, bleeding, arrhythmias, hypotension, numbness or tingling in fingers, toes, and area surrounding the mouth *Hypercalcemia:* lethargy, headache, muscle flaccidity, nausea, vomiting, anorexia, constipation, hypertension, polyuria

Understanding electrolytes *(continued)*

ELECTROLYTE	PRINCIPAL FUNCTIONS	SIGNS AND SYMPTOMS OF IMBALANCE
Chloride (Cl^-) ◆ Major anion found in ECF ◆ Normal serum level: 96 to 106 mEq/L	◆ Maintains serum osmolarity (along with Na^+) ◆ Combines with major cations to create important compounds, such as sodium chloride (NaCl), hydrogen chloride (HCl), potassium chloride (KCl), and calcium chloride ($CaCl_2$)	*Hypochloremia:* increased muscle excitability, tetany, decreased respirations *Hyperchloremia:* stupor; rapid, deep breathing; muscle weakness
Phosphorus (P) ◆ Major anion found in ICF ◆ Normal serum phosphate level: 2.5 to 4.5 mg/dl	◆ Helps maintain bones and teeth ◆ Helps maintain cell integrity ◆ Plays a major role in acid-base balance (as a urinary buffer) ◆ Promotes energy transfer to cells ◆ Plays essential role in muscle, red blood cell, and neurologic function	*Hypophosphatemia:* paresthesia (circumoral and peripheral), lethargy, speech defects (such as stuttering or stammering), muscle pain and tenderness *Hyperphosphatemia:* renal failure, vague neuroexcitability to tetany and seizures, arrhythmias and muscle twitching with sudden rise in phosphate level
Magnesium (Mg^{++}) ◆ Major cation found in ICF (closely related to Ca^+ and P) ◆ Normal serum level: 1.5 to 2.5 mg/dl with 33% bound protein and remainder as free cations	◆ Activates intracellular enzymes; active in carbohydrate and protein metabolism ◆ Acts on myoneural vasodilation ◆ Facilitates Na^+ and K^+ movement across all membranes ◆ Influences Ca^{++} levels	*Hypomagnesemia:* dizziness, confusion, seizures, tremor, leg and foot cramps, hyperirritability, arrhythmias, vasomotor changes, anorexia, nausea *Hypermagnesemia:* drowsiness, lethargy, coma, arrhythmias, hypotension, vague neuromuscular changes (such as tremor), vague GI symptoms (such as nausea), peripheral vasodilation, facial flushing, sense of warmth, slow, weak pulse

the other, and any solution given I.V. can affect a patient's fluid and electrolyte balance.

◆ Major intracellular electrolytes are:
- potassium
- phosphorus.

◆ Major extracellular electrolytes are:
- sodium
- chloride.

◆ Intracellular fluid (ICF) and extracellular fluid (ECF) contain different electrolytes because the cell membranes separating the two compartments have selective permeability — that is, only certain ions can cross those membranes.

◆ Although ICF and ECF contain different solutes, the concentration levels

Understanding I.V. solutions

Solutions used for I.V. therapy may be isotonic, hypotonic, or hypertonic. The type you give a patient depends on whether you want to change or maintain his body fluid status.

Isotonic solution

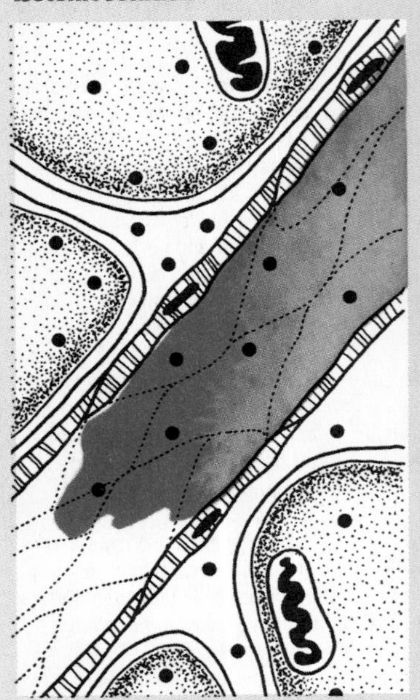

An isotonic solution has an osmolarity about equal to that of serum. Because it stays in the intravascular space, it expands the intravascular compartment.

Hypotonic solution

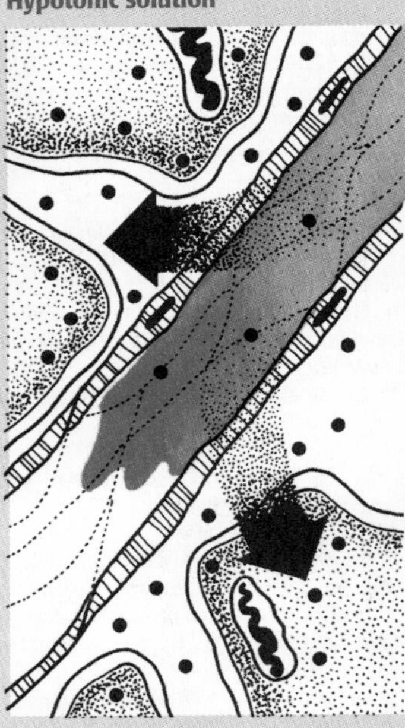

A hypotonic solution has an osmolarity lower than that of serum. It shifts fluid out of the intravascular compartment, hydrating the cells and the interstitial compartments.

of the two fluids are about equal when balance is maintained. (See *Understanding I.V. solutions*, and *Quick guide to I.V. solutions*, pages 436 and 437.)

Peripheral I.V. catheter insertion

◆ A peripheral catheter allows administration of fluids, drugs, blood, and blood components and maintains I.V. access to the patient.
◆ Peripheral I.V. catheter insertion involves several steps:

Hypertonic solution

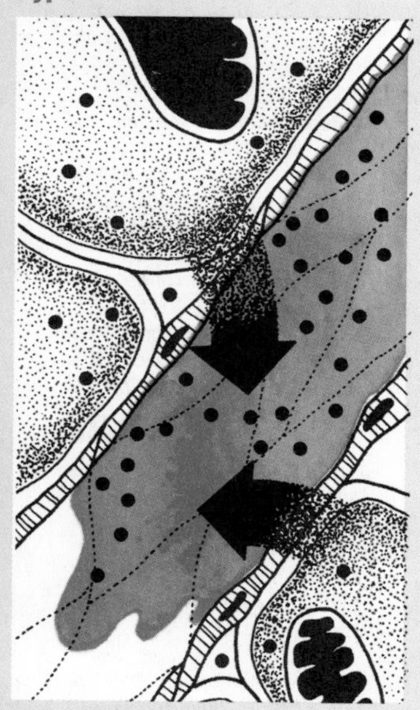

A hypertonic solution has an osmolarity higher than that of serum. It draws fluid into the intravascular compartment from the cells and the interstitial compartments.

- selection of a venipuncture device
- selection of an insertion site
- application of a tourniquet
- preparation of the site
- venipuncture.

◆ Selection of a venipuncture device and site depends on several considerations, including:

- type of solution to be used
- frequency and duration of infusion
- patency and location of accessible veins
- patient's age, size, and condition
- when possible, patient preference.

◆ If possible, the chosen vein should be in the patient's nondominant arm or hand.

◆ Preferred venipuncture sites are the cephalic and basilic veins in the lower arm and the veins in the dorsum of the hand. (See *Peripheral veins and drug delivery,* page 438.)

◆ The least favorable sites are the veins in the leg and the foot because of the increased risk of thrombophlebitis.

◆ Antecubital veins can be used if no other venous access is available. (See *Comparing peripheral venipuncture sites,* pages 439 and 440.)

◆ Insertion is contraindicated in certain situations:

- a sclerotic vein
- an edematous or impaired arm or hand
- a postmastectomy arm with axillary node dissection
- a limb with burns or an arteriovenous fistula.

◆ Subsequent venipunctures should be performed proximal to a previously used or injured vein.

Equipment

Alcohol pads or other approved antimicrobial solution such as chlorhexidine swabs ◆ gloves ◆ disposable tourniquet (latex-free tubing) ◆ I.V. access devices ◆ I.V. solution with attached and primed administration set ◆ I.V. pole ◆ sharps container ◆ transparent semipermeable dressing ◆ 1″ hypoallergenic tape ◆ adhesive bandage ◆ optional: arm board, roller gauze, and warm packs; commercial venipuncture kit with or without an I.V. access device (see *Comparing venipuncture devices,* page 441.)

Quick guide to I.V. solutions

A solution is isotonic if its osmolarity falls within (or near) the normal range for serum (240 to 340 mOsm/L). A hypotonic solution has a lower osmolarity; a hypertonic solution, a higher osmolarity. This chart lists common examples of the three types of I.V. solutions and provides key considerations for administering them.

OSMOLARITY	SOLUTION EXAMPLES	NURSING CONSIDERATIONS
Isotonic	◆ Lactated Ringer's (275 mOsm/L) ◆ Ringer's (275 mOsm/L) ◆ Normal saline (308 mOsm/L) ◆ Dextrose 5% in water (D_5W) (260 mOsm/L) ◆ 5% albumin (308 mOsm/L) ◆ Hetastarch (310 mOsm/L) ◆ Normosol (295 mOsm/L)	◆ Because isotonic solutions expand the intravascular compartment, closely monitor the patient for signs of fluid overload, especially if he has hypertension or heart failure. ◆ Because the liver converts lactate to bicarbonate, don't give lactated Ringer's solution if the patient's blood pH exceeds 7.5. ◆ Avoid giving D_5W to a patient at risk for increased intracranial pressure (ICP) because it acts like a hypotonic solution. (Although usually considered isotonic, D_5W is actually isotonic only in the container. After administration, dextrose is quickly metabolized, leaving only water – a hypotonic fluid.)
Hypotonic	◆ Half-normal saline (154 mOsm/L) ◆ 0.33% sodium chloride (103 mOsm/L) ◆ Dextrose 2.5% in water (126 mOsm/L)	◆ Give cautiously. Hypotonic solutions cause a fluid shift from blood vessels into cells. This shift could cause cardiovascular collapse from intravascular fluid depletion and increased ICP from fluid shift into brain cells. ◆ Don't give hypotonic solutions to patients at risk for increased ICP from stroke, head trauma, or neurosurgery. ◆ Don't give hypotonic solutions to patients at risk for third-space fluid shifts (abnormal fluid shifts into the interstitial compartment or a body cavity) – for example, patients suffering from burns, trauma, or low serum protein levels from malnutrition or liver disease.

Quick guide to I.V. solutions *(continued)*

OSMOLARITY	SOLUTION EXAMPLES	NURSING CONSIDERATIONS
Hypertonic	◆ Dextrose 5% in half-normal saline (406 mOsm/L) ◆ Dextrose 5% in normal saline (560 mOsm/L) ◆ Dextrose 5% in lactated Ringer's (575 mOsm/L) ◆ 3% sodium chloride (1,025 mOsm/L) ◆ 25% albumin (1,500 mOsm/L) ◆ 7.5% sodium chloride (2,400 mOsm/L)	◆ Because hypertonic solutions greatly expand the intravascular compartment, administer them by I.V. pump and closely monitor the patient for circulatory overload. ◆ Hypertonic solutions pull fluid from the intracellular compartment, so don't give them to a patient with a condition that causes cellular dehydration – for example, diabetic ketoacidosis. ◆ Don't give hypertonic solutions to a patient with impaired heart or kidney function – his system can't handle the extra fluid.

Implementation

◆ In many facilities, venipuncture equipment is kept on a tray or cart, allowing a choice of the correct access devices and easy replacement of contaminated items.
◆ Check the information on the label of the I.V. solution container, including:
- patient's name and identification number
- type of solution
- date and time of its preparation
- preparer's name
- ordered infusion rate.

◆ Compare the physician's orders with the solution label to make sure the solution is correct.
◆ Select the smallest-gauge device that's appropriate for the infusion (unless later therapy will require a larger one). Smaller gauges cause less trauma to the veins, allow greater blood flow around their tips, and reduce the risk of phlebitis. (See *Comparing needle and catheter gauges*, page 442.)
◆ Open the catheter device package to allow easy access.
◆ Place the I.V. pole in the proper slot in the patient's bed frame. If you're using a portable I.V. pole, position it close to the patient.
◆ Hang the I.V. solution with the attached primed administration set on the I.V. pole.
◆ Verify the patient's identity by comparing information on the solution container with the patient's wristband. In addition to the patient's name, check a second identifying characteristic (for example, date of birth, address). Don't use the patient's room number as the second identifier.
◆ Wash your hands thoroughly.
◆ Explain the procedure to the patient to ensure his cooperation and reduce anxiety. Anxiety can cause a vasomotor response that results in venous constriction.

Peripheral veins and drug delivery

This illustration shows the location of the veins most commonly used in peripheral venous therapy.

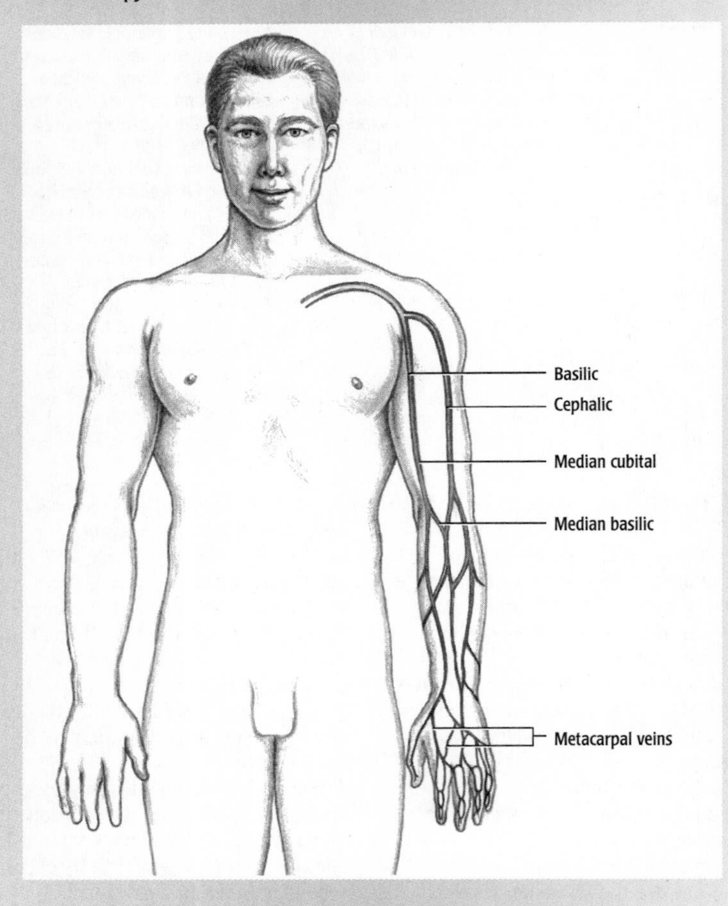

Selecting the site

- Select the puncture site.
- If long-term therapy is anticipated, start distal on the selected vein so that you can move proximally, as needed, for later I.V. insertion sites.
- For infusion of an irritating drug, choose a large vein.
- Make sure the intended vein can accommodate the I.V. access device.
- Place the patient in a comfortable, reclining position, leaving the arm in a

Comparing peripheral venipuncture sites

Venipuncture sites located in the hand, forearm, foot, and leg offer various advantages and disadvantages. This chart includes some of the major benefits and drawbacks of common venipuncture sites.

SITE	ADVANTAGES	DISADVANTAGES
Digital veins Along lateral and dorsal portions of fingers	◆ May be used for short term therapy ◆ May be used when other means aren't available	◆ Requires splinting fingers with a tongue blade, which decreases ability to use hand ◆ Uncomfortable for patient ◆ Significant risk of infiltration ◆ Not used if veins in dorsum of hand already used ◆ Won't accommodate large volumes or fast I.V. rates
Metacarpal veins On dorsum of hand; formed by union of digital veins between knuckles	◆ Easily accessible ◆ Lie flat on back of hand; more difficult to dislodge ◆ In adult or large child, bones of hand act as splint	◆ Wrist movement limited unless short catheter is used ◆ Painful insertion likely because of large number of nerve endings in hands ◆ Phlebitis likely at site
Accessory cephalic vein Along radial bone as a continuation of metacarpal veins of thumb	◆ Large vein excellent for venipuncture ◆ Readily accepts large gauge needles ◆ Doesn't impair mobility ◆ Doesn't require an arm board in an older child or adult	◆ Some difficulty positioning catheter flush with skin ◆ Discomfort during movement due to location of device at bend of wrist
Cephalic vein Along radial side of forearm and upper arm	◆ Large vein excellent for venipuncture ◆ Readily accepts large gauge needles ◆ Doesn't impair mobility	◆ Decreased joint movement due to proximity of device to elbow ◆ Possible difficulty stabilizing vein
Median antebrachial vein Rising from palm and along ulnar side of forearm	◆ Holds winged needles well ◆ A last resort when no other means are available	◆ Painful insertion or infiltration damage possible due to large number of nerve endings in area ◆ High risk of infiltration in this area

(continued)

Comparing peripheral venipuncture sites *(continued)*

SITE	ADVANTAGES	DISADVANTAGES
Basilic vein Along ulnar side of forearm and upper arm	◆ Takes large-gauge needle easily ◆ Straight, strong vein suitable for venipuncture	◆ Inconvenient position for patient during insertion ◆ Painful insertion due to penetration of dermal layer of skin where nerve endings are located ◆ Possible difficulty stabilizing vein
Antecubital veins In antecubital fossa (median cephalic, on radial side; median basilic, on ulnar side; median cubital, which rises in front of elbow joint)	◆ Large vein; facilitates drawing blood ◆ Commonly visible or palpable in children when other veins won't dilate ◆ May be used in an emergency or as a last resort	◆ Difficult to splint elbow area with arm board ◆ Veins may be small and scarred if blood has been drawn frequently from this site
Dorsal venous network On dorsal portion of foot	◆ Suitable for infants and toddlers	◆ Difficult to see or find vein if edema is present ◆ Difficult to walk with device in place ◆ Increased risk of deep vein thrombosis
Scalp veins	◆ Suitable for infants ◆ Commonly visible and palpable in infants ◆ May be used as a last resort	◆ Difficult to stabilize ◆ May require clipping hair at site ◆ Increased infiltration risk due to vein fragility

dependent position to increase venous fill of the lower arms and hands.

◆ If the patient's skin is cold, warm it by rubbing and stroking the arm, covering the entire arm with warm packs, or submerging it in warm water for 5 to 10 minutes.

Applying the tourniquet

◆ Apply a tourniquet above the antecubital fossa to dilate the vein.

◆ Check for a radial pulse. If it isn't present, release the tourniquet and reapply it with less tension to prevent arterial occlusion.

◆ To locate veins, lower the arm below heart level. Have the patient pump his fist. Tap gently over the intended vein.

◆ Lightly palpate the vein with the index and middle fingers of your nondominant hand.

◆ After the vein is identified and secure, stretch the skin to anchor the vein.

◆ If the vein feels hard or ropelike, select another vein.

Comparing venipuncture devices

Here's a comparison of the two major types of venous access devices.

Over-the-needle catheter

Purpose

◆ Long-term therapy for the active or agitated patient

Advantages

◆ Inadvertent puncture of vein less likely than with a winged steel needle set
◆ More comfortable for the patient
◆ Radiopaque thread for easy location
◆ Syringe attached to some units that permits easy check of blood return and prevents air from entering the vessel on insertion
◆ Safety needles that prevent accidental needle sticks
◆ Activity-restricting device, such as arm board, rarely required

Disadvantages

◆ Difficult to insert
◆ Extra care required to ensure that needle and catheter are inserted into vein

Winged steel needle set

Purpose

◆ Short-term therapy (such as a single-dose infusion) for cooperative adult patient
◆ Therapy of any duration for an infant or child or for an elderly patient with fragile or sclerotic veins

Advantages

◆ Easiest intravascular device to insert because needle is thin-walled and extremely sharp
◆ Ideal for nonirritating I.V. push drugs
◆ Available with catheter that can be left in place like over-the-needle catheter

Disadvantage

◆ Infiltration easily caused if rigid needle winged infusion device is used

Over-the-needle catheter

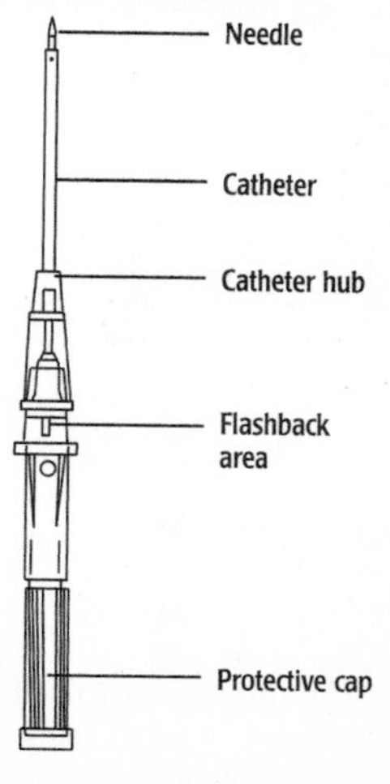

Winged steel needle set

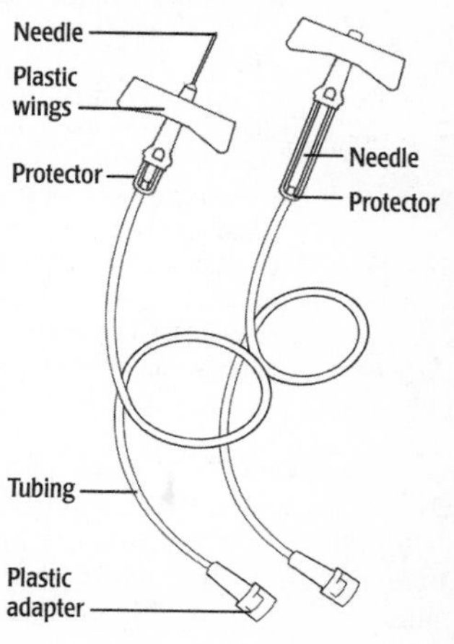

Comparing needle and catheter gauges

How do you know which gauge needle and catheter to use for your patient? The answer depends on the patient's age, his condition, and the type of infusion he's receiving. This chart lists the uses and nursing considerations for various gauges.

GAUGE	USES	NURSING CONSIDERATIONS
16	◆ Adolescents and adults ◆ Major surgery ◆ Trauma ◆ Whenever large amounts of fluids must be infused rapidly	◆ Painful insertion ◆ Requires large vein
18	◆ Older children, adolescents, and adults ◆ Administration of blood and blood components and other viscous infusions ◆ Routinely used preoperatively	◆ Painful insertion ◆ Requires large vein
20	◆ Children, adolescents, and adults ◆ Suitable for most I.V. infusions, blood, blood components, and other viscous infusions	◆ Commonly used
22	◆ Toddlers, children, adolescents, and adults (especially elderly) ◆ Suitable for most I.V. infusions	◆ Easier to insert into small veins ◆ Commonly used for most infusions
24, 26	◆ Neonates, infants, toddlers, school-age children, adolescents, and adults (especially elderly) ◆ Suitable for most infusions, but flow rates are slower	◆ For extremely small veins – for example, small veins of fingers or veins of inner arms in elderly patients ◆ Possible difficulty inserting into tough skin

◆ Leave the tourniquet in place for no longer than 3 minutes. If you can't find a suitable vein and prepare the site in that time, release the tourniquet for a few minutes. Then reapply it and continue the procedure.

Preparing the site

◆ Put on gloves.

◆ Clip the hair around the insertion site, if needed.

◆ Clean the site with alcohol pads or a chlorhexidine swab using a vigorous side-to-side motion to remove flora that would otherwise enter the vascular system with the venipuncture. Allow the antimicrobial solution to dry.

◆ If ordered, administer a local anesthetic.

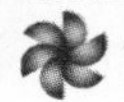
Alert Make sure the patient isn't sensitive to lidocaine.

Inserting the device

◆ Lightly press the vein with the thumb of your nondominant hand about 1½" (3.8 cm) from the intended insertion site. The vein should feel round, firm, fully engorged, and resilient.

◆ Grasp the access cannula.

– If you're using a winged infusion set, hold the short edges of the wings (with the bevel of the needle facing upward) between the thumb and forefinger of your dominant hand. Squeeze the wings together.

– If you're using an over-the-needle cannula, grasp the plastic hub with your dominant hand, remove the cover, and examine the cannula tip. If the edge isn't smooth, discard and replace the device.

◆ To stabilize the vein, use the thumb of your nondominant hand to stretch the skin taut below the puncture site, as shown below.

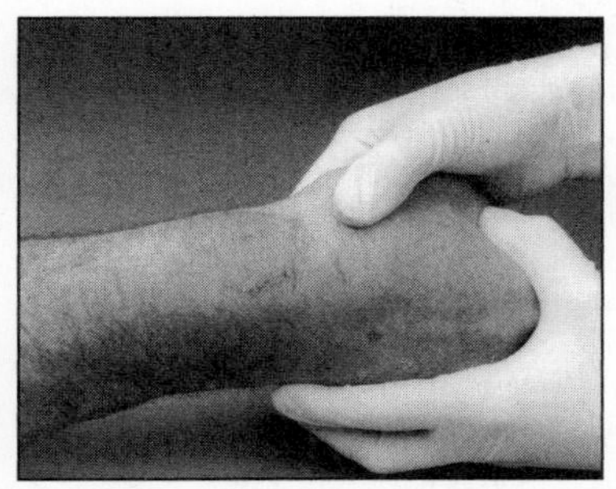

◆ Tell the patient that you're about to insert the device.

◆ Hold the needle with the bevel up and enter the skin directly over the vein at a 0- to 15-degree angle, as shown below.

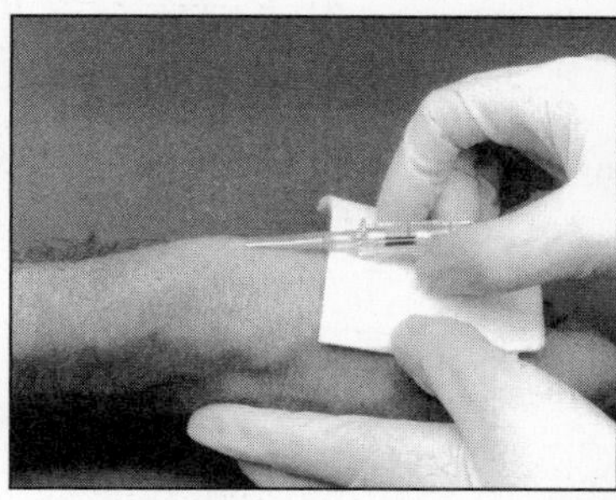

◆ Smoothly push the needle directly through the skin about 1¼" (1 cm) and into the vein in one motion.

After insertion

◆ Check the flashback chamber behind the hub for blood return, signifying that the vein has been properly accessed. You may not see blood return in a small vein.

◆ Level the insertion device slightly by lifting its tip to prevent puncturing the back wall of the vein with the access device.

◆ If you're using a winged infusion set, advance the needle fully, if possible, and hold it in place. Release the tourniquet, open the administration set clamp slightly, and check for free flow or infiltration.

◆ If you're using an over-the-needle cannula, advance the device to at least half its length to ensure that the cannula itself — not just the introducer needle — has entered the vein. Remove the tourniquet.

◆ Grasp the cannula hub to hold it in the vein and withdraw the needle. As you withdraw it, press lightly on the catheter tip to prevent bleeding.

◆ Advance the cannula up to the hub or until you meet resistance.

Methods of taping a venous access site

When using tape to secure the venous access device to the insertion site, use one of the basic methods described below. Only sterile tape should be used under a transparent semi-permeable dressing.

Chevron method

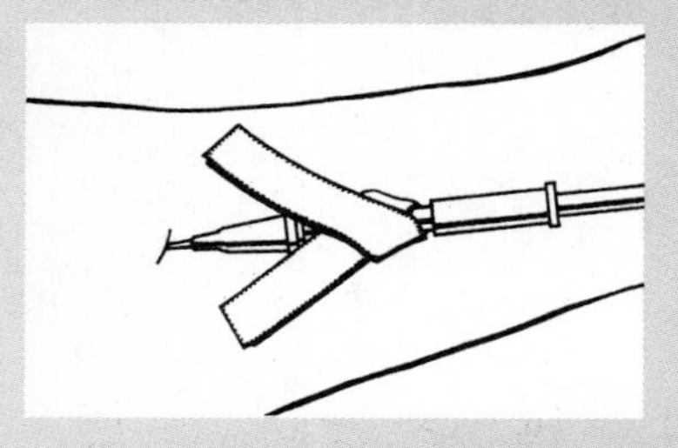

◆ Cut a long strip of ¼″ tape. With the sticky side up, place it under the cannula.
◆ Cross the ends of the tape over the cannula so that the tape sticks to the patient's skin (as shown).
◆ Apply a piece of 1″ tape across the two wings of the chevron.
◆ Loop the tubing, and secure it with another piece of 1″ tape. When the dressing is secured, apply a label. On the label, write the date and time of insertion, the type and gauge of the needle, and your initials.

U method

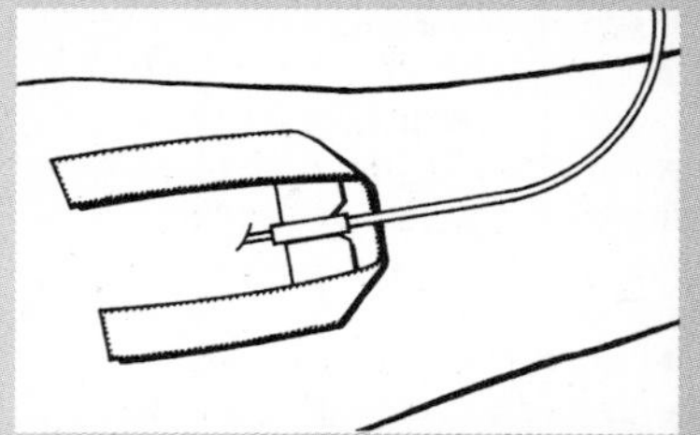

◆ Cut a 2″ (5-cm) strip of 1″ tape. With the sticky side up, place the tape under the hub of the cannula.
◆ Bring each side of the tape up, folding it over the wings of the cannula in a U shape (as shown). Press it down parallel to the hub.
◆ Apply tape to stabilize the catheter.
◆ When a dressing is secured, apply a label. On the label, write the date and time of insertion, the type and gauge of the needle or cannula, and your initials.

◆ To advance the cannula while infusing I.V. solution, release the tourniquet and remove the inner needle.
- Using sterile technique, attach the I.V. tubing and begin the infusion.
- Stabilize the vein with one hand and use the other to advance the catheter into the vein.
- When the catheter is advanced, decrease the I.V. flow rate.
- This method lessens the risk of puncturing the opposite wall of the vein because the catheter is advanced without the steel needle and because the rapid flow dilates the vein.

◆ To advance the cannula before starting the infusion, release the tourniquet.
- Stabilize the vein with one hand and use the other hand to advance the catheter up to the hub.
- Remove the inner needle and, using sterile technique, quickly attach the I.V. tubing.
- This method typically results in less blood being spilled.

Dressing the site

◆ After the venous access device has been inserted, clean the skin completely.

H method

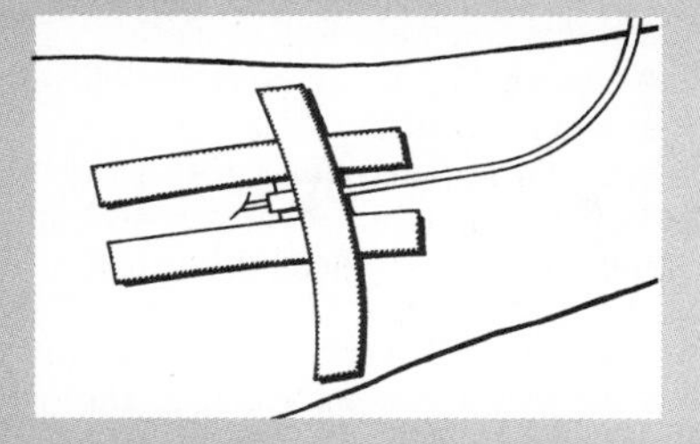

◆ Cut three strips of ½″ tape.
◆ Place one strip of tape over each wing, keeping the tape parallel to the cannula (as shown).
◆ Place the other strip of tape perpendicular to the first two strips. Put it either directly on top of the wings or just below the wings, directly on top of the tubing.
◆ Make sure that the cannula is secure. Then apply a dressing and a label. On the label, write the date and time of insertion, the type and gauge of the needle or cannula, and your initials.

X method

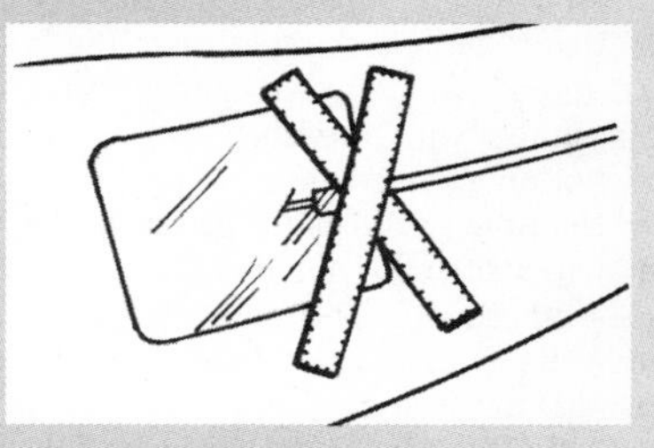

◆ Place a transparent semipermeable dressing over the insertion site.
◆ Cut two 2″ strips of ½″ tape.
◆ Place one strip diagonally, over the hub of the cannula.
◆ Place the second strip diagonal to the hub in the opposite direction, forming an X with the first strip (as shown).

◆ If needed, dispose of the stylet in a sharps container.
◆ Regulate the flow rate.
◆ You may use a transparent semipermeable dressing to secure the device. If you don't use a transparent dressing, cover the site with a sterile gauze pad.
◆ Loop the I.V. tubing on the patient's limb and secure the tubing with hypoallergenic tape. The loop allows some slack to prevent tension on the line from dislodging the cannula. (See *Methods of taping a venous access site*.)
◆ Label the last piece of tape with:
- type and gauge of the needle
- length of the cannula
- date and time of insertion
- your initials.

◆ Adjust the flow rate as ordered.
◆ If needed, place an arm board under the joint and secure it with roller gauze or tape to provide stability.
◆ Make sure the insertion site is visible and that the tape isn't constricting the patient's circulation.

Removing a peripheral I.V. catheter

◆ A peripheral I.V. catheter is removed for cannula site changes, for suspected infection or infiltration, and at the end of therapy.

◆ The procedure usually requires gloves, a sterile gauze pad, and an adhesive bandage.
◆ To remove the I.V. catheter, clamp the I.V. tubing to stop the flow of solution.
◆ Gently remove the transparent dressing and all tape from the skin.
◆ Using sterile technique, open the gauze pad and adhesive bandage and place them within reach.
◆ Put on gloves.
◆ Hold the sterile gauze pad over the puncture site with one hand and use your other hand to withdraw the cannula slowly and smoothly, keeping it parallel to the skin.
◆ Inspect the tip of the cannula; if it isn't smooth, check the patient immediately and notify the physician.
◆ Using the gauze pad, apply firm pressure over the puncture site for 1 to 2 minutes after removal or until bleeding has stopped.
◆ Clean the site and apply the adhesive bandage or, if blood oozes, apply a pressure bandage.
◆ If drainage appears at the puncture site, swab the tip of the cannula across an agar plate and send it to the laboratory to be cultured, according to facility policy.
◆ Clean the area, apply a sterile dressing and notify the physician.
◆ Instruct the patient to restrict activity for about 10 minutes and to leave the dressing in place for at least 1 hour.
◆ If the patient has lingering tenderness at the site, apply warm packs and notify the physician.

Special considerations

Age alert Apply the tourniquet carefully to avoid pinching the skin. If needed, apply it over the patient's gown. Make sure that skin preparation materials are at room temperature to avoid vasoconstriction from lower temperatures.
◆ If the patient is allergic to chlorhexidine, clean the skin with alcohol.
◆ If you don't see blood flashback, remove the cannula and try again, or proceed according to facility policy.
◆ Change a gauze or transparent dressing when it's dirty or loose.
◆ Rotate the I.V. site every 72 hours or according to facility policy.

Patient teaching tip If you're caring for a patient who's going home with a peripheral line, teach him how to care for the I.V. site and how to identify certain complications. If the patient has movement restrictions, make sure he understands them. Teach the patient how to examine the site. Tell him to notify the physician or home care nurse if he has redness, swelling, or discomfort, or if the dressing becomes moist. Tell the patient to report all problems with the I.V. line (for instance, if the solution stops infusing or if an alarm goes off on an infusion pump). Explain that a home care nurse will change the I.V. site at established intervals. If the patient is using an intermittent infusion device, teach him how and when to flush it. Teach the patient about possible complications of peripheral lines.

Documentation

◆ Record the date and time of the venipuncture (in your notes or on the appropriate I.V. sheets).
◆ Note the type, gauge, and length of the cannula.
◆ Note the anatomic location of the insertion site.
◆ Indicate the reason the site was changed.
◆ Note the number of attempts at venipuncture.
◆ Record the type and flow rate of I.V. solution.

◆ Record the name and amount of drug in the solution (if any).
◆ Note all adverse reactions.
◆ Note actions taken to correct adverse reactions.
◆ Note patient teaching and evidence of patient understanding.
◆ Include your initials.

Peripheral I.V. line maintenance

◆ Routine maintenance of I.V. sites and systems includes regular examination and rotation of the site and periodic changes of the dressing, tubing, and solution.
◆ These measures help prevent complications, such as thrombophlebitis and infection. They should be performed according to facility policy.
◆ Typically, I.V. dressings are changed when the device is changed or when the dressing becomes wet, soiled, or nonocclusive.
◆ I.V. tubing is changed every 72 hours or according to facility policy.
◆ I.V. solution is changed every 24 hours or as needed.
◆ The site should be checked every 4 hours if a transparent semipermeable dressing is used. Otherwise, it should be checked with every dressing change and should be rotated every 72 hours.

Equipment

For dressing changes

Gloves ◆ chlorhexidine or alcohol pad ◆ sterile 2″ × 2″ 20 gauze pad or transparent semipermeable dressing ◆ 1″ adhesive tape

For solution changes

Solution container as ordered (bag or bottle) ◆ alcohol pad

For tubing changes

I.V. administration set ◆ gloves ◆ sterile 2″ × 2″ gauze pad ◆ adhesive tape for labeling ◆ hypoallergenic tape

For I.V. site changes

◆ Commercial kits containing the equipment for dressing changes are available.

Implementation

◆ If the facility keeps I.V. equipment and dressings in a tray or cart, have it nearby, if possible, because you may need to select a new venipuncture site, depending on the condition of the current site.
◆ If you're changing the solution and tubing, attach and prime the I.V. administration set before you enter the patient's room.
◆ Wash your hands thoroughly to prevent the spread of microorganisms.
◆ Wear gloves whenever you're working near a venipuncture site.
◆ Explain the procedure to the patient to allay his fears and ensure cooperation.

Changing the dressing

◆ Remove the old dressing, open all supply packages, and put on gloves.
◆ Hold the cannula in place with your nondominant hand to prevent accidental movement or dislodgment, which could puncture the vein and cause infiltration.
◆ Check the venipuncture site for evidence of infection (redness and pain), infiltration (coolness, blanching, and edema), and phlebitis (redness, firmness, pain along the path of the vein, and edema).
– If such evidence is present, cover the area with a sterile 2″ × 2″ gauze pad and remove the catheter or needle.
– Apply pressure to the area until the bleeding stops and apply a bandage.

- Start the I.V. line in another appropriate site, preferably on the opposite limb.
- Change the I.V. solution and tubing.

◆ If the venipuncture site is without complications, stabilize the cannula and carefully clean around the puncture site with a chlorhexidine swab or an alcohol pad, using a vigorous side-to-side motion.

◆ Let the area dry completely.

◆ Cover the site with a transparent semipermeable dressing. This type of dressing allows visibility of the insertion site and maintains sterility. It's placed over the insertion site to halfway up the cannula.

Changing the solution

◆ Wash your hands.

◆ Inspect the new solution container for cracks, leaks, and other damage.

◆ Check the solution for discoloration, turbidity, and particulates.

◆ Note the date and time that the solution was mixed, as well as its expiration date.

◆ When inverting the tubing, clamp it to prevent air from entering.

◆ Keep the drip chamber half full.

◆ If you're replacing a bag, remove the seal or tab from the new bag and remove the old bag from the pole. Remove the spike, insert it into the new bag, and adjust the flow rate.

◆ If you're replacing a bottle, remove the cap and seal from the new bottle and wipe the rubber port with an alcohol pad. Clamp the line, remove the spike from the old bottle, and insert the spike into the new bottle. Then hang the new bottle, and adjust the flow rate.

Changing the tubing

◆ Reduce the I.V. flow rate, remove the old spike from the container, and hang it on the I.V. pole.

◆ Place the cover of the new spike loosely over the old one.

◆ Keeping the old spike in an upright position above the patient's heart level, insert the new spike into the I.V. container.

◆ Prime the system.

◆ Hang the new I.V. container and the primed set on the pole and grasp the new adapter in one hand.

◆ Stop the flow rate in the old tubing.

◆ Put on gloves.

◆ Place a sterile gauze pad under the needle or cannula hub to create a sterile field. Press one finger over the cannula to prevent bleeding.

◆ Gently disconnect the old tubing, taking care to avoid dislodging or moving the I.V. device.

- If you have trouble disconnecting the old tubing, use a hemostat to hold the hub securely while you twist the tubing to remove it.
- Alternatively, use one hemostat on the venipuncture device and another on the hard plastic end of the tubing and pull the hemostats in opposite directions. Don't clamp the hemostats shut; this could crack the tubing adapter or the venipuncture device.

◆ Remove the protective cap from the new tubing and connect the new adapter to the cannula. Hold the hub securely to avoid dislodging the needle or the cannula tip.

◆ Observe for blood backflow into the new tubing to verify that the needle or cannula is still in place. (You may not be able to do this with small-gauge cannulas.)

◆ Adjust the clamp to maintain the appropriate flow rate.

◆ Retape the cannula hub and I.V. tubing and recheck the I.V. flow rate because taping may alter it.

◆ Label the new tubing and container with the date and time. Label the solution container with a time strip.

Special considerations

◆ Check the prescribed I.V. flow rate before each solution change to prevent errors.

◆ If you crack the adapter or hub or accidentally dislodge the cannula from the vein, remove the cannula. Apply pressure and an adhesive bandage to stop bleeding. Perform a venipuncture at another site and restart the I.V. line.

Documentation

◆ Record the time, date, rate, and type of solution and any additives (in the I.V. flowchart).

◆ Note any dressing or tubing changes (in your notes).

◆ Note the appearance of the site.

Giving I.V. drugs

◆ Before you give an I.V. drug to your patient, you need to prepare the drug for delivery and select the right equipment.

Preparing drugs

◆ Most I.V. drug solutions are prepared in the pharmacy by pharmacists or pharmacy technicians. Occasionally, however, you may have to prepare I.V. drug solutions yourself.

◆ When you're preparing a drug for I.V. use, make sure to take some basic safety measures.

◆ Maintain sterile technique.

– Always wash your hands before mixing and avoid contaminating any part of the vial, ampule, syringe, needle, or container that must remain sterile.

– When you're inserting the needle into the vial and withdrawing it, make sure that the needle tip doesn't touch any part of the vial that isn't sterile.

– Make sure you don't inadvertently puncture your finger; to keep your hands steady, brace one against the other while you're inserting and withdrawing the needle.

◆ When drawing up the drug before adding it to the primary solution, make sure to use a syringe that's large enough to hold the entire dose.

◆ The needle should be at least 1″ long to penetrate the inner seal of the port on an I.V. bag.

◆ In many facilities, practitioners use a 5-micron filter needle for mixing drug powder or withdrawing drugs from glass ampules. This needle is then removed, a sterile 1″ needle is attached to the syringe, and the drug is then admixed.

◆ In many facilities, premixed doses are drawn up into a syringe in the pharmacy. A 24-hour supply is delivered to the nursing unit where the drug is stored in a refrigerator. The nurse then administers the dose using a syringe pump that delivers the drug over a predetermined period.

Reconstituting powdered drugs

Many I.V. drugs are supplied in powder form and have to be reconstituted with liquid diluents.

◆ Common diluents include:

– normal saline solution

– sterile water for injection

– dextrose 5% in water.

◆ Note the manufacturer's instructions about the appropriate type or amount of diluent. Some drugs should be reconstituted with diluents that contain preservatives.

◆ Some drugs come in double-chambered vials that contain powder in the lower chamber and a diluent in the upper one. To combine the contents, press the rubber stopper on top of the vial to dislodge the rubber plug separating the compartments. The diluent then mixes with the drug in the bottom chamber.

Diluting liquid drugs

◆ Liquid drugs may be packed in:
- single-dose ampules or vials
- multidose vials
- prefilled syringes
- disposable cartridges.

◆ Liquid drugs don't need reconstitution, but they commonly need further dilution.

◆ Several methods can be used to add a drug to an I.V. container. Additive vials of a drug can be attached directly to administration tubing. If the vial contains a drug powder, reconstitute it first. Then you can infuse the drug solution directly from the vial, using dedicated vented tubing.

Labeling solution containers

◆ A container prepared in the pharmacy has a label showing:
- patient's full name
- patient's room number
- date
- name and amount of the I.V. solution and drugs
- other vital information, such as the infusion rate.

◆ If you prepare the drug solution, be sure to label the container with the same information provided by a pharmacy. Also, note the date and time you mixed the drug solution, and sign or initial the label.

◆ Make sure that your label doesn't cover the manufacturer's label.

◆ If you use a time strip, label it with the patient's name and room number and the infusion rate (in milliliters per hour, drops per minute, or both).

Selecting equipment

◆ Selection of appropriate equipment depends on the answers to these and other questions:
- Which drug has been prescribed?
- What's the ordered drip rate?
- Is your patient an adult or a child?
- Which equipment options are available?

Preparing for drug delivery

Before you give I.V. drugs by any method, take time to properly prepare the patient and the drug. Follow these steps:

◆ Confirm the patient's identity by checking his full name and facility identification number on his wristband.

◆ Ask him to identify himself verbally, if possible. If the patient can't identify himself, ask another nurse to corroborate his identity.

◆ Check his history for allergies and explain the procedure to him.

◆ Make sure you know some key information about the drug you're giving, including:
- normal dosage
- possible infusion methods
- expected effects
- adverse reactions
- contraindications
- drug interactions. (See *Comparing infusion methods*.)

◆ If you're unfamiliar with the drug and don't have access to the package insert or a drug reference book, ask your pharmacist any drug-related questions.

◆ Follow the Centers for Disease Control and Prevention (CDC) guidelines to protect yourself and your patient from blood-borne pathogens and infection. These guidelines require you to wear

Comparing infusion methods

This chart reviews the indications, advantages, and disadvantages of common I.V. administration methods.

METHODS AND INDICATIONS	ADVANTAGES	DISADVANTAGES
Direct injection		
Into a vein (no infusion line) ◆ When a nonvesicant drug with low risk of immediate adverse reaction is required for a patient with no other I.V. needs (for example, an outpatient requiring I.V. contrast injections for radiologic examinations or a cancer patient receiving chemotherapeutic agents)	◆ Eliminates the risk of complications from an indwelling venipuncture device ◆ Eliminates the inconvenience of an indwelling venipuncture device	◆ Can only be given by a physician or specially certified nurse ◆ Requires venipuncture, which can cause patient anxiety ◆ Requires two syringes – one to give the drug and one to flush the vein after administration ◆ Risk of infiltration from steel needle ◆ Drug can't be diluted and delivery can't be interrupted if irritation occurs ◆ Carries risk of clotting with administration of a drug over a long period and with a small volume
Through existing infusion line ◆ When a drug is incompatible with the I.V. solution and must be given as bolus injection ◆ When a patient requires immediate high blood levels (for example, regular insulin, dextrose 50%, atropine, and antihistamines) ◆ In emergencies, for immediate drug effect	◆ Doesn't require time or authorization to perform venipuncture because the vein is already accessed ◆ Doesn't require a needle puncture, which can cause patient anxiety ◆ Allows the use of I.V. solution to test the patency of the venipuncture device before drug administration ◆ Allows continued venous access in case of adverse reactions	◆ Carries the same inconveniences and risk of complications associated with indwelling venipuncture device (such as infection, infiltration, and pain)

(continued)

Comparing infusion methods *(continued)*

METHODS AND INDICATIONS	ADVANTAGES	DISADVANTAGES
Intermittent infusion		
Piggyback method ◆ Commonly used with drugs given over short periods at varying intervals (for example, antibiotics and gastric-secretion inhibitors)	◆ Avoids multiple needle injections required by I.M. route ◆ Permits repeated administration of drugs through a single I.V. site ◆ Provides high drug blood levels for short periods without causing drug toxicity	◆ May cause periods when the drug blood level becomes too low to be clinically effective (for example, when peak and trough times aren't considered in the medication order)
Saline lock ◆ When a patient requires constant venous access but not a continuous infusion	◆ Provides venous access for patients with fluid restrictions ◆ Provides better patient mobility between doses ◆ Preserves veins by reducing venipunctures ◆ Lowers cost if used with a limited number of drugs	◆ Requires close monitoring during administration so the device can be flushed on completion
Volume control set ◆ When a patient requires a low volume of fluid	◆ Requires only one large volume container ◆ Prevents fluid overload from a runaway infusion ◆ Allows the chamber to be reused	◆ High cost ◆ Carries a high risk of contamination ◆ If there is no membrane to block air passage when empty, flow clamp must be closed when the set empties
Continuous infusion		
Through primary line ◆ To maintain continuous serum levels, if the infusion isn't likely to be stopped abruptly	◆ Maintains steady serum levels ◆ Presents less risk of rapid shock and vein irritation because of a large volume of fluid diluting the drug	◆ Risk of incompatibility increases with drug contact time ◆ Restricts patient mobility ◆ Carries an increased risk of infiltration

Comparing infusion methods *(continued)*

METHODS AND INDICATIONS	ADVANTAGES	DISADVANTAGES
Continuous infusion *(continued)*		
Through secondary line ◆ When a patient requires continuous infusion of two or more compatible admixtures administered at different rates ◆ When there's a significant chance of abruptly stopping one admixture without infusing the remaining drug in I.V. tubing	◆ Allows primary infusion and each secondary infusion to be given at different rates ◆ Allows primary line to be totally shut off and kept on stand-by to maintain venous access in case secondary line must be abruptly stopped ◆ Short contact time before infusion may allow the administration of incompatible admixtures – something not possible with long contact time	◆ Can't be used for drugs with immediate incompatibility ◆ Carries an increased risk of vein irritation or phlebitis from an increased number of drugs ◆ Use of multiple I.V. systems (for example, primary lines with secondary lines attached), especially with electronic pumps, can create physical barriers to patient care and limit patient mobility

gloves (and possibly a gown and mask) when exposed to body fluids.

Infusion through a secondary line

◆ A secondary I.V. line is a complete I.V. set that's connected to the lower Y-port (secondary port) of a primary line instead of to the I.V. catheter or needle.
◆ It features an I.V. container, long tubing, and either a microdrip or macrodrip system.
◆ It can be used for continuous or intermittent drug infusion. When used continuously, it permits drug infusion and titration while the primary line maintains a constant total infusion rate.
◆ A secondary line used only for intermittent drug administration is called a piggyback set.
◆ In this case, the primary line maintains venous access between drug doses.
◆ A piggyback set includes a small I.V. container, short tubing, and usually a macrodrip system. It connects to the upper Y-port (piggyback port) of the primary line.

Equipment

Patient's medication record and chart ◆ prescribed I.V. drug ◆ diluent, if needed ◆ prescribed I.V. solution ◆ administration set with a secondary injection port ◆ needleless adapter ◆ alcohol pads ◆ 1" adhesive tape ◆ time tape ◆ labels ◆ infusion pump ◆ extension hook and solution for intermittent piggyback infusion

Implementation

◆ Wash your hands.
◆ Inspect the I.V. container for cracks, leaks, or contamination, and check compatibility with the primary solution.
◆ See if the primary line has a secondary injection port.

◆ If needed, add the drug to the secondary I.V. solution.
– To do so, remove any seals from the secondary container and wipe the main port with an alcohol pad.
– Inject the prescribed drug and agitate the solution to mix the medication.
– Label the I.V. mixture.
– Insert the administration set spike.
– Open the flow clamp and prime the line.
– Close the flow clamp.
◆ Some drugs come in vials for hanging directly on an I.V. pole. In this case, inject the diluent directly into the drug vial. Then spike the vial, prime the tubing, and hang the set.
◆ If the drug is incompatible with the primary I.V. solution, replace the primary I.V. solution with a fluid that's compatible with both solutions, and flush the line before starting the drug infusion.
◆ Hang the container of the secondary set and wipe the injection port of the primary line with an alcohol pad.
◆ Insert the needleless adapter from the secondary line into the injection port and tape it securely to the primary line.
◆ To run the container of the secondary set by itself, lower the container of the primary set with an extension hook. To run both containers simultaneously, place them at the same height.
◆ Open the slide-clamp and adjust the drip rate.
– For continuous infusion, set the secondary solution to the desired drip rate and adjust the primary solution to the desired total infusion rate.
– For intermittent infusion, wait until the secondary solution is completely infused and adjust the primary drip rate, as required.
◆ If the tubing for the secondary solution is being reused, close the clamp on the tubing and follow facility policy: Either remove the needleless adapter and replace it with a new one, or leave it taped in the injection port and label it with the time that it was first used.
◆ Leave the empty container in place until you replace it with a new dose of drug at the prescribed time.
◆ If the tubing won't be reused, discard it appropriately with the I.V. container.

Special considerations

◆ If facility policy allows, use a pump for drug infusion.
◆ Put a time tape on the secondary container to help prevent an inaccurate administration rate.
◆ When reusing secondary tubing, change it according to facility policy, usually every 48 to 72 hours.
◆ Inspect the injection port for leakage with each use; change it more often, if needed.
◆ Except for lipids, don't piggyback a secondary I.V. line to a total parenteral nutrition line because of the risk of contamination.

I.V. bolus injection

◆ I.V. bolus injection allows rapid I.V. drug delivery to quickly achieve peak levels in the bloodstream.
◆ It may be used for drugs that can't be given I.M. because they're toxic, or for a patient with a reduced ability to absorb these drugs.
◆ This method may also be used to deliver drugs that can't be diluted.
◆ Bolus doses may be injected directly into a vein, through an existing I.V. line, or through an implanted vascular access port (VAP).

Equipment

Patient's medication record and chart ◆ prescribed drug ◆ 20G needle and syringe ◆ diluent, if needed ◆ disposable tourniquet ◆ chlorhexidine swab

◆ alcohol pad ◆ sterile 2″ × 3″ gauze pad ◆ gloves ◆ adhesive bandage ◆ tape ◆ optional: winged-tip needle with catheter and second syringe (and needle) filled with normal saline solution, noncoring needle for VAP

Implementation

◆ Draw the drug into the syringe and dilute it, if needed.
◆ Wash your hands and put on gloves.

Direct injection

◆ Select the largest suitable vein to dilute the drug and minimize irritation.
◆ Apply a tourniquet above the site to distend the vein. Clean the site with an alcohol or chlorhexidine swab, working in a side-to-side motion.
◆ If you're using the needle of the drug syringe, insert it at a 0- to 15-degree angle, with the bevel up. The bevel should reach 1/4″ (6 mm) into the vein.
◆ Insert a winged-tip needle with the bevel up. Tape the wings in place when you see blood return and attach the syringe containing the drug.
◆ Check for blood backflow.
◆ Remove the tourniquet and inject the drug at the ordered rate.
◆ Check for blood backflow to make sure the needle remained in place and that all of the injected drug entered the vein.
◆ For a winged-tip needle, flush the line with normal saline solution from the second syringe to ensure complete delivery.
◆ Withdraw the needle and apply pressure to the site with the sterile gauze pad for 3 minutes, or until the bleeding stops, to prevent a hematoma.
◆ Use an adhesive bandage when the bleeding stops.

Existing I.V. line

◆ Check the compatibility of the drug.
◆ Close the flow clamp, wipe the injection port with an alcohol pad, and inject the drug as you would a direct injection.
◆ Open the flow clamp and readjust the flow rate.
◆ If the drug is incompatible with the I.V. solution, flush the line with normal saline solution before and after the injection.

VAP

◆ Wash your hands, put on gloves, and clean the site three times with an alcohol or povidone-iodine pad.
◆ Palpate for the septum, anchor the port between your thumb and the first two fingers of your nondominant hand and give the injection.

Special considerations

◆ If the existing I.V. line is capped, making it an intermittent infusion device, verify the patency and placement of the device before injecting the drug. Flush the device with normal saline solution, give the drug and follow with the appropriate flush.
◆ Immediately report signs of acute allergic reaction or anaphylaxis.
◆ If extravasation occurs, stop the injection, estimate the amount of infiltration and notify the physician.
◆ When giving diazepam or chlordiazepoxide through a winged-tip needle or an I.V. line, flush with bacteriostatic water to prevent precipitation.

Administering total parenteral nutrition

◆ Total parenteral nutrition (TPN) may be delivered in one of two ways: continuously or cyclically.
◆ With continuous delivery, the patient receives the infusion over a 24-hour period. The infusion begins at a slow rate and increases to the opti-

mal rate as ordered. This type of delivery may prevent complications such as hyperglycemia caused by a high dextrose load.

◆ With cyclic delivery, the patient receives the entire 24-hour volume of parenteral nutrition solution over a shorter period, perhaps 8, 10, 12, 14, or 16 hours.
- Home care parenteral nutrition programs have boosted the use of cyclic therapy.
- This type of therapy may be used to wean the patient from TPN.

◆ TPN solutions must be infused in a central vein, using one of the following methods:
- peripherally inserted central catheter, with its tip lying in the superior vena cava
- central venous catheter
- implanted vascular access device.

◆ The location of the catheter tip in the superior vena cava is confirmed by X-ray.

◆ Long-term therapy requires the use of one of the following devices:
- tunneled CV catheter, such as a Hickman, Broviac, or Groshong catheter
- implanted vascular device, such as Infus-A-Port or Port-a-Cath.

◆ Because TPN fluid has about six times the solute concentration of blood, peripheral I.V. administration can cause sclerosis and thrombosis. To ensure adequate dilution, the central venous catheter is inserted into the superior vena cava, a wide-bore, high-flow vein.

Preparing the equipment

◆ Gather the TPN solution, a pump, an administration set with a filter, alcohol swabs, gloves, and an I.V. pole.

◆ Wash your hands before preparing the TPN solution for administration and prepare the administration set in a clean area.

◆ Always use tubing with a filter when administering TPN. Filters are required by the Food and Drug Administration.

◆ Remove the bag or bottle of TPN solution from the refrigerator about 60 minutes before hanging it to let it warm. Infusion of a chilled solution can cause discomfort, hypothermia, venous spasm, and venous constriction.

Checking the order

◆ Check the written order against the label on the bag or bottle.

◆ Make sure the volumes, concentrations, and additives are included in the solution.

◆ Check the infusion rate.

◆ Careful inspection of the infusate should be a habit.
- Check for clouding, floating debris, or a change in color. Any of these could indicate contamination, problems with the integrity of the solution, or a pH change.
- If you see anything suspicious, notify the pharmacy.
- Inform the physician that there may be a delay in hanging the solution; he may want to order $D_{10}W$ until a new container of TPN solution is available.
- Also, be prepared to return the solution to the pharmacy.

◆ Most TPN solutions contain lipid emulsions, which call for special precautions.

Starting the infusion

◆ When the infusion begins, watch for swelling at the catheter insertion site.

◆ Swelling may indicate extravasation of the TPN solution, which can cause necrosis (tissue damage).

◆ If the patient reports discomfort at the start of the infusion, the catheter may be malpositioned or impaired, which requires a follow-up by a physician.

Maintaining the infusion

◆ If the patient tolerates the solution well the first day, the physician usually increases intake to the goal rate by the second day.

◆ To maintain a TPN infusion, follow these key steps:

- Check the order provided by the physician against the label on the TPN container.
- Label the container with the expiration date, time at which the solution was hung, glucose concentration, and total volume of solution. (If the bag or bottle is damaged and you don't have an immediate replacement, you can approximate the glucose concentration until a new container is ready by adding 50% glucose to $D_{10}W$.)
- Maintain flow rates as prescribed, even if the flow falls behind schedule.
- Don't let TPN solutions hang for more than 24 hours.
- Change the tubing and filter every 24 hours, using strict sterile technique. Make sure all tubing junctions are secure.
- Perform site care and dressing changes according to your facility's policy and protocol.
- Check the infusion pump's volume meter and time tape to monitor for irregular flow rate. Gravity should never be used to administer TPN.

◆ Record the patient's vital signs when therapy starts and every 4 to 8 hours thereafter (or more often, if needed). Be alert for increased body temperature — one of the earliest signs of catheter-related sepsis.

◆ Monitor your patient's glucose levels as ordered using glucose fingersticks or serum tests.

◆ Accurately record the patient's daily fluid intake and output, specifying the volume and type of each fluid. This record is a diagnostic tool that you can use to assure prompt, precise replacement of fluid and electrolyte deficits.

◆ Check the patient's physical status daily. Weigh him at the same time each morning (after voiding), in similar clothing, using the same scale. Suspect fluid imbalance if the patient gains more than 1 lb (0.45 kg) per day. If ordered, obtain anthropometric measurements.

◆ Monitor the results of routine laboratory tests, such as serum electrolyte, blood urea nitrogen, and glucose levels, and report abnormal findings to the physician so appropriate changes can be made in the TPN solution.

◆ Check serum triglyceride levels, which should be in the normal range during continuous TPN infusion. Typically, alanine aminotransferase, aspartate aminotransferase, alkaline phosphatase, cholesterol, triglyceride, plasma-free fatty acid, and coagulation tests are performed weekly.

◆ Monitor the patient for signs and symptoms of nutritional aberrations, such as fluid and electrolyte imbalances and glucose metabolism disturbances. Some patients need supplementary insulin throughout TPN therapy; the pharmacy usually adds regular insulin directly to the TPN solution.

Special considerations

◆ Provide emotional support. Keep in mind that patients commonly associate eating with positive feelings and become disturbed when it's eliminated.

◆ Provide frequent mouth care for the patient.

◆ Document all examination findings and nursing interventions.

◆ Avoid using a TPN infusion port for another infusion.
– When using a single-lumen CV catheter, don't use the line to piggyback or infuse blood or blood products, give a bolus injection, administer simultaneous I.V. solutions, measure CV pressure, or draw blood for laboratory tests.
– In unavoidable circumstances, the TPN port may be used for electrolyte replacement or insulin drips because these infusions are commonly additives to the solution.
– Never add drugs to a TPN solution container.
– Avoid using add-on devices, which increase the risk of infection.

◆ For a patient with hypothyroidism who's receiving long-term TPN therapy, you may need to give thyroid-stimulating hormone (TSH). TSH affects lipase activity and may prevent triglycerides from accumulating in the vascular system.

◆ Patients receiving lipid emulsions commonly report a feeling of fullness or bloating; occasionally, they experience an unpleasant metallic or greasy taste.

◆ Early adverse reactions to lipid emulsion therapy occur in fewer than 1% of patients. These reactions may include:
– fever
– difficulty breathing
– cyanosis
– nausea
– vomiting
– headache
– flushing
– sweating
– lethargy
– dizziness
– chest and back pain
– slight pressure over the eyes
– irritation at the infusion site.

Preparing for home care

◆ To increase compliance, make sure that the patient understands the purpose of treatment and enlist his help throughout the course of therapy.

◆ Understanding TPN and its goals helps a home care patient assume a greater role in administering, monitoring, and maintaining therapy. When instructing a home care patient, focus your teaching on signs and symptoms of:
– fluid, electrolyte, and glucose imbalances
– vitamin and trace element deficiencies and toxicities
– catheter infection, such as fever, chills, discomfort on infusion, and redness or drainage at the catheter insertion site.

◆ To help prevent glucose imbalance, teach the home care patient receiving his first I.V. bag of TPN how to regulate the flow rate so he maintains the prescribed rate.

◆ Explain that a gradual increase in the flow rate allows the pancreas to establish and maintain the increased insulin production needed to tolerate this treatment.

◆ When the goal rate of the TPN infusion is met, there should be no reason to adjust the rate.

◆ Finally, review the details of the administration schedule, the equipment the patient will use and, to avoid incompatibilities, the prescribed and over-the-counter drugs he takes.

◆ To safely maintain this therapy, the patient and his caregivers must adhere to the prescribed regimen. Your teaching efforts and return demonstrations by the patient help boost compliance in all aspects of TPN therapy.

Administering partial parenteral nutrition

◆ Using an amino acid, dextrose, and lipid emulsion solution, partial parenteral nutrition (PPN) fulfills a patient's basic calorie needs without the risks involved in central venous access.
◆ PPN is administered through a peripheral vein.
◆ Because PPN solutions have lower tonicity than TPN solutions, a patient receiving PPN must be able to tolerate infusion of large volumes of fluid.

Preparing the patient

◆ Make sure that the patient understands what to expect before, during, and after therapy.
◆ Select the patient's largest available vein as the insertion site. Using a large vein enables the blood to adequately dilute the PPN solution, which can help avoid irritation.
◆ When using a short-term catheter, rotate the site every 48 to 72 hours, or according to your facility's policy and procedures.

Preparing the equipment

◆ To administer PPN, gather the needed equipment, including:
- ordered PPN solution (at room temperature)
- infusion pump
- administration set
- alcohol swabs
- I.V. pole
- venipuncture equipment, if needed.

Checking the order

◆ Check the written order against the written label on the bag.
◆ Make sure the solution is intended for peripheral infusion and that the volumes, concentrations, and additives are included in the solution.
◆ Check the infusion rate.
◆ In PPN therapy, lipid emulsions may be part of the solution.
- When giving lipids, use controllers that can accommodate lipid emulsions.
- If given separately, piggyback the lipid emulsion below the in-line filter close to the insertion site to avoid having lipids clog the filtration system.

Starting the infusion

◆ Start the PPN infusion as ordered.
◆ Watch for swelling at the peripheral insertion site. Swelling may indicate infiltration or extravasation of the PPN solution, which can cause tissue damage.

Maintaining the infusion

◆ Caring for a patient receiving a PPN infusion involves the same steps required for any patient receiving a peripheral I.V. infusion.
◆ You need to maintain the infusion rate and care for the tubing, dressings, infusion site, and I.V. devices.

Special considerations

◆ In addition, monitor the patient for signs or symptoms of sepsis, including:
- glucose in the urine (glycosuria)
- chills
- malaise
- increased white blood cells (leukocytosis)
- altered level of consciousness
- elevated glucose levels, measured by fingerstick or serum chemistry
- elevated temperature (usually higher than 100.4° F [38° C], according to the Centers for Disease Control and Prevention).

◆ Because the synthesis of lipase (a fat-splitting enzyme) increases insulin requirements, the insulin dosage of a diabetic patient may need to be increased as ordered. Insulin is one of the additives that may be adjusted in the formulation of the PPN solution.

◆ Some patients develop allergic reactions to the fat emulsion.

◆ Early adverse reactions to lipid emulsion therapy occur in fewer than 1% of patients. These reactions may include:
- fever
- difficulty breathing
- cyanosis
- nausea
- vomiting
- headache
- flushing
- sweating
- lethargy
- dizziness
- chest and back pain
- slight pressure over the eyes
- irritation at the infusion site.

◆ Changes in laboratory test results may also reveal problems when a patient receives lipid emulsions, including:
- hyperlipidemia
- hypercoagulability
- thrombocytopenia.

◆ The doctor monitors the patient's lipid emulsion clearance rate. Lipid emulsion may clear from the blood at an accelerated rate in a patient with severe burns, multiple trauma, or a metabolic imbalance.

14 Dosage calculation

Reviewing ratios and proportions

◆ A ratio is a mathematical expression of the relationship between two things.
◆ A ratio may be expressed with a fraction, such as ⅓, or with a colon, such as 1:3.
◆ A proportion is a set of two equal ratios.
◆ When ratios are expressed as fractions in a proportion, their cross products are equal.

Proportion

$$\frac{2}{4} \times \frac{5}{10}$$

Cross products

$$2 \times 10 = 4 \times 5$$

◆ When ratios are expressed using colons in a proportion, the product of the means (middle two values) equals the product of the extremes (beginning and end values).

Proportion

means
↓ ↓
3 : 30 :: 4 : 40
↑ extremes ↑

Product of means and extremes

$$30 \times 4 = 3 \times 40$$

◆ Whether fractions or ratios are used in a proportion, they must appear in the same order on both sides of the equal sign.
◆ When proportions are expressed as fractions, the units in the numerators (above the line) must be the same and the units in the denominators (below the line) must be the same (although they don't have to be the same as the units in the numerators).

$$\frac{mg}{kg} = \frac{mg}{kg}$$

◆ If the ratios in a proportion are expressed with colons, the units of the first term on the left side of the equal sign must be the same as the units of the first term on the right side. In other words, the units of the mean on one side of the equal sign must match the units of the extreme on the other side.

mg : kg :: mg : kg

Tips for simplifying dosage calculations

Incorporate units of measure

◆ Incorporating units of measure into the dosage calculation helps prevent one of the most common errors made in dosage calculation — using the incorrect unit of measure.
◆ Keep in mind that the units of measure that appear in both the numerator and denominator cancel each other out, leaving the correct unit of measure in the answer.
◆ The following example uses units of measure in calculating a drug with a usual dose of 4 mg/kg for a 55-kg patient.

1. State the problem as a proportion.

4 mg : 1 kg :: *X* : 55 kg

2. Solve for *X* by applying the principle that the product of the means equals the product of the extremes.

$$1\ kg \times X = 4\ mg \times 55\ kg$$

3. Divide and cancel out the units of measure that appear in the numerator and denominator.

$$X = \frac{4 \text{ mg} \times 55 \cancel{\text{kg}}}{1 \cancel{\text{kg}}}$$

$$X = 220 \text{ mg}$$

Check zeros and decimal places

◆ Suppose that you receive an order to give 0.1 mg of epinephrine subcutaneously, but the only epinephrine on hand is a 1-ml ampule that contains 1 mg of epinephrine. To calculate the volume for injection, use the ratio-and-proportion method.

◆ State the problem as a proportion.

$$1 \text{ mg} : 1 \text{ ml} :: 0.1 \text{ mg} : X$$

◆ Solve for X by applying the principle that the product of the means equals the product of the extremes.

$$1 \text{ ml} \times 0.1 \text{ mg} = 1 \text{ mg} \times X$$

◆ Divide and cancel out the units of measure that appear in both the numerator and the denominator, carefully checking the decimal placement.

$$\frac{1 \text{ ml} \times 0.1 \cancel{\text{mg}}}{1 \cancel{\text{mg}}} = X$$

$$0.1 \text{ ml} = X$$

Recheck results that seem unusual

◆ Carefully recheck any figures that seem unusual.

◆ If, for example, your calculation indicates that you should give 25 tablets, you've probably made an error.

◆ If you still have doubts after checking your work, review the calculations with another health care professional.

Determining the number of tablets to give

◆ Calculating the number of tablets to give lends itself to the use of ratios and proportions. To perform the calculation, follow this process:

1. Set up the first ratio with the known tablet (tab) strength.

2. Set up the second ratio with the unknown quantity.

3. Use these ratios in a proportion.

4. Solve for X, applying the principle that the product of the means equals the product of the extremes.

◆ For example, suppose that a drug order calls for 100 mg of propranolol P.O. q.i.d., but only 40-mg tablets are available. To determine the number of tablets to give, follow these steps:

1. Set up the first ratio with the known tablet (tab) strength.

$$40 \text{ mg} : 1 \text{ tab}$$

2. Set up the second ratio with the desired dose and the unknown number of tablets.

$$100 \text{ mg} : X$$

3. Use these ratios in a proportion.

$$40 \text{ mg} : 1 \text{ tab} :: 100 \text{ mg} : X$$

4. Solve for X by applying the principle that the product of the means equals the product of the extremes.

$$1 \text{ tab} \times 100 \text{ mg} = 40 \text{ mg} \times X$$

$$\frac{1 \text{ tab} \times 100 \cancel{\text{mg}}}{40 \cancel{\text{mg}} \times X} = X$$

$$2\tfrac{1}{2} \text{ tab} = X$$

Determining the amount of liquid to give

◆ You can also use ratios and proportions to calculate the amount of liquid drug to give. Simply follow the same four-step process used in determining the number of tablets to give.

◆ For example, suppose that a patient is to receive 750 mg of amoxicillin oral suspension. The label reads Amoxicillin (amoxicillin trihydrate) 250 mg/5 ml and the bottle contains 100 ml. To determine how many milliliters of amoxicillin solution the patient should receive, follow these steps:

1. Set up the first ratio with the known strength of the liquid drug.

$$250 \text{ mg} : 5 \text{ ml}$$

2. Set up the second ratio with the desired dose and the unknown quantity.

$$750 \text{ mg} : X$$

3. Use these ratios in a proportion.

$$250 \text{ mg} : 5 \text{ ml} :: 750 \text{ mg} : X$$

4. Solve for *X* by applying the principle that the product of the means equals the product of the extremes.

$$5 \text{ ml} \times 750 \text{ mg} = 250 \text{ mg} \times X$$

$$\frac{5 \text{ ml} \times 750 \cancel{\text{mg}}}{250 \cancel{\text{mg}}} = X$$

$$15 \text{ ml} = X$$

Giving drugs of varied concentration

◆ Because drugs — such as epinephrine, heparin, and allergy serums — come in varied concentrations, consider the concentration of the drug when calculating a drug dosage to avoid a potentially lethal mistake. To avoid a dosage error, make sure that drug concentrations are part of the calculation.

◆ For example, a drug order calls for 0.2 mg of epinephrine subcutaneously stat and the ampule is labeled as 1 ml of 1:1,000 epinephrine. Use these steps to calculate the correct drug volume.

1. Determine the strength of the solution based on its unlabeled ratio.

$$1{:}1{,}000 \text{ epinephrine} = 1 \text{ g}/1{,}000 \text{ ml}$$

2. Set up a proportion with this information and the desired dose.

$$1\text{g} : 1{,}000 \text{ ml} :: 0.2 \text{ mg} : X$$

– Before you can perform this calculation, however, you must convert grams to milligrams by using the conversion

$$1\text{g} = 1{,}000 \text{ mg.}$$

3. Restate the proportion with the converted units, and solve for *X*.

$$1{,}000 \text{ mg} : 1{,}000 \text{ ml} :: 0.2 \text{ mg} : X$$

4. Solve for *X* by applying the principle that the product of the means equals the product of the extremes.

$$1{,}000 \text{ ml} \times 0.2 \text{ mg} = 1{,}000 \text{ mg} \times X$$

$$\frac{1{,}000 \text{ ml} \times 0.2 \cancel{\text{mg}}}{1{,}000 \cancel{\text{mg}}} = X$$

$$0.2 \text{ ml} = X$$

Calculating I.V. drip and flow rates

◆ To compute the drip and flow rates, set up a fraction with the volume of solution to be delivered over the prescribed duration. For example, if a patient is to receive 100 ml of solution within 1 hour, the fraction is:

$$\frac{100\text{ ml}}{60\text{ minutes}}$$

◆ Next, multiply the fraction by the drip factor (the number of drops contained in 1 ml) to determine the drip rate (the number of drops per minute to be infused).
◆ The drip factor varies among I.V. sets; it appears on the package containing the I.V. tubing administration set.
◆ Following the manufacturer's directions for the drip factor is crucial. Standard sets have drip factors of 10, 15, or 20 gtt/ml. A microdrip (minidrip) set has a drip factor of 60 gtt/ml.

Use the following equation to determine the drip rate:

$$\frac{\text{total ml}}{\text{total minutes}} \times \text{drip factor} = \text{gtt/minute}$$

◆ For example, the patient receiving 100 ml of solution within 1 hour with an infusion set drip factor of 20 gtt/min, use the following equation:

$$X = \frac{100\ \cancel{\text{ml}}}{60\text{ min}} \times \frac{20\text{ gtt}}{1\ \cancel{\text{ml}}}$$

$$X = \frac{2000\text{ gtt}}{60\text{ min}}$$

◆ To solve for X, divide the numerator by the denominator after cancelling units:

$$X = \frac{100 \times 20\text{ gtt}}{60\text{ min}}$$

$$X = \frac{2000\text{ gtt}}{60\text{ min}}$$

$$X = 33.34\text{ gtt/min (rounded to 33)}$$

◆ The equation applies to solutions that are infused over many hours as well as to small-volume infusions such as those used for antibiotics, which are given for less than 1 hour.
◆ You can modify the equation by first determining the number of milliliters to be infused over 1 hour (the flow rate). Then, divide the flow rate by 60 minutes. Next, multiply the result by the drip factor to determine the number of drops per minute.
◆ The previous problem would be calculated this way by the modified equation:

$$X = \frac{100\text{ ml}}{1\ \cancel{\text{hr}}} \div \frac{1\ \cancel{\text{hr}}}{60\text{ min}}$$

$$X = \frac{1.67\text{ ml}}{\text{min}}$$

◆ Now multiply by the drip factor:

$$X = 1.67 \times 20$$

$$X = 33.4\text{ gtt/min (rounded to 33)}$$

◆ You'll also use the flow rate when working with infusion pumps to set the number of milliliters to be delivered in 1 hour.

Quick calculations of drip rates

◆ In addition to using the equation and its modified version, quicker computation methods are available.
◆ To give solutions using a microdrip set, adjust the flow rate (ml/hour) to equal the drip rate (gtt/minute). Using the equation, divide the flow rate by 60 minutes and multiply the result by the drip factor, which also equals 60. Because the flow rate and the drip factor are equal, the two arithmetic operations cancel each other out. For example, if the flow rate is 125 ml/hour, the equation would be:

$$\frac{125 \text{ ml}}{60 \text{ minutes}} \times 60 = \text{drip rate } (125)$$

◆ Instead of spending the time solving the equation, you can simply use the number assigned to the flow rate as the drip rate.
- For sets that deliver 20 gtt/ml, the flow rate divided by 3 equals the drip rate.
- For sets that deliver 15 gtt/ml, the flow rate divided by 4 equals the drip rate.
- For sets with a drip factor of 10, the flow rate divided by 6 equals the drip rate.

◆ To determine how many micrograms of a drug are in a milliliter of solution, use the following equation:

$$\text{mcg/ml} = \text{mg/ml} \times 1{,}000$$

◆ To express drip rates in micrograms per kilogram per minute (mcg/kg/minute), you must know the concentration of the solution (mcg/ml), the patient's weight (kg), and the infusion rate (ml/hour):

$$\text{mcg/kg/min} = \frac{\text{mcg/ml} \times \text{ml/min}}{\text{body weight (kg)}}$$

◆ To find the milliliters per minute (ml/minute), divide the number of milliliters per hour (ml/hour) by 60.

◆ You can also convert milliliters per hour (ml/hour) from a dosage given in micrograms per kilograms per minute (mcg/kg/min) as follows:

$$\text{ml/hr} = \frac{\text{wt (kg)} \times \text{mcg/kg/min}}{\text{mcg/ml}} \times 60$$

Dimensional analysis

◆ Dimensional analysis (also known as factor analysis, or factor labeling) is an alternative method of solving mathematical problems. It eliminates the need to memorize formulas and requires only one equation to determine an answer. To compare the ratio-and-proportion method and dimensional analysis at a glance, read the following problem and solutions.

◆ The physician prescribes 0.25 g of streptomycin sulfate I.M. The vial reads "2 ml = 1 g." How many milliliters should you give?

Dimensional analysis

$$\frac{0.25 \text{ g}}{1} \times \frac{2 \text{ ml}}{1 \text{ g}} = 0.5 \text{ ml}$$

Ratio and proportion

$$1 \text{ g} : 2 \text{ ml} :: 0.25 \text{ g} : X$$

$$2 \text{ ml} \times 0.25 \text{ g} = 1 \text{ g} \times X$$

$$\frac{2 \text{ ml} \times 0.25 \text{ g}}{1 \text{ g}} = X$$

$$0.5 \text{ ml} = X$$

◆ Dimensional analysis involves arranging a series of ratios, called factors, into a single fractional equation.

◆ Each factor, written as a fraction, consists of two quantities and their units of measurement that are related to each other in a given problem. For instance, if 1,000 ml of a drug should be given over 8 hours, the relationship between 1,000 ml and 8 hours is expressed by this fraction:

$$\frac{1{,}000 \text{ ml}}{8 \text{ hours}}$$

◆ When a problem includes a quantity and its unit of measurement that are unrelated to any other factor in the problem, they serve as the numerator of the fraction, and 1 (implied) becomes the denominator.

◆ Some mathematical problems contain all of the information needed to identify the factors, set up the equation, and find the solution. Other problems require the use of a conversion factor.

- Conversion factors are equivalents (for example, 1 g = 1,000 mg) that can be memorized or obtained from a conversion chart.
- Because the two quantities and units of measurement are equivalent, they can serve as the numerator or the denominator.
- Thus, the conversion factor 1 g = 1,000 mg can be written in fraction form as:

$$\frac{1{,}000 \text{ mg}}{1 \text{ g}} \text{ or } \frac{1 \text{ g}}{1{,}000 \text{ mg}}$$

◆ The factors given in the problem plus any conversion factors needed to solve the problem are called knowns. The quantity of the answer, of course, is unknown.

◆ When setting up an equation in dimensional analysis, work backward, beginning with the unit of measurement of the answer. After plotting all of the knowns, find the solution by following this sequence:

1. Cancel similar quantities and units of measurement.
2. Multiply the numerators.
3. Multiply the denominators.
4. Divide the numerator by the denominator.

◆ Mastering dimensional analysis can take practice, but you may find your efforts well rewarded.

◆ To understand more fully how dimensional analysis works, review the following problem and the steps taken to solve it.

◆ The physician prescribes *x* grains (gr) of a drug. The pharmacy supplies the drug in 300-mg tablets (tab). How many tablets should you administer?

1. Write down the unit of measurement of the answer, followed by an "equal to" symbol (=).

$$\text{tab} =$$

2. Search the problem for the quantity with the same unit of measurement (if one doesn't exist, use a conversion factor); place this in the numerator and its related quantity and unit of measurement in the denominator.

$$\text{tab} = \frac{1 \text{ tab}}{300 \text{ mg}}$$

- Separate the first factor from the next with a multiplication symbol (×).

$$\text{tab} = \frac{1 \text{ tab}}{300 \text{ mg}} \times$$

- Place the unit of measurement of the denominator of the first factor in the numerator of the second factor.
- Search the problem for the quantity with the same unit of measurement (if there's no common measurement, as in this example, use a conversion factor).
- Place this in the numerator and its related quantity and unit of measurement in the denominator; follow with a multiplication symbol.
- Repeat this step until all known factors are included in the equation.

$$\text{tab} = \frac{1 \text{ tab}}{300 \text{ mg}} \times \frac{60 \text{ mg}}{1 \text{ gr}} \times \frac{10 \text{ gr}}{1}$$

◆ Alternatively, you can treat the equation as a large fraction, using these steps.

1. First, cancel similar units of measurement in the numerator and the denominator. What remains should be what you began with — the unit of measurement of the answer; if not, recheck your equation to find and correct the error.
2. Multiply the numerators and then the denominators.
3. Divide the numerator by the denominator.

$$\text{tab} = \frac{1 \text{ tab}}{300 \cancel{\text{mg}}} \times \frac{60 \cancel{\text{mg}}}{1 \cancel{\text{gr}}} \times \frac{10 \cancel{\text{gr}}}{1}$$

Estimating body surface area in adults

Use this nomogram to plot an adult patient's height and weight to determine the patient's body surface area (BSA). To estimate the BSA, place a straightedge from the patient's height in the left-hand column to his weight in the right-hand column. The intersection of this line with the center scale shows the BSA.

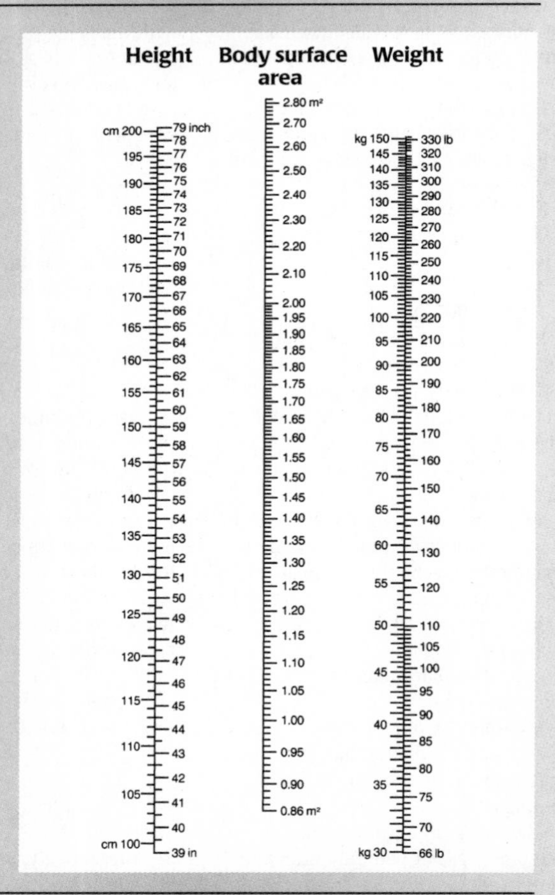

Adapted with permission from *Geigy Scientific Tables,* 8th ed., 1990. Vol. 5, p. 105. ©Novartis.

$$= \frac{60 \times 10 \text{ tab}}{300}$$

$$= \frac{600 \text{ tab}}{300}$$

$$= 2 \text{ tablets}$$

Body surface area estimation

◆ Body surface area (BSA) is a critical component of calculation of dosages for drugs that must be given in precise amounts. (See *Estimating body surface area in adults* and *Estimating body surface area in children.*)

Estimating body surface area in children

For an average-sized child, find the weight and the corresponding body surface area (BSA) in the box. Otherwise, to use the nomogram, place a straightedge on the correct height and weight points for the patient and note the point at which the line intersects on the scale.

Note: Don't base drug dosages for premature or full-term neonates on BSA; instead, use body weight.

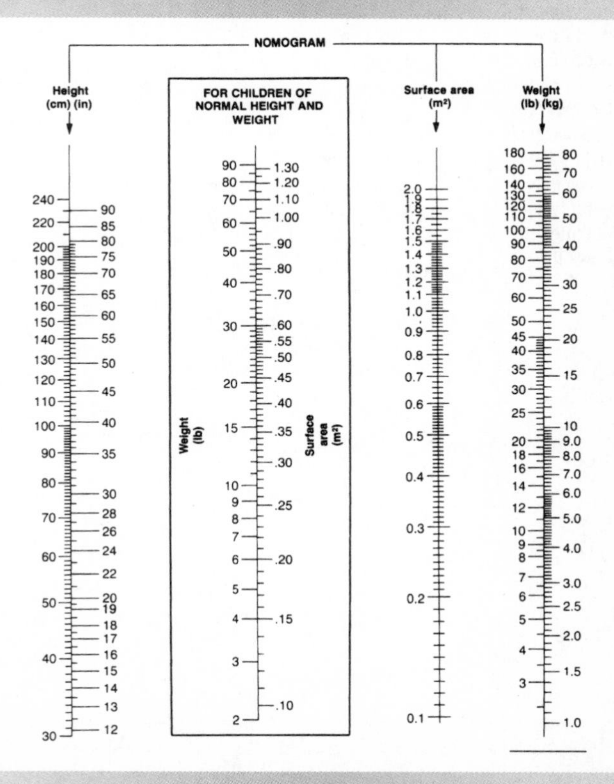

15 Elder care

Understanding the geriatric population

◆ People ages 65 and older need health care more often than people in any other age group.
◆ Older adults account for more than one-third of all hospital stays and over one-third of the country's total personal health care expenditures.
◆ Because so much of the health care population is elderly, it's important to understand some general concepts about this important group.

Societal attitudes and beliefs

◆ As a group, older adults in our society are stereotyped.
– Aging is a natural process, but the changes associated with it are rarely viewed as natural or positive.
– Health care professionals commonly describe such changes as "losses," such as a loss of tissue elasticity or a decrease in blood flow.
– In general, society regards aging as a series of inevitable, negative events that a person must tolerate.
– In addition, health care professionals often mention age-related changes and disease conditions in the same breath.
◆ Some of the myths, misconceptions, and negative stereotypes about older people stem from cultural values and beliefs.
– A youth-oriented society values intelligence, strength, self-reliance, and productivity — characteristics rarely attributed to older adults.
– Many people perceive older adults as senile, sick, and incapable of making worthwhile contributions to society.
– Portrayals of elderly people in movies, television, advertisements, and other media compound this sense.
◆ Such images perpetuate stereotypes and can reinforce negative ideas about aging.
◆ Health care workers aren't immune to perpetuating these errors, and the quality of health care that older adults receive can be affected as well. (See *Dispelling common myths about aging,* pages 472 and 473.)
◆ Stereotyping can influence many aspects of elder care, including the following:
– Planning and implementation — for example, a nurse might regularly delay her response to an older patient's call bell
– Salaries — nurses working in nursing homes typically make less money than those working in other facilities

Age-related adjustments and transitions

◆ The aging process is accompanied by role changes and transitions. Some roles — spouse, employee — may be lost, while new roles — widow, volunteer — may arise.
◆ Such changes require role adjustment. Factors that influence role adjustment include age, sex, beliefs, attitudes, income, health, culture, and past experiences.

Role changes

◆ With aging, changes in the marital role may occur.
– After retirement, the division of labor and household management may change.
– One spouse may become the primary caregiver if the other becomes ill.
– If a spouse dies, social relations for the survivor may change.
◆ As a result, spouses may need to renegotiate household roles as well as leisure and social activities.

Dispelling common myths about aging

Here are some common misconceptions about aging and facts to help dispel them.

Myth: Most older people are senile or demented.
Senility is a vague term commonly used inappropriately to refer to disease-related dementias. Most people age 65 and older aren't mentally disturbed or suffering from dementia. Significant, progressive, cognitive impairments are consequences of disease and affect less than 5% of people ages 65 to 74 and about 25% of people older than age 85.

Myth: Most older people feel miserable and depressed.
Studies of happiness, morale, and life satisfaction reveal that most older people are just as happy as they were when they were younger. Only about one-third of older people show signs of depression.

Myth: Older people can't work as effectively as younger people.
Studies show that older workers produce more consistent output and have less job turnover, fewer accidents, and less absenteeism than younger workers.

Myth: Older people experience a decline in intellectual ability and can't learn new skills.
Older adults are capable of learning new things, but the speed at which they process information is slower. Healthy older adults show no decline and sometimes show improvement in such cognitive skills as wisdom, judgment, creativity, and common sense. Most show a slight and gradual decline in other cognitive skills, such as abstraction, calculation, and verbal comprehension.

- Gradual erosion of the independent-adult role is linked to the aging person's growing need for assistance.

Retirement

- Retirement brings a major role change because it alters the way a person manages time and daily activities.
- Retirement alters identity, power, status, and friendships.
- The retiree may need to find new relationships and activities.
- Retirement is viewed as the beginning of old age.
- A person's income, health, and desire to retire predict his satisfactory adjustment to retirement.

Multiple losses

- Aging comes with major physical, psychological, and sociologic losses as well as a reduced ability to adapt to and compensate for stressors.
- Loss of loved ones, income, and perhaps decent transportation and housing, added to multiple or chronic diseases and their resulting limitations, can increase the older adult's sense of vulnerability and deplete coping resources.
- Older adults may lose a sense of control because of such factors as physical decline, status and role changes, negative cultural attitudes and mass media portrayals, and crime victimization.

Loneliness

- Any loss — such as death of a spouse, retirement, poor health, or inactivity — that creates a deficit in intimacy and interpersonal relationships can lead to loneliness.
- Loneliness can provoke or aggravate physical symptoms, sleep disturbances, and shortened survival.

Myth: Most older people are sick and need help with daily activities.
In fact, 80% of older people are healthy enough to carry on their normal lifestyles. About 15% have chronic health conditions that interfere with their daily lives, and another 5% are institutionalized.

Myth: Older people are set in their ways and can't change.
People tend to become more stable in their attitudes as they age, but they still adapt to many social changes and changes in lifestyle. In fact, older people may be required to change more frequently than they did when they were younger because of major events in their lives.

◆ The older adult needs caring, personal contact, and confidants in other age groups.
◆ It takes a satisfying relationship with frequent contact to prevent loneliness. However, some older people choose to be alone.

Depression and suicide
◆ Depression increases in likelihood and intensity with age.
◆ Changes in neurotransmitters, multiple losses, and decreased internal and external resources contribute to its occurrence.
◆ Depression may include complaints of physical symptoms and sleep disturbance. It may also occur in early stages of dementia, making depression the most common psychiatric problem among older adults.
◆ Risk factors for depression include:
- a recent major loss
- feelings of rejection by or isolation from family or friends
- feelings of hopelessness
- absence of an identifiable role in life
- loss of a partner or sexual function
- disability.

◆ With depression comes an increased risk of suicide.
◆ The suicide rate for older men is seven times that for older women.
◆ Risk factors for suicide include:
- alcoholism
- bereavement (especially within 1 year after a loss)
- loss of health
- loss of role
- living alone
- children having married and moved away.

Fear of death
◆ While some older people avoid the topic, many older adults think and talk about death, and many have less fear of death than of dependency, pain, and loss of function and control.
◆ Fear of death may involve such concerns as separation from loved ones and questions about divine judgment and afterlife.
◆ However, fear of the process of dying, the ultimate loss of self, and the unknown may lead to denial.
◆ Denying death can keep a person from valuing life, and it can negate the positive developmental process of preparing for death.

Variables affecting data collection

◆ Data collection may take place in a variety of settings, including:
- an acute care facility
- the patient's home
- a senior center
- an adult day care center
- a long-term care facility.

Age-related changes affecting mobility

The following major physical changes in five body systems affect the mobility of older people.

Musculoskeletal
- Changes in joint surfaces, ligaments, tendons, and connective tissues
- Decreased bone density (increases vulnerability for fractures)
- Decreased number and size of muscle fibers
- Atrophy of muscle tissue; replaced with fibrous tissue

Pulmonary
- Loss of elastic lung recoil
- Increased airway resistance
- Reduced vital capacity
- Decreased chest wall compliance
- Decreased gas exchange

Cardiovascular
- Increased blood pressure
- Decreased stroke volume
- Decreased cardiac reserve (ability to respond to stress)

Neurologic
- Reduced nerve conduction speed
- Decreased rate and magnitude of reflex response
- Decreased sensory activity
- Decreased myoneural transmission
- Decreased muscle contraction speed
- Increased postural sway (contributes to balance problems)

Skin
- Decreased subcutaneous adipose tissue
- Decreased elasticity of connective tissue
- Loss of sweat and sebaceous glands

Adapted with permission from Stone, J.T., et al. *Clinical Gerontological Nursing*, 2nd Ed., Philadelphia: Elsevier, Inc., 1998.

- The setting and the patient's age don't affect the specific methods used to collect data, but other factors may affect the overall atmosphere of trust, caring, and confidentiality, including these:
  - the time needed for data collection
  - the patient's energy level
  - the environment
  - the patient's consent
  - language or communication deficits
  - the patient's attitude
  - the nurse's attitude about aging.

Time and energy level
- Be sure to allow enough time for the examination.
- Older adults possess a wealth of information but may process information more slowly than a younger adult.
- The patient may need extra time, or even several shorter sessions, if such problems as fatigue or discomfort limit the amount of time he can participate meaningfully.

Deficits
- Sensory deficits, such as hearing and vision losses, are common in older people.
- Other impairments, such as musculoskeletal or neurologic deficits, appear frequently. (See *Age-related changes affecting mobility*.)

◆ All of these can significantly interfere with accurate data collection.

Language

◆ When talking with an older patient, tailor the language you use to that individual.
◆ Consider the patient's educational level, culture, and other languages he may speak.

The patient's attitude

◆ Try to determine the patient's attitude toward his body and health.
◆ An older person may have a distorted perception of his health problems, dwelling on them needlessly or dismissing them as normal signs of aging.
◆ He may ignore a serious problem because he doesn't want his fears confirmed.
◆ If an older patient is seriously ill, the subjects of dying and death may come up during the health history interview.
- Listen carefully to what the patient says about dying, and ask about his religious affiliation and spiritual needs; many older people find comfort in their religious beliefs and practices.
- Ask the patient whether he has or wants help with a living will.

◆ The health history can serve as a life review for an older person by allowing him to recount his history in a purposeful, systematic manner.

The nurse's attitude

◆ Communicating with an older adult may challenge you to confront your personal attitude about aging and older people.
◆ Any prejudices revealed will probably interfere with efforts to communicate because older people are especially sensitive to others' reactions and can easily detect negative attitudes and impatience.
◆ You should examine your feelings and decide in advance how you'll handle them.

Nutritional status

◆ In many ambulatory care settings, nutritional assessment consists mainly of obtaining a 24-hour dietary recall and comparing it to standard dietary guidelines. This obtains, at best, a cursory review of food intake over a limited time period.
◆ In the acute care setting, nutrition assessments are usually a part of the nurse's admission assessment and are rather superficial — they're sometimes limited to food preferences and allergies. Daily food intake is documented on flow sheets and the dietitian is consulted as needed.
◆ Few data collection instruments are specific to older people.
- A nutritional component is included as part of the assessment and care screening Minimum Data Set for nursing home residents.
- The Nutrition Screening Initiative (NSI), a joint venture of the American Academy of Family Physicians, the American Dietetic Association, and the National Council on Aging, includes screening methods and interventions to prevent and remedy nutritional deficiencies specifically in older adults.

◆ The NSI is widely used in outpatient settings. This program begins with a self-administered questionnaire that highlights areas of known risk for nutritional deficiencies.
◆ After the questionnaire is scored, at-risk patients are referred for more extensive screening. This screening includes another questionnaire administered by a health professional. It further explores the known risk areas using the mnemonic device DETERMINE:
- Disease
- Eating poorly

Preventing dehydration in elderly patients

To maintain adequate hydration, an elderly patient needs 1,000 to 3,000 ml of fluid daily. Less than 1,000 ml daily may lead to constipation, which can contribute to urinary incontinence. It may also result in more concentrated urine, which predisposes the patient to urinary tract infections. Follow these guidelines to make sure the patient is adequately hydrated.

Monitoring

◆ Monitor intake and output. Ensure an intake of at least 1,500 ml of oral fluids and urine output of 1,000 to 1,500 ml per 24 hours.
◆ Check skin turgor and mucous membranes.
◆ Monitor vital signs, especially pulse rate, respiratory rate, and blood pressure. An increase in pulse and respiratory rates with decreased blood pressure may indicate dehydration.
◆ Monitor laboratory test results, such as serum electrolyte, blood urea nitrogen, and creatinine levels; hematocrit; and urine and serum osmolarity. Check for signs of acidosis.
◆ Weigh the patient at the same time daily, using the same scale and with the patient wearing the same type of clothes.
◆ Auscultate bowel sounds for any increase in activity. Monitor stools for character: Hard stools may indicate dehydration; loose, watery stools indicate loss of water.
◆ Be aware of diagnostic tests that affect intake and output (for example, laxative or enema use, which cause fluid loss), and replace any lost fluids.

Providing fluids

◆ Provide fluids often throughout the day, for example, every hour and with a bedtime snack.
◆ Provide modified cups that the patient can handle; help those who have difficulty.
◆ Offer fluids other than water; find out the types of beverages the patient likes and the preferred temperatures (for example, ice cold or room-temperature drinks).
◆ Monitor coffee intake; coffee acts as a diuretic and may cause excessive fluid loss.
◆ If the patient is unable to take oral fluids, request an order for I.V. hydration.

- Tooth loss or mouth pain
- Economic hardship
- Reduced social contact and interaction
- Multiple drugs
- Involuntary weight loss or gain
- Need for assistance with self-care
- Elder at an advanced age.

◆ Hydration status may affect an older patient's ability to maintain nutritional status as well. (See *Preventing dehydration in elderly patients*.)

◆ Once a nurse determines the patient's nutritional status, she can begin to formulate interventions.

Age-related changes and drug therapy

◆ Drug therapy for older people presents special problems because age-related physiologic changes affect drug absorption, distribution, metabolism, and excretion. These changes may facilitate adverse reactions, which then interfere with compliance.

◆ Close monitoring and careful dosage adjustments are crucial to ensuring safe, effective elder care.

◆ The aging process alters body composition and triggers changes in the digestive system, liver, and kidneys. These changes, in turn, affect drug metabolism, which alters dosage and administration techniques. (See *How drug action is altered in older adults*, pages 478 and 479.)

◆ In addition, normal physiologic changes in the older person may be altered or accelerated by acute or chronic disease. Together, these factors can increase the risk of drug toxicity and adverse reactions. (See *Age-related risk factors for adverse drug reactions,* page 480.)

Mental and emotional needs of older patients

◆ The overall health of an older person is determined by a composite of the person's lifestyle, physical health, social support network, coping skills, and cognitive abilities.

◆ Mental health problems in older adults commonly contribute to decreased self-esteem, diminished quality of life, and impaired social functioning.

◆ As people age, issues they have grappled with their entire lives (or possibly tried to ignore), such as alcoholism, family dysfunction, abuse, and other stressors, tend to impact their health.

◆ Good mental health implies a capacity to manage life stresses to achieve a state of emotional homeostasis.

◆ Keep in mind that the far-reaching physical changes of aging commonly have profound psychological effects. Many older adults who seek mental health services have an underlying physical illness. Emotional difficulties may also cause physical symptoms.

Retirement

◆ The earlier a person has prepared for retirement, the better his outlook and quality of life tends to be.

◆ For an older patient who is preparing for retirement, the following teaching needs should be addressed:

- Structuring leisure time
- Planning to live within a fixed, limited budget
- Getting to know one's spouse again now that retirement approaches
- Meeting new friends outside of work, such as through clubs, volunteer work, religious affiliations, and hobbies

Widowhood

◆ One of the most profound losses a person can experience is the death of a spouse.

◆ In addition, widowhood can seriously affect a person's financial status, social network, and physical and mental health.

◆ Make the patient aware of counseling services, support groups, and other resources that are available to help him cope with the loss of a spouse. If the affected person is a caregiver, inform her about respite care services that are available.

Death of an adult child

◆ Refer an older patient who must cope with the loss of an adult child to an appropriate community resource, such as Interfaith, a clergyman, a social worker, or a grief therapist.

Family estrangement

◆ Older people may become estranged from family members for many reasons, such as drug or alcohol abuse, disagreements over religion, sexual orientation, choice of marriage partner,

How drug action is altered in older adults

Absorption
◆ Change in quality and quantity of digestive enzymes
◆ Increased gastric pH
◆ Decreased number of absorbing cells
◆ Decreased GI motility
◆ Decreased intestinal blood flow
◆ Decreased GI emptying time

Distribution
◆ Decreased cardiac output and reserve
◆ Decreased blood flow to target tissues, liver, and kidneys
◆ Decreased distribution space and area
◆ Decreased lean body mass
◆ Increased adipose stores
◆ Decreased plasma protein (decreases protein binding)
◆ Decreased total body water

inheritance issues, or business dealings.
◆ Estrangement from grandchildren and great-grandchildren can be especially painful.
◆ Referring such a patient to family therapy can be very effective.

Changes in body image
◆ Older adults may go through the grieving process and may become depressed after experiencing alterations in body image from normal aging, trauma, or serious illness, such as a stroke or coronary artery disease. What's more, physical changes that impact lifestyle can be devastating to the self-esteem and sexuality.
◆ You can gauge the patient's response to a changed body image by encouraging discussion.
◆ If indicated, refer the patient to a psychotherapist for follow-up.

Financial loss
◆ Many older people face serious financial hardships after retirement, especially if they must depend on Social Security as their primary, or sole, source of income.
◆ Older people are particularly vulnerable to financial scams. Report suspected abuses to the local Office on Aging or county department of human services.

Common psychiatric problems

◆ Older adults don't usually develop new mental illnesses late in life; most are chronic, having started when the person was significantly younger.
◆ Some forms of mental illness, such as depression and schizophrenia, run in families.
◆ With support from family and friends, a person with a mental health problem can develop coping skills that allow him to function for years, sometimes without treatment.
◆ The following are some common mental health disorders among older adults.

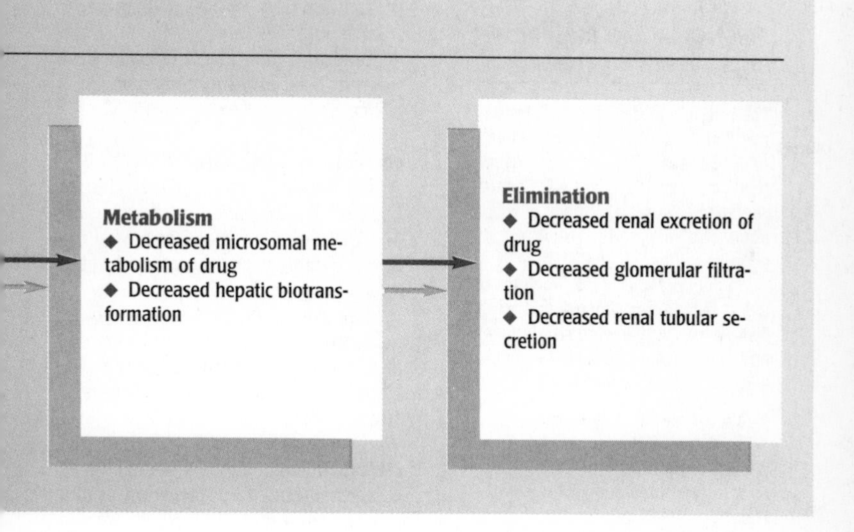

Anxiety

◆ In many cases, the symptoms of anxiety resemble those of depression; a person who is depressed is likely to be anxious as well.

◆ Many psychosocial stressors, such as an impending serious diagnostic test, a sudden financial reversal, or the severe illness of a family member, can trigger a normal anxiety reaction.

◆ Many physical disorders are marked by symptoms of anxiety.

◆ The best way to assist the anxious older adult is to refer him to an available mental health professional or social worker.

◆ Teaching the patient some simple relaxation techniques may be helpful as well.

Alert Alcohol is a common self-treatment for anxiety, but not a benign one. Ask the patient about his alcohol use — what type he drinks (beer, wine, whiskey), about how much per day, and for how long.

Depression

◆ Depression is the most common psychiatric illness affecting older adults, but regarding it as a normal response to aging is a mistake.

◆ The term depression is used to describe a mood, symptom, or disease.

◆ Physical, hormonal, psychological, and social factors profoundly contribute to its development in older people.

◆ Several nonpsychotropic drugs may produce depression as an adverse effect.

Alert Depression may be more common among older adults than the general population because of such factors as loss of friends and relatives, decline in health, and reduced independence.

◆ Many nursing interventions can help the depressed older patient without requiring a physician's order.

- Exercise, such as walking and swimming, is a natural means of treating depression; it helps replace certain depleted brain chemicals, such as serotonin and norepinephrine.

Age-related risk factors for adverse drug reactions

The physiologic changes of aging make older adults more susceptible to drug-induced illnesses and adverse reactions than younger adults. Other conditions common to many older patients also increase the risk of adverse reactions.

To help prevent these problems or detect them early, check the patient's history for the following risk factors, any of which can increase the likelihood of adverse reactions:

- ◆ altered mental status
- ◆ financial problems
- ◆ frail health
- ◆ history of previous adverse reactions
- ◆ history of allergies
- ◆ multiple chronic illnesses
- ◆ living alone
- ◆ polypharmacy or complex drug regimens
- ◆ poor nutritional status
- ◆ renal failure
- ◆ small build
- ◆ treatment by several physicians.

– Gardening therapy is effective for treating people with mental illness.

◆ Provide a safe environment, find out if the patient has suicidal thoughts or plans, and implement appropriate suicide precautions.

Bipolar disorder

◆ Formerly known as cyclical depression and manic-depressive illness, bipolar disorder is characterized by cyclical mood changes from mania (which may range from elation to psychosis) to deep depression.

◆ Managing an older adult with bipolar disorder includes monitoring drug levels and adverse drug reactions.

◆ Lithium is the primary drug used to treat bipolar disorder.

◆ Lithium blood levels must be monitored at least monthly to screen for toxicity.

Obsessive-compulsive disorder

◆ Obsessive-compulsive disorder is marked by repetitive performance of acts or rituals, such as hand-washing, house cleaning, checking doorknobs, and making lists.

◆ This rigid behavior, which usually develops over a lifetime and may start at any stage in adulthood, may worsen if the person experiences a serious stressful event.

Delirium

◆ Characterized by alteration in attention, orientation, intellectual function, and affect that may be accompanied by fear or agitation.

◆ Also called acute confusional state, acute encephalopathy, and altered mental status, delirium isn't a disease but a symptom of an underlying problem, such as:

- infection
- blood sugar imbalance
- pain
- electrolyte imbalances
- sleep deprivation
- head injury
- surgical procedure, anesthesia
- sudden change in physical surroundings
- drug interaction or withdrawal.

◆ Someone must stay with the patient while the physician is notified of the patient's change in mental status.

◆ Obtain the most recent laboratory results and specimens for any newly ordered laboratory tests.

◆ Reorient the patient and decrease noise, light, and other environmental stimuli.

◆ Use restraints, if ordered, as a last resort after other methods have failed to protect the patient.
◆ Delirium may resolve with treatment of the underlying problem, or it may progress and become chronic.

Dementia

◆ Characterized by a progressive or permanent alteration in intellectual function including orientation and judgment. The condition interferes with usual social function and self-care.
◆ Although there's some controversy about the differences between dementia and delirium, dementia is generally thought to be more chronic in nature and irreversible.
◆ There are many forms of dementia. Some types of dementia are reversible, such as the dementia that occurs with pernicious anemia, which responds to vitamin B_{12} therapy. Other types of dementia aren't reversible.
◆ Alzheimer's disease is the most common form of dementia.
◆ Other conditions related to dementia include hydrocephalus, AIDS, multiple small brain infarcts, Huntington's disease, and Parkinson's disease.
◆ Provide appropriate care, as needed.
- Protect the patient from injury.
- Decrease environmental stimuli, such as noise, excessive artificial light, and television use.
- Speak to the patient in a soft, calm, low-pitched voice.
- Use validation therapy when the patient talks about an event that isn't happening or people who are no longer alive, affirming the emotions of the patient without adding to or refuting the fantasy.
- In many cases, referral to health care professionals skilled in caring for these patients is appropriate.

Elements of elder care

Fall prevention

◆ By focusing on preventing falls, you can make tremendous gains in preserving life; helping patients maintain functional abilities, independence, and quality of life; and conserving health care dollars.
◆ Proactive interventions to meet the needs of geriatric patients in an acute care setting could reduce falls by more than 80%.
◆ To be effective, a prevention program must consist of an accurate analysis of the problem, clearly stated goals, practical and efficient interventions, and a strong commitment by all participants to make it work.

Data collection findings

◆ By learning the causes of falls and evaluating an older person for risk factors, you can predict and thus prevent many falls.
◆ A thorough consideration of fall risk should include a review of:
- history of falls
- drug regimens
- medical history
- cognitive status
- social history
- nutritional status
- elimination patterns
- environmental factors
- present status.

Risk identification

◆ Identifying risk factors, followed by timely and appropriate interventions, is the key to a successful program of preventing falls.
◆ Risk factors for falls usually fit one of three categories:
- Intrinsic (physiologic, or within the body)

– Extrinsic (external, or outside the body)
– Iatrogenic (resulting from medical care or treatment)
◆ Unclassified or idiopathic falls are those with no identifiable cause.
◆ Although the categories overlap, they help to identify those factors that can be eliminated or reduced and those that can only be managed.
◆ In older people, falls usually result from a combination of risk factors.

Intrinsic factors

The following physiologic factors increase the risk of falls:
◆ *Age and sex* — The risk of falls increases markedly at age 75, with people ages 80 to 89 at highest risk.
◆ *Sensory deficits* — Vision and hearing problems are a major contributing factor in falls.
◆ *Medical conditions* — Many neurologic, cerebrovascular, cardiovascular, and musculoskeletal conditions cause seizures, drop attacks, and syncopal episodes that result in falls. People with cancer or other progressive, debilitating diseases have a high risk of falling, as do those with multiple or chronic conditions.
◆ *Gait and balance changes* — Gait and balance disorders are the second most common cause of falls, after environmental hazards. This can be attributed to the following:
– a decrease in lean muscle mass
– degenerative changes in the spine, causing stooped posture and a change in the center of gravity
– slowed neurologic response times
– decreased muscle strength and range of motion. (See *Consequences of falls*.)

Alert A fall can be the sole indicator that an elderly person has an acute illness or that a chronic illness is worsening.

Extrinsic factors

The following external factors increase the risk of falls.
◆ *Environmental hazards* — The most common causes of falls are objects in the immediate environment. Electrical cords, throw rugs, loose carpeting, toys, pets, stools, or other low furniture can all be hazards. Wet floors, bathtubs, or showers and objects left on the floor can lead to a slip. Dim lighting, overly bright lighting, uneven or highly patterned floors, and steep stairs can all pose a danger to elderly people.
◆ *Assistive devices* — Many falls stem from improper use of assistive devices, such as canes and walkers. Many elderly people buy such devices without learning how to use them and fail to maintain them properly (for example, replacing worn rubber tips on canes or walkers).
◆ *Alcohol abuse* — Alcohol is a significant cause of falls in elderly people, especially those who live alone. Symptoms of alcohol abuse are easy to overlook because of their similarity to other medical problems. Such symptoms include GI disorders, malnutrition, hypoglycemia, poor sleep patterns, peripheral neuropathies, tremors, abnormal gait, and cognitive impairments and depression, which commonly lead to self-neglect.

Care settings and levels of care

◆ Many care and service options, including those described below, are available to elderly people to help them maintain their independence and to provide care when they can no longer care for themselves.

Multipurpose senior centers

◆ These centers provide a wide variety of services to active, independent adults in the community, including health screening and promotion pro-

Consequences of falls

Falls can lead to a vicious cycle that results in more falls, as shown below.

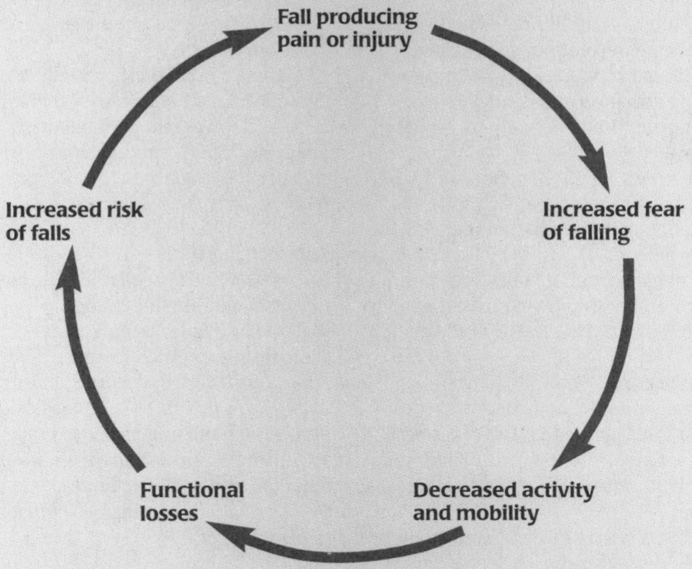

grams, social and recreational programs, tax assistance, and educational programs.

Homemaker services

◆ These services help with such activities as light cleaning, cooking, shopping, and laundry.
◆ A discount may be available through an Area Agency on Aging.

Home maintenance and repair

◆ These services provide help with home repairs and chores for those unable to perform tasks independently.
◆ Cost is sometimes underwritten by an Area Agency on Aging.
◆ These services may be provided by service groups, such as church youth groups, Scouts, or adult volunteer groups.

Check-in service

◆ This service offers telephone check-in to ascertain patient status and provide social contact through volunteers from senior centers, churches, and other community agencies.
◆ It provides periodic scheduled visits from friendly visitors to provide social contact, assistance with correspondence and, possibly, transportation to a community activity.

Community-based adult day care

◆ This option offers numerous services for frail or cognitively compromised older adults in a variety of settings.
◆ It provides structured activities, personal care, recreation, socialization, nutritional support, and health monitoring; social services and caregiver support are frequently a part of these programs.
◆ It allows family members and other caregivers to maintain their jobs and to postpone or avoid institutionalizing an older person.
◆ Charges commonly are based on patient's ability to pay and may be underwritten by an Area Agency on Aging.

Respite care

◆ Trained individuals provide relief (for a brief, limited period of a few hours, days, or weeks) for family members who care for an elderly patient at home.
◆ This service can be offered in the home, through a day-care program, or in a facility.

Hospice care

◆ This service may be offered in an institutional or home setting for a terminally ill patient and the caregivers or family.
◆ Hospice care is covered by most medical insurance companies, Medicare, and Medicaid.
◆ Hospice care is regulated by state and federal agencies.
◆ Care is provided by a team of nurses, physicians, social workers, pharmacists, volunteers, and spiritual counselors, typically through a home health agency or in-patient hospice center.
◆ Bereavement services for the grieving family are a mandated part of the care.
◆ Hospice emphasizes palliative care and freedom from discomfort for the patient in a setting that maintains freedom, dignity, and personal choice.

Acute care

◆ The hospital setting provides care for acute illness or acute exacerbations of chronic illness.
◆ Geriatric units with specially trained interdisciplinary staff (nurses, pharmacists, social workers, rehabilitation therapists, and mental health professionals) are available in some hospitals.

Subacute care

◆ This service is available in some hospitals and nursing homes.
◆ Usually it is for people who need short-term care, such as those recuperating from surgery or illness and those with a chronic illness that needs short-term skilled nursing care.
◆ Subacute care usually includes rehabilitation and social activities.
◆ The goal is to discharge the patient to his home.

Home health care

◆ Services are provided by Medicare, Medicaid, and private insurers to those who meet eligibility criteria for skilled nursing or therapeutic care.
◆ Services may include an RN or supervised LPN; a physical, occupational, or speech therapist; a home health aide; or a social worker on short-term episodic basis.
◆ Maintenance level programs provide personal care services and periodic nursing assessments to support the frail elderly in the home setting. Costs are usually covered by local Area Agency on Aging programs or long-term care insurance.

Assisted living

◆ This option allows the elderly person to remain in a home-like setting.

◆ It provides meals, assistance with activities of daily living (ADLs), health care, 24-hour supervision, and other supportive systems.
◆ Assisted living isn't regulated by the federal government; licensing guidelines are developed by each state.
◆ The goal is to maintain the patient's independence, individuality, freedom of choice, privacy, and dignity.
◆ Fees usually are paid by the patient or, in some cases, by long-term care insurance.

Long-term care

◆ This service provides around-the-clock nursing care for chronically ill or cognitively impaired people, most of whom have four or five limitations in performing ADLs.
◆ Long-term care is regulated by state and federal governments.
◆ Fees are paid by Medicare, Medicaid, the patient, and insurance companies.

Elderly patient rights

◆ The concept of patient rights is a fundamental ethical and legal issue. Competent individuals have the right to make their own decisions about health care issues, including whether or not to be hospitalized or subjected to lifesaving devices and measures, unless the state can show that its interests outweigh that right. Examples of overriding state interests include:
- protecting third parties, especially minor children
- preserving life, especially that of minors and incompetents
- protecting society from the spread of disease.

◆ Ethicists call this right *autonomy*; the legal profession refers to it as *informed consent* and *self-determination*.
◆ The concept of self-determination — the right of a person to decide what will or will not happen to his body — has its origins in both constitutional (legal) rights and autonomy (ethical) rights. This concept is most often evoked in cases involving death and dying, but it applies to all aspects of consent and refusal.
◆ These rights are not lost merely because a person is older or has diminished capacity, and there are several ways in which the patient's wishes can be honored.
◆ To ensure that his wishes are known and respected, the patient should declare those wishes while he's still competent.
◆ In some states, oral wishes are upheld by the judiciary.
◆ The best way to elicit this information is to have the patient prepare a document that encompasses his values and expectations.

Role of consent

◆ Generally, the health care provider's right to treat a patient — except in emergencies and other unanticipated situations — is based on an agreement that arises through the mutual consent of the parties to the relationship.
◆ Consent is the voluntary authorization by a patient or the patient's legal representative to do something to the patient.
◆ The keys to valid consent are the patient's comprehension of the procedure and full disclosure of all significant consequences.
◆ Consent concerns the health care provider's right to treat an individual, not the manner in which treatment is delivered. Thus, one can deliver safe, competent care and still be sued for lack of consent.
◆ A health care provider has a duty to obtain consent before treating a patient.

◆ Consent isn't implied by a patient's request for information or clarification; it must be actively sought by the health care practitioner who will be performing the procedure.
◆ The right to consent or refuse consent is based on a long-recognized, common-law right of people to be free from harmful or offensive touching of their bodies.

Advance directives

◆ To prevent needless worry by patients about relying on others to make decisions should they become unable to speak for themselves, patients must be informed about advance directives, a document that expresses the patient's wishes in writing while he's competent.
◆ Many states recognize more than one form of advance directive, giving patients choices to suit their individual needs and circumstances.
◆ Experts estimate that the numbers of advance directives presented to health care providers will dramatically increase in the next 10 years as more people, particularly competent older people, decide to convey their wishes about future care should they become incompetent.

Living wills

◆ A living will, one type of advance directive, is written by a competent individual to medical personnel and family members regarding the treatment the individual is to receive if he becomes seriously ill and unable to convey his wishes.
◆ A living will isn't applicable while the patient is competent and capable of making his wishes known.
◆ Typically, the language of a living will is broad, dealing only with items such as cardiopulmonary resuscitation, use of a ventilator, blood products, tube feedings, dialysis, and antibiotics. It gives little direction to the health care provider concerning the many varying circumstances that can arise in health care nor the actual time that the patient wishes the living will to be honored.
◆ Most living wills do not provide for the patient to designate a surrogate to act on their behalf if they are no longer able to communicate their wishes. There are several variants, such as the Durable Power of Attorney for Healthcare Decisions that do provide for this designation and help ensure that the patient's wishes are followed.
◆ Living wills, where legally mandated by a state, are typically enforceable legally, although the actual practice of knowing when to implement a living will can be difficult.
– Medical practitioners usually choose to abide by the patient's wishes if they are aware of them, but may ignore them under strong disagreement by family members.
– Because these documents don't protect practitioners from criminal or civil liability, many physicians have refused to follow a living will's direction for fear that family members or the state would file charges of wrongful death.
◆ No matter which state you work in, know the laws of your state and check your facility's policy and procedures manual.

Legal guardian determination

◆ A legal guardian or representative is a person who is legally responsible for giving or refusing consent for an incompetent adult.
◆ To appoint a legal guardian or representative, the court must first declare an adult incompetent. The court then appoints either a temporary or permanent guardian. If the court has reason to believe the adult is only temporarily incapacitated, it appoints a guardian to

act until the adult is able to resume managing personal affairs.

◆ Because the language and requirements for guardianships vary from state to state, health care providers should ensure that their state requirements are met before relying on the guardianship papers as presented.

◆ A guardian is usually selected from a patient's family in the belief that such a person has the patient's best interests at heart and is in a position to best know the patient's desires. The order of selection in cases involving older patients is usually:

1. spouse
2. adult children or grandchildren
3. adult brothers and sisters
4. adult nieces and nephews.

◆ Three types of guardians may be appointed:

- *Guardianship of property* — permits guardian to make only financial decisions (not medical).
- *Guardianship of person* — permits guardian to make only medical decisions (not financial).
- *Plenary guardianship* — permits guardian to make all types of decisions about the incompetent person's medical and financial needs.

Elder abuse and neglect

◆ Definitions and categories of elder abuse and neglect vary from state to state and among agencies.

- Abuse always involves a specific action that's committed knowingly and that causes harm.
- Neglect involves the failure to provide treatment, care, goods, or a service, which then leads to harm.

◆ Abuse and neglect are serious and prevalent problems for older people in home, community, and institutional settings. (See *Types of elder abuse*.)

◆ Older people are given inadequate care for reasons beyond abuse and neglect, such as ignorance, disability, poverty, lack of access to care, and poor caregiver training. It's up to professionals who care for aging adults to determine when inadequate care is actually due to abuse or neglect.

Alert About 10% of adults over age 65 have been victims of abuse or neglect. Adults over age 80 are at highest risk for neglect. In most cases, the abuser is an adult child or spouse.

Types of elder abuse

Elder abuse can come in a number of forms, some of which are easier to detect and prevent than others. Here are the most common forms of elder abuse.

Physical abuse

◆ Physical abuse is any use of force resulting in bodily injury, physical pain, or physical impairment.

◆ It may involve such acts of violence as striking, pushing, shoving, shaking, slapping, kicking, pinching, and burning.

◆ It may also include the inappropriate use of medication, restraints, force-feeding, and physical punishment of any kind.

Sexual abuse

◆ Sexual contact with any person incapable of giving consent is considered sexual abuse.

◆ It may include unwanted touching or any type of sexual assault or battery, including rape, sodomy, coerced nudity, and sexually explicit photographing.

(continued)

Types of elder abuse *(continued)*

Emotional or psychological abuse

◆ Emotional abuse is the infliction of pain or distress through verbal or nonverbal acts.

◆ Emotional and psychological abuse may involve the abusive use of language, silence, or isolation.

◆ It may include verbal assaults, insults, threats, intimidation, humiliation, and harassment.

Neglect

◆ Neglect is the refusal or failure to fulfill any part of a person's obligations to an elder.

◆ Neglect may also include failure of a person who has financial responsibility to provide care or the failure on the part of a service provider to provide needed care.

◆ Neglect typically means the refusal or failure to provide life necessities such as food, water, clothing, shelter, personal hygiene, medicine, comfort, personal safety, and other essentials included in an implied or agreed-upon responsibility to an elder.

Abandonment

◆ Abandonment is the desertion of an elderly person by an individual who has assumed responsibility for providing care or by a person with physical custody.

Financial or material exploitation

◆ This type of exploitation involves the illegal or improper use of an elder's funds, property, or assets.

◆ It may involve the use of funds without permission; forging a signature; misusing or stealing possessions; coercing or deceiving the elder into signing any document; and the improper use of conservatorship, guardianship, or power of attorney.

Self-neglect

◆ Self-neglect is behavior by an elderly person that threatens his own health or safety.

◆ This includes any patient who isn't mentally or physically capable of self-care but excludes the mentally competent older person who fully understands the consequences of his decisions and has made a conscious choice to engage in acts that threaten his health or safety.

16 Home care

Basic principles

What is home care?

◆ Home care is a component of comprehensive health care in which services are provided to patients of all ages and their families in their homes to restore, maintain, or promote health and to minimize the effects of illness and disability.
◆ Based on the patient's needs, the appropriate care is planned, coordinated, and supplied by a home care agency.
◆ Home care nursing requires a nurse to have a broad-based knowledge of all facets of health care.
◆ With the speedy discharge of patients from hospitals (the "quicker and sicker" syndrome), the increasing number of elderly patients, and the availability of safe, easily operated health care equipment, home care has a bright future.
◆ Dramatic changes in home care regulations have occurred since the Balanced Budget Act of 1997.
– These legislative changes included prospective pay and the implementation of a standardized assessment tool (OASIS) when providing home care.
– In addition, the Health Care Financing Administration (HCFA) investigated billing practices and how care was being provided, which resulted in the closing of more than 20% of home care agencies since 1996.
◆ The home care industry may conceivably become one of the primary suppliers of health care in the United States. Currently, long-term care is the primary supplier of health care.
◆ Because skilled nursing service lies at the heart of any successful home care program, it's important for you to understand home care principles and practices.

Certification and accreditation

◆ Home care agencies serving Medicare patients, except for some hospices and home health aide (HHA) agencies, are regulated by the Medicare Conditions of Participation.
– These standards are accepted for use by many other private insurance companies and the Medicaid system as well.
– Hospices are certified as Medicare providers under a separate federal standard.
◆ Federal agencies ensure compliance with standards by providing audits by health surveyors employed and licensed by state department agencies.
– These health surveyors have moved from annual inspections to more frequent visits, commonly related to service complaints.
– The inspectors determine if an agency can be "certified" under HCFA regulations for Medicare. For more information, see "Managing and improving care," page 502.
◆ In addition to Medicare certification, agencies may opt for accreditation by the Joint Commission on Accreditation of Healthcare Organizations (JCAHO) or the National League for Nursing's Community Health Accreditation Program (CHAP).
– Although JCAHO and CHAP accreditation aren't required, many managed care and private insurance companies mandate this accreditation for their contracted agencies.
– Home care agencies not Medicare-certified or JCAHO- or CHAP-accredited can still serve the needs of privately paying clients and those who need only the services of a certified nurse's aide or a homemaker.

- However, they may be required to meet standards of the Area Agency of Aging to serve clients supported by those programs.

◆ An agency applying for accreditation must show compliance with established standards.

◆ Every 3 years, the accrediting body reviews the agency's operations, policies, and procedures; interviews staff; and evaluates home visits and compliance with clinical practice standards.

Determining the patient's eligibility

◆ The provider must recognize the patient as being homebound (able to leave the home infrequently, primarily for medical care) and requiring intermittent *skilled care* services (nursing, physical therapy, and speech therapy) for him to be eligible for home care covered by Medicare, Medicaid, and many private insurance companies.

◆ Nursing services are broken down into:

- services provided only by an RN, such as completing the OASIS tool
- services that can be delegated to an LPN or certified HHA under the supervision of an RN every 14 days.

◆ HHA services, occupational therapy, and medical social services are *ancillary* services that can only be provided when a skilled care service provider is already in the home.

◆ Other services may be offered at home, such as nutrition and respiratory services, but these aren't considered skilled care. (See *Understanding skilled and ancillary home care services*, pages 492 and 493.)

◆ Patients are referred for home care services mainly by facility discharge planners. They may also be referred by physicians, their families, community agencies, skilled nursing facilities, or insurance case managers.

◆ The home care agency must obtain a physician's order before starting service, and the physician must review a progress report and recertify the need for continued skilled service every 2 months (not more than 62 days).

Continuing developments

Several major trends are emerging as the home care industry continues to evolve:

◆ *Accountability pressures* — Today, home care services are reimbursed by Medicare, Medicaid, and managed care private insurers. More and more private insurers are requiring that home care services be preauthorized. This cost-conscious environment confronts the nurse with challenges ranging from loss of control over patient care to ethical dilemmas and quality improvement issues.

◆ *Emphasis on outcomes* — Disease-specific management programs — such as those now in place for diabetes and heart failure — will require home care agencies to develop critical pathways that incorporate patient outcome analysis. In the future, an agency's quality will be measured by outcome data.

◆ *Computerizing care* — Increasingly, home care nurses are coping with an expanding paperwork load by using laptop computers. These are equipped with software that speeds clinical documentation to develop the care plan, formulate goals, monitor patient progress, update drugs, and generate visit notes. This technology expedites the exchange of current clinical data and other information among physicians, other care providers, and reimbursers.

◆ *Financial stability* — As reimbursement moves from cost-based to prospective pay, greater emphasis will be placed on streamlining care, triaging admissions, and improving efficiency.

Understanding skilled and ancillary home care services

This table shows examples of skilled and ancillary services used in home health care and how they may be reimbursed

SERVICES	INDICATIONS AND EXAMPLES	CONSIDERATIONS
Physical therapy (skilled service)	Indicated for functional limitations and deficits in safety, mobility, strength, and range of motion; examples: gait training, strengthening exercises	Some states allow trained physical therapists to perform wound debridement. A physical therapist (PT) may be the sole professional on a home care case and may complete all OASIS tools. A certified physical therapy assistant may be used by the PT for some visits but must be supervised by the PT every 15 visits or 30 days, whichever comes first.
Speech therapy (skilled service)	Indicated for dysphasia and dysphagia; examples: assessment and evaluation, diagnostic testing, teaching and training, aural rehabilitation, maintenance therapy	Medicare won't reimburse for repetition and reinforcement, work-related therapy, or a nondiagnostic or nontherapeutic routine. Speech therapists may also complete OASIS data and be the sole provider in the home.
Occupational therapy (ancillary service)	Indicated for functional limitation of activities of daily living that relates to the primary or secondary diagnosis; examples: therapeutic activities, energy-conservation methods, task simplification	Skilled nursing, physical therapy, or speech therapy must be ordered and provided for occupational therapy services to be reimbursed. The occupational therapist (OT) can complete the discharge OASIS tool and be the sole provider left in a home on recertifications. A certified occupational therapy assistant may be used by the OT if supervised according to regulations.
Medical social service (ancillary service)	Indicated for social or emotional difficulties of the patient or caregiver that affect treatment or rate of recovery; examples: referrals, counseling, long-term care planning	Skilled nursing, physical therapy, or speech therapy must be ordered and provided for medical social service to be reimbursed. OASIS forms may not be completed by medical social service representatives.

Understanding skilled and ancillary home care services *(continued)*

SERVICES	INDICATIONS AND EXAMPLES	CONSIDERATIONS
Home health aide (HHA) care (ancillary service)	Determined by the home care nurse, usually at the initial visit; HHA assistance with personal hygiene, patient transfers, light meal preparation, light housekeeping and, possibly, drugs (for drugs, check state laws)	Skilled nursing, physical therapy, or speech therapy must be ordered and provided for HHA care services to be reimbursed.

◆ *Client satisfaction* — Home care agencies have always focused on client satisfaction. However, given the potential that a single complaint can turn into a full agency survey, many home care agencies are extending their response to service complaints.

Ethical and legal aspects of home care

◆ The Code for Nurses of the American Nurses Association (ANA) includes standards of ethical conduct and practice that are relevant to home care.
◆ As in any other health care setting, you're expected to provide services while respecting the patient's human dignity and uniqueness without regard to his socioeconomic status, personal attributes, or nature of the health problem.
◆ Specific ethical principles include autonomy, beneficence, veracity, fidelity, justice, and respect for others. Each of these principles helps to define the quality and adequacy of health care delivered in the home setting. (See *Applying ethical principles in home health nursing,* page 494.)
◆ Many factors can complicate ethical decisions, such as the legal right of a competent adult to refuse care, increasing patient sophistication, living wills, confidentiality issues, and limited financial resources.
◆ Ethical concerns are strongly emphasized in the home care field. In its accreditation process, JCAHO directs agencies to establish committees that handle ethical issues that arise in the home.
◆ Ethical guidelines are supported by a network of federal and state laws relating to home nursing care.
- For example, you won't lose your nursing license if you fail to abide by the ANA's Code for Nurses — a voluntary guide document.
- However, you may lose your license if you violate your state's nurse practice act, which sets legal practice standards in your state.

◆ Federal and state laws relevant to home care are briefly reviewed here.

Federal legislation

◆ Federal legislation sets requirements for all home health care nurses.
◆ The Omnibus Budget Reconciliation Act (OBRA), as amended in 1987, substantially changed the law relating to participating Medicare agencies. The law requires that:

Applying ethical principles in home health nursing

PRINCIPLE	MEANING	EXAMPLE OF NURSING APPLICATION
Autonomy	Personal freedom	Allowing the patient to decide when to implement care or to refuse treatment
Beneficence	Duty to promote good	Allowing the patient to die without life-sustaining treatment if that's what he desires
Veracity	Being truthful	Providing the patient with enough information to allow him to make informed choices about care
Fidelity	Keeping one's promise	Not promising the patient that you or another health care worker will be at the bedside when death comes (a promise you may not be able to keep)
Justice	Treating others fairly	Ensuring that you'll provide the care that the patient needs even if there are other, more seriously ill patients that you need to see
Respect for others	Right of individuals to be treated equally	Treating all patients with the same level of empathy and competent care, even when they're noncompliant or of another culture or race

- patients be screened for eligibility
- they be informed of their legal rights before signing the home care contract
- they be fully informed in advance about the agency's care plan and about changes in care or treatment that may affect their well-being, as well as any costs they may incur in addition to what their insurance pays.

◆ The law gives the patient a voice in planning his care and treatment and addresses confidentiality and grievance issues.

◆ The specific scope of practice for an LPN in home health care is mandated by the individual agency, within the guidelines of state and federal regulations.

◆ A separate OBRA provision sets strict criteria for HHAs, who typically provide a large share of hands-on patient care.

◆ An agency may not use any individual who isn't a licensed health care professional unless that person has successfully completed a training program that meets minimum federal standards and is deemed competent to provide assigned services. For more information, see "Working with home health aides," page 500.

◆ The Older Americans Act was amended in 1987 to strengthen home care consumer protections such as the rights of developmentally disabled persons.

◆ The Patient Self-Determination Act of 1991 requires federally funded home care agencies to abide by the terms of a patient's living will or other special directive such as a durable power of attorney. If a patient lacks such an instrument but wants to obtain it, the agency must instruct the patient how to do so.

◆ Since 1999, home care agencies have been required to collect specific information on each patient who is older than age 18 and not receiving services related to childbirth.

- An Outcome and Assessment Information Set (OASIS), made up of 79 data elements, helps this process by allowing the agency to submit completed information electronically to the HCFA.
- In addition to the initial OASIS assessment, a repeat assessment is done if the patient is admitted to a health care facility, has a significant change in his condition, is recertified for ongoing care, or is discharged.
- OASIS helps home care agencies determine patient needs, plan care, assess care over the course of treatment, and learn how to improve the quality of that care.
- It incorporates all information regarding the patient's health, functional status, health service use, living conditions, and social supports.
- It allows quality to be monitored and is essential for accurate payment under the new home health prospective payment system (PPS) instituted on October 1, 2000.
- Timely and accurate completion of the OASIS is essential so that the employer can review the guidelines and identify the specifications of the OASIS.

◆ The PPS sets an amount of money per patient and care is reviewed per episode rather than per number of visits.

◆ Patients who don't have a caregiver may not be admitted if their care needs are generally expected to exceed the government reimbursement rate.

◆ Although the exact impact of the PPS is unknown, it's generally agreed that home care will offer fewer visits with increased emphasis on patient teaching for most patients.

State legislation

◆ As you might expect, your state's nurse practice act governs the standards of practice and standards of care in the patient's home as in other health care settings.

◆ You should be aware of your state's laws in such areas as tenants' rights, protection of uninsured persons, and abused or homeless persons. For example, you should know how and when to report cases of suspected abuse.

◆ Familiarize yourself with family law issues, such as guardians' rights, durable power of attorney, and consent to perform procedures on minors or incompetent persons.

Common legal issues

Verbal orders

◆ If you are legally required to obtain a verbal order, JCAHO and most agencies require that the order be documented and read back to the physician completely for verification.

◆ Have the physician co-sign it as soon as possible and insert the signed copy in the patient's record to replace the verbal copy.

◆ If a patient is injured while you were relying on a verbal order and no documentation of the order can be found, you may have trouble proving that you accurately implemented the physician's order.

◆ Be sure you've obtained the verbal order and had it approved *before* the approved care plan expires. Medicare won't cover care that the patient's physician hasn't fully described and authorized.
◆ Because home care is reimbursed through prospective pay, all reimbursement for each episode, rather than for each visit, is jeopardized by irregularities in authorization.

Contracts
◆ Home health nurses must honor contracts made with patients.
◆ Contracts include written and oral agreements of understanding made between the agency and the prospective patient.
◆ Services described in the agency's brochures and other advertisements can be construed as part of the formal contract.
◆ A home care plan of care contract, generally referred to as the "HCFA-485," should specify these elements:
- provider's and patient's respective roles and responsibilities
- duration, type, frequency, and limitations of services
- discharge planning, cost, and payment schedules
- provisions for obtaining informed consent from the patient or patient's surrogate for specific interventions.
◆ This form serves as the physician's order sheet and must be signed by the physician and updated every 60 days if care is to continue.
◆ Before any agency Consent to Treat form is signed, the patient should be informed about the availability of 24-hour staffing, the way to contact staff during off-hours, the reasons this service may be needed, and how the services are covered financially.
◆ If needed, a patient may be transferred to another site by the agency after the contract has been signed. All aspects of a transfer (physical, psychological, and financial) should be discussed with the patient beforehand.
◆ The agency must develop and implement a satisfactory discharge plan to avoid liability in the event of perceived patient "abandonment" or "dumping" at termination or discharge.
◆ Discharge planning should be started with the initial patient evaluation and the patient should be involved in the plan throughout the care period.
◆ When a patient is to be discharged, he must be given reasonable notice (at least 5 days per JCAHO) and adequate health care services up to the discharge date. The final OASIS form is completed from the last visit.
◆ The agency isn't obligated to provide ongoing services without compensation. Nor must the agency continue to care for a patient who is a threat to the physical safety of the staff.

Confidentiality
◆ As a general rule, you must protect the confidentiality of the patient's medical record. For more information, see *Patient rights under HIPAA*, pages 538 and 539.
- In most states, all health care records — including clinical data obtained from examinations, treatments, observations, and conversations — are confidential.
- Specific state laws may restrict disclosure of this information.
◆ The implementation of OASIS has brought issues of confidentiality to the forefront of home care. At the center of the controversy is the government's right to OASIS assessment data when the patient isn't insured by the federal government.
◆ You may have to share the patient's record with other members of the home care team and with third-party payers.

- You may be legally required to disclose confidential information in exceptional instances, such as child abuse cases, matters of public health and safety, and criminal cases.
- To address these issues, obtain written consent from your patient beforehand, preferably at contract signing.
  - If no provision was made for sharing of information, have the patient sign a release form.
  - This form should specify what information is to be released, to whom it will be given, and the time period during which the release is valid.
- Because the patient may request information from the record, the agency should have a written policy concerning release of information to the patient or patient's surrogate. Although the original record is the property of the agency, a copy may be given to the patient for his records.
- Other common confidentiality problems include:
  - listening to voice messages on the office speaker phone when other staff is present
  - leaving patient files where they may be viewed by others, such as in a car
  - taking other patient folders or a schedule with patient names on it into the patient's home
  - talking to neighbors about the location of the patient
  - talking on a cell phone while in the patient's or others' presence unless the call is specific to the patient
  - leaving voice mails on patient or caregivers home phone systems
  - documenting on a patient chart while in a public place
  - leaving voicemail for healthcare staff, especially a physician leaving a verbal order
  - using a speaker phone instead of the handset.

Refusal of care

- An issue of growing concern is the patient's right to refuse treatment.
- Even if the patient has previously consented to treatment, a mentally competent patient can later withdraw consent if the patient has been fully informed about his medical condition and the likely consequences of refusal.
- Verbal withdrawal of consent is adequate; this should be immediately communicated to other members of the home care team including the physician.
- The patient's refusal or withdrawal of consent must be documented, along with any patient education measures, and placed in the patient's medical record.

Implementation

Ensuring safe home care visits

- When providing patient care in the home, you're faced with two challenges that don't normally arise in a hospital setting:
  - making sure you aren't harmed before, during, and after the home visit
  - making sure the patient can receive care in a safe home environment.
- This section will help you meet these challenges.

Personal safety guidelines

- Most home care agencies have specific policies and procedures to ensure staff safety.
- Discuss any safety concerns with your supervisor as soon as they arise so that the appropriate corrective action can be taken. (See *Personal safety pointers*, page 498.)

Personal safety pointers

As a home health care nurse, you'll serve many patients who may be scattered over a wide area in various settings. The suggestions here will help you to avoid problems.

Before you go

- ◆ Know your agency's safety protocols.
- ◆ Verify where the patient lives; call the family or use a map. Use a public telephone or mobile telephone so that your home address can't be tracked by the patient.
- ◆ Leave a copy of your itinerary at the office.
- ◆ If the patient lives in an unsafe area, try planning your visit early in the day; if possible, bring a nurse "buddy" along.
- ◆ If you don't wear a uniform, dress in business clothes, wear a name tag, and carry agency identification; make it easy for the patient to identify you.
- ◆ Carry an extra set of keys with you (in case you lock yourself out of your car), bring just enough money for emergency calls and transportation, and have a list of important phone numbers (agency, police, fire).

On the road

- ◆ Make sure your car runs well and fill the gas tank before a visit. Consider joining an automobile club for quick access to road service.
- ◆ Always use your seat belt; practice defensive driving.
- ◆ If you're taking public transportation, make sure you know the route; if you must walk, don't accept rides from strangers.
- ◆ Be prepared for poor weather and delays on the road. Have a flashlight, blanket, and snacks handy.

When you arrive

- ◆ Don't park your car near the patient's home if it's in an unsafe area. Instead, park in a public area and walk to the home along well-lit streets. If you must visit in the evening, park in an open, well-lit area.
- ◆ Before you get out of your car, look around. If you feel unsafe, drive to a safe place to phone the agency about your concern.
- ◆ If you have doubts about the safety of entering the patient's home or building, don't enter. Immediately contact the agency.
- ◆ If the patient doesn't answer the door, call the patient from a pay phone or mobile phone or have the agency contact the patient.
- ◆ When entering the home, look for all the exits. If you're uneasy or if you suspect anyone in the home is using alcohol or drugs, do what you need to do and leave. If this isn't possible, leave immediately.
- ◆ If a pet is hostile or poses safety problems, politely ask that it be moved to another room. Always be respectful of the patient's attachment to the pet. After your visit, document the animal's presence in the home to warn other caregivers.
- ◆ Be alert to the presence of guns in the house and use your judgement about whether care can be provided safely if a gun is visible. When in doubt, leave and call the agency.
- ◆ If you are sexually harassed or receive threats of physical violence, leave and report these incidents immediately to the agency supervisor.

Assessing the home environment

◆ You're legally responsible for ensuring that the home is indeed the best place for your patient to receive prescribed care and treatment.
◆ Begin checking the patient's home environment for actual and potential safety problems at your first visit.
◆ Document your findings regarding room layout, accessibility, bathroom facilities, storage areas, provision for medical waste disposal, emergency exit routes, smoke detectors, and availability of support persons.
◆ Check for and correct safety concerns for the duration of the contract period.
◆ Teach the patient and his family about specific safety measures to implement in your absence.
◆ The information below will help you assess possible safety hazards and provide appropriate teaching.

General safety

◆ Make sure stairs have secure railings and nonslip tread surfaces.
◆ Ensure good lighting in halls and stairways.
◆ Install a bedside telephone or access to a portable phone.
- Provide phone numbers of emergency contact persons, the physician, 911 (local fire and police), and the agency (agencies must be accessible 24 hours a day).
- If needed, install a telephone alert system.

◆ Make sure pathways are clear and unobstructed; rugs, if used, should have nonslip backings. Avoid using rugs in high-traffic areas.
◆ Provide nonskid slippers or shoes for the patient to use when out of bed.
◆ Have a plan for natural disasters, such as fires, earthquakes, tornadoes, and hurricanes.

Bathroom safety

◆ Adjust water heater temperature to below 120° F (48.9° C); instruct the patient or family member to check water temperature before getting into the tub or shower.
◆ Advise the patient and his family to install rubber mats or nonslip strips in the tub and shower.
◆ Advise the patient and his family to install grab bars in the tub and shower, and near toilets if needed.

Patient care safety

◆ Determine availability of support persons.
◆ Demonstrate safe storage of drugs, out of the reach of children, and disposal of old or expired drugs.
◆ Instruct the patient to keep wheelchair brakes locked and footrests out of the way when transferring to a wheelchair.
◆ If ordered, apply patient restraints properly and teach caregivers how to check and remove restraints to avoid circulatory or other complications.
◆ Advise the patient to set electrical heating pads on low to medium, to use a cover over them, and to remove them before settling down to sleep or every 20 to 30 minutes, whichever comes first.
◆ Place personal and safety items within the patient's reach when they are in bed or in a chair.
◆ Institute and teach infection-control measures to the patient and caregiver.

Fire safety

◆ Warn the patient against smoking in bed or while using oxygen and tell him to make sure all cigarettes and matches are extinguished before throwing them away.
◆ Advise installation of smoke or heat detectors on each level of the home.

◆ Place portable heaters in well-ventilated areas.
◆ Make sure electrical cords are intact, not frayed or split, and have straight plug prongs.
◆ Make sure an evacuation plan is in place and practiced and that the local fire company is aware that a resident may need help to evacuate.

Medical equipment
◆ Instruct the patient and family regarding the function, proper use, and routine care of prescribed equipment, the audible and visual warning alarms on the equipment, and the reporting of malfunctions.
◆ Explain possible hazards related to electrical, mechanical, and fire safety aspects of equipment.
◆ Store medical gases, supplies, and drugs in a safe, protected area.

Medical waste disposal
◆ Make sure appropriate containers are available for disposal of needles, syringes, and other contaminated medical supplies.
◆ Teach proper handling of medical waste.

Documenting your actions
◆ Document your home care safety recommendations.
◆ Enclose a statement in the patient's record listing what was taught or recommended and record instances of the patient's or family's refusal or failure to follow your recommendations. For example, they may balk at the extra expense of installing smoke detectors or a tub rail. Or, the patient may continue to smoke when oxygen is being used.
◆ Notify the caregiver or family member, the physician, and possibly protective services or a medical social worker if a patient refuses to implement a safety recommendation.
◆ Carefully documenting noncompliance will help protect you and your agency from possible liability.

Working with home health aides

◆ If the patient's condition and situation warrant it, a paraprofessional home health aide (HHA) may be assigned to help the patient intermittently with personal care and activities of daily living.
◆ The HHA's role is crucial because she may spend more time with the patient and family than any other member of the health care team.
◆ Typically, the need for HHA services will be determined during the initial home visit.

Criteria for home health aide services
◆ For planning and reimbursement purposes, the use of HHAs is considered an ancillary (not a skilled care) service.
◆ The National Association for Home Care has identified three levels of HHA services.
- An HHA I performs housekeeping services only, this service may be identified as homemaker care.
- An HHA II performs nonmedical personal care as well as level I tasks, and may be identified as an attendant care or personal care aide.
- An HHA III performs medically supervised tasks, such as providing nonsterile wound care, assisting with prescribed rehabilitation therapy, and assisting the patient to self-administer medications, in addition to performing levels I and II tasks, and may be called a certified nurse's aide (CNA).

◆ Medicare will reimburse a home care agency only for care provided by a certified level III HHA.

◆ An HHA III may become certified after completing a training program of at least 75 hours, 16 of which must be in laboratory and clinical settings.
◆ To justify HHA III services, the agency must be able to demonstrate that skilled care is being provided on an intermittent basis, thereby creating a need for hands-on personal care and assistance with the patient's treatment.
◆ Under Medicare and most insurers, the continued need for HHA services must be documented following a supervisory visit at least every 2 weeks.
- The physician must confirm the type and frequency of HHA service in the care plan.
- The physician must recertify the order for HHA service every 2 months.
◆ Patients receiving level I to III services through private insurance or the Area Agency on Aging must have supervisory visits every 30 days to verify that safe, effective care is being given and is still required.
◆ Explain to the patient and family that HHA services will only be reimbursed by Medicare or Medicaid if these criteria are met.
◆ Patients and their families can become dependent on the HHA and have trouble adjusting when HHA services stop. Referrals can be made for private home health aide assistance or the Area Agency on Aging for ongoing assistance as appropriate.

What home health aides do

◆ Most of the tasks of an HHA III involve assisting with the patient's personal care. This includes:
- bathing
- changing bed linens for an incontinent patient
- dressing
- grooming
- oral hygiene
- routine foot care
- shaving
- skin care.

◆ The HHA may help with feeding and elimination; she may empty catheters and colostomy appliances and help the patient replace an ostomy bag if instructed by a nurse on the procedure.
◆ The HHA can assist the patient with ambulation, changing position in bed, and transfers.
◆ Examples of reimbursable HHA services include:
- a dressing change that doesn't require skilled care, such as a dry, nonsterile dressing change
- helping a competent patient to self-medicate (such as open a cap as directed by the patient)
- helping with activities related to skilled therapy services that don't require the therapist to be present, such as maintenance exercises and speech exercises
- performing routine care of prosthetic and orthotic devices.

◆ The HHA may perform other activities during a home visit, but these aren't reimbursable unless they're performed during that same visit. Such activities, labeled by Medicare as "incidental," may include:
- light housekeeping
- light cleaning of the patient's immediate area
- meal preparation and cleanup
- laundry related to the patient's care
- essential grocery shopping and errands
- taking out the trash.

Supervising home health aides

◆ When HHA services are ordered, plan to meet with the aide during one of your home care visits. This allows the aide and the patient to get acquainted and discuss the care plan established by the RN.

◆ The care plan will specify the HHA's duties. At the end of the visit, leave a copy with the patient.
◆ Typically, you're responsible for communicating with the HHA about any changes in the patient's condition or care and communicating with the patient and family about the care provided. However, if another skilled service (such as physical or speech therapy) is involved and skilled nursing isn't, you can delegate supervisory responsibility to the therapist.
◆ An RN must monitor the HHA's performance during a home visit while the aide is present to directly observe, to instruct the HHA, and to make recommendations and suggestions for care.
◆ Plan a visit when the HHA isn't present so that you can get additional feedback. The patient may be reluctant to say anything about the HHA while she is present.
◆ Managed care organizations and private insurers have reimbursement and supervisory criteria for HHA services similar to Medicare's. Consult your case manager about specific requirements.

Documenting home health aide services

◆ Most home care agencies use a standardized form for documenting HHA supervision. These data should also be entered in the patient's care record.
◆ Information about the patient's health status, rapport of the patient and HHA, and determination of goal achievement should be included.
◆ Include in your visit notes any recommendations and suggestions from the data you collected and any comments made by the patient and report these findings to the supervising RN.
◆ If teaching is involved, document what was taught and the HHA's response to the teaching, including a return demonstration, if appropriate.

Managing and improving care

◆ Case management and quality improvement are concepts central to providing professional home care services. They are intended to provide a structure for care according to standards established by government regulation, voluntary accreditation agencies, professional organizations, third-party payers, and individual agencies.

Case management

◆ Case management involves prioritizing care among the patients in a caseload and delivering that care according to procedural steps that ensure successful patient outcomes. The home-care RN is the designated case manager; the LPN assists in implementing the care plan.
◆ These steps are based on the nursing process and include information gathering and assessment, establishing a multidisciplinary care plan, and implementing and evaluating the care plan.
◆ At its best, external case management matches the home care nurse's strengths — knowledge of the patient and the community resources available — with the case manager's strengths — knowledge of reimbursement procedures and efficient use of available resources.
◆ Case management may pose challenges.
– A managed care environment may alter your agency's flexibility in responding to changing patient needs and it may alter your decision-making authority.
– A single patient may have several case managers from different managed

care organizations with different policies and procedures.
- Case managers, for their part, may be frustrated by the need to constantly explain and justify their role when they feel they should be treated as valued customers.
◆ Effective communication can reduce the level of mutual distrust and frustration.

Quality improvement

◆ Health care agencies' quality control efforts have advanced from static reviews of patient care documentation to ongoing integration of quality improvement measures into all procedures.
◆ The original term *quality assurance* evolved to total quality management, followed by total quality improvement, continuous quality improvement and, finally, outcome-based quality improvement (OBQI).
◆ The OBQI process can be seen as yet another variation of the nursing process.
- Data is gathered.
- Problems are defined.
- Goals are set.
- Actions are selected.
- Evaluations are made using structure, process, and outcome indicators.
- Variances are identified.
- A new round of the OBQI process begins.

◆ The process begins with the OASIS assessment tool and outcomes determined from that assessment.
◆ Nurses have multiple opportunities to become involved in the OBQI process. If chosen to participate on a quality improvement committee, you would work with other caregivers to set the course for the OBQI program for a significant time period. Many agencies have a quality improvement coordinator or director who chairs the committee.
◆ On another quality front, many health care providers are developing sets of standard interventions, based on medical diagnoses or surgical procedures, to ensure that patients receive care that's standardized for the specific condition.
- These standard interventions are known as clinical paths, critical paths, care tracks, and coordinated care guides.
- Clinical paths resemble standardized nursing care plans in some respects.
- They're multidisciplinary tools that need to be accepted by all involved in the patient's care, particularly the physician.
- Clinical paths can reduce documentation requirements and streamline the quality improvement process.

Medicare site visits

◆ When home care agencies are reviewed to certify them for Medicare reimbursement, the aspects of care that are examined are determined by the conditions of participation in the Medicare program documented in the Home Health Agency Health Insurance Manual.
◆ To prepare for a Medicare site visit, agency personnel should review all practices to make sure Medicare guidelines are followed for every Medicare-reimbursed case:
- Check admission practices to ensure that the patient and family understand the conditions of Medicare eligibility, their rights with regard to Medicare service, and the way to access information about these rights.
- Document that a copy of the patient's bill of rights was given to the patient and place a copy in the patient's record.

– Document that the patient's wishes with regard to advance medical directives were discussed.
– Review the patient's record for adherence to standards of timeliness of documentation, for visit frequency, and for completion of all necessary forms, particularly physician's orders (HCFA-485).
– Make sure that visit records reflect the skilled care given, the homebound status of the patient, and the coordination of all services provided by the agency.
– Perform supervision of HHAs according to the agency's policy. Document the patient's or caregiver's satisfaction with the service, the rationale for continued HHA service, and the nurse's recommendation to continue or modify the service.
– Review patient knowledge of and input into the care plan as outlined on the HCFA-485.
– Review safety issues in the home and patient understanding and response.

Working with families

◆ Your relationships with family members can sometimes be as important as those with patients.
◆ Although technically a home care visit is intended to provide care for a sick person, in reality, you usually will be working with the patient's family as well.
◆ When someone is sick, family members worry. They usually want to know something about what's wrong with the patient. Often, they want to help care for the patient. Sometimes they have to care for the patient when you can't be there.

Starting a relationship

◆ Family members start forming an impression about you, as a person and as a professional, as soon as they meet you.
◆ Above all, you want them to see right from the start that they can rely on you to give good care to their loved one. You can do this in several ways.
– Look neat and professional when you arrive at a patient's home.
– Make sure you're wearing your name tag.
– When someone answers the door, introduce yourself with confidence and a smile.
– Offer a firm handshake as you tell the person your first and last name, your agency's name, and the reason for your visit.
– Show your I.D. if the person asks for it.
◆ Once you get inside the home, remember that you're a guest.
◆ Introduce yourself to the other family members and be respectful of the patient and his family.
◆ When you come back for other visits, greet family members warmly and ask how they're doing.
◆ If they talk about things you aren't trained to handle, ask your supervisor for help.

Encouraging help

◆ Family members can help support the patient — and you — if you let them.
– For instance, they can tell you what the patient likes and dislikes.
– They may be able to tell you what the patient is saying if he's difficult to understand.
– They can tell you about the patient's daily routines.
◆ Getting this information from the family can save you a lot of time and

energy. It helps build a special bond between you and family members.

◆ Letting them help you care for their loved one builds bonds. Remember that many family members feel helpless when a loved one gets sick. Don't assume that family members know how to care for a sick person, though, or even that they want to.

◆ If a family member wants to pitch in, show him how to help with feeding or bathing. If a family member feels unwilling or unable to help, be careful not to make comments that make him feel guilty.

Supporting caregivers

◆ Usually, family members do help care for their ill loved ones and they may spend lots of time and energy doing it. In fact, family members may be under great stress from trying to carry out their own usual roles while also caring for a sick person. A caregiver who doesn't have help can easily burn out.

◆ Often the job of caring for a sick person falls mainly on a female family member such as the wife, mother, daughter, daughter-in-law, or sister of the patient. This person may have to shop, cook, run errands, do laundry, and even hold a job while also trying to care for the patient when you aren't there. If the patient has a long-term illness, this caregiver could be facing years of hard work.

◆ That's why one of your most helpful roles is to support family caregivers. You can do this in many ways. For one, you can urge the caregiver to talk about how she's holding up. Ask her to talk about herself and how she's feeling. Use empathic instead of sympathetic techniques when working with the patient and caregivers. (See *Empathy versus sympathy*.)

Empathy versus sympathy

When caring for patients, use empathy, not sympathy. Here's the difference.

Empathy

◆ Help patients or families know how they are feeling.

◆ Stay emotionally and intellectually sensitive to the feelings expressed.

◆ Stay objective.

◆ Use sentences such as, "Tell me what you are feeling."

Sympathy

◆ Take on the patient's or family's feelings.

◆ Get upset along with the patient or family.

◆ Identify with what the patient or family says.

◆ Use phrases such as, "I know how you're feeling."

◆ Ask the caregiver who can help her. Does she have a friend or someone from church who could watch the kids, help with laundry, or sit with the patient while she rests or does something fun?

◆ As much as possible, help the caregiver learn safe, quick ways to care for the patient by watching you. Make sure she uses safe body positions to keep from getting hurt. Praise her and help her feel good about herself and her abilities as she cares for the patient.

◆ Urge her to take care of herself. That means eating right, exercising, and trying to relax whenever possible. Local services may be available to help her, such as support groups, respite care, Meals On Wheels, and groups for people with specific illnesses, such as diabetes or cancer.

◆ Tell your supervisor if you think the patient's main caregiver is getting exhausted, angry, or resentful. Be on the lookout for sadness, depression, and any mention of suicide or "giving up." Use her exact words or your observations to do this rather than giving your opinion. Use the services of a medical social worker to help caregivers with emotional and financial needs whenever possible.

17 End-of-life care

The experience of dying is unique for each patient and family. Nurses must discover what each dying patient and his family need. What are they afraid of? What do they need to know? What will help them? It's important to help both the patient and his family prepare for the dying process.

The dying process

- The dying process is total body system failure.
- Although each patient's death progresses differently, the dying process usually occurs over 10 to 14 days, but can take as little as 24 hours.
- The following is a summary of the effect of the dying process on each body system.

Cardiovascular system

- Decreasing need for food and drink
- Dehydration
- Initial increase in heart rate, followed by a decrease as hypoxia develops
- Decrease in blood pressure and the volume of Korotkoff sounds

Integumentary system

- Perspiration
- Cold, clammy skin
- Pale, ashen, or mottled skin
- Darkened skin at the sacrum and lower back
- Blanching of the skin when touched

Respiratory system

- Diminished or adventitious breath sounds
- Moist-sounding respirations
- Dyspnea or air hunger
- Tachypnea
- Irregular breathing, or Cheyne-Stokes respirations

Musculoskeletal system

- Muscle weakness
- Drooping of the mouth
- Difficulty swallowing
- Relaxation of the tissues of the soft palate
- Decline in the gag reflex and reflexive clearing of the oropharynx

Renal system

- Decreased urine output
- Urinary incontinence

Other signs and symptoms

- Moaning and grunting with breathing
- Agitation and restlessness
- Decreased communication ("transitional withdrawal" as a result of the body failing)
- Decreased hearing and vision
- Confusion
- Difficulty rousing the patient
- Visions of people and things not visible to others

Five signs of impending death

- Clouding of consciousness
- Rattling sound from secretions deep in the throat, heard with respiration
- Mandibular movement on respiration
- Cyanosis of the extremities
- No pulse in the radial artery

Meeting patient and family needs

Meeting patient needs

Stages of grief

◆ Grief is a process that lets a person gradually accept a difficult life change that he can't control — such as death.
◆ Experts say that grief usually has five phases: denial, anger, bargaining, depression, and acceptance.
– Most people don't move in order from one of these phases to the next.
– Some people may go back and forth between phases a few times, and some don't even experience all of the phases. (See *Responding to grief*.)

Denial

◆ At first, a patient who learns that he's dying may not believe it.
◆ Some people never do accept the fact and they die without moving to later stages of the grief process.

Anger

◆ Once the person begins to realize that he's going to die, he may get angry, resentful, impatient, irritable, and difficult.

Bargaining

◆ In this phase, the patient is looking for a way out. He may pray for miracles or promise to be a better person if he lives.

Depression

◆ As the person begins to face the reality of his death, he may withdraw and become quiet and sad.
◆ He may talk about what he'll miss about his life.

Acceptance

◆ In this stage, the patient has accepted that he'll die soon.
◆ He talks about being emotionally ready.
◆ He shares his feelings with his family and he may be able to talk about the illness itself.
◆ Many patients never get to this stage.

Responding to grief

If your patient or a family member is grieving, your response can help him work through whatever phase he's experiencing.

◆ Be mentally available when the patient wants to talk.
◆ Listen as the patient talks.
◆ Don't interrupt the patient or try to "correct" any feelings expressed.
◆ Don't offer false hope by saying things such as, "Everything will be okay."
◆ If the patient is angry, don't get angry back.
◆ Support the patient with words and gestures. Touch or hugging is useful if the patient is comfortable with it.
◆ Talk to your nursing supervisor and the physician if the person expresses suicidal thoughts or plans.

Meeting family needs

◆ Meeting family needs is as important as meeting the needs of the dying patient.
◆ In many cases they may not be prepared for the loss of their loved one, particularly in sudden accidents or the death of a young person. In other cases, as with long illnesses, the family may be more prepared.
◆ Regardless, ask the family members what their specific needs are. Do this

early and make sure to include all family members.
- Does the family have questions about the benefits and disadvantages of artificial nutrition and hydration?
- Do they have concerns about pain relief for the patient?
- Do they want to be present at the time of death?
- How involved do they want to be with the patient's physical care?
- What do they need to know?

Teaching

◆ Discuss the signs of imminent death with the family before they occur.
◆ Encourage family members to stay with the patient if they wish.
◆ Teach the family simple techniques to help keep the patient comfortable, such as helping to turn the patient, using pillows for positioning, giving mouth care, and performing gentle massage. Offer this teaching only if the family is comfortable with it.
◆ When the patient's words and statements are unclear, work with family members to determine what the patient is trying to communicate.
◆ Explain to the family that some dying patients appear to see and hear someone or something that isn't visible or audible to others in the room. Often, dying patients see visions of someone who has died or of comforting figures.

Care after death

◆ Ask if the family needs the support of a clergy member.
◆ Express sympathy for the family.
◆ Bathe and handle the body according to the family's wishes. Some cultures have rules and rituals for treatment of the body.
◆ Always treat the body with respect.
◆ Ask if the family needs assistance in contacting the funeral director.
◆ Don't remove the body until the RN or physician has initiated a death certificate and the family is ready.
◆ Make sure that the patient's personal possessions and valuables are given to the family.

18 Alternative and complementary therapies

Aromatherapy

◆ Aromatherapy is the inhalation or application of essential oils distilled from various plants.
◆ Those who use aromatherapy say that it's effective in reducing stress, preventing disease, and even treating certain illnesses — both physical and psychological.
◆ Aromatherapy is popular in Europe, where dilutions of essential oils are inhaled, massaged into the skin, or placed in bath water to create pleasant sensations, promote relaxation, or treat specific ailments.
◆ Aromatherapy can be used — either alone or with such therapies as massage or herbal therapy — to treat bacterial and viral infections, anxiety, pain, muscle disorders, arthritis, herpes simplex, herpes zoster, skin disorders, premenstrual syndrome, headaches, and indigestion.
◆ When absorbed by body tissues, these oils are believed to interact with hormones and enzymes to produce changes in blood pressure, pulse rate, and other physiologic functions. (See *Therapeutic uses of essential oils*.)
◆ Aromatherapy may be administered by a trained aromatherapist or may be self-administered.
- In the United States, where interest has skyrocketed, many people self-administer.
- Administration training and certification programs are available for practitioners.
- These organizations can provide information to interested lay people and health care providers, referrals to aromatherapists, and sources for obtaining essential oils.

◆ Nurses who are trained in aromatherapy may recommend specific oils as adjuncts to conventional therapies, teach patients how to use them, and administer treatment themselves.

Implementation

◆ In addition to the appropriate essential oil, aromatherapy may require other supplies, depending on how the oil is being administered (for example, massage, inhalation, bath, or diffusion).
◆ Massage requires a carrier oil and full-body massage requires a massage table. Massage involves diluting the essential oil in the appropriate carrier oil and applying it to the exposed body part or the entire body using massage techniques.
◆ Inhalation requires a bowl of hot water and a large towel. The patient leans over a bowl of steaming water that contains a few drops of the essential oil. With the towel draped over his head and the bowl to concentrate the steam, the patient inhales the vapors for a few minutes.
◆ A bath requires a tub filled with warm water. The patient adds a few drops of essential oil to the surface of the bath water and then soaks in the tub for 10 to 20 minutes, inhaling the vapors as he soaks.
◆ Diffusion requires a micromist or candle diffuser or a ceramic ring that can be placed on a light bulb. This method involves placing a few drops of the essential oil in the diffuser and turning on the heat source to diffuse microparticles of the oil into the air. The average treatment is 30 minutes.

Special considerations

◆ Citrus oils shouldn't be applied before exposure to the sun.
◆ Cinnamon and clove oil shouldn't be applied to the skin.
◆ Certain oils — such as basil, fennel, lemongrass, rosemary, and verbena —

Therapeutic uses of essential oils

This table shows some popular essential oils and the traditional indications for which practitioners use them.

ESSENTIAL OIL	TRADITIONAL THERAPEUTIC USES
chamomile *(Anthemis nobilis)*	◆ Anti-inflammatory, antifungal, and antibacterial effects ◆ Relieving mental or physical stress ◆ Balancing body and mind
eucalyptus *(Eucalyptus radiata)*	◆ Antiviral and expectorant effects ◆ Coughs, colds, and asthma ◆ Clearing the sinuses ◆ Boosting the immune system ◆ Relieving muscle tension
geranium *(Pelargonium x asperum)*	◆ Antiviral and antifungal effects ◆ Stimulating metabolism in the skin ◆ Improving cell regeneration ◆ Balancing hormones in women ◆ Relieving pain ◆ Both relaxing and uplifting
lavender *(Lavandula angustifolia)*	◆ Anti-inflammatory and antibacterial effects ◆ Treating burns, insect bites, and minor injuries ◆ Soothing stomachache and colic ◆ Relieving toothache and teething pain ◆ Relieving mental or physical stress
peppermint *(Mentha piperita)*	◆ Antibacterial and antiviral effects ◆ Treating headaches and muscle aches ◆ Relieving nausea and motion sickness ◆ Soothing irritable bowel
rosemary *(Rosmarinus officinalis)*	◆ Antibacterial, antifungal, and antiviral effects ◆ Restoring energy and alleviating stress ◆ Improving cell regeneration ◆ Treating wounds and infection
tea tree *(Melaleuca alternifolia)*	◆ Anti-inflammatory, antibacterial, and antiviral effects ◆ Treating burns, insect bites, and minor injuries ◆ Providing calmness and sedation

may cause irritation if the patient has sensitive skin. If irritation develops, advise the patient to stop using these oils.

◆ High doses of certain oils — such as aniseed, camphor, cedar wood, cinnamon, clove, fennel, lemon, sage, thyme, and wintergreen — can cause nonlethal poisoning.

◆ Different administration methods require specific safety precautions.

– When using inhalation therapy, the patient should keep his face far enough from the surface of the water to avoid a burn injury.
– When using the diffusion method, he should be at least 3′ (0.9 m) away from the diffuser.
◆ Aromatherapy is contraindicated during pregnancy because it poses a toxic risk to the mother and fetus.
◆ It should be used with caution in infants and children younger than age 5 because many essential oils are toxic to patients in this age-group.
◆ Caution patients to keep essential oils away from the eyes and mucous membranes to avoid irritation. If contact occurs, the patient should flush the area with plenty of water; if flushing doesn't relieve the pain, he should seek medical attention.

Art therapy

◆ Art therapy is the creative use of various expressive media to help a patient process subconscious thoughts, emotions, life changes, personal issues, and conflicts.
◆ The concept behind art therapy is that by externalizing feelings through art, the patient can discover meaning and insight, which supports growth, change, healing, and integration of the whole person.
◆ Creative activities include drawing, painting, sculpting, collaging, and puppetry. Mask making is another powerful and popular form of expression that is often used in groups and in individual healing rituals. Photography, videography, and computer-generated art are newer forms of art therapy.
◆ Art therapy is useful in patients with posttraumatic stress disorder, substance abuse, addictions, catastrophic illness (for example, cancer or acquired immunodeficiency syndrome), chronic pain or disease, prolonged hospitalization or treatment, or extensive surgery. This therapy may help patients who have lost their voices (through surgery, tracheostomy, or intubation) and may benefit those who have an age-related decrease in function, chronic fatigue syndrome, or immune dysfunction syndrome.

Implementation

◆ Explain the creative procedure to the patient and make sure that he's willing to participate.
◆ Make sure that the patient is physically capable of carrying out the artistic activity. Medications, weakness, inflamed or painful joints in the hands or fingers, or neurologic damage can impair the patient's ability.
◆ Assess the patient's need for special equipment or other accommodations.
◆ Collect and prepare the necessary materials.
◆ Provide a quiet, comfortable environment, and arrange a clean, flat work surface.
◆ Reassure the patient that he doesn't need any previous knowledge or training in art. For example, if the patient is drawing, he can use stick figures.
◆ Give the patient adequate time to complete the project to his satisfaction. Sometimes it's important for the patient to attend to every small detail and search for just the right color.
◆ When the project is complete, allow the patient to show it to you and tell you about it.
◆ Support the patient's efforts and summarize the experience for him.
◆ If a patient is especially proud of his artwork, arrange to have it displayed, if possible, so that others may admire it.
◆ Someone who is physically unable to manipulate the materials may still participate in collaging. For example,

the patient can choose pictures, words, or materials for someone else to cut and paste or can indicate the position of cutouts and colors. Computer programs may be available to allow patients to create art with adapted controls.

Special considerations

◆ Some patients may not wish to participate in art therapy, either because they're shy and self-conscious or because they aren't interested. Don't insist; instead, work on building a trusting therapeutic relationship. The patient may be willing to participate in the future.
◆ Praise all efforts and be careful not to make suggestions about colors or forms. Remain nonjudgmental and supportive.
◆ If the patient has signs and symptoms of a disease, encourage him to draw a picture representing himself in relation to the disease. You may suggest that the patient draw himself before the disease, with the disease, and after treatment.
◆ Listen attentively. There may be a healing story involved, or the patient may reach new insights. You may want to point out certain details of his artwork.
◆ Restate what the patient has said to validate his message.
◆ Notice how the patient represents his size in relation to other figures or objects. Is the entire body drawn? What are the dominant colors and shapes? Does the face show a smile or frown? What is the overall mood?
◆ Strong emotions may surface as a patient explores and connects with underlying emotions. If the patient shows signs of agitation or uncontrolled emotion, end the session and reassure him that it's normal to have strong feelings and it's appropriate to express them.

Refer the patient to other health care professionals, as appropriate.

Biofeedback

◆ Biofeedback is any modality that measures and immediately reports information about the patient's physiologic processes. It lets the patient learn to influence the measured body function consciously, such as heart rate or blood pressure.
◆ The goal of biofeedback is to help the patient improve his overall health by consciously regulating bodily functions that are usually controlled unconsciously.
◆ With this procedure, electrodes are attached to specific areas of the body to monitor such functions as skeletal muscle activity, heart or brain wave activity, body temperature, or blood pressure.
◆ The electrodes feed information into a small monitoring box that reports the results with a sound or light that varies in pitch or brightness as the body function increases or decreases ("feedback").
◆ A biofeedback therapist leads the patient in mental exercises to help him regulate body functions, such as temperature, blood pressure, bladder control, or muscle tension, to achieve the desired result.
◆ The patient eventually learns to control the inner mechanisms of the body through mental processes.
◆ The most common forms of biofeedback involve measuring muscle tension, skin temperature, electrical conductance or resistance in the skin, brain waves, and respiration.
◆ As advances in technology have made measurement devices more sophisticated, the applications of biofeedback have expanded. Sensors can now measure the activity of the internal and

external rectal sphincters, the activity of the detrusor muscle of the bladder, esophageal motility, and stomach acidity.

◆ Some biofeedback treatments are accepted in traditional medicine. The American Medical Association, for instance, has endorsed electromyogram biofeedback training for the treatment of muscle-contraction headaches.

◆ Biofeedback has a vast range of preventive and restorative applications.
- It's most successful when psychological factors play a role in the patient's health problems, such as sleep disorders and stress-related disorders.
- Patients with disorders that arise from poor muscle control, such as incontinence, postural problems, back pain, and temporomandibular joint syndrome, also benefit.
- Biofeedback training benefits patients who have lost control of function as a result of brain or nerve damage or chronic pain disorders.
- Improvement is seen in patients with heart dysfunctions, GI disorders, swallowing difficulties, esophageal dysfunction, tinnitus, eyelid twitching, fatigue, and cerebral palsy.

◆ Biofeedback isn't recommended for severe structural problems, such as broken bones or slipped disks.

Implementation

◆ Provide a private environment that's free from noise or other distractions.

◆ Gather the necessary equipment and wash your hands.

◆ Explain the procedure to the patient and answer his questions. If relaxation techniques or imagery will be used at the same time, review them with the patient.

◆ Depending on the body function that will be monitored, clean and prepare the skin and attach the electrodes according to the manufacturer's instructions.

◆ Place the monitor where both you and the patient can see the results easily.

◆ Set a goal for the session with the patient and review the information he'll be seeing on the monitor.

◆ Turn on the monitor, and establish a baseline for the targeted body function.

◆ If goggles will be used, help the patient place them comfortably over his eyes.

◆ When the patient is ready, begin the session by starting the relaxation tapes or imagery sequence.

◆ At the end of the session, disconnect the monitor and remove the electrodes.

◆ Clean the patient's skin, as needed.

Special considerations

◆ You'll probably work with a trained biofeedback practitioner when conducting the session.

◆ Reassure the patient that biofeedback isn't a test that he has to pass, but a learning experience.

◆ The patient may have local skin irritation from the electrodes used in biofeedback monitoring. Wash the skin well with soap and water to remove leftover irritants and pat it dry.

Dance therapy

◆ Also known as dance movement therapy, dance therapy capitalizes on the direct relationship between body movement and the mind.
- Specific aspects of dance therapy, such as music, rhythm, and synchronous movement, alter mood states, recall memories and feelings, and reduce isolation.

- Additionally, dance therapy organizes thoughts and actions and helps the patient to establish relationships.
- Used in a group setting, dance therapy is believed to create the emotional intensity needed for behavioral change.

◆ Dance therapy is used for various purposes.

- It's used to help emotionally disturbed patients express their feelings, gain insight, and develop relationships.
- With physically disabled people, dance therapy increases movement and self-esteem while providing an enjoyable, creative outlet.
- In groups of older people, dance therapy is used to help participants maintain physical function, enhance self-worth, develop relationships, and express fear and grief.

◆ A wide variety of disorders and disabilities can be treated with dance therapy.

- Typically, the target patient has social, emotional, cognitive, or physical problems.
- Dance therapy is even being used to prevent disease and promote health among healthy people.
- Additionally, caregivers and patients with cancer, acquired immunodeficiency syndrome, and Alzheimer's disease use it to reduce stress.

◆ Dance therapy promotes flexibility, strengthens muscles, improves cardiovascular function, and improves pulmonary function. It also provides touch, socialization, and a sense of connectedness.

◆ Group dance, probably the most common form of dance therapy, allows people of different physical abilities to participate. By simply tapping their toes or patting their thighs in time to the music, patients can participate. Dance routines range from simple clapping and swaying movements to intricate aerobic sessions.

◆ The music should be appropriate for the group in both its pace and its aesthetic appeal. Fast rock music is probably less enjoyable for a group of agile senior citizens than a fast polka might be.

◆ Use faster music to stimulate group members and slower music to calm them.

Implementation

◆ Arrange the space so that participants can move freely.

◆ Arrange chairs around the periphery for those who can't stand or who become tired during the session.

◆ Assess the group for risk factors. The presence of one or more risk factors doesn't preclude group members from participating, but may influence the type of dance and the length of the session. Risk factors to consider include:

- poor cardiovascular status
- a history of chronic obstructive pulmonary disease
- degenerative musculoskeletal problems.

◆ Explain the purpose of the session and encourage everyone to participate as fully as possible.

◆ When the group is ready, start the music and position yourself so you're facing the group.

◆ If a structured routine is being used, demonstrate the movements and encourage the group to mimic them.

◆ If free expression is the goal, circulate through the group, providing encouragement and motivation to those who are hesitant.

◆ Praise the participants' efforts and encourage them to discuss the feelings they experienced while dancing.

◆ After the session, document the type of activity and the group's response.

Special considerations

- Because dancing is an aerobic activity, watch participants for signs of cardiovascular compromise, such as dizziness, flushing, profuse sweating, and disorientation.
- Rapid motion may result in dizziness.
- If a participant becomes dizzy, help him to a seat, and check his vital signs.

Imagery

- Imagery is a mind-body technique in which patients use the imagination to promote relaxation, relieve symptoms (or cope with them more effectively), and heal disease.
- Imagery can be used for many purposes, such as:
  - to control pain and enhance immune function
  - as adjunct therapy for several diseases
  - in patients with cancer, to help mobilize the immune system, alleviate nausea and vomiting from chemotherapy, relieve pain and stress, and promote weight gain (in concert with traditional cancer treatment)
  - to assist in cardiac rehabilitation programs
  - to assist centers specializing in chronic pain
  - to help patients to tolerate medical procedures.
- According to imagery advocates, people with strong imaginations, those who can literally "worry themselves sick," are excellent candidates for imagery.
- Two popular imagery techniques are palming and guided imagery.
  - In palming, the patient places his palms over his closed eyes and tries to fill his entire field of vision with only the color black. He then tries to picture the black changing to a color that he associates with stress, such as red, and then mentally replaces that color with one he finds soothing, such as pale blue.
  - In guided imagery, the patient is asked to visualize a goal that he wants to achieve and then to picture himself taking action to achieve it.
- As an active means of relaxation, imagery is a central part of almost all stress-reduction techniques. Additionally, it's a useful self-care tool.
- With proper instruction, patients can use imagery to relieve stress, enhance their immune function (for example, to fight a cold virus), and improve their sense of well-being.

Implementation

- Provide a private, quiet environment that's free from distractions. Make sure there's a comfortable place in which the patient can lie down.
- If you're using a taped imagery sequence, make sure the tape player is working and that the room has an electrical outlet.
- Help the patient into a comfortable position and explain the exercise. Answer any questions.
- When the patient is comfortable, instruct him to close his eyes. Dim the lights, if possible.
- Use a low, steady, soothing voice throughout the exercise.
- Instruct the patient to take a few deep breaths and to imagine that, with each breath, he's taking in calmness and peacefulness and releasing tension, discomfort, and worry. Tell him to let his breath find its own rate and rhythm and to continue to breathe in calmness and peacefulness and breathe out tension and worry.
- Help the patient to relax.

– Instruct him to imagine that he's breathing calmness into his feet and legs and releasing tension with each exhalation.
– Continue this sequence, moving from feet to head, having him breathe calmness into each successive body part.
◆ As you complete this portion of the exercise, remind the patient to let his whole body sink into a peaceful, relaxed state.
◆ Tell the patient to imagine himself in a peaceful, beautiful place — perhaps somewhere he has visited or a special place he would like to be.
– Encourage him to notice the details of the place, such as the colors, shapes, and living things found there.
– Tell him to think about the sounds and smells of the place and to pay attention to his feelings of peacefulness and relaxation.
◆ Remain quiet and let the patient spend as long as he wants in this place. Tell him that, when he's ready, he should allow the images to fade and slowly bring himself back to the present world.
◆ If the patient is willing, discuss the experience with him, concentrating on his feelings of relaxation and peace.
◆ Document the length of the session, the imagery path used, and the patient's response.

Special considerations

◆ Imagery is contraindicated in patients with psychosis.
◆ To enhance the effects of imagery, consider adding a smell to trigger the image that the patient is trying to experience.
◆ Occasionally, an imagery session leads a patient to remember an unpleasant time or event. If this occurs, stop the session and encourage the patient to tell you what he was seeing and feeling. If the patient becomes upset, stay with him. When possible, notify the physician.
◆ Patients with breathing problems may have trouble controlling their breathing.

Magnetic field therapy

◆ Magnetic field therapy (also called biomagnetic therapy, magnet therapy, or magnetotherapy) involves the use of magnetic fields to prevent and treat disease and to treat injuries. Its goal is to restore a person's internal bioelectromagnetic balance.
◆ With successful therapy, the patient should learn to maintain this internal balance without the need for continued external intervention.
◆ One theory of magnetic therapy suggests that diseased cells have lost their magnetic equilibrium and that topically applied magnets work on a molecular level to restore this equilibrium in the cells. This restoration of equilibrium benefits the surrounding cells and the entire organism.
◆ Another theory, based on the magnetic nature of red blood cells, supposes that there's a magnetically induced increase in the blood and oxygen supply to diseased tissues. This improved circulation helps to adjust the pH, increase the availability of nutrients, and relieve congestion and pain.
◆ Practitioners of magnetic field therapy range from self-healing lay people to licensed health care professionals, including massage therapists, nurses, physician assistants, acupuncturists, chiropractors, physical therapists, physicians, and dentists.
◆ Practitioners claim that therapeutic magnets benefit a wide range of conditions that range from acute and chronic pain, strains, and swelling to systemic illness. Magnetic field therapy is recog-

nized in sports medicine for its effectiveness in relieving sprains and strains. It's used in conjunction with other therapies, such as nutrition, herbs, and acupuncture.

◆ Practitioners agree that biomagnetic therapy effectively relieves pain, swelling, and discomfort, but they disagree as to whether the therapeutic effects are best obtained using the bionorth (2) pole, the biosouth (1) pole, or both. They disagree about which gauss strengths are most appropriate.

Implementation

◆ Magnets used for magnetic field therapy should be high-quality medical magnets.

◆ True bionorth and biosouth poles can be determined by using a simple compass. The bionorth pole is attracted to the biosouth, or positive, pole; the biosouth pole, to the bionorth, or negative, pole. Gauss meters are available for measuring the external field strength of the magnet.

◆ Handbooks of magnetic field therapy describe the best placement and magnet strength for self-treatment of various illnesses.

◆ The simplest home remedy for pain involves applying a low- to medium-gauss (800-gauss or less) magnet to the area of discomfort and leaving it in place until well after the discomfort disappears.

– The longer the treatment, the quicker the healing and the greater the relief of symptoms.

– If pain decreases with treatment, the magnet is oriented correctly; if it increases, even if the bionorth side of the magnet is facing the patient, the magnet must be turned over.

◆ Magnetic therapy may be of short duration (1 to 2 hours), or the therapy may be used overnight or for 24 hours or longer for maximum effect.

Special considerations

◆ Because of the experimental nature of magnetic field therapy, it isn't recommended for children younger than age 5 or for pregnant women.

◆ Positive (biosouth) magnetic energy should be used only under medical supervision. Some investigators believe that the brain can become overstimulated, producing seizures, hallucinations, insomnia, hyperactivity, and magnetic addiction. It has been claimed that positive magnetic energy may stimulate the growth of tumors and microorganisms.

◆ Magnets may alter the function of magnetic instruments, such as pacemakers, battery-powered wristwatches, hearing aids, and other equipment that may be in use around a patient.

◆ Keep magnets away from magnetic resonance imaging machines and away from patients who have metallic parts in their body. Post signs above the patient's bed to warn other staff and visitors.

◆ Patients with a pacemaker or defibrillator shouldn't use magnetic beds, and no magnets should be placed closer than 6″ (15 cm) from a pacemaker or defibrillator, to avoid interfering with their function.

◆ Inform the patient to avoid using magnets on the abdomen for 60 to 90 minutes after meals to allow peristalsis to take place.

◆ Because magnet polarity is important in treatment, caution the patient to use a magnetometer or compass to check the poles on the magnets that he plans to use.

◆ Because of the complex range of symptoms that many elderly patients experience, encourage these patients to continue to seek conventional treatment and to report any alternative therapies that they're using.

◆ Monitor a patient who is undergoing magnetic field therapy for potential adverse effects. If adverse effects occur, you may need to decrease or discontinue his magnetic therapy.
◆ Inform the patient that with magnetic field therapy, more and stronger magnets aren't necessarily better.
◆ Warn the patient to remove all magnets before undergoing surgery because they may cause life-threatening instrument malfunction.
◆ If the patient is treating himself with magnets, teach him about safe magnet use. Inform him that magnets may alter the function of magnetic instruments (such as pacemakers and hearing aids), that magnets shouldn't be banged or dropped, that they shouldn't be heated to more than 500° F (260° C) because heat can decrease their strength, and that magnets of different sizes shouldn't be kept together because doing so can alter their strength.
◆ Tell the patient to keep magnets away from computer hard drives and magnetic media — such as disks, recording tapes, credit or bank cards, videotapes, and compact disks — to prevent damage or erasure of contents.

Meditation

◆ The ancient art of meditation involves focusing attention on a single sound or image or on the rhythm of the person's own breathing.
◆ By directing attention away from worries about the future or preoccupation with the past, meditation reduces stress, which is a major contributing factor in many health problems.
◆ Stress reduction has a wide range of physiologic and mental health benefits — from decreased oxygen consumption, heart rate, and respiratory rate to improved mood, spiritual calm, and heightened awareness.
◆ Most approaches to meditation involve one of two techniques: concentrative meditation and mindful meditation.
- Concentrative meditation involves focusing on an image, a sound (called a mantra), or the person's own breathing to achieve a state of calm and heightened awareness. Transcendental meditation is a form of concentrative meditation in which the person repeats a mantra over and over while sitting in a comfortable position. When other thoughts enter his mind, he's instructed to notice them and return to the mantra. Concentrating on the mantra prevents distracting thoughts.
- Mindful meditation takes the opposite approach. Instead of focusing on a single sensation or sound, the individual is aware of all sensations, feelings, images, thoughts, sounds, and smells that pass through his mind without actually thinking about them. The goal is a calmer, clearer, nonreactive state of mind.
◆ Meditation has a wide variety of indications.
- It's used to enhance immune function in patients with cancer, acquired immunodeficiency syndrome, and autoimmune disorders.
- It has been successful in treating drug and alcohol addiction as well as posttraumatic stress disorder.
- Anxiety disorders, pain, and stress are commonly treated with meditation.
- Meditation can also be used, along with dietary and lifestyle changes, in patients with hypertension or heart disease.

Implementation

◆ Provide a private, quiet environment that's free from distractions and offers a comfortable place for the patient to sit or recline.

◆ Explain the procedure and answer the patient's questions. Tell him that he can stop the exercise if he becomes uncomfortable.

◆ Help him into a comfortable position. If he's in a sitting position, ask him to keep his back straight and to let his shoulders droop.

◆ Using a low, calm, soothing voice, instruct the patient to close his eyes if doing so feels comfortable.

◆ Tell him to focus on his abdomen, feeling it rise each time he inhales and fall each time he exhales.

◆ Tell him to concentrate on his breathing. Explain that if his mind wanders, he should simply return to concentrating on his breathing, regardless of what the thought was.

◆ Have the patient practice the exercise for 15 minutes every day for a week; then evaluate its benefits with him.

◆ Document the session, the instructions you gave the patient, and his response.

Special considerations

◆ Meditation may elicit negative emotions, disorientation, or unpleasant memories. If this occurs, ask the patient about the unpleasant feeling or memory, and direct him to a safer, more pleasant thought or memory. If this isn't possible, stop the session, notify the physician, and stay with the patient until he's calm and controlled.

◆ Meditation should be used cautiously in patients with schizophrenia or attention deficit hyperactivity disorder.

◆ Remind the patient that meditation isn't a substitute for medical treatment. If he's taking a prescribed drug, such as an antihypertensive, tell him to continue taking it.

◆ Patients with respiratory problems may have trouble with meditation techniques that focus on breathing.

Music therapy

◆ Music therapy uses the universal appeal of rhythmic sound to communicate, explore, and heal. It can take the form of creating music, singing, moving to music, or just listening to music.

◆ Music therapy benefits patients with developmental disabilities, mental health disorders, substance addictions, and chronic pain. Studies show the positive effects of music in reducing pain and procedural anxiety as well as in dental anesthesia.

◆ Patients who listen to classical music before surgery and then again in the recovery room report minimal postoperative disorientation.

◆ Music has been used successfully to communicate with patients with Alzheimer's disease and those with head trauma when other approaches have failed.

- In a study of the effects of music on patients with Alzheimer's disease, those who listened to big band music during the day were more alert and happier and had better long-term recollection than the control group.
- Throughout the illness, music can reorient confused patients.
- In the final stages of the disease, it provides psychological comfort.

Implementation

◆ Provide a comfortable environment.

◆ Choose music that's appropriate for the patients and the objectives of the session. The music should be meaningful to the participants.

◆ For sessions that involve making music, collect instruments that are appropriate for the group.

◆ For sessions that involve singing, choose music that's familiar to the group members. Provide words for the songs, either in writing or by repeating them to the group.
◆ Introduce the participants to one another. Explain the purpose of the session and encourage everyone to participate as he feels able.
◆ When the group is ready, start the music and position yourself so that you're facing the group.
◆ If the group will be listening to music, watch the reactions of the participants. If they're making music, circulate among the group members and offer individual support.
◆ Encourage the participants to discuss the feelings they experienced while listening to or making music. Praise their efforts.
◆ After the session, document the type of activity and the group's response.

Special considerations

◆ Music is especially effective as a means of reminiscence therapy for older people. For many of them, the music that they enjoyed in their youth hasn't been part of their lives for decades.

Pet therapy

◆ A pet can help a patient combat loneliness and can help to bridge the gap between the patient and the health care provider.
◆ Commonly used in long-term care facilities, pet therapy helps an older patient who's apathetic and depressed and often improves his interaction with others.
◆ Some facilities adopt a pet as a mascot; the residents share responsibility for its care, thus helping to build a sense of community.

Implementation

◆ Select a pet that's well behaved and has a good temperament. Pets that have completed obedience training are ideal.
◆ Make sure that the pet has been examined by a veterinarian and is current on immunizations.
◆ Let the patient play with and hold the pet. Encourage him to talk to the animal and, if appropriate, reminisce about pets he once had.
◆ Provide as much time as the patient needs, if possible.

Special considerations

◆ Make sure that the environment is appropriate for pet therapy.
– The facility should have an area where the pet can retreat when necessary.
– The animal must be kept away from patients who are allergic to animals, have no interest in pets, or are afraid of them.
◆ If the pet is chosen as a mascot for the facility, have a responsible person make a schedule for residents who are interested in participating in the animal's care. Assign someone to make sure that care is provided as scheduled.
◆ If the pet isn't a permanent resident of the facility, arrange for a volunteer from an animal shelter to accompany the pet to ensure the safety of the animal and the patients.

Prayer and mental healing

◆ Throughout the ages, humans have used prayer and mental healing to seek assistance from a higher being for a wide range of problems.
◆ The underlying beliefs of those who use prayer for healing are the same for all religions. They include:

- the belief that a higher power exists
- the belief that humans can communicate with this higher being through prayer
- the belief that this deity can hear human prayers and intervene in human affairs, including healing the sick.

◆ In prayer, the person communicates directly with the divine being, asking the being to intervene to heal the patient. In mental healing, the power of the divine being is channeled through a healer.

◆ There are two main types of mental healing.
- In type 1 healing, the healer enters into a spiritual level of consciousness in which he views himself and the patient as a single being. No physical contact with the patient is necessary.
- Type 2 mental healing requires the healer to touch the patient in an attempt to transfer energy from the healer's hands to the diseased parts of the patient's body.

◆ Most people who use prayer for healing view it as an adjunct to conventional medical treatment.

◆ Although the therapeutic uses of prayer and mental healing are limitless, the reliability of these practices still needs to be established.

◆ Proponents of prayer argue that even if prayer can't cure disease, it can at least relieve some of its effects, enhance the effectiveness of conventional medical treatments, and provide meaning and comfort to the patient.

Implementation

◆ Provide the patient with privacy in a quiet, distraction-free environment.

◆ Facilitate the use of prayer and mental healing by asking the patient such questions as "Is religion or spirituality important to you?" and "Does religion or spirituality help you to cope with your illness?"

◆ If religion or spirituality is important to the patient, explore his usual practices with him to identify ways to incorporate them into his current situation.

◆ Determine whether the patient would like to discuss his faith with the facility chaplain, another clergy member, or some other spiritual guide and assist in making arrangements.

Special considerations

◆ Patients who have attempted prayer and haven't seen the results they expected may express disappointment when spirituality is discussed. If this occurs and if it's possible, arrange for a trusted spiritual adviser to explore the patient's feelings with him.

◆ Remain nonjudgmental when implementing the exercise.

◆ Some prayer rituals may not be suitable for a health care facility. Rites involving incense, large groups, or loud music and dance may be beyond the capacity of most facilities.

◆ Although it's important to be sensitive to the patient's religious beliefs, sometimes a compromise is needed. For example, you could suggest that the patient be wheeled to an outside area of the facility if incense is involved or taken to a conference room during off-hours if noise is an issue or if a prayer vigil involves a large number of people.

◆ Ethical questions arise if prayer and mental healing are used without the patient's knowledge. Additionally, some are concerned that prayer and mental healing may be used to harm an individual instead of healing him.

◆ Advise the patient to consider prayer a complementary therapy, not a substitute for conventional medical care. If a patient's religion advocates the use of prayer as the sole form of treatment, make sure that he understands the consequences of forgoing conventional medical treatment so that he can make an informed decision.

Reflexology

◆ Reflexology is a widely practiced form of manual therapy that involves applying pressure to specific parts of the body, usually the soles (sometimes the palms).
◆ It's based on the theory that these parts of the body correspond to — and can therapeutically affect — various organs and glands. For example, the top of the big toe is said to connect to the brain, and the arch area corresponds to the solar plexus.
◆ Some practitioners believe that these points follow the same meridians that are used in acupuncture.
◆ The roots of reflexology can be traced back 3,000 years to folk medicine traditions in China, India, and Egypt. The current revival of interest in this technique began in the early 1900s, when an American ear, nose, and throat specialist, William Fitzgerald, discovered that his patients felt less pain when he applied pressure to specific points on their soles or palms before surgery.
◆ In the 1930s, Eunice Ingham, a physical therapist, expanded on Fitzgerald's work. Ingham believed that applying varying levels of pressure to certain areas could not only decrease pain but also provide other health benefits. She mapped the specific reflex zones on the feet that reflexologists use today. (See *Right foot reflex zones,* page 526.)
◆ Reflexologists, most of whom are massage therapists, physical therapists, or nurses with special training, say that the technique works by reducing the amount of lactic acid in the feet and breaking up calcium crystal deposits that accumulate in the nerve endings and block the flow of energy.
◆ Many health clubs and spas offer reflexology treatments. No specific license or certification is needed to practice reflexology.
◆ Like full-body massage, reflexology relieves stress and muscle tension and produces relaxation. Reflexologists claim that they can treat numerous conditions, including skin disorders (eczema and acne), GI disorders (diarrhea and constipation), hypertension, migraines, anxiety, and asthma.

Implementation

◆ Reflexology requires only a treatment table or chair or a stool to elevate the feet. A quiet environment is preferred.
◆ The patient is either seated comfortably in a reclining chair or placed in a supine position on a treatment table with the feet raised and supported. The therapist is seated facing the patient's soles.
◆ After an initial assessment of the patient's feet to detect alterations in skin thickness and abnormalities in foot structure, the therapist feels for tender areas and signs of tension or thickening on the sole.
◆ A treatment session typically begins with relaxation techniques designed to release tension and make the patient comfortable with the manipulation of his feet.
◆ The therapist uses thumbs and fingers to apply gentle, firm pressure to the reflex zones of the foot, paying more attention to zones that are tender to the touch. Working systematically, the therapist begins with the toes and proceeds in small, creeping movements proximally toward the heel. (For therapy using the hand, the therapist starts with the fingers and moves proximally toward the wrist.)

Right foot reflex zones

This illustration, which shows the organs and body parts associated with specific regions of the right foot, serves as a map that guides reflexologists in performing therapy.

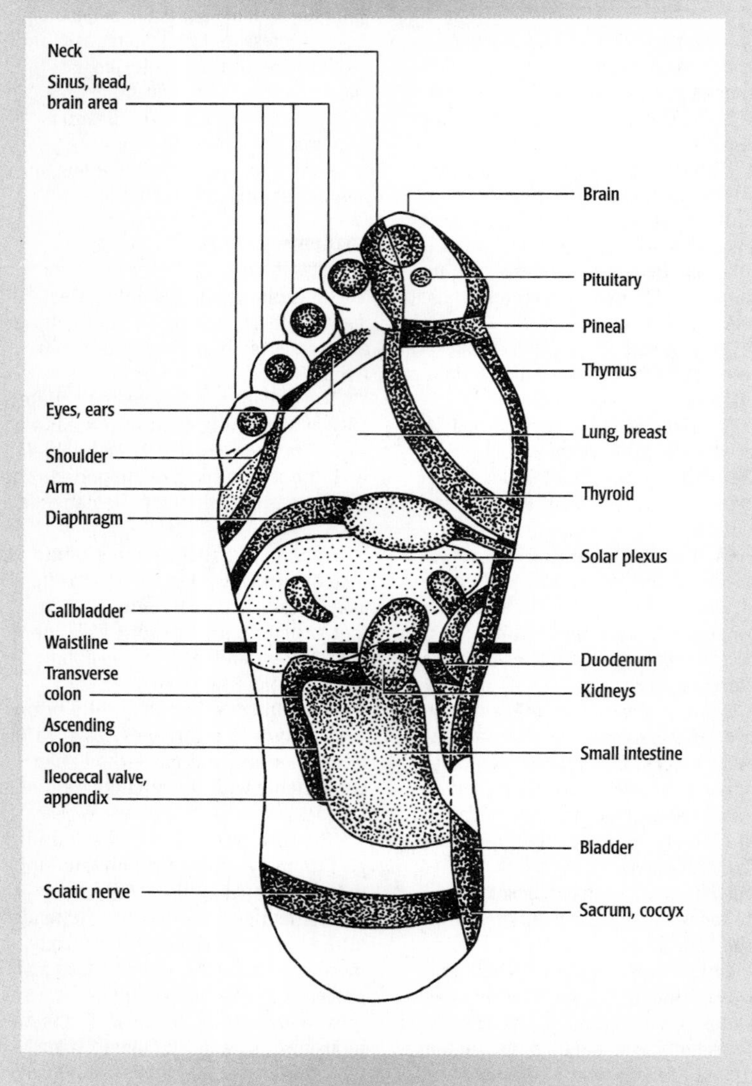

◆ A typical session lasts 20 to 60 minutes.

Special considerations

◆ Advise the patient to postpone reflexology treatments if he has cuts, boils, bruises, or other injuries on his feet.

Alert If the patient has diabetes, peripheral vascular disease, or another vascular problem in his legs, such as thrombosis or phlebitis, instruct him to consult his physician before trying reflexology.

Alert If the patient is pregnant, advise her to obtain her physician's consent before trying reflexology.

◆ Many people who claim to practice reflexology are actually performing a simple foot massage. If your patient wants treatment for a specific symptom, he should make sure that the practitioner has been trained in reflexology.

Reiki

◆ Reiki is a Japanese healing therapy that uses emotional, spiritual, and universal energy.

◆ Although its origins trace back to ancient Buddhist practices, Reiki as a modern healing method was introduced in the late 19th century by Dr. Mikao Usui, a Japanese Buddhist monk.

◆ The word Reiki refers to the universal life energy; it's derived from the Japanese words *rei,* which means spirit, and *ki,* meaning energy life force.

◆ Reiki therapy is the transference of energy through the practitioner to the patient; this healing therapy isn't a passive practice.

– The Reiki practitioner uses specific healing techniques to restore and balance the natural life force energy within the body.

– The Reiki practitioner places his hands on or above the patient and the patient draws energy from the practitioner as needed.

◆ The patient becomes an active agent in his healing by identifying his needs — body, mind, and spirit — and using energy to achieve restoration and balance.

◆ The goal of Reiki therapy is to help restore the body's energy balance and enhance its natural ability to heal itself. It may produce deep relaxation and help relieve pain.

◆ Reiki has been studied as primary pain treatment and as adjuvant therapy with opioids.

◆ In patients who are terminally ill, Reiki therapy has been linked to increased quality of life and relief from pain, anxiety, dyspnea, and edema.

◆ Reiki also benefits patients with autoimmune illness, including multiple sclerosis, lupus, and rheumatoid arthritis.

◆ Reiki is used in patients with pancreatitis, fibromyalgia, heart failure, emphysema, and cancer.

Implementation

◆ Reiki treatments vary from a full-body treatment, which may last about 45 minutes, to treatment of an isolated body area (such as a shoulder or knee), which can last about 10 minutes.

◆ After an initial consultation, the patient (who remains fully clothed) is positioned on a table, mat, or couch.

◆ The Reiki practitioner places his hands on or above the patient. The energy is then channeled through the practitioner to the patient in a series of hand positions over the main energy centers of the body (chakras), starting at the head and moving down the body.

- ◆ During Reiki treatments, patients may feel the flow of energy in various ways.
  - They may report a feeling of warmth from the practitioner's hands.
  - Some patients experience a tingling sensation.
  - Patients sometimes report a feeling of deep meditation.
  - Some patients recall past experiences.
  - Sometimes spontaneous emotional release occurs from areas that were blocked.
  - Some patients don't feel a physical sensation but describe mental or emotional changes, such as a sense of calmness or peace.
  - Nearly everyone experiences the treatment as deeply relaxing.

Special considerations

- ◆ Only trained Reiki practitioners should perform the treatment.
  - Training involves three degrees of learning and attainment of Reiki skills.
  - Training may take several years to complete.
- ◆ Reiki practitioners don't diagnosis illness or prescribe treatment. If the patient wasn't referred for treatment by his primary care practitioner, the Reiki practitioner should advise the patient to follow up with his primary care provider.

Therapeutic massage

- ◆ Massage, the process of stroking, rubbing, and kneading the body, has played an important role in traditional medical systems through the centuries.
- ◆ It's used mainly for stress reduction and relaxation, but it can also serve as a complementary therapy for a wide range of conditions. These include:
  - chronic pain
  - circulatory problems
  - digestive disorders
  - inflammation
  - intestinal disorders
  - joint mobility disorders
  - muscle tension
  - overstimulation or understimulation of the nervous system
  - skin conditions
  - swelling.
- ◆ The main physiologic effect of therapeutic massage is improved blood circulation.
  - As the muscles are kneaded and stretched, blood return to the heart increases, and toxins, such as lactic acid, are carried out of the muscle tissue for excretion.
  - Improved circulation results in increased perfusion and oxygenation of tissues.
  - Improved oxygenation of the brain helps the patient to think more clearly and feel more alive.
  - Improved perfusion and oxygenation of other organ systems leads to improved digestion and elimination as well as faster wound healing.
  - Massage also appears to trigger the release of endorphins, the body's natural pain relievers.
- ◆ Five basic massage techniques are used.

Effleurage

- ◆ This is a long, gliding stroke performed with the entire hand or the thumb as a warm-up technique.
- ◆ The gliding stroke, which always moves toward the heart, improves circulation.

Pétrissage

- ◆ This is a kneading and compressing motion in which the muscles are grabbed and lifted.

◆ This motion relieves sore muscles by clearing away lactic acid and increasing circulation to the muscle tissue.

Friction

◆ Here the therapist uses the thumbs and fingertips to work around the joints and the thickest parts of the muscles.
◆ Circular motions are used to break down adhesions; they may also help make soft tissues and joints more flexible.
◆ For larger muscles, the palm or heel of the hand may be used.

Tapotement

◆ The therapist uses the sides of the hands, fingertips, cupped palms, or slightly closed fists to make chopping, tapping, and beating motions.
◆ These motions invigorate and stimulate the muscles, resulting in a burst of energy.
◆ When muscles are cramped, strained, or spastic, tapotement can worsen the problem if performed for more than about 10 or 15 minutes.

Vibration

◆ The therapist presses the fingers or flattened hands firmly into the muscle and then "vibrates" (transmits a trembling motion) the area rapidly for a few seconds.
◆ This motion is repeated until the entire muscle has been vibrated.
◆ This technique helps to stimulate the nervous system and may increase circulation and improve gland function.

Implementation

◆ Massage therapy requires a sturdy massage table, lubricating oil or lotion, and a quiet room with relaxing music to induce relaxation.
◆ Have the patient undress in private, lie on the table, and cover himself with a sheet or towel.
◆ To respect the patient's modesty, keep the body fully draped, exposing only the area that's being worked on at the moment.
◆ A scented oil or lotion is usually used to prevent friction between the therapist's hands and the patient's skin while he kneads various muscle groups in a systematic way from head to toe.

Special considerations

◆ A trained massage therapist pays close attention to the patient's body language as well as his comments, to avoid causing pain or discomfort.
◆ Massage is contraindicated in patients with diabetes or varicose veins or other blood vessel disorders because it may dislodge a blood clot. Massage shouldn't be performed on patients with pitting edema.
◆ Avoid massaging the abdomen of a patient with hypertension or gastric or duodenal ulcers, and massage at least 6″ (15 cm) away from bruises, cysts, broken bones, and breaks in skin integrity.
◆ Advise a patient who's seeking a massage therapist to obtain recommendations from people who have been satisfied with their treatment. He should also make sure that the therapist is properly trained and licensed and belongs to a professional organization.

Therapeutic Touch

◆ Developed in the 1970s, Therapeutic Touch is a widely used complementary therapy. It was developed by nurses for nurses in an attempt to bring a more humane and holistic approach to their practice.

◆ This technique focuses on "healing" rather than "curing" and is built on the belief that all healing is basically self-healing.
◆ Central to Therapeutic Touch is the concept of a universal life force that practitioners believe permeates space and sustains all living organisms. Practitioners believe that, in healthy people, this vital energy flows freely in and through the body in a balanced way that nourishes all body organs and that when people become ill it's because their energy field is out of equilibrium.
◆ By using their hands to manipulate the energy field above the patient's skin, practitioners say that they can restore equilibrium, thereby reactivating the mind-body-spirit connection and empowering the patient to participate in his own healing.
◆ Intention is an important aspect of therapeutic touch. The practitioner's intent to facilitate healing by restoring the patient's energy field must be present during the treatment.
◆ Despite its name, Therapeutic Touch doesn't require actual physical contact. In most cases the nurse's hands remain several inches above the patient's body.
◆ Therapeutic Touch is widely used by practitioners of holistic nursing and other health professionals. It's practiced in many hospitals, hospices, long-term care facilities, and other settings.
◆ Although most practitioners are nurses, other health care professionals (massage therapists, physical therapists, dentists, and physicians) and nonprofessionals have incorporated this therapy into their practice. According to practitioners, anyone can study this technique and apply it to himself.
◆ Therapeutic Touch can be used as a complementary therapy for virtually all medical and nursing diagnoses as well as surgical procedures.
– Practitioners say that it's especially helpful for patients with wounds or infections because it eases discomfort and speeds the healing process.
– The technique is best known for its ability to relieve pain and anxiety, making it helpful in treating stress-related disorders, such as tension headaches, hypertension, ulcers, and emotional problems.
– It's also used in Lamaze classes and delivery rooms to induce relaxation and in neonatal intensive care units to help speed the growth of premature infants.

Implementation

◆ Select an environment that will allow the patient to relax and the nurse to concentrate. This may include a comfortable chair, bed, or massage table for the patient and, possibly, soothing music to help create a relaxing atmosphere.
◆ The nurse achieves a calm, meditative state that allows her to remain sensitive to the patient's signs and symptoms. This heightened sensitivity is needed to perceive subtle changes in the patient's energy field.
◆ After becoming centered, the nurse begins her assessment by slowly moving her hands over the patient's body, 2″ to 4″ (5 to 10 cm) away from the skin surface, to detect alterations in the energy field, such as feelings of cold or heat, vibration, or blockages.
◆ Depending on the assessment findings, the nurse then performs interventions aimed at balancing the energy field and removing obstructions. Possible interventions include "unruffling" a chaotic and tangled field, eliminating "congestion," and acting as a conduit to direct the "life energy" from the environment into the patient.
◆ Throughout the treatment the patient remains quiet and relaxed. Ac-

cording to practitioners, it isn't necessary for the patient to believe consciously in the power of the procedure.
◆ To effectively channel energy into the patient, the nurse must have "conscious intent"—that is, the intent to become a calm, focused instrument of healing, enabling the patient's body ultimately to heal itself.

Special considerations

◆ Care must be taken to moderate the length and strength of treatment for small children and elderly people because their bodies are more fragile. A common sign of overtreatment in these patients is restlessness during or after the treatment.
◆ Other patients who warrant extra sensitivity and shorter treatment periods include pregnant women, patients with head injuries or psychosis, emaciated patients, and patients who are in shock.
◆ Respect the patient's personal preferences. People have different tolerances for touch and some regard energy work as an invasion of their personal space.

Yoga

◆ Among the oldest known health practices, yoga (meaning "union" in Sanskrit) is the integration of physical, mental, and spiritual energies to promote health and wellness. It can be practiced by young and old alike, either individually or in groups, and can be started at any age.
◆ Based on the idea that a chronically restless or agitated mind causes poor health and decreased mental strength and clarity, yoga outlines specific regimens for lifestyle, hygiene, detoxification, physical activity, and psychological practices. By integrating these practices, yoga aims to increase physical vitality and spiritual awareness.
◆ There are several styles of yoga. The most common in the West is Hatha yoga. It combines physical postures and exercises (called asanas), breathing techniques (called pranayamas), relaxation, diet, and "proper thinking."
◆ Asanas fall into two categories, meditative and therapeutic.
– Meditative asanas promote proper blood flow through the body by bringing the spine and body into perfect alignment. The mind and body are brought into a state of relaxation and stillness, which facilitates concentration during meditation. These asanas keep the heart, glands, and lungs properly energized.
– Therapeutic asanas are commonly prescribed for joint pain. The "cobra," "locust spinal twist," and "shoulder stand" positions are examples.
◆ The goal of a properly executed asana is to create a balance between movement and stillness, which is the state of a healthy body. Very little movement is needed. Instead, the mind provides discipline, awareness, and a relaxed openness to maintain the posture and execute the asana properly.
◆ Using these asanas, the individual learns to regulate such autonomic functions as heartbeat and respirations while relaxing physical tensions.
◆ Pranayamas focus on disciplined breathing. Pranayama exercises regulate the flow of prana (breath and electromagnetic force), keeping the person healthy.
◆ Pranayama aids digestion, regulates cardiac function, and alleviates various physical ailments. It can be especially effective in reducing the frequency of asthma attacks.
◆ The goal of breathing in yoga is to make the process as smooth and regular as possible. The assumption is that

A simple pranayama exercise

This pranayama exercise is called purification of the channels (*nadi shodhana* [channel cleansing], or *sweet breath*), which involves alternate nostril breathing. You can easily teach it to a patient.

◆ Have the patient sit upright on a cushion or in a firm chair, with his head, neck, and body aligned.
◆ Tell him to breathe from his diaphragm, in a relaxed fashion, taking care to keep his inhalations and exhalations slow, steady, and full.
◆ Instruct him to begin by using his right thumb to close his right nostril and inhale through his left nostril.
◆ Then close his left nostril with his ring finger and exhale through his right nostril.
◆ Next, while still holding his left nostril closed, inhale through his right nostril, and then close his right nostril with his thumb and exhale through his left nostril.
◆ This completes one cycle of *nadi shodhana.* Instruct the patient to complete 3 cycles of the exercise.
◆ As the patient practices this technique, instruct him to try to lengthen his inhalations and exhalations, always keeping them even.
◆ Encourage him to practice *nadi shodhana* twice each day, in the morning and evening.

the rhythm of the mind is mirrored in the rhythm of breathing. By keeping respirations steady and rhythmic, the mind will remain calm and focused.
◆ Samadhi, or spiritual realization, is an additional component of Eastern yoga. Yoga practitioners compare Samadhi to a fourth state of consciousness, separate from the normal states of waking, dream, and sleep.
◆ The technique called HongSau uses meditation to develop the powers of concentration. Thought and energy are withdrawn from outer distractions and focused on a goal or problem chosen by the individual.
◆ The Aum technique expands the person's awareness beyond the limitations of the body and mind, allowing him to experience what is called "Divine Consciousness," which is believed to underlie and uphold all life. "Aum" is the sound that occurs with every inhaled breath. The sounds of inhalation are "a" through the mouth and "um" through the nose. Taken together, these sounds form the sound "aum." To achieve Divine Consciousness, the user alters his breathing and focuses on sounding out the "a" and "um" sounds.
◆ Among the measured benefits of yoga are improvement in health, vitality, and peace of mind.
– Yoga is successfully used to alleviate stress and anxiety, lower blood pressure, relieve pain, improve motor skills, treat addictions, increase auditory and visual perception, and improve metabolic and respiratory function.
– Yoga is effective in treating lung ailments because it can increase lung capacity and lower the respiratory rate.
– Yoga has been credited with decreasing serum cholesterol levels and increasing histamine levels in the treatment of allergies.
– Its ability to help regulate blood flow is being studied in cancer therapy. Scientists are investigating whether restricted blood flow to the region will slow tumor growth.

Implementation

◆ Provide a private, quiet environment that's free from distractions.

- Allow adequate room for participants to move without touching or distracting other members.
- Each participant will need a small blanket or large towel to use in some of the postures.
- Explain the purpose of the session and describe the planned exercises and their benefits. (See *A simple pranayama exercise.*)
- Answer the participants' questions and remind participants that they don't have to engage in any posture that may be uncomfortable.
- When the group is ready, talk the participants through the positions or breathing techniques, demonstrating each one.
- After the participants have assumed the position, begin the breathing pattern, and circulate among the participants to assess and adjust their technique, as needed.
- Praise all of their efforts.
- After you've led the group through all of the planned exercises, end the session by having everyone take slow, deep breaths.
- Document the session, the techniques used, and the participants' responses.

Special considerations

- Some of the more physical aspects of yoga positions can cause muscle injury if they aren't performed properly. Injury may occur if an older adult attempts to force his body into position.
- Caution patients to attempt the various techniques and postures cautiously and remind them that very few people can perform all of the postures in the beginning.
- There are yoga techniques to meet the needs of all people, regardless of their physical condition. Individuals who can't perform some of the more physically demanding postures can still benefit from the breathing or meditation techniques.

19 Documentation

Legal and ethical implications of documentation

◆ Accurately and completely documenting the nature and quality of your nursing care helps the other members of the health care team confirm their impressions of the patient's condition and progress — or may signal the need for adjustments in the therapeutic regimen.

◆ The clinical account of a patient's condition, treatment, and responses is also used as evidence in the courtroom — for example, in malpractice suits, workers' compensation litigation, personal injury cases and, possibly, criminal cases.

- If you think of the medical record first and foremost as a clinical communication that you documented carefully, you need not panic if the court subpoenas it.
- However, if you think only of legal implications or document to protect yourself, your part of the medical record will sound self-serving and defensive.
- Such documentation tends to have a negative impact on a judge and jury.

Standards of documentation

◆ The type of nursing information that appears in a medical record isn't dictated by standards set by the courts. It's governed by standards developed over the years by the nursing profession and by state laws.

◆ Documentation that meets these standards communicates the patient's status, medical treatment, and nursing care.

◆ Professional organizations such as the American Nurses Association (ANA) and regulatory agencies, such as the Joint Commission on Accreditation of Healthcare Organizations (JCAHO) and the Centers for Medicare and Medicaid Services (CMS), have established that documentation must include ongoing data collection, interventions made, patient teaching, responses to therapy, and relevant statements made by the patient.

◆ Although documentation goals have changed little since their inception, documentation methods have changed dramatically.

- For example, nurses no longer need to spend valuable time writing long narrative notes. Instead, many facilities today use such methods as flow sheets, graphic records, checklists, and charting by exception (in which only exceptions from articulated standards of care are charted).
- While flow sheets save valuable nursing time, they've been criticized as being too abbreviated and lacking important narrative information about the patient's condition. If used prudently, however, flow sheets can trigger or remind a nurse what actions are indicated.

Errors and omissions

◆ Errors and omissions can severely undermine your credibility in court.

- A jury could reasonably conclude that you didn't perform a function if it wasn't charted.
- If you failed to chart something and need to enter a late entry, date it the day you entered it.

◆ In the case of *Anonymous v. Anonymous*, Suffolk Superior Court, Boston (1993), failure to chart led to a $1 million settlement.

- A 2-year-old was admitted to Children's Hospital for correction of a congenital urinary defect.
- Postoperative orders required blood pressure, pulse, and temperature readings to be taken every 4 hours, and

respiratory rate and reaction to analgesia every hour.
- The child's care wasn't charted for 5 hours.
- The child was found in cardiorespiratory arrest and died from an overdose of an opioid infusion.
- The responsible nurse admitted failing to assess the child strictly according to the orders; she also claimed that she had assessed the child adequately but had been "too busy" to chart her observations.

◆ Failure to comply with a facility's policy can constitute an omission.
- In *Wallace v. Sacred Heart Hospital,* Escambia County, Florida (1997), a nurse failed to apply Posey restraints to a patient who had a history of stroke and seizure disorder and was at high risk for falls.
- Early one morning, the patient was discovered trying to walk to the bathroom.
- A nurse found her and assisted her back to bed but neglected to apply physician-ordered restraints.
- One hour later, the patient was found on the floor with a fractured left hip.
- The nurses involved failed to follow the facility's policy for patients at high risk for falls and the physician's order for restraints.
- A confidential settlement was reached during mediation.

Timely communication

◆ The purpose of charting is communication, with an emphasis on timeliness.

◆ When the patient's condition deteriorates or changes in therapy are clearly indicated, you must not only chart this information but also contact the physician as soon as possible and chart the fact that you contacted the physician, the time the contact was made, and the physician's response.

◆ If the physician isn't responding appropriately in your opinion, you must contact the next individual in the chain of command. Failure to do so is a breach of duty to the patient and leaves you vulnerable to a malpractice lawsuit.

◆ There are numerous legal cases involving failure of a nurse to notify a physician of changes in the patient's condition. When such notification isn't documented, it's nearly impossible to prove that the physician was called in a timely manner and that all critical information was communicated. These cases are often extremely serious, resulting in death or permanent disability.

◆ In a California case, *Malovec v. Santa Monica Hospital,* Los Angeles County, California Superior Court, Case No. SC 019-167 (1994), a woman in labor repeatedly asked the charge nurse to call the chief of obstetrics because her obstetrician refused to perform a cesarean delivery despite guarded fetal heart tracings. The charge nurse refused, and the baby was born with cerebral palsy and spastic quadriplegia. A confidential settlement was reached.

Corrections and alterations

◆ Any needed corrections to the medical record should be made *only* by drawing a line through the initial charting, signing it, and dating it. Then you can proceed to supply the proper entry.

Alert Never erase, obliterate, or otherwise alter a record.

◆ Completely defensible malpractice cases have been lost because of chart alterations. The jury simply concluded the nurse was covering up something.

◆ Never try to make the record "better" after you learn a malpractice case has been filed. Attorneys have methods

Tips for writing an incident report

When a malpractice lawsuit reached the courtroom in years past, the plaintiff's attorney wasn't allowed to see incident reports. Today, however, the plaintiff in many states is legally entitled to a record of the incident if he requests it through proper channels.

When writing an incident report, keep in mind the people who may read it, and follow these guidelines.

Write objectively
Record the details of the incident in objective terms, describing exactly what you saw and heard. For example, unless you actually saw a patient fall, write: "Found patient lying on the floor." Then describe only the actions you took to provide care at the scene, such as helping the patient get back into bed or checking him for injuries.

Include only essential information
Document the time and place of the incident and the name of the physician who was notified.

Avoid opinions
Don't write your opinions into an incident report. Rather, verbally share your suggestions or opinions on how an incident may be avoided with your supervisor and risk manager.

Assign no blame
Don't admit to liability, and don't blame or point your finger at colleagues or administrators. Steer clear of such statements as "Better staffing would have prevented this incident." State only what happened.

Avoid hearsay and assumptions
Each staff member who knows about the incident should write a separate incident report. If one of your patients is injured in another department, the staff members in that department are responsible for documenting the details of the incident.

File the report properly
Don't file the incident report with the medical record. Send the report to the person designated to review it according to your facility's policy.

for analyzing papers and inks and can easily detect discrepancies.

Completing incident reports

◆ An incident report is a formal report, written by physicians, nurses, or other staff members, that informs facility administrators about an adverse event suffered by a patient.
◆ Incident reports are continually being revised, and some may be computerized. (Computer processing permits classifying and counting of incidents to indicate trends.)
◆ If you're filing an incident report and need more room than the form allows, check your facility's policy; additional blank pages may not be protected from disclosure to a patient's attorney. (See *Tips for writing an incident report*.)
◆ State, federal, and military statutes protect performance improvement and peer review documents from disclosure to a patient's attorney on the grounds that health care providers should be allowed to freely and thoroughly investigate claims of adverse events without having to worry about being sued for what they discover; however, incident reports may not be thus protected.
◆ Because the patient's attorney may be able to obtain a copy of an incident

Patient rights under HIPAA

The goal of the Health Insurance Portability and Accountability Act (HIPAA) is to provide safeguards against the inappropriate use and release of personal medical information, including all medical records and identifiable health information in any form (electronic, paper, or oral).

Patients are the beneficiaries of this privacy rule, which includes the following six rights:

- the right to give consent before information is released for treatment, payment, or health care operations
- the right to be educated to the provider's policy on privacy protection
- the right to access their medical records
- the right to request that their medical records be amended for accuracy
- the right to access the history of non-routine disclosures (those disclosures that didn't occur in the course of treatment, payment, or health care operations, or those not specifically authorized by the patient)
- the right to request that the provider restrict the use and routine disclosure of information he has (providers aren't required to grant this request, especially if they think the information is important to the quality of care for the patient, such as disclosing HIV status to another medical provider who is providing treatment).

Enforcement of HIPAA

Enforcement of HIPAA regulation resides with the United States Department of Health and Human Services (HHS) and is based primarily on significant financial fines. HHS can impose civil penalties up to $25,000 a year per plan for unintentional violations. With hundreds of requirements, fines could quickly add up. Criminal penalties can also be imposed for intentional violations, including fines up to $250,000, 10 years of imprisonment, or both.

Impact on nursing practice

Keep in mind that HIPAA regulations aren't intended to prohibit health care providers from talking to one another or to patients. Instead, they exist to help ease the communication process. The regulations require organizations to make

report, the document should be factual and succinct.

- Keep in mind that although names of individuals who know about the incident are important, placing those names on the report may result in their being called to testify or give a deposition regarding the incident.
- Still, the goal of completing the incident report is to be truthful, timely, and objective.
- Historically, nurses have been reluctant to complete incident reports for such events as medication errors because they feared retribution. The problem with this is that failure to complete a report may create the appearance that you're intentionally hiding information.

Documenting an incident in the medical record

- When documenting an incident in the patient's medical record, keep the following in mind:
  - Write a factual account of the incident, including the treatment and follow-up care provided and the patient's response. If you don't document the incident, the plaintiff's lawyer might think you're hiding something. This documentation shows that the patient

"reasonable" accommodations to protect patient privacy and to employ "reasonable" safeguards to prevent inappropriate disclosure. Changes in nursing practice will likely be needed to meet these reasonable accommodations and safeguards.

Employers must provide education to nurses regarding the policies and procedures to be followed at their individual institutions. Nurses should be aware of how infractions will be handled because they, as well as the institution, face penalties for violations. Some safeguards nurses can enact in their everyday practice include:
◆ ensuring that computer passwords are protected
◆ making sure computer screens aren't in public view
◆ keeping patient charts closed when not in use
◆ immediately filing loose patient records
◆ not leaving faxes and computer printouts unattended
◆ properly disposing of unneeded patient information in accordance with the facility's procedure.

was closely monitored after the incident. If the case goes to court, the jury may be asked to determine whether the patient received appropriate care after the incident.
– Include in the progress notes and in the incident report anything the patient or his family says about their role in the incident, for example, "Patient stated, 'The nurse told me to ask for help before I went to the bathroom, but I decided to go on my own.'" This kind of statement helps the defense attorney prove that the patient was guilty of contributory or comparative negligence.

◆ Contributory negligence is conduct that contributed to the patient's injuries.
◆ Comparative negligence involves determining the percentage of each party's fault. For example, the nurse might be found 25% negligent and the patient 75% negligent.

Confidentiality

◆ One of your documentation responsibilities includes protecting the confidentiality of the patient's medical record.
◆ Usually, you can't reveal confidential information without the patient's permission.
◆ The Health Insurance Portability and Accountability Act (HIPAA), signed into law in 1996, has components to protect patient privacy. Most clinical entities had until April 14, 2003, to fully comply with privacy regulations. (See *Patient rights under HIPAA*.)
◆ Besides your legal responsibilities, you also have professional and ethical responsibilities (as specified by the ANA, JCAHO, and other professional bodies in their codes and standards) to protect your patient's privacy. (See *Ethical codes for nurses*, pages 540 and 541.)
◆ Nurses assume a primary role in maintaining confidentiality and in safeguarding the privacy of medical records.
– Breaches in confidentiality can result from unintentional release of information, unauthorized entry into a patient's record, or even a casual conversation that's overheard by others.
– In fact, breaches of patient confidentiality on the part of nursing staff are more likely to occur through inadvertent conversations in cafeterias and

(Text continues on page 542.)

Ethical codes for nurses

Licensed practical and vocational nurses (LPNs and LVNs) have an ethical code, which is set forth in each state by the state's nurses association. The National Federation of Licensed Practical Nurses also has a code of ethics for its members. In addition, the International Council of Nurses, an organization based in Geneva, Switzerland that seeks to improve the standards and status of nursing worldwide, has published a code of ethics. One of the most important ethical codes for registered nurses is the American Nurses Association (ANA) code. Summaries of these codes appear below.

Code for LPNs and LVNs

The code of ethics for LPNs and LVNs seeks to provide a motivation for establishing, maintaining, and elevating professional standards. It includes the following imperatives:

- Know the scope of maximum utilization of the LPN and LVN, as specified by the nurse practice act, and function within this scope.
- Safeguard the confidential information acquired from any source about the patient.
- Provide health care to all patients regardless of race, creed, cultural background, disease, or lifestyle.
- Refuse to give endorsement to the sale and promotion of commercial products or services.
- Uphold the highest standards in personal appearance, language, dress, and demeanor.
- Stay informed about issues affecting the practice of nursing and delivery of health care and, where appropriate, participate in government and policy decisions.
- Accept the responsibility for safe nursing by keeping oneself mentally and physically fit and educationally prepared to practice.
- Accept responsibility for membership in the National Federation of Licensed Practical Nurses and participate in its efforts to maintain the established standards of nursing practice and employment policies that lead to quality patient care.

International Council of Nurses code of ethics

According to the International Council of Nurses, the fundamental responsibility of the nurse is fourfold: to promote health, to prevent illness, to restore health, and to alleviate suffering.

The International Council of Nurses further states that inherent in nursing is respect for life, dignity, and human rights and that nursing is unrestricted by considerations of nationality, race, creed, color, age, sex, politics, or social status. The key points of the code appear below.

Nurses and people

- The nurse's primary responsibility is to those who require nursing care.
- The nurse, in providing care, respects the beliefs, values, and customs of the individual.
- The nurse holds in confidence personal information and uses judgment in sharing this information.

Nurses and practice

- The nurse carries personal responsibility for nursing practice and for maintaining competence by continual learning.
- The nurse maintains the highest standards of nursing care possible within the reality of a specific situation.
- The nurse uses judgment in relation to individual competence when accepting and delegating responsibilities.

Ethical codes for nurses *(continued)*

◆ The nurse, when acting in a professional capacity, should at all times maintain standards of personal conduct that would reflect credit upon the profession.

Nurses and society

◆ The nurse shares with other citizens the responsibility for initiating and supporting action to meet the health and social needs of the public.

Nurses and coworkers

◆ The nurse sustains a cooperative relationship with coworkers in nursing and other fields.

◆ The nurse takes appropriate action to safeguard the individual when his care is endangered by a coworker or any other person.

Nurses and the profession

◆ The nurse plays a major role in determining and implementing desirable standards of nursing practice and nursing education.

◆ The nurse is active in developing a core of professional knowledge.

◆ The nurse, acting through the professional organization, participates in establishing and maintaining equitable social and economic working conditions in nursing.

ANA code of ethics

The ANA views both nurses and patients as individuals who possess basic rights and responsibilities and who deserve respect for their values and circumstances at all times. The ANA code provides guidance for carrying out nursing responsibilities consistent with the ethical obligations of the profession. According to the ANA code, the nurse is responsible for the following actions:

◆ To provide services with respect for human dignity and the uniqueness of the patient unrestricted by considerations of social or economic status, personal attributes, or the nature of health problems.

◆ To safeguard the patient's right to privacy by judiciously protecting information of a confidential nature.

◆ To safeguard the patient and the public when health care and safety are affected by the incompetent, unethical, or illegal practice of any person.

◆ To assume responsibility and accountability for individual nursing judgments and actions.

◆ To maintain competence in nursing.

◆ To exercise informed judgment and use individual competence and qualifications as criteria in seeking consultation, accepting responsibilities, and delegating nursing activities to others.

◆ To cooperate in activities that contribute to the ongoing development of the profession's body of knowledge.

◆ To participate in the profession's efforts to implement and improve standards of nursing.

◆ To take part in the profession's efforts to establish and maintain conditions of employment conducive to high-quality nursing care.

◆ To share in the profession's efforts to protect the public from misinformation and misrepresentation and to maintain the integrity of nursing.

◆ To collaborate with members of the health care professions and other citizens in promoting community and national efforts to meet the health needs of the public.

elevators than through a specific request for a patient's chart.
- The best way to prevent such breaches is to avoid discussing patient concerns in areas where you can be overheard.
◆ Most requests for copies of the medical record will go through the medical records department rather than through nursing staff.
- If you're asked for a copy of the record or an opportunity to view it, don't release the record without the documented consent of a competent patient.
- Increasing use of computers for documentation creates a new avenue for unauthorized release of patient information.
- All patient information is confidential, even information that may seem innocent. The release of certain information — for example, mental health records as well as information about drug and alcohol abuse and infectious diseases — is further constrained by state statutes.
◆ In the case of *Anonymous v. Chino Valley Medical Center,* San Bernardino County, California Superior Court (1997), a 35-year-old disabled inpatient underwent a blood test for human immunodeficiency virus (HIV).
- He specifically told the physician that he didn't want the results to be given to anyone but him.
- On the day of discharge, his sister was present in the hospital room. A nurse asked the sister to come into the hall so she could tell her about the patient's diet instructions upon discharge.
- In the hallway, the nurse told the sister that the patient had a positive HIV test. A few moments later, the physician approached them and also conveyed the test results.
- No action was filed against the physician. The nurse denied releasing the information.
- A trial court imposed a $5,000 statutory civil penalty against the medical center.
◆ In the case of *Hobbs v. Lopes,* 645 N.E.2d 1261, Ohio App. 4 DST. (1994), a 21-year-old Ohio woman was found to be pregnant after consulting a physician for another medical problem.
- Options, including abortion, were discussed.
- The physician instructed a nurse to call the woman to find out what option she had chosen.
- The nurse called the woman's parents' home and disclosed the fact that their daughter was pregnant and had sought advice about an abortion.
- The daughter sued for medical malpractice, invasion of privacy, breach of privilege, and infliction of emotional distress.
◆ Both of these cases underscore the importance of documenting the patient's consent or nonconsent to release of information.
- The patient's consent to release information should be on an official facility form.
- This form is handled not by the nurse but by the medical records department or hospital attorney.
◆ Keep in mind that the law requires you to disclose confidential information in certain situations — for example, in instances of alleged child abuse, matters of public health and safety, and criminal cases.

Informed consent

◆ Required before most treatments and procedures, *informed consent* means that the patient understands the proposed therapy and its risks and agrees to undergo it by signing a consent form.
◆ The physician (or other practitioner) who will perform the procedure is

legally responsible for obtaining the patient's informed consent.

◆ In some situations, the duty may be delegated to a nurse; however, the responsibility remains with the physician or practitioner.

◆ Depending on your facility's policy, you may be asked to witness the patient's signature.

Legal requirements

◆ For informed consent to be legally binding, the patient must be mentally competent and the physician must:
- explain the patient's diagnosis as well as the nature, purpose, and likelihood of success of the treatment or procedure
- describe the risks and benefits associated with the treatment or procedure
- explain the possible consequences of not undergoing the treatment or procedure
- describe alternative treatments and procedures
- inform the patient that he has the right to refuse the treatment or procedure without having other care or support withdrawn; this includes withdrawing his consent after giving it
- identify who will perform the procedure
- identify who is responsible for the patient's care
- obtain consent without coercing the patient.

◆ Informed consent has two elements, the information and the consent.
- To be *informed*, the patient must be provided with a description of the treatment or procedure, the name and qualifications of the person who will perform it, and an explanation of risks and alternatives — all in language the patient can understand.
- Based on this, the patient may *consent* to the treatment or procedure.

◆ JCAHO mandates the elements of informed consent.

◆ In addition, most states have statutes that set out specific elements of informed consent.
- In a few states, the physician can explain the procedure and simply ask whether the patient has any questions.
- If the patient has none, the physician isn't obligated by state law to discuss alternatives and risks unless the patient requests the information.
- Although this policy is inconsistent with JCAHO guidelines, keep in mind that those guidelines aren't the law; they're a set of requirements for licensure and accreditation.

◆ In life-threatening emergencies, informed consent may not be required. In such cases, the law assumes that every individual wants to live and allows the physician to intervene to save life without obtaining consent.

◆ In many cases, a patient may attempt to clarify issues with a nurse after giving the physician his informed consent.
- If you're questioned in this way, be aware that you aren't obligated to answer the patient's questions; however, if you do, be careful to document your answers.
- You should notify the physician and document that you have done so, including the date and time.

Witnessing informed consent

◆ When you witness the patient signing an informed consent document, you're *not* witnessing that he received or understood the information. You're simply witnessing that the person who signed the consent form is in fact the person he says he is.
- For this purpose, check the patient's armband to ensure that he is in fact the correct patient.

– You don't need to be present when the physician gives the information because you're only witnessing that the patient is signing the document, not that the information was given.
◆ Before a procedure is performed, make sure the patient's record contains a signed informed consent form.
◆ If the patient appears to be concerned about the procedure or the physician's explanation of it, notify your supervisor or the physician, and chart that you've done this.
◆ If the patient wants to change his mind, contact the physician as soon as possible and chart the patient's comments, the date and time you contacted the physician, and the physician's response.

20 Bioterrorism readiness

A terrorist attack that involves biological weapons, chemicals, or radiation may cause a sudden increased demand on facility services and, depending on the weapon involved, may pose a threat to health care workers. Effective management of patients after such an attack can pose a multitude of challenges.

Biological weapons

- As a nurse, you may be the first to recognize that a patient has been exposed to a biological weapon.
- Rapid recognition and response can help decrease danger to the patient and to others.
- Exposure to a biological weapon may not be easy to identify because symptoms may mimic those of common diseases or may be delayed. (See *Signs and symptoms of exposure to biological weapons*.)

Signs and symptoms of exposure to biological weapons

Listed below are conditions that could be caused by biological weapons and the major associated signs and symptoms.

CONDITION	MAJOR SIGNS AND SYMPTOMS
Anthrax (cutaneous)	◆ Fever ◆ Headache ◆ Lymphadenopathy ◆ Malaise ◆ Papular rash
Anthrax (GI)	◆ Abdominal pain ◆ Bloody diarrhea ◆ Fever ◆ Hematemesis ◆ Nausea ◆ Vomiting
Anthrax (inhalation)	◆ Chest pain ◆ Chills ◆ Cough ◆ Decreased blood pressure ◆ Decreased stridor ◆ Dyspnea ◆ Fever ◆ Weakness

Signs and symptoms of exposure to biological weapons *(continued)*

CONDITION	MAJOR SIGNS AND SYMPTOMS
Botulism	◆ Diplopia ◆ Dysarthria ◆ Dysphagia ◆ Dyspnea ◆ Ptosis ◆ Weakness
Cholera	◆ Decreased blood pressure ◆ Decreased skin turgor ◆ Muscle spasms (cramps) ◆ Oliguria ◆ Tachycardia ◆ Vomiting ◆ Watery diarrhea ◆ Weakness
Plague (bubonic and septicemic)	◆ Chills ◆ Fever ◆ Lymphadenopathy
Plague (pneumonic)	◆ Chest pain ◆ Chills ◆ Cough ◆ Dyspnea ◆ Fever ◆ Headache ◆ Hemoptysis ◆ Myalgia ◆ Tachypnea
Smallpox	◆ Abdominal pain ◆ Back pain ◆ Fever ◆ Headache ◆ Malaise ◆ Papular rash
Tularemia	◆ Chest pain ◆ Chills ◆ Cough ◆ Dyspnea ◆ Fever ◆ Headache ◆ Myalgia

Secondary contamination

◆ Patients covered with liquid or solid biologicals may contaminate facility personnel by direct contact. These patients should undergo a decontamination process that involves:
- removing all clothing
- flushing the skin with plain water and mild soap
- irrigating irritated eyes with saline
- if the agent was ingested, giving 4 to 8 ounces of water to dilute the stomach contents.

◆ Until the identity of the biologic agent is determined, consider sec-

Treatment for biological weapons exposure

Listed below are potentially threatening biological (bacterial and viral) agents and the treatments and vaccines that are currently available to combat them.

Implement standard precautions for all cases of suspected exposure. For smallpox, institute airborne precautions for the duration of the illness and until all scabs fall off. For pneumonic plague, institute droplet precautions for 72 hours after initiation of effective therapy.

BIOLOGICAL AGENTS (CONDITIONS)	TREATMENTS AND VACCINES
Bacillus anthracis **(anthrax)**	◆ Ciprofloxacin, doxycycline, or penicillin ◆ Vaccine: Limited supply available; recommended only for people exposed to anthrax
Clostridium botulinum **(botulism)**	◆ Supportive: Endotracheal intubation and mechanical ventilation ◆ Passive immunization with equine antitoxin to lessen nerve damage ◆ Vaccine: Postexposure prophylaxis with equine botulinum antitoxin; botulinum toxoid available from Centers for Disease Control and Prevention; recombinant vaccine under development
Francisella tularensis **(tularemia)**	◆ Gentamicin or streptomycin; alternatively, doxycycline, chloramphenicol, or ciprofloxacin ◆ Vaccine: Live, attenuated vaccine currently under investigation and review by the Food and Drug Administration (FDA)
Variola major **(smallpox)**	◆ No FDA-approved antiviral available; cidofovir may be therapeutic if administered 1 to 2 days after exposure ◆ Vaccine: Prophylaxis within 3 to 4 days of exposure
Yersinia pestis **(pneumonic plague)**	◆ Streptomycin or gentamicin; alternatively, doxycycline, ciprofloxacin, or chloramphenicol ◆ Vaccine: No longer available

ondary contamination of facility personnel a real risk.

◆ If possible, before patients arrive, make sure personal protective equipment has been distributed and put on and that areas that could become contaminated are cleared and secured.

Treatment

◆ When managing patients after a possible biological attack, follow a systematic approach.
- Use standard precautions, including precautions for cleaning, disinfection, and sterilization of equipment and environment.
- Follow additional precautions based on the biological agent used and the degree of infection.
- Wear protective equipment.
- Wash your hands with antimicrobial soap.

◆ If many patients arrive at once, group those with similar symptoms in a designated area.

◆ Limit transport of infected people.

◆ Don't discharge patients with bioterrorism-related infections until they're no longer infectious. (See *Treatment for biological weapons exposure.*)

Chemical weapons

◆ As with biological weapons, you may be the first to recognize that a patient has been exposed to a chemical agent, although the difficulty of pinpointing signs and symptoms is similar. (See *Signs and symptoms of exposure to chemical weapons.*)

◆ Clues that might suggest covert release of a chemical agent include:

(Text continued on page 554.)

Signs and symptoms of exposure to chemical weapons

Examples of signs and symptoms of related to selected chemical agents are listed below.

CHEMICAL AGENTS	SIGNS AND SYMPTOMS
Acrylamide	◆ Ataxia ◆ Delirium ◆ Depressed or absent deep tendon reflexes (DTRs) ◆ Encephalopathy ◆ "Glove and stocking" sensory loss ◆ Memory loss ◆ Muscle weakness and atrophy
Arsenic	◆ Abdominal pain ◆ Hypotension ◆ Multisystem organ failure (possible) ◆ Profuse diarrhea (possibly bloody) ◆ Vomiting

(continued)

Signs and symptoms of exposure to chemical weapons *(continued)*

CHEMICAL AGENTS	SIGNS AND SYMPTOMS
Arsenic (inorganic)	◆ Ataxia ◆ Delirium ◆ Depressed or absent DTRs ◆ Encephalopathy ◆ "Glove and stocking" sensory loss ◆ Memory loss ◆ Muscle weakness and atrophy
Barium	◆ Abdominal pain ◆ Hypokalemia ◆ Hypotension ◆ Multisystem organ failure (possible) ◆ Profuse diarrhea (possibly bloody) ◆ Vomiting
Carbamate (insecticides and medicinal)	◆ Altered mental status ◆ Bradycardia or tachycardia ◆ Bronchorrhea ◆ Diaphoresis ◆ Diarrhea ◆ Fasciculations ◆ Hypotension or hypertension ◆ Increased urination ◆ Lacrimation ◆ Miosis ◆ Salivation ◆ Seizures ◆ Weakness
Carbon monoxide	◆ Altered mental status ◆ Dyspnea ◆ Headache ◆ Hypotension ◆ Metabolic acidosis ◆ Nausea ◆ Seizures ◆ Vomiting
Caustics (acids and alkalies)	◆ Lip, mouth, and pharyngeal ulcerations and burning pain
Colchicine	◆ Abdominal pain ◆ Hypotension ◆ Profuse diarrhea (possibly bloody) ◆ Multisystem organ failure (possible) ◆ Vomiting

Signs and symptoms of exposure to chemical weapons *(continued)*

CHEMICAL AGENTS	SIGNS AND SYMPTOMS
Cyanide	◆ Altered mental status ◆ Bitter almond odor ◆ Dyspnea ◆ Headache ◆ Hypotension ◆ Metabolic acidosis ◆ Nausea ◆ Seizures ◆ Vomiting
Diquat	◆ Lip, mouth, and pharyngeal ulcerations and burning pain
Hydrogen sulfide	◆ Altered mental status ◆ Dyspnea ◆ Headache ◆ Hypotension ◆ Metabolic acidosis ◆ Nausea ◆ Seizures ◆ Vomiting
Inorganic mercuric salts	◆ Lip, mouth, and pharyngeal ulcerations and burning pain
Lead	◆ Ataxia ◆ Delirium ◆ Depressed or absent DTRs ◆ Encephalopathy ◆ "Glove and stocking" sensory loss ◆ Memory loss ◆ Muscle weakness and atrophy
Mercury (organic)	◆ Ataxia ◆ Delirium ◆ Depressed or absent DTRs ◆ Encephalopathy ◆ "Glove and stocking" sensory loss ◆ Memory loss ◆ Muscle weakness and atrophy ◆ Paresthesia ◆ Vision disturbances

(continued)

Signs and symptoms of exposure to chemical weapons *(continued)*

CHEMICAL AGENTS	SIGNS AND SYMPTOMS
Methemoglobin-causing agents	◆ Altered mental status ◆ Dyspnea ◆ Headache ◆ Hypotension ◆ Metabolic acidosis ◆ Nausea ◆ Seizures ◆ Vomiting
Mustards	◆ Lip, mouth, and pharyngeal ulcerations and burning pain
Nicotine	◆ Altered mental status ◆ Bradycardia or tachycardia ◆ Bronchorrhea ◆ Diaphoresis ◆ Diarrhea ◆ Fasciculations ◆ Hypotension or hypertension ◆ Increased urination ◆ Lacrimation ◆ Miosis ◆ Salivation ◆ Seizures ◆ Weakness
Organophosphate insecticides	◆ Altered mental status ◆ Bradycardia or tachycardia ◆ Bronchorrhea ◆ Decreased acetylcholinesterase activity ◆ Diaphoresis ◆ Diarrhea ◆ Fasciculations ◆ Hypotension or hypertension ◆ Increased urination ◆ Lacrimation ◆ Miosis ◆ Salivation ◆ Seizures ◆ Weakness
Paraquat	◆ Dyspnea and hemoptysis secondary to pulmonary edema or hemorrhage; can progress to pulmonary fibrosis over days to weeks ◆ Lip, mouth, and pharyngeal ulcerations and burning pain

Signs and symptoms of exposure to chemical weapons *(continued)*

CHEMICAL AGENTS	SIGNS AND SYMPTOMS
Ricin	◆ Abdominal pain ◆ Hypotension ◆ Multisystem organ failure (possible) ◆ Profuse diarrhea (possibly bloody) ◆ Severe respiratory illness (if inhaled) ◆ Vomiting
Sodium azide	◆ Altered mental status ◆ Dyspnea ◆ Headache ◆ Hypotension ◆ Metabolic acidosis ◆ Nausea ◆ Seizures ◆ Vomiting
Sodium monofluoroacetate	◆ Altered mental status ◆ Dyspnea ◆ Headache ◆ Hypocalcemia or hypokalemia ◆ Hypotension ◆ Metabolic acidosis ◆ Nausea ◆ Seizures ◆ Vomiting
Strychnine	◆ Hypertension ◆ Intact sensorium ◆ Seizure-like, generalized muscle contractions or painful spasms (neck and limbs) ◆ Tachycardia
Thallium	◆ Ataxia ◆ Delirium ◆ Depressed or absent DTRs ◆ Encephalopathy ◆ "Glove and stocking" sensory loss ◆ Memory loss ◆ Muscle weakness and atrophy

Adapted from the Centers for Disease Control and Prevention. Available at: *www.cdc.gov/mmwr/preview/mmwrhtml/mm5239a3.htm.*

- a sudden and unusual increase in the number of patients with illnesses that could be chemical-related
- unexplained deaths among young and otherwise healthy people
- emissions of unexplained odors by patients
- clusters of illness in persons with common characteristics, such as drinking water from the same source
- rapid onset of symptoms after exposure to a potentially contaminated medium
- unexplained death of plants or wildlife
- a syndrome similar to a disease caused by known chemical exposure.

◆ Immediately report the release of chemicals, whether intentional or accidental, to your state health department and the Centers for Disease Control and Prevention.

Secondary contamination

◆ Patients exposed only to gas or vapor and who have no gross deposition of a chemical on their clothing or skin aren't likely to pose a secondary contamination risk.

◆ Patients covered with liquid or solid chemical or with condensed vapor may contaminate facility personnel by direct contact or by vapor. These patients should undergo a decontamination process that involves:
- removing all clothing
- flushing of the skin with plain water and mild soap
- irrigating irritated eyes with saline
- if the agent was ingested, giving 4 to 8 ounces of water to dilute the stomach contents.

◆ Until the identity of the chemical agent is determined, consider secondary contamination of facility personnel a real risk.

◆ If possible, before patients arrive, make sure personal protective equipment has been distributed and donned and that areas that could become contaminated are cleared and secured.

◆ Most patients will be transferred and treated in an intensive care unit.

Treatment

◆ At all times, pay attention to the patient's respiratory and cardiovascular status.
- Ensure a patent airway.
- Make sure the patient is intubated and ventilated as needed.
- If needed, support breathing and circulation through cardiopulmonary resuscitation.

◆ Patients who are comatose, hypotensive, or have seizures or ventricular arrhythmias should be treated in the usual medical manner for those conditions.

Radiation weapons

◆ Radiation is energy that exists in different forms.

◆ Everyone is exposed to small amounts of radiation daily from natural and man-made sources.

◆ Exposure to radiation can affect the body in a number of ways, but it may take several years before the adverse effects of exposure develop.

◆ Exposure to large doses of radiation because of an accidental or terrorist event is considered a medical emergency; death can occur in a few days or months.

Secondary exposure

◆ When treating patients with radiation exposure, facility personnel should follow these guidelines:
- Use standard precautions.
- Wear two pairs of gloves for added protection.

- Change gloves often.
- Establish multiple receptacles for contaminated waste.
- Use radiation survey meters to locate contaminated areas and measure exposure rate.

Treatment

◆ The first course of action is to medically stabilize the patient, if needed, before starting any significant decontamination procedures.

◆ Immediately remove and bag contaminated clothing, then decontaminate wounds and intact skin with one of these recommended cleaning solutions:
- soap and water
- hexachlorophene 3% detergent and water
- povidone iodine and water.

◆ Wash the patient's hair with shampoo and no conditioner.

◆ Obtain nasal swabs and urine and stool specimens as early as possible to check for internal contamination.

◆ Assist in treating internal contamination to reduce the radiation dose and the risk of long-term effects from absorbed radionuclides.

◆ Immediate treatments include these:
- gastric lavage for ingestion of radioactive material within 2 hours of exposure
- antacids for ingested radionuclides
- cathartics for large ingestions
- increased fluid intake for tritium contamination
- oral potassium iodide for radioiodine contamination
- Prussian blue for cesium contamination
- chelating agents, such as calcium or zinc diethylene-triaminepenta-acetate for plutonium and transuranics contamination
- oral aluminum phosphate or barium sulfate for strontium ingestion.

◆ Use a radiation survey meter to monitor the progress of decontamination.

Appendices
Selected references
Index

Cultural considerations in patient care

Regardless of the setting in which you work, as a health care professional you'll typically interact with a diverse, multicultural patient population and you should base your care plan on the overall needs of the patient and his family. Generally, each culture has its own unique set of beliefs about health and illness, dietary practices, and other matters that you should consider when providing care.

Although negative stereotyping of different cultures must be avoided, it is important to learn about representative characteristics of different groups. However, you should be aware that people have widely varying beliefs that are sometimes based only in part on

CULTURAL GROUP	HEALTH CARE BELIEF AND ILLNESS PHILOSOPHY
African Americans	◆ May believe that illness is related to supernatural causes ◆ May seek advice and remedies from faith or folk healers ◆ May show stoic response to pain until it's unbearable and then seek emergency care ◆ May be family oriented – customary for many family members to remain with a dying patient in the hospital ◆ May express grief by crying, screaming, praying, singing, and reading scripture
Arab Americans (major populations include those from Egypt, Iran, Iraq, Lebanon, Palestine, and Syria)	◆ May remain silent about some health problems such as sexually transmitted diseases, substance abuse, mental illness ◆ A devout Muslim may interpret illness as the will of Allah, a test of faith, representing a type of fatalistic view ◆ May rely on ritual cures or alternative therapies before seeing a health care provider ◆ May have strong respect for the elderly and feel obliged to take care of elderly relatives ◆ May express pain freely ◆ After death, the family or community members may want to prepare the body by washing and wrapping the body in unsewn white cloth ◆ Postmortem examinations are discouraged unless required by law

cultural heritage. Health care professionals should try to understand each person and be sensitive to and respectful of individual beliefs.

This appendix summarizes some health care beliefs and practices relating to dietary, communication, family roles, death rituals, health care practices, and folk health practices for five cultural groups that are common in the United States. These include African Americans, Arab Americans, Asian Americans, Latino Americans, and Native Americans. The predominant Western Culture health care beliefs and practices are also summarized.

DIETARY PRACTICES	OTHER CONSIDERATIONS
◆ May have food restrictions based on religious beliefs (such as not eating pork, if Muslim) ◆ Have a higher incidence of high blood pressure and obesity, which may be diet related ◆ High incidence of lactose intolerance with difficulty digesting milk and milk products ◆ May view cooked greens as good for health ◆ Traditional "soul" food diet is high in protein and fat	◆ Predominant values: Family bonding, matriarchal, present orientation, and spiritual orientation ◆ Tend to be affectionate, as shown by touching and hugging friends and loved ones ◆ Many Muslim women must keep their heads covered at all times ◆ Primary religions: Baptist and other Protestant denominations, Muslim (Islam)
◆ May choose foods based on the humoral theory of balancing hot and cold ◆ May prefer dairy products, rice, and wheat breads ◆ May avoid pork and alcohol if Muslim ◆ Islamic patients observe month long fast of Ramadan (begins approximately mid October); those who are suffering chronic illness and women who are pregnant, breast-feeding, or menstruating don't fast ◆ May avoid mixing milk and fish, sweet and sour, or hot and cold ◆ May avoid using ice in drinks ◆ May believe that hot soup can help recovery	◆ Predominant values: Family patriarchal and hierarchical, respect for elders, modesty, respectability, and politeness ◆ Muslim women may avoid eye contact as a show of modesty ◆ Many Muslim women wear the traditional hijab (head cover) ◆ Respect for higher education and advanced degrees ◆ Use same-sex family members as interpreters ◆ Preventive care among adults isn't highly valued ◆ Primary religions: Catholic, Greek Orthodox, Muslim (Islam), Protestant

CULTURAL GROUP	HEALTH CARE BELIEF AND ILLNESS PHILOSOPHY
Asian Americans (major populations include those from Cambodia, China, India, Indonesia, Korea Pakistan, Philippines, Thailand, and Vietnam)	◆ Asian Americans have differing health views depending in part on their particular subculture – Chinese: May believe illness results when a person fails to act in harmony with nature, such as yin and yang – Filipino: May believe dying is God's plan and that neither the client nor the health care provider should interfere with God's will – Korean: May adhere to traditional values that dictate that client should die at home – Japanese: May believe that illness is karma, resulting from behavior in the current life or a past life ◆ May value ability to endure pain and grief with silent stoicism ◆ Typically family oriented; extended family should be involved in care of dying patient
Latino Americans (major populations include those from the Caribbean, Central and South America, and Mexico)	◆ May view illness as a sign of weakness, punishment for evil doing or retribution for shameful behavior ◆ May use the terms "hot" and "cold" in reference to vital elements needed to restore equilibrium to the body ◆ May consult with a curandero (healer) or voodoo priest (Caribbean) ◆ May view pain as a necessary part of life and believe that enduring pain is a sign of strength (especially men) ◆ May have open expression of grief, such as praying for the dead, saying the rosary ◆ May use various amulets to protect individual from evil ◆ Family members are typically involved in all aspects of decision making such as terminal illness
Native Americans	◆ May turn to a medicine man to determine the true cause of an illness, such as why a person is out of harmony with nature ◆ May value the ability to endure pain or grief with silent stoicism ◆ May view death as part of life cycle ◆ Burial practices vary among tribal groups. Example: Navajos fear death and distance themselves from death and may avoid touching a dead or dying person. ◆ May believe that the spirit of a dying person can't leave his body until the family is there ◆ Grief tends to be family oriented with all members assuming roles in the grieving process

DIETARY PRACTICES	OTHER CONSIDERATIONS
◆ Hot/cold theory (yin and yang) often involved. Example: Curing a "hot" disease such as arthritis may require cold foods or medicines ◆ Hindu religious food practices include refraining from eating meat from cows; some are lacto-vegetarians eating only milk products and vegetables ◆ Chinese patients may use an herbalist or acupuncturist before seeking medical help; may eat rice with most meals and may use chopsticks ◆ Sodium intake is generally high because of salted and dried foods and use of condiments	◆ Predominant values: Group orientation, submission to authority, respect for elders, respect for past, modesty, conformity, and tradition ◆ May believe that prolonged eye contact is rude and an invasion of privacy ◆ Tend to be very modest; prefer same sex clinicians ◆ May nod without necessarily understanding (especially elderly Japanese patients) ◆ May prefer to maintain a comfortable physical distance between the patient and the health care provider ◆ Primary Religions: Buddhist, Catholic, Confucianism, Hindu and Islam (India), Protestant, Shinto (Japanese), Taoism, Zen Buddhism
◆ May use herbal teas and soup to aid in recuperation ◆ Traditional diet is basically vegetarian with emphasis on corn, corn products, beans, rice, and breads ◆ Select beans and tortillas are staples and may be eaten at every meal ◆ Typically eat a lot of fresh fruits and vegetables; however, variety in diet may be limited ◆ High prevalence of obesity, particularly central obesity, that raises the risk of diabetes and heart disease	◆ Predominant values: Group emphasis, extended family, fatalism, present orientation ◆ May have fatalistic view of life ◆ May see no reason to submit to mammograms or vaccinations ◆ May need private room where grief can be expressed openly ◆ May be modest (especially women) ◆ Use same sex family members as interpreters ◆ Primary religion: Roman Catholic
◆ Diet may be deficient in vitamin D and calcium because many suffer from lactose intolerance or don't drink milk ◆ Obesity and diabetes are major health concerns ◆ Herbs are used in the treatment of many illnesses to cleanse the body of ill spirits or poisons	◆ Predominant values: Bonding to family or group, sharing with others, present orientation, extended family, cooperation and acceptance of nature ◆ May divert their eyes to the floor when they are praying or paying attention ◆ Raised to be reserved and noncommittal, may respond to assessment questions with silence or monosyllables ◆ Belief system: Characterized by intense relationship with nature

CULTURAL GROUP	HEALTH CARE BELIEF AND ILLNESS PHILOSOPHY
Western Culture (primarily of European background)	◆ May value technology almost exclusively in the struggle to conquer disease ◆ May have strong shared belief in the biomedical approach, which may result in serious barriers to communication with other cultures who choose to use alternative or complementary therapies ◆ Health is generally understood to be the absence, minimization, or control of disease processes ◆ Hospitalization may foster an atmosphere that requires the patient and family to be compliant, dependent, and vulnerable to get needs met ◆ Health care emphasis is shifting from treating diseases to disease prevention and health promotion

DIETARY PRACTICES	OTHER CONSIDERATIONS
◆ Health care facilities frequently have standard dietary guidelines, which may or may not consider cultural variations ◆ Eating utensils primarily consist of knife, fork, and spoon ◆ Three daily meals is typical ◆ Values convenience and may substitute ready-to-eat (fast food) items, which are generally low in nutrition and health benefits; meals eaten out tend to be higher in calories, fat, and sodium ◆ Growing incidence of obesity	◆ Predominant values: Independence, self-reliance and individualism, resistance to authority, nuclear/blended family, innovation, emphasis on youth, future orientation, competition ◆ Health care is a culture of its own rituals and language often incomprehensible to patients or their families of other cultures ◆ Belief systems widely varied

Quick guide to potential agents of bioterrorism

Listed below are examples of biological agents that may potentially be used as biological weapons and the major signs and symptoms associated with each.

	MAJOR ASSOCIATED SIGNS AND SYMPTOMS													
POTENTIAL AGENTS	Abdominal pain	Back pain	Blood pressure, decreased	Chest pain	Chills	Cough	Diarrhea, bloody	Diarrhea, watery	Diplopia	Dysarthria	Dysphagia	Dyspnea	Fever	Headache
Anthrax (cutaneous)													●	●
Anthrax (GI)	●						●						●	
Anthrax (inhalation)			●	●	●	●						●	●	
Botulism									●	●	●	●		
Cholera			●					●						
Plague (bubonic and septicemic)					●								●	
Plague (pneumonic)				●	●	●						●	●	●
Smallpox	●	●											●	●
Tularemia				●	●	●						●	●	●

Hematemesis	Hemoptysis	Lymphadenopathy	Malaise	Muscle spasms (muscle cramps)	Myalgia	Nausea	Oliguria	Papular rash (skin lesions)	Ptosis	Skin turgor, decreased	Stridor	Tachycardia	Tachypnea	Vomiting	Weakness
		●	●					●							
●						●								●	
											●				●
									●						●
				●			●			●		●		●	●
		●													
	●				●								●		
			●					●							
					●										

Web sites of selected organizations

Agency for Healthcare Research and Quality
www.ahrq.gov

American Association of Critical-Care Nurses
www.aacn.org

American Burn Association
www.ameriburn.org

American Cancer Society
www.cancer.org

American Diabetes Association
www.diabetes.org

American Heart Association
www.americanheart.org

American Holistic Nurses Association
www.ahna.org

American Lung Association
www.lungusa.org

American Nurses Association
www.nursingworld.org

American Pain Society
www.ampainsoc.org

Centers for Disease Control and Prevention
www.cdc.gov

Drugs @ FDA
www.accessdata.fda.gov/scripts/cder/drugsatfda

Infusion Nurses Society
www.ins1.org

Joint Commission on Accreditation of Healthcare Organizations
www.jcaho.com

LPN Central – The Practical Nurse's Station
www.lpncentral.com

National Institutes of Health
www.nih.gov

National Kidney Foundation
www.kidney.org

National League for Nursing
www.nln.org

National Library of Medicine
www.nlm.nih.gov

National Parkinson Foundation
www.parkinson.org

Sigma Theta Tau International – Honor Society of Nursing
www.nursingsociety.org

Wound Ostomy and Continence Nurses Society
www.wocn.org

Dangerous abbreviations

The Joint Commission on Accreditation of Healthcare Organizations has agreed upon a list of dangerous abbreviations, acronyms, and symbols. Using this list should help protect patients from the effects of miscommunication in clinical documentation.

ABBREVIATION	DANGER	PREFERRED USE
U or u (for "unit")	Mistaken for the numbers 0 or 4 (for example, 4U seen as 40 or 4u seen as 44). Also mistaken for "cc" (for example, 4u seen as 4cc).	Write "unit."
IU (for "international unit")	Mistaken for I.V. (intravenous) or 10 (ten).	Write "international unit."
q.d. (Latin abbreviation for "every day")	Mistaken for q.i.d., especially if the period after the "q" or the tail of the "q" could be seen as an "i."	Write "daily" or "once daily."
q.o.d. (Latin abbreviation "every other day")	Mistaken for q.d. ir q.i.d. if the "I" is poorly written.	Write "every other day."
Trailing zero (such as 1.0 mg)	Decimal point may be missed (for example, 1.0 may be seen as 10).	Never write a zero by itself after a decimal point (1 mg rather than 1.0 mg).
Lack of leading zero (such as .5 mg)	Decimal point may be missed (for example, 0.5 may be seen as 5).	Always write a zero before a decimal point (0.5 mg rather than .5 mg).
MS or MSO_4 (morphine sulfate)	Mistaken for magnesium sulfate.	Write "morphine sulfate."
$MgSO_4$ (magnesium sulfate)	Mistaken for morphine sulfate.	Write "magnesium sulfate."

Outcomes and interventions for common nursing diagnoses

After exploring a patient's chief complaint, you can compile a list of applicable nursing diagnoses (also called a problem list) and develop a care plan. For each diagnosis, you'll need to specify patient outcomes and the interventions needed to achieve them, as these examples show.

Risk for activity intolerance related to immobility

Definition

Accentuated risk of extreme fatigue or other physical symptoms during or following simple activity

Key outcomes

Record appropriate patient outcomes on the care plan. Possible outcomes include these:

- Patient maintains muscle strength and range-of-motion (ROM), as indicated by use of functional mobility scale.
- Patient carries out isometric exercise regimen.
- Patient communicates understanding of rationale for maintaining activity level.
- Patient avoids risk factors that may lead to activity intolerance.
- Patient performs self-care activities to tolerance level.
- Vital signs remain within prescribed range during periods of activity (specify).

Nursing interventions

Document interventions related to:

- patient's expressed motivation to maintain maximum activity level within restrictions imposed by illness
- patient's physiologic response to increased activity (times and dates of vital signs: blood pressure, respirations, heart rate and rhythm)
- patient repositioning and turning (including times and assistive devices used)
- patient's functional level (use a functional mobility scale)
- prescribed ROM and other exercises (including times and assistive devices used such as trapezes)
- patient teaching (including reason for treatment regimen and signs and symptoms of overexertion, such as dizziness, chest pain, and dyspnea) and patient's response
- patient's ability to perform activities of daily living (ADLs)
- evaluation of expected outcomes.

Ineffective airway clearance related to decreased energy or fatigue

Definition

Anatomic or physiologic obstruction of the airway that interferes with the maintenance of a clear airway.

Key outcomes

Record appropriate patient outcomes on the care plan. Possible outcomes include these:
- ◆ Airway remains patent.
- ◆ Adventitious breath sounds are absent.
- ◆ Chest X-ray shows no abnormality.
- ◆ Oxygen level is in normal range.
- ◆ Patient breathes deeply and coughs to remove secretions.
- ◆ Patient expectorates sputum.
- ◆ Patient demonstrates controlled coughing techniques.
- ◆ Ventilation is adequate.
- ◆ Patient shows no signs of pulmonary compromise.
- ◆ Patient demonstrates skill in conserving energy while attempting to clear airway.
- ◆ Patient states understanding of changes needed to diminish oxygen demands.

Nursing interventions

Document interventions related to:
- ◆ patient's perception of ability to cough
- ◆ observed respiratory status and other physical findings
- ◆ patient positioning and repositioning (including times)
- ◆ airway and pulmonary clearance maneuvers (such as coughing and deep breathing, suctioning to stimulate cough and clear airways, aerosol treatments, postural drainage, percussion and vibration) and patient's response
- ◆ sputum characteristics (including amount, odor, consistency)
- ◆ prescribed drug administration (including expectorants, bronchodilators, and other drugs)
- ◆ amount of fluid intake to help liquefy secretions
- ◆ oxygen administration (including times, dates, equipment, and supplies)
- ◆ test results, including arterial blood gas (ABG) levels and hemoglobin values, and reportable deviations from baseline levels
- ◆ endotracheal (ET) intubation
- ◆ patient teaching
- ◆ evaluation of expected outcomes.

Anxiety related to situational crisis

Definition

Feeling of threat or danger to self arising from an unidentifiable source

Key outcomes

Record appropriate expected outcomes on the care plan. Possible outcomes include these:
- ◆ Patient identifies factors that elicit anxious behaviors.
- ◆ Patient discusses activities that tend to decrease anxious behaviors.
- ◆ Patient practices progressive relaxation techniques ____ times per day.
- ◆ Patient copes with current medical situation (specify) without demonstrating severe signs of anxiety (specify for individual).

Nursing interventions

Document interventions related to:
- ◆ patient's expressions of anxiety and feelings of relief
- ◆ observed signs of patient's anxiety
- ◆ time spent with patient, duration of anxious episodes, and emotional support given to patient and family
- ◆ comfort measures
- ◆ patient teaching (including clear, concise explanations of anything about to occur and relaxation techniques, such as guided imagery, progressive muscle relaxation, and meditation)

- referrals to community or professional mental health services
- patient's involvement in making decisions related to care
- evaluation of expected outcomes.

Disturbed body image

Definition

Negative perception of self that makes healthful functioning more difficult

Key outcomes

Record appropriate expected outcomes on the care plan. Possible outcomes include these:

- Patient acknowledges change in body image.
- Patient communicates feelings about change in body image.
- Patient participates in decision making about his care (specify).
- Patient talks with someone who has experienced the same problem.
- Patient demonstrates ability to practice two new coping behaviors.
- Patient expresses positive feelings about self.

Nursing interventions

Document interventions related to:

- patient's observed coping patterns and responses to change in structure or function of body part (such as touching or not touching)
- patient's participation in self-care
- patient's perception of self, prostheses, adaptive equipment, and limitations
- patient's focus on or denial of specific body parts
- patient's involvement in decision making related to care
- patient's response to nursing interventions
- patient teaching (including information on how bodily functions are improving or stabilizing and specific coping strategies)
- referrals to a mental health professional, a support group, or another person who has had a similar problem
- positive reinforcement of patient's efforts to adapt and use coping strategies
- evaluation of expected outcomes.

Ineffective breathing pattern related to decreased energy or fatigue

Definition

Change in rate, depth, or pattern of breathing that alters normal gas exchange

Key outcomes

Record appropriate expected outcomes on the care plan. Possible outcomes include these:

- Patient's respiratory rate stays within 5 breaths of baseline.
- ABG levels return to baseline.
- Patient reports feeling comfortable when breathing.
- Patient reports feeling rested each day.
- Patient demonstrates diaphragmatic pursed-lip breathing.
- Patient achieves maximum lung expansion with adequate ventilation.
- Patient demonstrates skill in conserving energy while carrying out ADLs.

Nursing interventions

Document interventions related to:

- patient's expressions of comfort in breathing, emotional state, understand-

ing of medical diagnosis, and readiness to learn
◆ physical condition related to pulmonary status (including respiratory rate and depth, breath sounds, and reportable changes)
◆ test results such as ABG levels
◆ prescribed drug and oxygen administration (including dates, times, dosages, routes, adverse effects, equipment, and supplies)
◆ comfort measures (including supporting upper extremities with pillows, providing an overbed table with a pillow to lean on, or elevating the head of the bed)
◆ airway suctioning to remove secretions
◆ patient teaching (including pursed-lip breathing, abdominal breathing, relaxation techniques, drugs [dosage, frequency, reportable adverse effects], activity and rest, and diet)
◆ scheduling of activities to allow periods of rest
◆ evaluation of expected outcomes.

Decreased cardiac output related to reduced stroke volume as a result of mechanical or structural problems

Definition

Cardiovascular or respiratory symptoms resulting from insufficient blood being pumped by the heart

Key outcomes

Record appropriate expected outcomes on the care plan. Possible outcomes include these:
◆ Patient maintains hemodynamic stability: pulse not less than ____ and not greater than ____ beats/minute; blood pressure not less than ____ and not greater than ____ mm Hg.
◆ Patient has no arrhythmias.
◆ Skin remains warm and dry.
◆ Patient has no pedal edema.
◆ Patient achieves activity within limits of prescribed heart rate.
◆ Patient expresses sense of physical comfort after activity.
◆ Heart's workload diminishes.
◆ Patient maintains adequate cardiac output.
◆ Patient performs stress-reduction techniques every 4 hours while awake.
◆ Patient states understanding of signs and symptoms, prescribed activity level, diet, and drugs.

Nursing interventions

Document interventions related to:
◆ patient's needs and perception of problem
◆ observed physical findings (including level of consciousness [LOC], heart rate and rhythm, blood pressure, and auscultated heart and breath sounds)
◆ reports of abnormal findings (including times, dates, and names)
◆ intake and output measurements, daily weight
◆ observation of pedal or sacral edema
◆ interventions for life-threatening arrhythmias, as ordered
◆ skin care measures to enhance skin perfusion and venous flow
◆ increasing patient's activity level within limits of prescribed heart rate
◆ observed pulse rate before and after activity
◆ patient's response to activity
◆ dietary restrictions as ordered
◆ patient teaching (including desired skills related to diet, prescribed activity, and stress-reduction techniques; procedures and tests; chest pain and other reportable symptoms; drugs [name, dosage, frequency, therapeutic

and adverse effects]; and simple methods for lifting and bending)
- ◆ administration of and response to oxygen therapy
- ◆ evaluation of expected outcomes.

Impaired verbal communication related to decreased circulation to the brain

Definition

Deficient ability in processing a system of verbal symbols

Key outcomes

Record appropriate expected outcomes on the care plan. Possible outcomes include these:
- ◆ Staff consistently meets patient's needs.
- ◆ Patient maintains orientation.
- ◆ Patient maintains effective level of communication.
- ◆ Patient answers direct questions correctly.

Nursing interventions

Document interventions related to:
- ◆ patient's current level of communication, orientation, and satisfaction with communication efforts
- ◆ changes in speech pattern or level of orientation
- ◆ observed speech deficits, expressiveness and receptiveness, and ability to communicate
- ◆ diagnostic test results
- ◆ supplies or equipment used to promote orientation (television, radio, calendars, reality orientation boards)
- ◆ promoting effective communication and patient's response
- ◆ evaluation of expected outcomes.

Constipation related to personal habits

Definition

Interruption of normal bowel elimination pattern characterized by infrequent or absent stools or by dry, hard stools

Key outcomes

Record appropriate expected outcomes on the care plan. Possible outcomes include these:
- ◆ Elimination pattern returns to normal.
- ◆ Patient moves bowels every ____ day(s) without laxative or enema.
- ◆ Patient states understanding of causative factors of constipation.
- ◆ Patient gets regular exercise.
- ◆ Patient describes changes in personal habits to maintain normal elimination pattern.
- ◆ Patient states plans to seek help resolving emotional or psychological problems.

Nursing interventions

Document interventions related to:
- ◆ frequency of bowel movements and characteristics of stools
- ◆ administration of laxatives or enemas and their effectiveness
- ◆ patient's weight (weekly)
- ◆ referrals to or consultations with nutritional staff
- ◆ patient's expressions of concern about change in diet, activity level, use of laxatives or enemas, and bowel pattern
- ◆ establishment of daily schedule
- ◆ adherence to dietary recommendations
- ◆ observed diet, activity tolerance, and characteristics of stools

◆ patient teaching (high-fiber diet, increased fluid intake, exercise, importance of responding to urge to defecate, and long-term effects of laxatives or enemas)
◆ evaluation of expected outcomes.

Ineffective coping related to situational crisis

Definition

Inability to use adaptive behaviors in response to difficult life situations, such as loss of health, a loved one, or job

Key outcomes

Record appropriate expected outcomes on the care plan. Possible outcomes include these:
◆ Patient communicates feelings about the present situation.
◆ Patient becomes involved in planning own care.
◆ Patient expresses feeling of having greater control over present situation.
◆ Patient uses available support systems, such as family and friends, to aid in coping.
◆ Patient identifies at least two coping behaviors.
◆ Patient demonstrates ability to use two healthful coping behaviors.

Nursing interventions

Document interventions related to:
◆ patient's perception of current situation and what it means
◆ patient's efforts at self-care
◆ patient's coping behaviors and his evaluation of their effectiveness
◆ patient's verbal expression of feelings indicating comfort or discomfort
◆ observed patient behaviors
◆ nursing interventions to help patient cope and his responses
◆ patient teaching (about treatments and procedures)
◆ referrals to counselors and support groups
◆ patient's verbalization of factors that decrease the ability to cope
◆ evaluation of expected outcomes.

Ineffective denial related to fear or anxiety

Definition

The attempt to reduce concern or worry by the conscious or unconscious refusal to admit to the reality of a situation

Key outcomes

Record appropriate expected outcomes on the care plan. Possible outcomes include these:
◆ Patient describes knowledge and perception of present health problem.
◆ Patient describes lifestyle and reports recent changes.
◆ Patient expresses knowledge of stages of grief.
◆ Patient demonstrates behavior associated with grief process.
◆ Patient discusses present health problem with physician, nurses, and family members.
◆ Patient indicates by conversation or behavior an increased awareness of reality.

Nursing interventions

Document interventions related to:
◆ patient's perception of health problem, including its severity and potential impact on lifestyle
◆ patient's verbalization of feelings related to present problem

- mental status (baseline and ongoing)
- communications with physician (to determine what patient has been told about illness)
- patient's knowledge of grief process
- patient's behavioral responses
- interventions implemented to assist patient
- patient's response to nursing interventions
- patient teaching and patient's response
- evaluation of expected outcomes.

Diarrhea related to malabsorption, inflammation, or irritation of bowel

Definition

Passage of loose, unformed stools

Key outcomes

Record appropriate expected outcomes on the care plan. Possible outcomes include these:

- Patient controls diarrhea with drug therapy.
- Elimination pattern returns to normal.
- Patient regains and maintains fluid and electrolyte balance.
- Skin remains intact.
- Patient discusses causative factors, preventive measures, and changed body image.
- Patient practices stress-reduction techniques daily.
- Patient seeks persons with similar condition or joins a support group.
- Patient demonstrates ability to use ostomy devices if diarrhea results from colorectal surgery.

Nursing interventions

Document interventions related to:

- patient's expressions of concern about diarrhea, causative factors, and adaptation to changes in body image if diarrhea results from colorectal surgery
- administration and observed effects of antidiarrheal drugs
- intake and output measurements and daily weight
- observed stool characteristics and frequency of defecation
- skin condition (especially decreased skin turgor or excoriation)
- bowel sounds (auscultation findings)
- patient teaching (including causes, prevention, cleaning of perineal area and comfort, dietary restrictions, stress reduction, preoperative instruction about ileostomy or colostomy and abdominal surgery, and postoperative instructions about ostomy equipment)
- referrals to support groups (such as ostomy clubs) if appropriate
- evaluation of expected outcomes.

Deficient fluid volume related to active loss

Definition

Excessive loss of body fluid

Key outcomes

Record appropriate expected outcomes on the care plan. Possible outcomes include these:

- Vital signs remain stable.
- Skin color and temperature are normal.
- Electrolyte levels stay within normal range.
- Patient produces adequate urine volume.
- Patient has normal skin turgor and moist mucous membranes.

- Urine specific gravity remains between 1.005 and 1.010.
- Fluid and blood volume return to normal.
- Patient expresses understanding of factors that caused deficient fluid volume.

Nursing interventions

Document interventions related to:
- vital signs
- patient's complaints of thirst, weakness, dizziness, and palpitations
- interventions to control fluid loss and patient's response
- observed skin and mucous membrane condition and other physical findings (including signs of fluid and electrolyte imbalances, such as tachycardia, dyspnea, or hypotension)
- intake and output and significant changes (including amount and characteristics of urine, stools, vomitus, wound drainage, nasogastric drainage, chest tube drainage, or other output)
- urine specific gravity (including times and dates)
- administration of fluids, blood or blood products, or plasma expanders and patient's response
- patient's daily weight and abdominal girth
- patient teaching (about fluid loss and ways to monitor fluid volume at home such as by measuring intake and output and body weight daily)
- evaluation of expected outcomes.

Impaired gas exchange related to altered oxygen supply

Definition

Interference in cellular respiration resulting from inadequate exchange or transport of oxygen and carbon dioxide

Key outcomes

Record appropriate expected outcomes on the care plan. Possible outcomes include these:
- Patient maintains respiratory rate within 5 breaths of baseline.
- Patient expresses feeling of comfort.
- Patient coughs effectively.
- Patient expectorates sputum.
- Patient maintains sufficient fluid intake to prevent dehydration: ____ ml/24 hours.
- Patient performs ADLs to level of tolerance.
- Patient has normal breath sounds.
- Patient's ABG levels return to baseline: ____ pH; ____ Pao_2; ____ $Paco_2$.
- Patient performs relaxation techniques every 4 hours.
- Patient correctly uses breathing devices to improve gas exchange and increase oxygenation.

Nursing interventions

Document interventions related to:
- patient's complaints of dyspnea, headache, or restlessness or expression of well-being
- observed physical findings (including vital signs, auscultation results, pulmonary status, and cardiac rhythm)
- drug and oxygen administration (including times, dates, dosages, route, adverse effects, and equipment and supplies) and patient's response
- patient positioning and repositioning and times; bronchial hygiene measures, such as coughing, percussion, postural drainage, suctioning
- intake and output measurements
- reportable signs of dehydration or fluid overload
- test results, including ABG levels
- ET intubation and mechanical ventilation measures (including equipment and supplies used)

◆ patient teaching (including relaxation techniques and other measures to lower demand for oxygen)
◆ patient's ability to perform ADLs
◆ evaluation of expected outcomes.

Hopelessness related to failing or deteriorating physiologic condition

Definition

Subjective state in which an individual sees few or no available alternatives or personal choices and can't mobilize energy on own behalf

Key outcomes

Record appropriate expected outcomes on the care plan. Possible outcomes include these:
◆ Patient identifies feelings of hopelessness regarding current situation.
◆ Patient demonstrates more effective communication skills, including direct verbal responses to questions and increased eye contact.
◆ Patient resumes appropriate rest and activity pattern.
◆ Patient participates in self-care activities and in decisions regarding care planning.
◆ Patient participates in diversional activities (specify).
◆ Patient identifies social and community resources for continued assistance.

Nursing interventions

Document interventions related to:
◆ patient's mental status
◆ patient's verbal and nonverbal communication
◆ patient's medical regimen
◆ increasing patient's feelings of hope and self-worth and involvement in self-care and his response (including time spent communicating, talking, or sitting with patient)
◆ drug administration and comfort measures
◆ referrals to ancillary services, such as dietitian, social worker, clergy, mental health clinical nurse specialist, or support groups
◆ patient teaching (including diversional activities, self-care instruction, and discharge planning)
◆ patient's response to comfort measures
◆ evaluation of expected outcomes.

Functional urinary incontinence related to sensory or mobility deficits

Definition

Involuntary and unpredictable passage of urine in socially unacceptable situations

Key outcomes

Record appropriate expected outcomes on the care plan. Possible outcomes include these:
◆ Patient discusses impact of incontinence on self and others.
◆ Patient voids in appropriate situation using suitable receptacle.
◆ Patient voids at specific times.
◆ Patient has no wet episodes.
◆ Patient maintains fluid balance; intake equals output.
◆ Complications are avoided or minimized.
◆ Patient and family members demonstrate skill in managing incontinence.
◆ Patient and family members identify resources to assist with care following discharge.

Nursing interventions

Document interventions related to:
- ◆ patient's expression of concern about incontinence and motivation to participate in self-care
- ◆ voiding pattern
- ◆ intake and output
- ◆ hydration status
- ◆ bladder elimination procedures (including bladder training, commode use times, toileting regimen, episodic wetness or dryness, use of external catheter, and use of protective pads and garments)
- ◆ skin condition and care (including use of protective pads and garments)
- ◆ patient teaching (including toileting environment, time, and place; alcohol and fluid intake; techniques for stimulating voiding reflexes; and techniques for reducing anxiety)
- ◆ patient's response to treatment regimen and patient teaching
- ◆ referrals to appropriate counselors and support groups
- ◆ family involvement in assisting patient with toileting
- ◆ evaluation of expected outcomes.

Risk for infection related to external factors

Definition

Increased risk for invasion by organisms capable of producing disease

Key outcomes

Record appropriate expected outcomes on the care plan. Possible outcomes include these:
- ◆ Temperature stays within normal range.
- ◆ WBC count and differential stay within normal range.
- ◆ No pathogens appear in cultures.
- ◆ Patient maintains good personal and oral hygiene.
- ◆ Respiratory secretions are clear and odorless.
- ◆ Urine remains clear yellow and odorless and exhibits no sediment.
- ◆ Patient shows no evidence of diarrhea.
- ◆ Wounds and incisions appear clean, pink, and free from purulent drainage.
- ◆ I.V. sites show no signs of inflammation.
- ◆ Patient shows no evidence of skin breakdown.
- ◆ Patient consumes ____ ml of fluid and ____ g of protein daily.
- ◆ Patient states infection risk factors.
- ◆ Patient identifies signs and symptoms of infection.
- ◆ Patient remains free from all signs and symptoms of infection.

Nursing interventions

Document interventions related to:
- ◆ temperature readings (including dates and times and reporting of elevations)
- ◆ test procedures (including dates, times, and sites of obtained test specimens)
- ◆ test results (including white blood cell count and cultures of urine, blood, respiratory secretions, and wound drainage) and reporting of abnormal results
- ◆ skin condition and wound care
- ◆ preventive measures (including personal hygiene, oral hygiene, airway suctioning, coughing, and deep-breathing measures)
- ◆ catheter management procedures (including dates and times of all catheter insertions, removals, and site care)
- ◆ equipment and supplies (including particulars of humidification or nebulization of oxygen)

◆ sanitary measures (for example, providing tissues and disposal bag for expectorated sputum)
◆ fluid intake
◆ nutritional intake
◆ isolation and other precautions
◆ patient teaching (including toileting and hygiene, hand-washing technique, factors that increase infection risk, and infection signs and symptoms)
◆ patient's response to nursing interventions
◆ episodes of loose stools or diarrhea
◆ evaluation of expected outcomes.

Risk for injury related to sensory or motor deficits

Definition

Accentuated risk of physical harm cause by sensory or motor deficits

Key outcomes

Record appropriate expected outcomes on the care plan. Possible outcomes include these:
◆ Patient identifies factors that increase potential for injury.
◆ Patient assists in identifying and applying safety measures to prevent injury.
◆ Patient and family members develop strategy to maintain safety.
◆ Patient performs ADLs within sensorimotor limitations.

Nursing interventions

Document interventions related to:
◆ observed factors that may cause or contribute to injury
◆ safety measures (side rails, positioning, use of call button and bed controls, orienting patient to environment, keeping bed in low position, and close night watch)
◆ statements by patient and family members about potential for injury due to sensory or motor deficits
◆ observed or reported unsafe practices
◆ interventions to decrease risk of injury to patient and his response
◆ patient teaching (including safe ways to improve visual discrimination, to decrease risk of burns from sensory loss, to use hearing aids and mobility assistive devices, and to ensure household, automobile, and pedestrian safety)
◆ evaluation of expected outcomes.

Deficient knowledge (specify) related to lack of exposure

Definition

Inadequate understanding of information or inability to perform skills needed to practice health-related behaviors

Key outcomes

Record appropriate expected outcomes on the care plan. Possible outcomes include these:
◆ Patient communicates a need to know.
◆ Patient states or demonstrates understanding of what has been taught.
◆ Patient demonstrates ability to perform new health-related behaviors as they are taught, and lists specific skills and realistic target dates for each.
◆ Patient sets realistic learning goals.
◆ Patient states intention to make needed changes in lifestyle, including seeking help from health care professionals when needed.

Nursing interventions

Document interventions related to:
- patient's statements of known or unknown information and skills, expressions of need to know, and motivation to learn
- patient teaching (including learning objectives, teaching methods used, information imparted, skills demonstrated) and patient's responses
- referrals to resources or organizations that can continue instructional activities after discharge
- evaluation of expected outcomes.

Impaired physical mobility related to pain or discomfort

Definition

Limitation of physical movement

Key outcomes

Record appropriate expected outcomes on the care plan. Possible outcomes include these:
- Patient states relief from pain.
- Patient displays increased mobility.
- Patient shows no evidence of complications, such as contractures, venous stasis, thrombus formation, or skin breakdown.
- Patient attains highest degree of mobility possible within confines of disease.
- Patient or family member demonstrates mobility regimen.
- Patient states feelings about limitations.

Nursing interventions

Document interventions related to:
- patient's observed daily functional ability and changes (use functional mobility scale)
- patient's expressed feelings and concerns about immobility and its impact on his lifestyle, and his willingness to participate in care
- observed impairments and pain
- prescribed treatment regimen for underlying condition and patient's response to treatment and nursing interventions
- drug administration and other supportive measures (including padding extremities to prevent skin breakdown and ensuring correct height of crutches)
- prescribed range of motion (ROM) exercises
- patient repositioning (include times)
- progressive mobilization up to limits of patient's tolerance for pain (bed to chair to ambulation)
- patient and family teaching (including instructions for using crutches and walkers; practicing techniques to control pain, such as distraction and imaging; understanding need for mobility despite pain; performing ROM exercises, transfers, skin inspection, and mobility regimen) and patient's response
- referrals to counselor, support group, or social service agency
- evaluation of expected outcomes.

Noncompliance (specify) related to patient's value system

Definition

Full or partial nonadherence to practice prescribed health-related behaviors

Key outcomes

Record appropriate expected outcomes on the care plan. Possible outcomes include these:
- Patient identifies factors that influence noncompliance.

◆ Patient contracts with nurse to perform ____ (specify behavior and frequency).
◆ Patient uses support systems to modify noncompliant behavior.
◆ Patient demonstrates a level of compliance that doesn't interfere with physiologic safety.

Nursing interventions

Document interventions related to:
◆ patient's stated reasons for noncompliance
◆ observed specific noncompliant behaviors
◆ promoting compliance (including negotiations and terms agreed upon with patient as well as positive reinforcements provided) and patient's response
◆ daily progress in complying with treatment regimen
◆ referrals to counselors or support groups
◆ evaluation of expected outcomes.

Imbalanced nutrition: Less than body requirements related to inability to digest or absorb nutrients because of biological factors

Definition

Change in normal eating pattern that fails to meet metabolic needs

Key outcomes

Record appropriate expected outcomes on the care plan. Possible outcomes include these:
◆ Patient tolerates oral, tube, or I.V. feedings without adverse effects.
◆ Patient takes in ____ calories daily.
◆ Patient gains ____ lb weekly.
◆ Patient shows no further evidence of weight loss.
◆ Patient and family or significant other communicate understanding of special dietary needs.
◆ Patient and family or significant other demonstrate ability to plan diet after discharge.

Nursing interventions

Document interventions related to:
◆ daily weight
◆ daily fluid intake and output measurements (include volume and characteristics of any vomitus and stools — a clue to nutrient absorption)
◆ parenteral fluid administration
◆ daily food intake from prescribed diet
◆ electrolyte levels
◆ consultations with dietary department or nutritional support team
◆ abnormal findings.

If the patient receives tube feedings, document interventions related to:
◆ concentration and delivery of regular feeding formula or one containing food-coloring additives (especially in patient with altered level of consciousness or diminished gag reflex)
◆ use of supportive equipment such as an infusion pump
◆ degree of elevation of head of bed during feeding
◆ feeding tube placement.

If the patient receives total parenteral nutrition, document interventions related to:
◆ monitored blood glucose levels and urine specific gravity (at least once per shift)
◆ monitored bowel sounds (once per shift)
◆ oral hygiene
◆ patient teaching (including the reasons for the current treatment regimen, principles of nutrition suited to the patient's specific condition, meal plan-

ning, and preoperative instructions if applicable)
- evaluation of expected outcomes.

Acute pain related to physical, biological, or chemical agents

Definition

A disagreeable physical experience that arises from tissue damage, either actual or potential, that lasts for less than 6 months

Key outcomes

Record appropriate expected outcomes on the care plan. Possible outcomes include these:
- Patient identifies pain characteristics.
- Patient articulates factors that intensify pain and modifies behavior accordingly.
- Patient states and carries out appropriate interventions for pain relief.
- Patient expresses a feeling of comfort and relief from pain.

Nursing interventions

Document interventions related to:
- patient's description of physical pain, pain relief, and feelings about pain
- observed physical, psychological, and sociocultural responses to pain
- prescribed drug administration (including times, dates, dosages, routes, adverse effects) and comfort measures (such as massage, relaxation techniques, heat and cold applications, repositioning, distraction, and bathing)
- patient's response to nursing interventions
- patient teaching (about pain and pain-relief strategies) and patient's response
- evaluation of expected outcomes.

Risk for impaired skin integrity

Definition

Presence of risk factors for interruption or destruction of skin surface

Key outcomes

Record appropriate expected outcomes on the care plan. Possible outcomes include these:
- Patient maintains muscle strength and joint range of motion (ROM).
- Patient sustains adequate food and fluid intake.
- Patient maintains adequate skin circulation.
- Patient communicates understanding of preventive skin care measures.
- Patient and family demonstrate preventive skin care measures.
- Patient and family correlate risk factors and preventive measures.
- Patient experiences no skin breakdown.

Nursing interventions

Document interventions related to:
- skin condition and changes
- repositioning patient as scheduled and ordered (including dates and times)
- ambulation or active ROM exercises to improve circulation and mobility (including dates and times)
- use of skin care devices and supplies (such as foam mattress, sheepskin, alternating pressure mattress, lo-

tions and powders) and effectiveness of interventions
- ◆ nutritional intake
- ◆ hydration status
- ◆ weekly risk factor potential and score (use the Braden scale)
- ◆ patient teaching (including the need to implement preventive measures to promote skin integrity, good personal hygiene habits, signs of skin breakdown, patient and responsible caregiver's demonstrated skill in carrying out preventive skin care measures) and patient's response
- ◆ evaluation of expected outcomes.

Disturbed sleep pattern related to internal factors, such as illness, psychological stress, drug therapy, or biorhythm disturbance

Definition

Inability to meet individual need for sleep or rest arising from internal or external factors

Key outcomes

Record appropriate expected outcomes on the care plan. Possible outcomes include these:
- ◆ Patient identifies factors that prevent or disrupt sleep.
- ◆ Patient performs relaxation exercises at bedtime.
- ◆ Patient sleeps ____ hours a night.
- ◆ Patient reports feeling well rested.
- ◆ Patient shows no physical signs of sleep deprivation.
- ◆ Patient exhibits no sleep-related behavioral symptoms, such as restlessness, irritability, lethargy, or disorientation.

Nursing interventions

Document interventions related to:
- ◆ patient's complaints about sleep disturbances
- ◆ patient's report of improvement in sleep patterns
- ◆ observed physical and behavioral sleep-related disturbances
- ◆ interventions used to alleviate sleep disturbances (such as pillows, bath, food or drink, reading material, TV, soft music, quiet environment) and patient's response
- ◆ prescribed drug and patient's response
- ◆ patient teaching (including reason for treatment, relationship of regular exercise and sleep, and relaxation techniques, such as imagery, progressive muscle relaxation, and meditation)
- ◆ evaluation of expected outcomes.

Impaired swallowing related to neuromuscular impairment

Definition

Inability to move food, fluid, or saliva from the mouth through the esophagus

Key outcomes

Record appropriate expected outcomes on the care plan. Possible outcomes include these:
- ◆ Patient shows no evidence of aspiration pneumonia.
- ◆ Patient achieves adequate nutritional intake.
- ◆ Patient maintains weight.
- ◆ Patient maintains oral hygiene.
- ◆ Patient and responsible caregiver demonstrate correct eating or feeding techniques to maximize swallowing.

Nursing interventions

Document interventions related to:
- patient's expressed feelings about current condition
- observed and reported swallowing impairment, as evidenced by cyanosis, dyspnea, or choking
- nursing interventions and patient's response (include times of turning and repositioning and degree of elevation of head during mealtimes and for 30 minutes after)
- respiratory status and airway suctioning (including dates and times, instances of cyanosis, dyspnea, or choking)
- daily intake and output and weight measurements
- referrals to dietitian and other health services such as dysphagia rehabilitation team
- oral hygiene and comfort measures
- patient teaching (about positioning, dietary requirements, oral hygiene, and stimuli and feeding techniques to improve mastication, promote swallowing, and decrease aspiration)
- evaluation of expected outcomes.

Ineffective tissue perfusion (cardiopulmonary) related to decreased cellular exchange

Definition

Decrease in cellular nutrition and respiration due to decreased capillary blood flow

Key outcomes

Record appropriate expected outcomes on the care plan. Possible outcomes include these:
- Patient attains hemodynamic stability: pulse not less than ____ and not greater than ____ beats/minute; blood pressure not less than ____ and not greater than ____ mm Hg.
- Patient doesn't exhibit arrhythmias.
- Patient's skin remains warm and dry.
- Patient's heart rate remains within prescribed limits while he carries out ADLs.
- Patient maintains adequate cardiac output.
- Patient modifies lifestyle to minimize risk of decreased tissue perfusion.

Nursing interventions

Document interventions related to:
- patient's perception of health problems and health needs
- observed physical findings (including heart rate, blood pressure, central venous pressure, pulse rate, temperature, skin color, respiratory rate, and breath sounds)
- observed response to activity
- test procedures (including electrocardiogram to monitor heart rate and rhythm and results of creatine kinase, lactate dehydrogenase, and ABG analysis)
- prescribed drugs and oxygen therapy (including dates, times, dosages, routes, adverse effects, equipment, and supplies)
- patient positioning and repositioning to enhance vital capacity and to avoid lung congestion and skin breakdown
- patient teaching (about need for low-fat, low-cholesterol diet; nitroglycerin or other drugs, including possible adverse effects; activity level; stress management; risk factors for heart and lung disease; need to avoid straining with bowel movements; and benefits of quitting smoking)
- evaluation of expected outcomes.

Impaired urinary elimination related to sensory or neuromuscular impairment

Definition

Alteration or impairment of urine elimination

Key outcomes

Record appropriate expected outcomes on the care plan. Possible outcomes include these:

- Patient discusses impact of urologic disorder on self and others.
- Patient maintains fluid balance; intake equals output.
- Patient voices increased comfort.
- Complications are avoided or minimized.
- Patient and family members demonstrate skill in managing urinary elimination problem.
- Patient and family members identify resources to assist with care after discharge.

Nursing interventions

Document interventions related to:

- observed neuromuscular status
- observed voiding pattern
- patient's expression of concern about the urologic problem and its impact on body image and lifestyle
- patient's motivation to participate in self-care
- intake and output and fluid replacement therapy
- drug administration
- bladder training (including times and dates of commode use, Kegel exercises to strengthen sphincter)
- intermittent catheterization (record dates, times, volume eliminated spontaneously, volume eliminated via catheter, bladder balance)
- external catheterization of male patient (including time and date of condom catheter application and changes, supplies used, skin condition of penis, and hygiene)
- indwelling urinary catheterization (including time and date of catheter insertion and changes, condition and care of urinary meatus, type of drainage system used, and volume drained)
- suprapubic catheterization (including time and date of catheter insertion and changes, dressing changes, type of drainage system used, and supplies used)
- supportive care measures (including pain control and hydration, prompt response to call light, and bed in close proximity to bathroom), their effectiveness, and patient's response
- patient teaching (including signs and symptoms of full bladder, home catheterization techniques and management, signs and symptoms of autonomic dysreflexia, management of autonomic dysreflexia, and emergency measures)
- referrals of patient and family members to counselors and support groups
- evaluation of expected outcomes.

Selected references

American Association of Critical Care Nurses. *AACN Procedure Manual for Critical Care,* 5th ed. Edited by Lynn-McHale, D.J., and Carlson, K.K. Philadelphia: W.B. Saunders Co., 2005.

Bickley, L.S., and Hoekelman, R.A. *Bates' Guide to Physical Examination and History Taking,* 8th ed. Philadelphia: Lippincott Williams & Wilkins, 2003.

Braunwald, E., and Goldman, L. *Primary Cardiology,* 2nd ed. Philadelphia: W.B. Saunders Co., 2003.

Burke, M.M., and Laramie, J. *Primary Care of the Older Adult: A Multidisciplinary Approach,* 2nd ed. St. Louis: Mosby–Year Book, Inc., 2003.

Centers for Disease Control and Prevention (CDC). *Guidelines for Isolation Precautions in Hospitals,* November 2002.

Centers for Disease Control and Prevention (CDC). *Guidelines for Prevention of Intravascular Catheter Related Infections: MMWR Recommendations and Reports* 51(RR-10), 2002.

Cook, A.F., et al. "An Error by Any Other Name," *AJN* 104(6):32-43, June 2004.

Craven, R.F., and Hirnle, C.J. *Fundamentals of Nursing: Human Health and Function,* 4th ed. Philadelphia: Lippincott Williams & Wilkins, 2004.

ECG Cards, 4th ed. Philadelphia: Lippincott Williams & Wilkins, 2004.

Elkin, M.K., et al. *Nursing Interventions and Clinical Skills,* 3rd ed. St. Louis: Mosby–Year Book, Inc., 2003.

Fast Facts for Nurses. Philadelphia: Lippincott Williams & Wilkins, 2004.

Fauci, A.S., et al. *Harrison's Principles of Internal Medicine,* 16th ed. New York: McGraw-Hill Book Co., 2005.

Fischbach, F.T. *A Manual of Laboratory and Diagnostic Tests,* 7th ed. Philadelphia: Lippincott Williams & Wilkins, 2004.

Food and Drug Administration (FDA). *FDA Public Health Advisory: Reports of Blue Discoloration and Death in Patients Receiving Enteral Feedings Tinted with the Dye, FD&C Blue No.1,* September 2003.

Fortunato, N.H. *Berry and Kohn's Operating Room Technique,* 10th ed. St. Louis: Mosby–Year Book, Inc., 2004.

Handbook of Diagnostic Tests, 3rd ed. Philadelphia: Lippincott Williams & Wilkins, 2003.

Ignatavicius, D.D., and Workmann, M.L. *Medical-Surgical Nursing Critical Thinking for Collaborative Care,* 5th ed. Philadelphia: W.B. Saunders Co., 2005.

Infusion Nurses Society, Inc. *Core Curriculum for Infusion Nursing,* 3rd ed. Norwood, Mass., 2003.

Jarvis, C. *Pocket Companion for Physical Examination and Health,* 4th ed. Philadelphia: W.B. Saunders Co., 2003.

Joint Commission on Accreditation of Healthcare Organizations. *Comprehensive Accreditation Manual for Hospitals.* Oakbrook Terrace, Ill., 2005.

Joint Commission on Accreditation of Healthcare Organizations. *National Patient Safety Goals,* Oakbrook Terrace, Ill., 2006.

Kozier, B., et al. *Fundamentals of Nursing: Concepts, Process, and Practice,* 7th ed. Upper Saddle River, N.J.: Prentice Hall Health, 2003.

Muñoz, C.C., and Luckmann, J. *Transcultural Communication in Nursing,* 2nd ed. Clifton Park, N.Y.: Delmar Learning, 2005.

NANDA Nursing Diagnoses: Definitions and Classification 2005-2006. Philadelphia: North American Nursing Diagnosis Association, 2005.

Nursing Procedures, 4th ed. Philadelphia: Lippincott Williams & Wilkins, 2004.

Pierson, F.M. *Principles and Techniques of Patient Care,* 3rd ed. Philadelphia: W.B. Saunders Co., 2002.

Phillips, L.D. *I.V. Therapy Notes: Nurse's Clinical Pocket Guide.* Philadelphia: F.A. Davis Co., 2005.

Professional Guide to Diagnostic Tests. Philadelphia: Lippincott Williams & Wilkins, 2005.

Professional Guide to Diseases, 8th ed. Philadelphia: Lippincott Williams & Wilkins, 2005.

Professional Guide to Signs & Symptoms, 4th ed. Philadelphia: Lippincott Williams & Wilkins, 2004.

Rakel, R.E., and Bope, E.T., eds. *Conn's Current Therapy 2005.* Philadelphia: W.B. Saunders Co., 2005.

Smeltzer, S.C., and Bare, B.G. *Brunner and Suddarth's Textbook of Medical-Surgical Nursing,* 10th ed. Philadelphia: Lippincott Williams & Wilkins, 2003.

Sole, M.L., et al., eds. *Introduction to Critical Care Nursing,* 4th ed. Philadelphia: W.B. Saunders Co., 2005.

Varcarolis, E.M. *Foundations of Psychiatric Mental Health Nursing: A Clinical Approach,* 4th ed. Philadelphia: W.B. Saunders Co., 2002.

Index

i refers to an illustration; t refers to a table.

B

i refers to an illustration; t refers to a table.

i refers to an illustration; t refers to a table.

i refers to an illustration; t refers to a table.

D

i refers to an illustration; t refers to a table.

i refers to an illustration; t refers to a table.

i refers to an illustration; t refers to a table.

i refers to an illustration; t refers to a table.

i refers to an illustration; t refers to a table.

i refers to an illustration; t refers to a table.

i refers to an illustration; t refers to a table.

i refers to an illustration; t refers to a table.

---

i refers to an illustration; t refers to a table.

i refers to an illustration; t refers to a table.

---
i refers to an illustration; t refers to a table.

---

i refers to an illustration; t refers to a table.